UNDERSTANDING ANATOMY & PHYSIOLOGY

A Visual, Auditory, Interactive Approach

2nd edition

Your guide to...

UNDERSTANDING ANATOMY & PHYSIOLOGY

A Visual, Auditory, Interactive Approach

Gale Sloan Thompson

SECOND EDITION

Overcome your fears and build your confidence
The author listened to students like you. She designed a text that divides a seemingly huge volume of information into manageable sections.

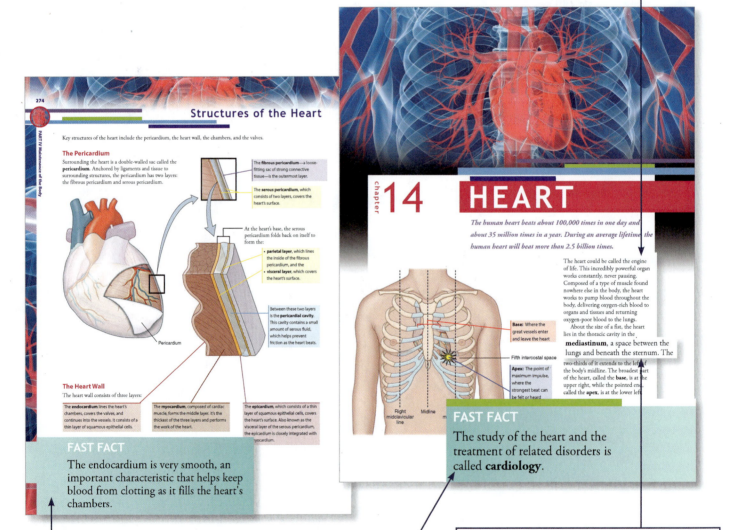

Expand your knowledge
"Fast Facts" are important points of information related to specific body systems that help you build a firm foundation in A&P.

Master the language of A&P
New terms are defined right in the text, making it easy for you to build an A&P vocabulary.

DESIGNED FOR HOW YOU LEARN

Welcome to the challenging but rewarding world of anatomy and physiology.

Whatever your learning style…looking, listening, doing, or a little bit of each… this interactive approach to anatomy & physiology is designed just for you.

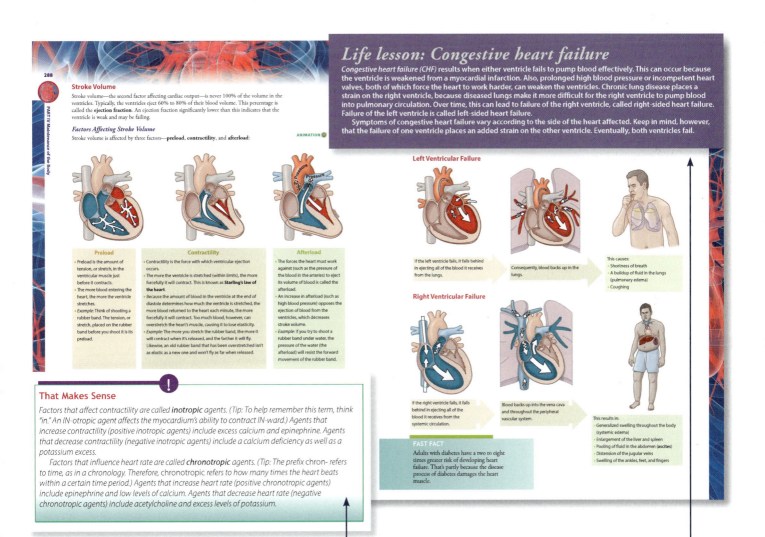

Retain what you've learned

"That Makes Sense" boxes use practical examples, restatements, and mnemonics to help you remember the material.

Explore real-life examples

"Life Lesson" boxes make anatomy and physiology pertinent to daily life by applying material to clinical situations.

Identify your strengths and weaknesses

Answer the "Test Your Knowledge" questions at the end of every chapter to make sure you understand the material while you assess your progress.

Build your vocabulary

A "Review of Terms" lets you quickly locate short definitions for the key terms in every chapter. Use the audio glossary online at **Davis*Plus*.com** to hear pronunciations of the terms.

291

Test Your Knowledge

1. The point of maximum impulse of the heart is at the:
   a. mediastinum.
   b. base.
   c. apex.
   d. aorta.

7. On an electrocardiogram, the QRS complex represents:
   a. atrial depolarization.
   b. ventricular depolarization.
   c. ventricular repolarization.
   d. impulse transmission from the atria to the ventricles.

Answers: Chapter 14

1. *Correct answer: c. The mediastinum is the space between the lungs in which the heart lies. The base*

2. The portion of the heart wall that lines the heart's chambers is the:

8. The cardiac cycle is:
   a. the amount of blood pumped

276

PART IV Maintenance of the Body

The Heart Valves

To ensure that blood moves in a forward direction through the heart, the heart contains four valves: one between each atrium and its ventricle and another at the exit of each ventricle. Each valve is formed by two or three flaps of tissue called **cusps** or **leaflets**.

The **atrioventricular (AV) valves** regulate flow between the atria and the ventricles.

- The right AV valve—also called the **tricuspid valve** (because it has three leaflets)—prevents backflow from the right ventricle to the right atrium.
- The left AV valve—also called the **bicuspid valve** (because it has two leaflets), or, more commonly, the **mitral valve**—prevents backflow from the left ventricle to the left atrium.

The **semilunar valves** regulate flow between the ventricles and the great arteries. There are two semilunar valves:

- The **pulmonary valve** prevents backflow from the pulmonary artery to the right ventricle.
- The **aortic valve** prevents backflow from the aorta to the left ventricle.

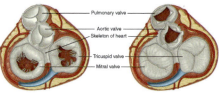

- Pulmonary valve
- Aortic valve
- Skeleton of heart
- Tricuspid valve
- Mitral valve

Ventricles relaxed   Ventricles contracted

The Heart Skeleton

A semi-rigid, fibrous, connective tissue called the **skeleton of the heart** encircles each valve. Besides offering support for the heart, the skeleton keeps the valves from stretching; it also acts as an insulating barrier between the atria and the ventricles, preventing electrical impulses from reaching the ventricles other than through a normal conduction pathway.

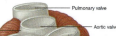

- Pulmonary valve
- Skeleton of heart, including fibrous rings around valves
- Aortic valve
- Tricuspid valve
- Mitral valve

Review of Key Terms

...rload: The forces that impede the ...w of blood out of the heart

...tic valve: Heart valve that prevents ...kflow from the aorta to the left ...tricle

...x: Pointed end of the heart, the ...ation of the point of maximum ...pulse

...ioventricular (AV) node: Group of ...emaker cells in the interatrial ...tum that relays impulses from the ...a to the ventricles

...ium: The upper chamber of each ...f of the heart

...omaticity: The unique ability of ...cardiac muscle to contract ...hout nervous stimulation

...oreceptors: Pressure sensors in the ...ta and carotid arteries that detect ...nges in blood pressure; also called ...soreceptors

...e: Broadest part of the heart; ...ere great vessels enter and leave

...diac cycle: The series of events that ...ur from the beginning of one ...rtbeat to the beginning of the next

...diac output: The amount of blood ...mped by the heart in 1 minute

...emoreceptors: Sensors in the aortic ...h, carotid arteries, and medulla ...t detect increased levels of carbon ...xide, decreased levels of oxygen, ...d decreases in pH

Chordae tendineae: Tendinous cords that connect the edges of the AV valves to the papillary muscles to prevent inversion of the valve during ventricular systole

Coronary arteries: Vessels that deliver oxygenated blood to the myocardium

Coronary sinus: Large transverse vein on the heart's posterior that returns blood to the right atrium

Diastole: The period of cardiac muscle relaxation

Electrocardiogram (ECG): Record of the electrical currents in the heart

Endocardium: The endothelial membrane that lines the chambers of the heart

Epicardium: The serous membrane on the surface of the myocardium

Mediastinum: Space between the lungs and beneath the sternum

Mitral valve: The valve that regulates blood flow between the left atrium and left ventricle

Myocardium: The middle layer of the heart wall; composed of cardiac muscle

Pericardial cavity: Space between the visceral and parietal layers of the serous pericardium that contains a small amount of serous fluid

Pericardium: The membranous fibroserous sac enclosing the heart and the bases of the great vessels

Preload: The amount of tension, or stretch, in the ventricular muscle just before it contracts

Proprioceptors: Sensors in muscles and joints that signal the cardiac center of changes in physical activity

Pulmonary valve: Heart valve that prevents backflow from the pulmonary artery to the right ventricle

Purkinje fiber: Nerve-like processes that extend from the bundle branches to the ventricular myocardium; form the last part of the cardiac conduction system

Rhythmicity: Term applied to the heart's ability to beat regularly

Semilunar valves: The two valves that regulate flow between the ventricles and the great arteries

Sinoatrial node: The heart's primary pacemaker, where normal cardiac impulses arise

Stroke volume: The amount of blood ejected by the heart with each beat

Systole: Contraction of the chambers of the heart

Tricuspid valve: The right atrioventricular valve, which regulates flow between the right atrium and right ventricle

Ventricles: The two lower chambers of the heart

The Body AT WORK

Valves open and close in response to pressure changes within the heart. For example, when a ventricle relaxes, the pressure within that ventricle drops. The AV valve leaflets hang limply, allowing blood to flow through the open valve into the ventricle. As the ventricle fills, pressure in the ventricle rises. After filling, the ventricle begins to contract and the pressure rises even more. This increased pressure pushes against the cusps of the AV valve, causing it to snap closed. When pressure in the ventricle exceeds the pressure "downstream," the semilunar valve pops open, allowing blood to flow out into the area of lower pressure.

Own the Information

To make the information in this chapter part of your working memory, take some time to reflect on what you've learned. On a separate sheet of paper, write down everything you recall from the chapter. After you're done, log on to the Davis*Plus* website, and check out the Study Group podcast and Study Group Questions for the chapter.

Key Topics for Chapter 14:
- The size, location, and key structures of the heart
- Sounds made by the heart
- Heart chambers, valves, and great vessels
- Blood flow through the heart
- Coronary circulation
- Cardiac conduction and ECGs
- Cardiac cycle
- Cardiac output and the factors affecting cardiac output

Understand how the body functions

"The Body at Work" explains how physiological processes work.

Build a complete understanding of A&P

"Own the information" is a detailed plan of study that shows you how to absorb what you need to know about the most important concepts.

SEE, LISTEN, and DO...
Don't miss all of the ways to help you learn.

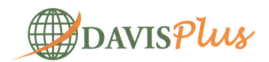

BEYOND THE TEXT...
There's so much more online to help you excel in class, on exams, and in the lab.

The *Plus* Code on the inside front cover unlocks a wealth of learning resources.

Visit **www.DavisPlus.com** today!

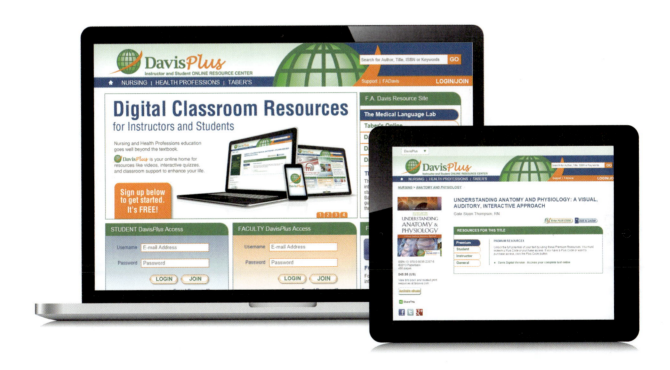

- **Animations**
  Watch the full-color animations that show you how physiological processes work while a narrator explains step by step.

- **Audio Glossary**
  Hear pronunciations of the key terms in the book.

- **Interactive Exercises**
  Complete the image-based "Body Language" labeling and matching exercises to find out what you know and don't know.

- **Davis Digital Version**
  Access your complete text online. Quickly search, highlight, and bookmark the information you need.

- **Flash Cards**
  Read each chapter and then "Test Yourself" to make sure that you understand the material.

- **Audio Podcasts**
  Listen to the "Chapter in Brief" summary for each chapter and to students in a "Study Group" as they quiz each other.

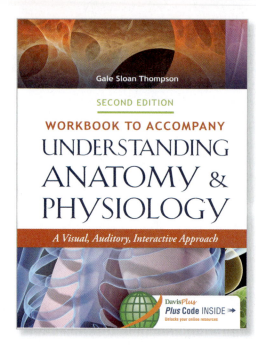
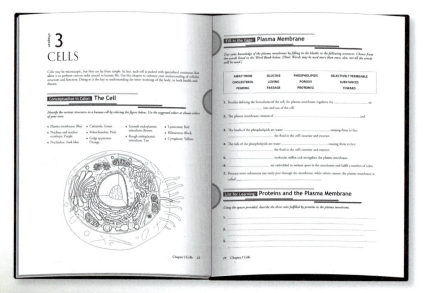

UNDERSTANDING ANATOMY & PHYSIOLOGY

A Visual, Auditory, Interactive Approach

2nd edition

Gale Sloan Thompson, RN

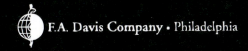

F.A. Davis Company • Philadelphia

F. A. Davis Company
1915 Arch Street
Philadelphia, PA 19103
www.fadavis.com

Printed in the United States of America

Last digit indicates print number: 10 9 8 7 6 5 4 3 2 1

Publisher, Nursing: Lisa B. Houck
Director of Content Strategy: Darlene D. Pedersen
Content Project Manager II: Victoria White
Illustration & Design Manager: Carolyn O'Brien
Project Manager, Digital Solutions: Kate Crowley

As new scientific information becomes available through basic and clinical research, recommended treatments and drug therapies undergo changes. The author(s) and publisher have done everything possible to make this book accurate, up to date, and in accord with accepted standards at the time of publication. The author(s), editors, and publisher are not responsible for errors or omissions or for consequences from application of the book, and make no warranty, expressed or implied, in regard to the contents of the book. Any practice described in this book should be applied by the reader in accordance with professional standards of care used in regard to the unique circumstances that may apply in each situation. The reader is advised always to check product information (package inserts) for changes and new information regarding dose and contraindications before administering any drug. Caution is especially urged when using new or infrequently ordered drugs.

Library of Congress Cataloging-in-Publication Data

Thompson, Gale Sloan.
  Understanding anatomy & physiology: a visual, auditory, interactive approach / Gale Sloan Thompson.—2nd edition.
    p. ; cm.
  Understanding anatomy and physiology
  Includes index.
  ISBN 978-0-8036-4373-4 — ISBN 0-8036-4373-X
  I. Title. II. Title: Understanding anatomy and physiology.
  [DNLM: 1. Anatomy—methods. 2. Physiology—methods. QS 4]
  QP38
  612—dc23

  2014044646

PREFACE

Even as you read this sentence, your body is performing amazing feats. Electrical impulses are rocketing through your brain at over 200 miles per hour. Hundreds of muscles continually tense and relax to keep you in an upright position and to allow your eyes to track across the words on this page. A specific muscle—your heart—is contracting and relaxing at regular intervals to propel blood throughout your body. In fact, your blood will make two complete trips around your body before you finish reading this preface.

Even more amazing is the fact that the vast array of cells, tissues, organs, and organ systems making up your body arose from just two simple cells—an egg and a sperm. Consider, too, that you are genetically unique: out of the over 6 billion people populating the earth, no two individuals are completely alike. That is reason to marvel.

Artists and scientists have long been captivated by the human body. For centuries, artists have studied the body's outward form, focusing on the movement and shape of muscles and bones when rendering works of art. Scientists, on the other hand, yearned to discover the mysteries inside the body. For almost 3,000 years, scientists have explored the depths of the human body: not just how it is put together, but how and why it functions as it does. Exploration continues today, with the latest discovery being that of the human microbiome. Indeed, this one discovery has set the medical community abuzz with its implications for human health.

For you, the journey to discovery begins with reading this book. Contained on these pages is information about which ancient scientists only dreamed. This information will enlighten you about your own body; what's more, it will arm you with knowledge that is foundational to any health- or sports-related career.

Truly, before you can understand a body in illness, you must understand how it functions in health. For example, without a thorough knowledge of fluid and electrolyte balance, how can you explain why chronic vomiting or diarrhea can cause irregular electrical activity in the heart? Without an understanding of how the cardiovascular and respiratory systems interrelate, how will you grasp why chronic lung disease can lead to heart failure? How can you appreciate the need for caution in administering antibiotics without an understanding of the human microbiome? Consequently, you must learn—really *learn* and not just memorize— the information contained in this book.

There is much to learn, to be sure; but don't be overwhelmed. *Understanding Anatomy & Physiology* breaks the information into "bite-sized" pieces, making topics easier to understand and also to remember. As you read the text—and you *must* read the text—you'll be drawn naturally to vibrant figures that will illuminate what you're reading. Being able to see a structure while you're reading about it will make learning easier. Also, consult the inside back cover of this book to discover your particular learning style; then take advantage of the ancillary materials most likely to help you learn.

You *can* learn this. By the end of this course, understanding the body's form and function can become second nature. While tackling this class may seem like an impossible marathon, you can indeed get to the finish line. As with any marathon, the keys are to follow a plan (read the book); don't skip workouts (review and study daily); and take it step by step (study each chapter in sequence). You *will* get there.

Gale Sloan Thompson

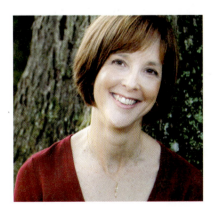

ACKNOWLEDGMENTS

Understanding Anatomy & Physiology, 2nd edition, remains a unique work in the field of anatomy and physiology textbooks. As always, I am grateful for the vision and forward-thinking of Lisa Houck, Publisher. Her commitment to making *Understanding Anatomy & Physiology* a leader in its field is illustrated by her push for a second edition so that we could include a chapter on the revolutionary discovery of the human microbiome. Thank you, Lisa, as always, for your tenacity, drive, and commitment to excellence.

I am also grateful to Victoria White, managing editor. Pulling off a second edition of a book with such a vast array of ancillary materials was no small task. Overseeing all aspects of this project—ranging from coordinating the schedules of myriad departments down to the minutiae of ensuring that each correction passed through every ancillary—required both skill and patience. Thank you, Victoria, for never compromising in your efforts to ensure that the second edition would surpass the first in both completeness and accuracy.

A special thanks, too, goes to Naomi Adams, for her invaluable review. Naomi scrutinized every page of the book and workbook and painstakingly reviewed each and every ancillary. I remain impressed by her breadth of knowledge of nursing and anatomy and physiology; I am, perhaps, even more impressed by her keen eye and attention to detail. Thank you, Naomi, for the obvious care and concern you took when reviewing this work; it is much better for having passed across your desk.

A book for visual learners would, obviously, not be effective without hundreds of vivid illustrations. Stretching the artists and compositors into new territory required that the text be integrated with the art during layout. As always, Carolyn O'Brien, Art Director, expertly led her team to incorporate all changes with precision.

The vast array of ancillary materials, including the animations, online quizzes, Body Language, Study Group, and Chapter in Brief depended upon the skills of many others. This talented group of individuals was headed up by Kate Crowley.

I would also like to thank the reviewers, who are listed separately, for their willingness to review various chapters. Their specialized knowledge of anatomy and physiology helped me improve the scope of the book and also hone the accuracy of the information presented. Having the input of those who work with students on a daily basis, and who understand the areas with which students struggle, was invaluable in helping me make the topic of anatomy and physiology more clear, concise, and relevant to the lives of students.

Last, but certainly not least, I want to thank Jaclyn Lux, Marketing Manager, and her entire sales force for their enthusiasm for this product. I appreciate their energy in not only exploring the attributes and unique features of this package but also in promoting those features to instructors at various schools and colleges. I look forward to hearing the feedback they receive from instructors and students as to how to make *Understanding Anatomy & Physiology* even better.

To Bob: Thank you for always believing, not just in my work, but in me. Your love, your support, and your encouragement mean the world.

CONSULTANTS

Naomi Adams, RN, AA, BN
Owner, Adams Medical-Legal Consulting
Woodbridge, VA

Bruce A. Fenderson, PhD
Professor of Pathology, Anatomy &
Cell Biology
Thomas Jefferson University
Philadelphia, PA

REVIEWERS

Tetteh Abbeyquaye, PhD
Assistant Professor
Quinsigamond Community College
Worcester, MA

Janice Ankenmann, RN, MSN,
CCRN, FNP-C
Professor
Napa Valley College
Napa, CA

Dan Bickerton, MS
Instructor
Ogeechee Technical College
Statesboro, GA

Anne L. Brown, RN, BSN
Nursing Instructor
Broome-Tioga BOCES
Binghamton, NY

Susan E. Brown, MS, RN
Faculty
Riverside School of Health Careers
Newport News, VA

Henry Steven Carter, MS, CRC, CVE
Coordinator of Continuing and
Workforce Education/Instructor
El Centro College
Dallas, TX

Thea L. Clark, RN, BS, MS
Coordinator Practical Nursing
Tulsa Technology Center
Tulsa, OK

Ginny Cohrs, RN, BSN
Nursing Faculty
Alexandria Technical College
Alexandria, MN

Tamera Crosswhite, RN, MSN
Nursing Instructor
Great Plains Technology Center
Frederick, OK

Fleurdeliza Cuyco, BS, MD
Dean of Education
Preferred College of Nursing, Los
Angeles
Los Angeles, CA

Judith L. Davis, RN, MSN, FNP
Practical Nursing Instructor
Delta-Montrose Technical College
Delta, CO

Carita Dickson, RN
LVN Instructor
San Bernadino Adult School LVN
Program
San Bernadino, CA

Teddy Dupre, MSN
Instructor
Capital Area Technical College
Baton Rouge, LA

Hisham S. Elbatarny, MB BCh, MSc,
MD
Professor
St. Lawrence College–Queen's
University
Kingston, Ontario

Alexander Evangelista
Adjunct Faculty
The Community College of
Baltimore County
Baltimore, MD

John Fakunding, PhD
Adjunct Instructor
University of South Carolina, Beaufort
Beaufort, SC

Kelly Fleming, RN, BN, MSN
Practical Nurse Facilitator
Columbia College
Calgary, Alberta

Ruby Fogg, MA
Professor
Manchester Community College
Manchester, NH

Cheryl S. Fontenot, RN
Professor
Acadiana Technical College
Abbeville, LA

Shena Borders Gazaway, RN, BSN,
  MSN
Lead Nursing/Allied Health Instructor
Lanier Technical College
Commerce, GA

Daniel G. Graetzer, PhD
Professor
Northwest University
Kirkland, WA

Dianne Hacker, RN, MSN
Nursing Instructor
Capital Area School of Practical
  Nursing
Springfield, IL

Leslie K. Hughes, RN, BSN
Practical Nursing Instructor
Indian Capital Technology Center
Tahlequah, OK

Constance Lieseke, CMA (AAMA),
  MLT, PBT (ASCP)
*Medical Assisting Faculty Program
  Coordinator*
Olympic College
Bremerton, WA

Julie S. Little, MSN
Associate Professor
Virginia Highlands Community
  College
Abingdon, VA

C. Kay Lucas, MEd, BS, AS
Nurse Educator
Commonwealth of Virginia
  Department of Health Professions
Henrico, VA

Barbara Marchelletta, CMA (AAMA),
  CPC, CPT
Program Director, Allied Health
Beal College,
Bangor, ME

Nikki A. Marhefka, EdM, MT
  (ASCP), CMA (AAMA)
Medical Assisting Program Director
Central Penn College
Summerdale, PA

Jean L. Mosley, CMA (AAMA), AAS,
  BS
Program Director/Instructor
Surry Community College
Dobson, NC

Elaine M. Rissel Muscarella, RN, BSN
LPN Instructor
Jamestown, NY

Brigitte Niedzwiecki, RN, MSN
*Medical Assistant Program Director and
  Instructor*
Chippewa Valley Technical College
Eau Claire, WI

Jill M. Pawluk, RN, MSN
Nursing Instructor
The School of Nursing at Cuyahoga
  Valley Career Center
Brecksville, OH

Kathleen Hope Rash, MSN, RN
*Curriculum & Instructional Resource
  Coordinator*
Riverside Schools of Nursing
Newport News, VA

Amy Fenech Sandy, MS, MS
Dean, School of Sciences
Columbus Technical College
Columbus, GA

Marianne Servis, RN, MSN
Nurse Educator/Clinical Coordinator
Career Training Solutions
Fredericksburg, VA

Glynda Renee Sherrill, RN, MS
Practical Nursing Instructor
Indian Capital Technology Center
Tahlequah, OK

Cathy Soto, PhD, MBA, CMA
El Paso Community College
El Paso, TX

Joanne St. John, CMA
Adjunct Instructor–Health Science
Indian River State College
Fort Pierce, FL

Diana A. Sunday, RN, BSN,
  MSN/ED
*Nurse Educator–Practical Nursing
  Program*
York County School of Technology
York, PA

Joyce B. Thomas, CMA (AAMA)
Instructor
Central Carolina Community College
Pittsboro, NC

Marianne Van Deursen, MS Ed,
  CMA (AAMA)
*Medical Assisting Program
  Director/Instructor*
Warren County Community College
Washington, NJ

Monna L. Walters, MSN, RN
Director of Vocational Nursing Program
Lassen Community College
Susanville, CA

Amy Weaver, MSN, RN, ACNS-BC
Instructor
Youngstown State University
Youngstown, OH

CONTENTS

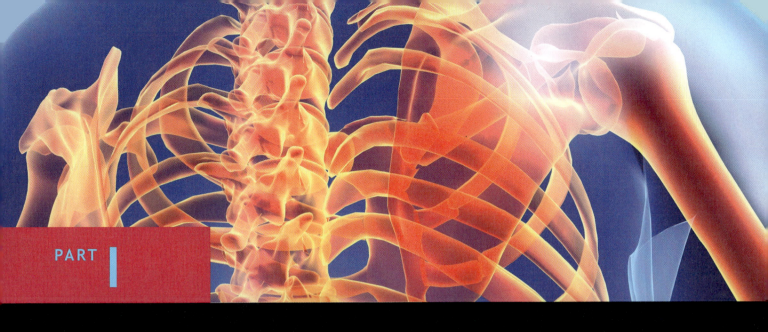

PART I

ORGANIZATION OF THE BODY

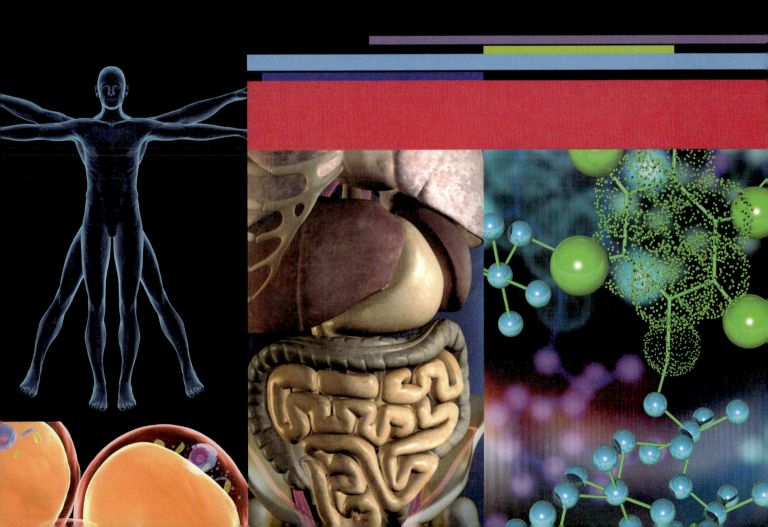

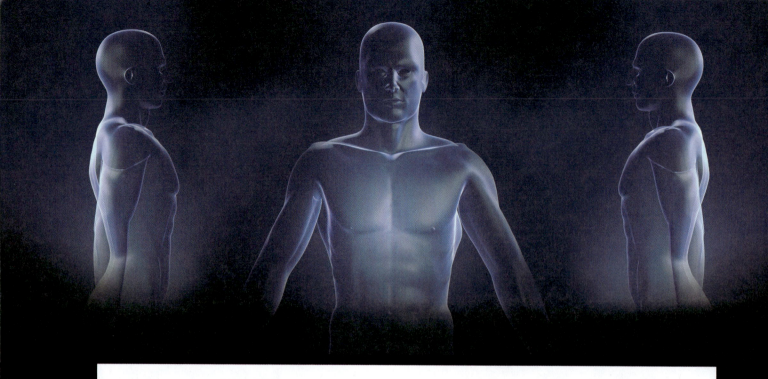

CHAPTER OUTLINE

Organization of the Body

Organ Systems

Anatomical Terms

Homeostasis

LEARNING OUTCOMES

1. Define anatomy and physiology.

2. Describe the organization of the body from the very simple to the very complex.

3. Name the 11 organ systems and identify key functions of each.

4. Define commonly used directional terms.

5. Name the body planes and describe how each dissects the body.

6. Identify common body regions.

7. Identify and describe the major body cavities.

8. Name the nine abdominal regions and identify organs found in each.

9. Name the four abdominal quadrants.

10. Define homeostasis.

11. Explain the process of homeostasis through both negative and positive feedback.

chapter 1

ORIENTATION TO THE HUMAN BODY

More than 6 billion human bodies currently reside on the earth. While each is individually unique, all have the same basic design and structure.

The structure of the body, **anatomy**, is closely entwined with how it functions, **physiology**. Once you learn the structure of a specific part of the body, you'll naturally want to know how it works. Learning normal anatomy and physiology will also help you grasp the changes and symptoms that occur with certain disease processes. The study of the processes that disturb normal function is called **pathophysiology**. (*Patho* means suffering or disease; therefore, *pathophysiology* refers to diseased functioning.)

As an example, in a later chapter, you'll learn that the lungs consist of a series of tubes, called bronchi, and that the smallest of these bronchi end in tiny sacs, called alveoli. That's a very basic description of the structure, or anatomy, of the lung. From there, you'll learn that oxygen is absorbed into the bloodstream through the alveoli. That's how the lung functions: its physiology. Armed with that information, you can then comprehend why someone becomes short of breath if the bronchi become narrowed (such as during an acute asthmatic attack) or blocked (such as from a tumor).

The human body is an amazing organism. It is intricate and complex, but all of its processes make sense. Embark on this journey to study anatomy and physiology as you would any great adventure: with interest, excitement, *and* determination. Remember: you're learning about *yourself!*

The Body AT WORK

We're all aware that people look different on the outside. But did you know that people can vary internally as well? The art in this book reflects the anatomy typical of most people. However, variations do occur. For example, some people are born with only one kidney; others have an extra bone in their feet; still others have carotid arteries that follow an atypical route. Perhaps the most extreme example of anatomical variation is called situs inversus. In this inherited condition—affecting about 1 in 10,000 people—the organs are reversed. Instead of the spleen, pancreas, sigmoid colon, and most of the heart being on the left, they're on the right. Likewise, the gallbladder, appendix, and most of the liver are on the left instead of on the right.

FAST FACT

Although Aristotle of Greece made the first recorded attempts to study anatomy in 380 B.C., the first atlas of anatomy wasn't published until 1543 A.D.

Organization of the Body

The human body is organized in a hierarchy, ranging from the very simple (a microscopic atom) to the very complex (a human being). Specifically:

ATOMS link together to form…

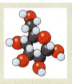

MOLECULES. Molecules are organized into various structures, including…

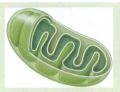

ORGANELLES, the metabolic units within a cell that perform a specific function necessary to the life of the cell. Examples include mitochondria—the powerhouses that furnish the cell's energy—and the cell's nucleus. Organelles are contained within…

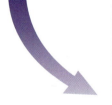

ORGANS, which are structures of two or more tissue types working together to carry out a particular function. Examples include the heart, stomach, and kidney. Organs then form…

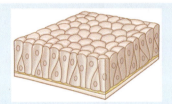

TISSUES, which are specialized groups of cells with similar structure and function. Tissues come together to form…

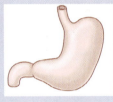

CELLS, the smallest living units that make up the body's structure. Cells group together to form…

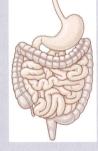

ORGAN SYSTEMS, which are groups of organs that all contribute to a particular function. All of the organ systems together form…

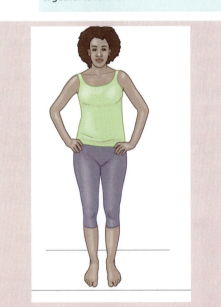

A HUMAN ORGANISM: one complete individual.

The Body AT WORK

The body contains four types of tissues:

- *Epithelial tissue* covers or lines body surfaces; examples include the outer layer of the skin, the walls of capillaries, and kidney tubules.
- *Connective tissue* connects and supports parts of the body; some transport and store materials; examples include bone, cartilage, and adipose tissues.
- *Muscle* contracts to produce movement; examples include skeletal muscles and the heart.
- *Nerve tissue* generates and transmits impulses to regulate body function; examples include the brain and nerves.

Organ Systems

The human body consists of 11 organ systems. The organs of each system contribute to a particular function. However, some organs belong to more than one system. Specifically, the pharynx is part of both the respiratory and the digestive systems, and the male urethra belongs to both the reproductive and urinary systems.

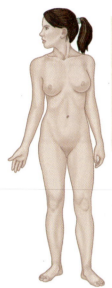

Consists of skin, hair, and nails

Key functions:
- Protection
- Temperature regulation
- Water retention
- Sensation

Integumentary system

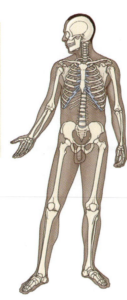

Consists of bones, cartilage, and ligaments

Key functions:
- Protection of body organs
- Support
- Movement
- Blood formation

Skeletal system

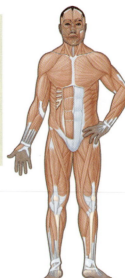

Consists primarily of skeletal muscles

Key functions:
- Movement
- Posture
- Heat production

Muscular system

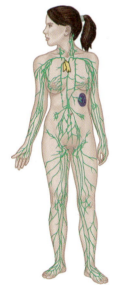

Consists of lymph nodes, lymphatic vessels, lymph, thymus, spleen, and tonsils

Key functions:
- Role in fluid balance
- Production of immune cells
- Defense against disease

Lymphatic system

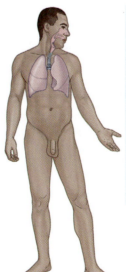

Consists of the nose, pharynx, larynx, trachea, bronchi, and lungs

Key functions:
- Absorption of oxygen
- Discharge of carbon dioxide
- Acid-base balance
- Speech

Respiratory system

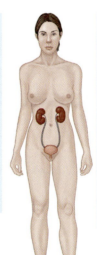

Consists of the kidneys, ureters, urinary bladder, and urethra

Key functions:
- Excretion of wastes
- Regulation of blood volume and pressure
- Control of fluid, electrolyte, and acid-base balance

Urinary system

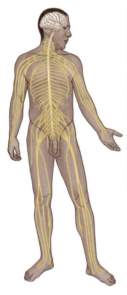

Consists of the brain, spinal cord, nerves, and sense organs

Key functions:
- Control, regulation, and coordination of other systems
- Sensation
- Memory

Nervous system

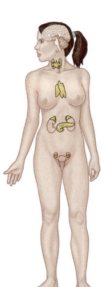

Consists of the pituitary gland, adrenals, pancreas, thyroid, parathyroids, and other organs

Key functions:
- Hormone production
- Control and regulation of other systems

Endocrine system

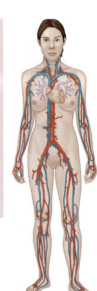
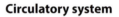

Consists of the heart, arteries, veins, and capillaries

Key functions:
- Distribution of oxygen, nutrients, wastes, hormones, electrolytes, immune cells, and antibodies
- Fluid, electrolyte, and acid-base balance

Circulatory system

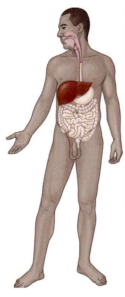

Consists of the stomach, small and large intestines, esophagus, liver, mouth, and pancreas

Key functions:
- Breakdown and absorption of nutrients
- Elimination of wastes

Digestive system

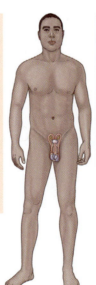
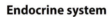

Consists of the testes, vas deferens, prostate, seminal vesicles, and penis

Key functions:
- Production and delivery of sperm
- Secretion of sex hormones

Male reproductive system

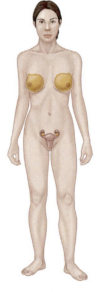

Consists of the ovaries, fallopian tubes, uterus, vagina, and breasts

Key functions:
- Production of eggs
- Site of fertilization and fetal development
- Birth
- Lactation
- Secretion of sex hormones

Female reproductive system

Terms are crucial for navigating your way around the human body. Besides being used to identify the location of various body parts, the use of proper terms ensures accurate communication between health-care providers.

Because the body is three-dimensional, a number of different terms are needed. These include directional terms as well as terms for body planes, body regions, and body cavities.

Directional Terms

Directional terms are generally grouped in pairs of opposites.

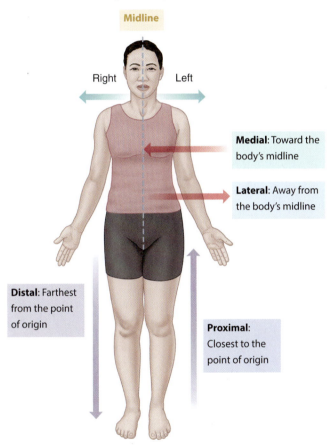

Midline

Right   Left

Medial: Toward the body's midline

Lateral: Away from the body's midline

Distal: Farthest from the point of origin

Proximal: Closest to the point of origin

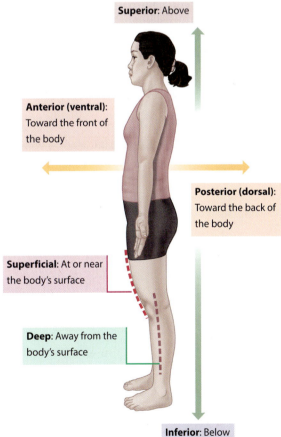

Superior: Above

Anterior (ventral): Toward the front of the body

Posterior (dorsal): Toward the back of the body

Superficial: At or near the body's surface

Deep: Away from the body's surface

Inferior: Below

FAST FACT

All terms are based on the body being in the anatomical position—standing erect, arms at the sides, with face, palms, and feet facing forward. Keep in mind, too, that the terms *right* and *left* always refer to the *patient's* right and left side.

Body Planes

Body planes divide the body, or an organ, into sections.

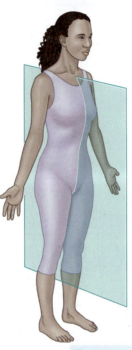

Sagittal Plane

- Divides the body lengthwise into right and left sides
- Called a *midsagittal* plane if the section is made exactly at midline
- Often used in illustrations to reveal the organs in the head or pelvic cavity

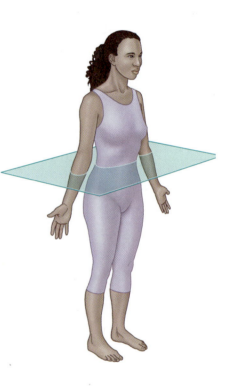

Transverse Plane

- Divides the body horizontally into upper (superior) and lower (inferior) portions
- Also called a *horizontal* plane
- Used by CT scanners to reveal internal organs

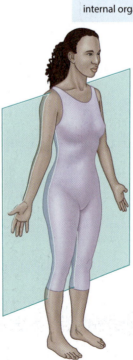

Frontal Plane

- Divides the body lengthwise into anterior and posterior portions
- Also called a *coronal* plane
- Often used in illustrations to show the contents of the abdominal and thoracic cavities

FAST FACT

The frontal plane is also called a coronal plane because the line of the plane crosses the top, or crown, of the head. The word *coronal* comes from a Latin word meaning crown.

Body Regions

The illustration below shows the terms for the different regions of the body. These terms are used extensively when performing clinical examinations and medical procedures.

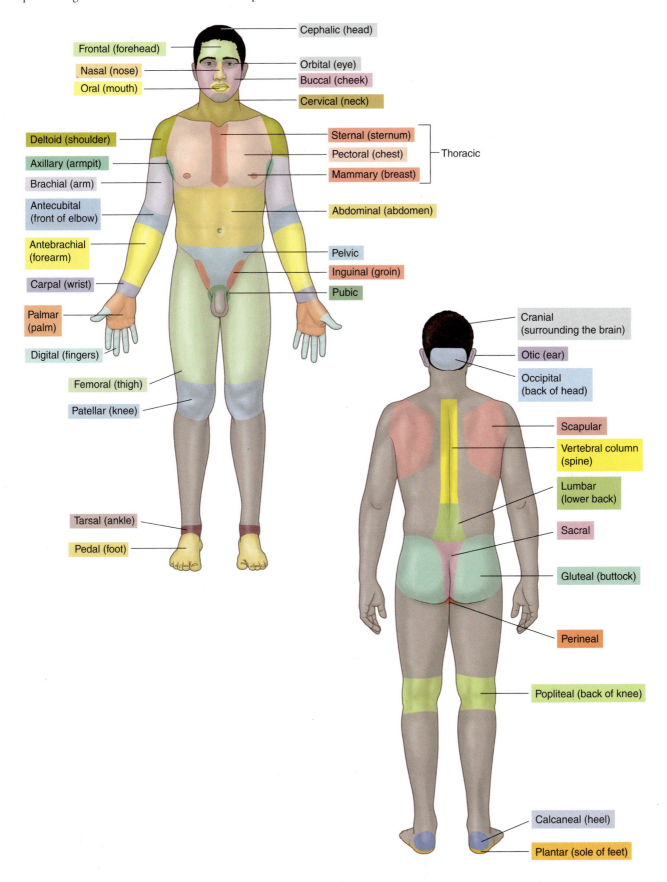

Cephalic (head)

Frontal (forehead)

Nasal (nose)

Oral (mouth)

Orbital (eye)

Buccal (cheek)

Cervical (neck)

Deltoid (shoulder)

Axillary (armpit)

Brachial (arm)

Antecubital (front of elbow)

Antebrachial (forearm)

Carpal (wrist)

Palmar (palm)

Digital (fingers)

Femoral (thigh)

Patellar (knee)

Sternal (sternum)

Pectoral (chest)

Mammary (breast)

} Thoracic

Abdominal (abdomen)

Pelvic

Inguinal (groin)

Pubic

Tarsal (ankle)

Pedal (foot)

Cranial (surrounding the brain)

Otic (ear)

Occipital (back of head)

Scapular

Vertebral column (spine)

Lumbar (lower back)

Sacral

Gluteal (buttock)

Perineal

Popliteal (back of knee)

Calcaneal (heel)

Plantar (sole of feet)

Body Cavities

The body contains spaces—called cavities—that house the internal organs. The two major body cavities are the **dorsal cavity** and the **ventral cavity**. Each of these cavities is subdivided further, as shown below.

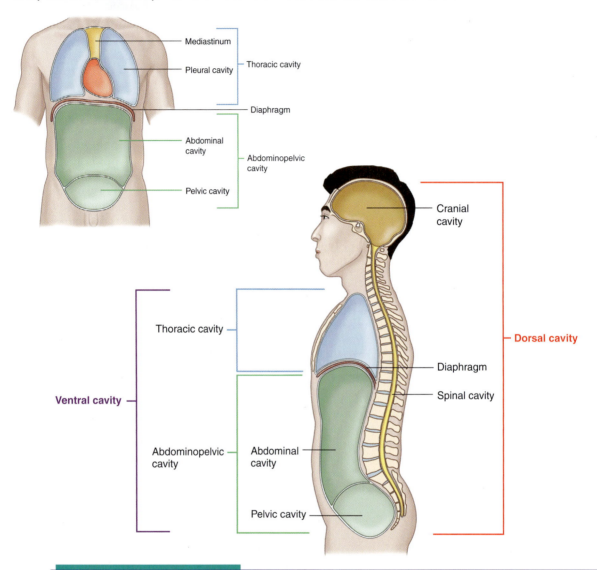

Ventral Cavity	Dorsal Cavity
• Located at the front of the body	• Located at the back of the body
• Consists of two compartments (the thoracic and abdominopelvic), which are separated by the diaphragm	• Contains two divisions but is one continuous cavity
Thoracic cavity	**Cranial cavity**
• Surrounded by ribs and chest muscles	• Formed by the skull
• Subdivided into two pleural cavities (each containing a lung) and the mediastinum	• Contains the brain
• The mediastinum contains the heart, large vessels of the heart, trachea, esophagus, thymus, lymph nodes, and other blood vessels and nerves	
Abdominopelvic cavity	**Spinal cavity**
• Subdivided into the abdominal cavity and the pelvic cavity	• Formed by the vertebrae
• The abdominal cavity contains the stomach, intestines, spleen, liver, and other organs	• Contains the spinal cord
• The pelvic cavity contains the bladder, some of the reproductive organs, and the rectum	

Abdominal Regions and Quadrants

Because the abdominopelvic cavity is so large, and because it contains numerous organs, it's divided further into regions (which are used to locate organs in anatomical studies) as well as quadrants (which are used to pinpoint the site of abdominal pain).

Abdominal Regions

The illustration below shows the location of the nine abdominal regions. The chart beside it lists some (but not all) of the organs found in each quadrant. Note that some organs, such as the liver, stretch over multiple quadrants.

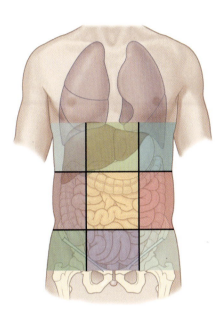

Right Hypochondriac Region	Epigastric Region	Left Hypochondriac Region
• Liver • Gallbladder • Right kidney	• Stomach • Liver • Pancreas • Right and left kidneys	• Stomach • Liver (tip) • Left kidney • Spleen
Right Lumbar Region	**Umbilical Region**	**Left Lumbar Region**
• Liver (tip) • Small intestines • Ascending colon • Right kidney	• Stomach • Pancreas • Small intestines • Transverse colon	• Small intestines • Descending colon • Left kidney
Right Iliac Region	**Hypogastric Region**	**Left Iliac Region**
• Small intestines • Appendix • Cecum and ascending colon	• Small intestines • Sigmoid colon • Bladder	• Small intestines • Descending colon • Sigmoid colon

Abdominal Quadrants

Probably used most frequently, lines intersecting at the umbilicus divide the abdominal region into four quadrants.

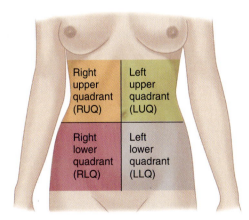

Life lesson: Abdominal pain

Abdominal pain is a common complaint, but diagnosing the cause can be difficult. While some conditions cause pain in a particular quadrant—for example, appendicitis typically causes pain in the right lower quadrant—many times abdominal pain results from a disorder in an entirely different area. For example, disorders in the chest, including pneumonia and heart disease, can also cause abdominal pain. This is called *referred pain*. Likewise, although the gallbladder is located in the right upper quadrant of the abdomen—and may cause pain in this region—it may also cause referred pain in the shoulder.

To function properly, the body must maintain a relatively constant internal environment despite changes in external conditions. This constancy, or balance, is called **homeostasis**. Because the body must make constant changes to maintain balance, homeostasis is often referred to as maintaining a **dynamic equilibrium**. (*Dynamic* means "active," and *equilibrium* means "balanced.") If the body loses homeostasis, illness or even death will occur.

Specifically, the body operates within a narrow range of temperature, fluids, and chemicals. This range of normal is called the **set point** or **set point range**. For example, the body's internal temperature should remain between 97° and 99° F (36°–37.2° C) despite the temperature outside the body. Likewise, blood glucose levels should remain between 65 and 99 mg/dl, even when you decide to indulge in an occasional sugar-laden dessert. Just as a gymnast must make constant physical adjustments to maintain balance on a balance beam, the body must make constant internal adjustments to maintain homeostasis.

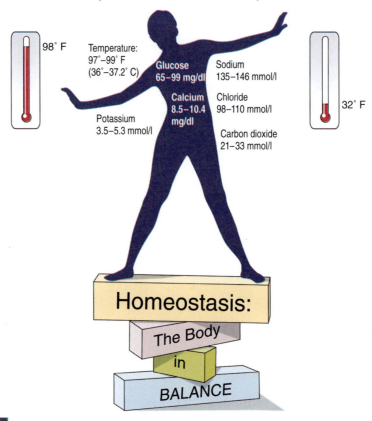

The Body AT WORK

Every organ system is involved in helping the body maintain homeostasis. None works in isolation. The body depends on all organ systems interacting together. In fact, a disruption in one body system usually has consequences in one or more other systems.

Consider how the following systems contribute to helping the body generate heat:

- **Nervous system**: The hypothalamus in the brain contains the body's "thermostat."
- **Cardiovascular system**: Blood vessels constrict to conserve heat.
- **Muscular system**: The muscles contract to cause shivering, which generates heat.
- **Integumentary system**: Sweat production stops and "goose bumps" form, which creates an insulating layer.
- **Endocrine system**: Thyroid hormone production increases metabolism, which raises body temperature.
- **Digestive system**: The metabolism of food and stored fat generates heat.

That Makes Sense

To grasp how homeostasis works, think of balancing a pencil on your finger. If you hold your finger still, the pencil will remain motionless and balanced. This reflects static (or nonmoving) equilibrium. If you move your finger slightly, the pencil will move. By making fine adjustments to your finger, you can keep the pencil balanced as it moves. This is dynamic equilibrium, just as homeostasis is a type of dynamic equilibrium. If the pencil veers too far to one side, it will fall. In the body, this type of shift results in disease.

Homeostatic Regulation

Maintaining a stable environment requires constant monitoring and adjustment as conditions change. This process of adjustment (called **homeostatic regulation**) involves:

1. a receptor (which receives information about a change in the environment),
2. a control center (which receives and processes information from the receptor), and
3. an effector (which responds to signals from the control center by either opposing or enhancing the stimulus).

The signal sent by the effector is called feedback; feedback can be either negative or positive.

- **Negative feedback**: when the effector *opposes* the stimulus (such as a dropping temperature) and *reverses* the direction of change (causing the temperature to rise)
- **Positive feedback**: when the effector *reinforces* the stimulus (such as uterine contractions during childbirth, which trigger the release of the hormone oxytocin) and *amplifies* the direction of change (causing even greater contractions and further release of oxytocin)

Most systems supporting homeostasis operate by negative feedback. Because positive feedback is stimulatory, there are only a few situations in which it is beneficial to the body (such as during childbirth or in blood clotting). More often, positive feedback is harmful (such as when a high fever continues to rise).

Homeostatic Regulation Through Negative Feedback

ANIMATION

Change in environment

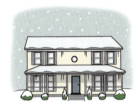

The outside temperature falls.

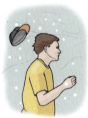

The outside temperature falls.

Receptor

A thermometer in the house detects the falling temperature and sends a message to the thermostat.

Temperature receptors in the skin detect the falling temperature and send a message to the brain.

Control center

The thermostat has been adjusted to a "set point" of 68°. When the temperature falls below that point, it sends a message to the furnace.

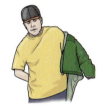

The hypothalamus in the brain receives the message that the body temperature is dropping below its "set point" and sends nerve impulses to the muscles.

Effector

The furnace then begins to generate heat, raising the indoor temperature.

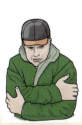

The muscles begin to shiver, causing the body temperature to rise.

Review of Key Terms

Anatomy: The study of the structure of the body

Anterior: Toward the front of the body

Distal: Farthest from the point of origin

Dorsal cavity: Located at the back of the body; contains the cranial and spinal cavities

Frontal plane: Divides the body lengthwise into anterior and posterior portions

Homeostasis: The state of dynamic equilibrium of the internal environment of the body

Inferior: Beneath or lower

Lateral: Away from the body's midline

Medial: Toward the body's midline

Negative feedback: When the effector opposes the stimulus and reverses the direction of change

Organ: Structures of two or more tissue types that work together to carry out a particular function

Organelle: Metabolic units (or "tiny organs") within a cell that perform a specific function necessary to the life of the cell

Pathophysiology: Functional changes resulting from disease

Physiology: The study of how the body functions

Positive feedback: When the effector reinforces the stimulus and amplifies the direction of change

Posterior: Toward the back of the body

Proximal: Closest to the point of origin

Sagittal plane: Divides the body into right and left sides

Superficial: At or near the body's surface

Superior: Situated above something else

Tissue: Specialized groups of cells with similar structure and function

Transverse plane: Divides the body into upper (superior) and lower (inferior) portions

Ventral cavity: Located at the front of the body; consists of the thoracic and abdominopelvic cavities

Own the Information

To make the information in this chapter part of your working memory, take some time to reflect on what you've learned. On a separate sheet of paper, write down everything you recall from the chapter. After you're done, log on to the Davis*Plus* website, and check out the Study Group podcast and Study Group Questions for the chapter.

Key Topics for Chapter 1:
- Organization of the body
- Organ systems
- Directional terms
- Body planes
- Body regions
- Body cavities
- Abdominal regions and quadrants
- Homeostasis and homeostatic regulation

Test Your Knowledge

1. The study of the structure of the body is:
   a. physiology.
   b. anatomy.
   c. pathophysiology.
   d. homeostasis.

2. Specialized groups of cells with similar structure and function are:
   a. tissues.
   b. organs.
   c. organelles.
   d. mitochondria.

3. The term used to describe something toward the body's midline is:
   a. lateral.
   b. superficial.
   c. medial.
   d. proximal.

4. The plane that divides the body into right and left sides is the:
   a. transverse plane.
   b. sagittal plane.
   c. lateral plane.
   d. frontal plane.

5. Which organ system functions to destroy pathogens that enter the body?
   a. Circulatory system
   b. Nervous system
   c. Immune system
   d. Respiratory system

6. The term *patellar* is used to identify which region of the body?
   a. Foot
   b. Palm
   c. Knee
   d. Armpit

7. What is the name of the major body cavity encompassing the front portion of the body?
   a. Pelvic
   b. Ventral
   c. Dorsal
   d. Thoracic

8. What is the term used to describe the abdominal region just under the breastbone?
   a. Hypogastric
   b. Hypochondriac
   c. Epigastric
   d. Iliac

9. What type of tissue covers or lines body surfaces?
   a. Muscular
   b. Connective
   c. Skeletal
   d. Epithelial

10. The process of homeostatic regulation operates most often through a system of:
    a. positive feedback.
    b. negative feedback.
    c. situs inversus.
    d. respiration.

Answers: Chapter 1

1. *Correct answer:* **b.** Physiology is the study of how the body functions. Pathophysiology is the study of the processes that disturb normal function. Homeostasis is the state of dynamic equilibrium of the internal environment of the body.

2. *Correct answer:* **a.** Organs are structures of two or more tissue types that work together to carry out a particular function. Organelles are the metabolic units within a cell. Mitochondria are a type of organelle.

3. *Correct answer:* **c.** Lateral refers to something away from the body's midline. Superficial means at or near the body's surface. Proximal means closest to the point of origin.

4. *Correct answer:* **b.** The transverse plane divides the body into upper and lower portions. The frontal plane divides the body into anterior and posterior portions. There is no lateral plane.

5. *Correct answer:* **c.** The circulatory system distributes oxygen and nutrients throughout the body. The nervous system controls and regulates the other body systems. The respiratory system absorbs oxygen and discharges carbon dioxide.

6. *Correct answer:* **c.** The term for foot is *pedal*. The term for palm is *volar*. The term for armpit is *axillary*.

7. *Correct answer:* **b.** The pelvic and thoracic cavities are contained within the ventral cavity. The dorsal cavity encompasses the posterior portion of the body.

8. *Correct answer:* **c.** The hypogastric region lies below the umbilicus. The hypochondriac regions lie to the right and the left of the epigastric region. The iliac regions lie in the lower portion of the abdomen, to the right and the left of the hypogastric region.

9. *Correct answer:* **d.** Muscular tissue produces movement. Connective tissue connects and supports parts of the body. Skeletal is a type of muscular tissue.

10. *Correct answer:* **b.** Positive feedback is rarely beneficial to the body, and therefore does not typically promote homeostasis. Situs inversus is a rare condition in which the organs are reversed. Respiration works with the other body systems to contribute to homeostasis, but it is not the means by which homeostasis is maintained.

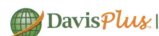

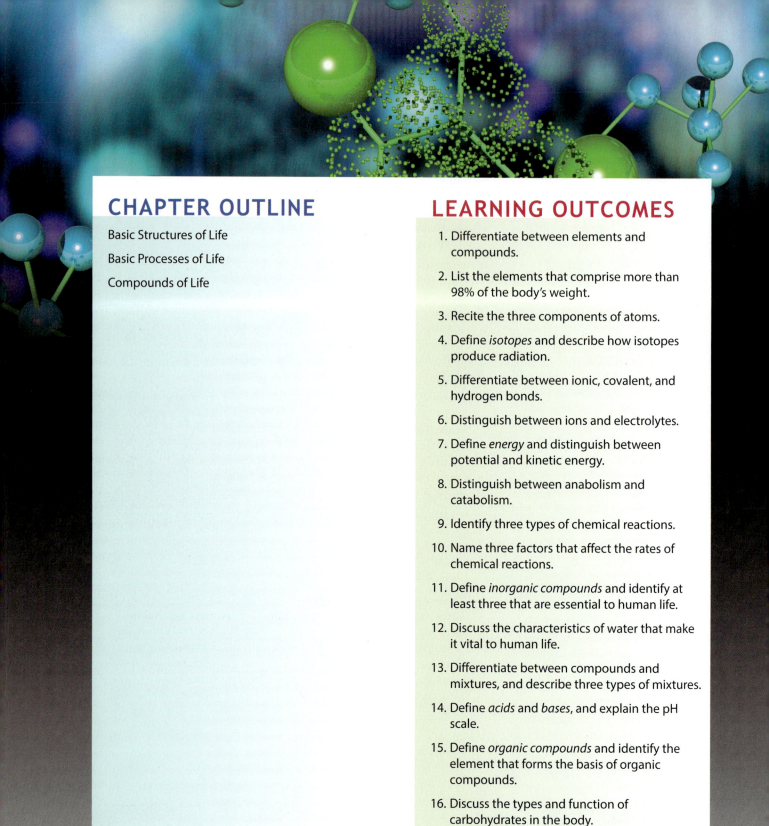

CHAPTER OUTLINE

Basic Structures of Life

Basic Processes of Life

Compounds of Life

LEARNING OUTCOMES

1. Differentiate between elements and compounds.

2. List the elements that comprise more than 98% of the body's weight.

3. Recite the three components of atoms.

4. Define *isotopes* and describe how isotopes produce radiation.

5. Differentiate between ionic, covalent, and hydrogen bonds.

6. Distinguish between ions and electrolytes.

7. Define *energy* and distinguish between potential and kinetic energy.

8. Distinguish between anabolism and catabolism.

9. Identify three types of chemical reactions.

10. Name three factors that affect the rates of chemical reactions.

11. Define *inorganic compounds* and identify at least three that are essential to human life.

12. Discuss the characteristics of water that make it vital to human life.

13. Differentiate between compounds and mixtures, and describe three types of mixtures.

14. Define *acids* and *bases*, and explain the pH scale.

15. Define *organic compounds* and identify the element that forms the basis of organic compounds.

16. Discuss the types and function of carbohydrates in the body.

17. Summarize the types and functions of lipids.

18. Describe the structure of protein and discuss the roles of protein in the body.

19. Explain the structure of ATP, its role in the body, and how it is formed.

20. Identify the body's two main types of nucleic acids.

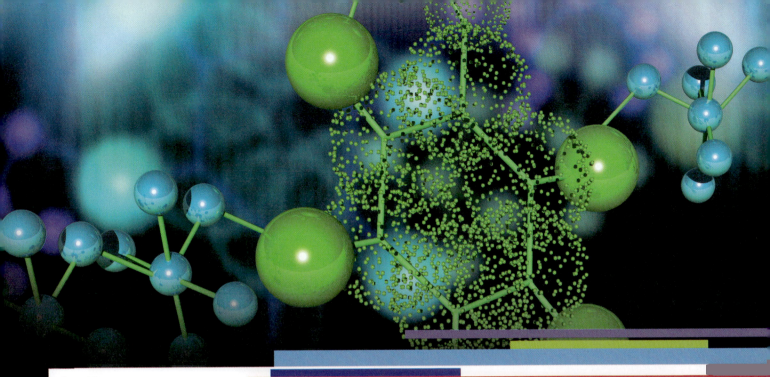

CHEMISTRY OF LIFE

Almost 60 chemical elements are found in the body, but the purpose for every one of those elements is still unknown.

We know a lot about the chemistry of life, but not everything. For example, we know that 96% of the human body consists of just four elements: oxygen, carbon, hydrogen, and nitrogen. Most of that is in the form of water. The remaining 4% consists of a sampling of various elements of the periodic table.

Life depends on a precise balance between all of those chemicals. Scientists may not know the exact purpose of every element in the body, but they do know they're all essential. The first step in understanding the human body is grasping how those chemicals interact. Without that knowledge, how can you explain why a potassium deficiency can cause an abnormal heartbeat? Or why too much sodium in the diet may lead to high blood pressure? What's more, how can you comprehend how medications (which are chemicals) can effectively treat disease?

MATTER
is anything that has mass and occupies space. In turn, matter consists of substances that can be either elements or compounds.

ELEMENTS
are pure substances: they can't be broken down or decomposed into two or more substances.

One example is oxygen; oxygen can't be broken down or decomposed into anything but oxygen.

COMPOUNDS
are chemical combinations of two or more elements.

(For example, water is a compound that results from the combination of hydrogen and oxygen. Hydrogen and oxygen are elements, each having their own unique properties; in turn, the properties of water are entirely different than those of either hydrogen or oxygen.)

Basic Structures of Life

Elements

Of the 92 elements known to exist in nature, 24 are found in the human body.

Major Elements

Name	Symbol	Percentage of Body Weight
Oxygen	O	65.0
Carbon	C	18.0
Hydrogen	H	10.0
Nitrogen	N	3.0
Calcium	Ca	1.5
Phosphorus	P	1.0

These six elements account for 98.5% of the body's weight.

Lesser Elements

Name	Symbol	Percentage of Body Weight
Sulfur	S	0.25
Potassium	K	0.20
Sodium	Na	0.15
Chlorine	Cl	0.15
Magnesium	Mg	0.05
Iron	Fe	0.006

These six elements account for 0.8% of the body's weight.

Trace Elements

Name	Symbol	Name	Symbol
Chromium	Cr	Molybdenum	Mo
Cobalt	Co	Selenium	Se
Copper	Cu	Silicon	Si
Fluorine	F	Tin	Sn
Iodine	I	Vanadium	V
Manganese	Mn	Zinc	Zn

These 12 elements—known as **trace elements**—comprise just 0.7% of the body's weight. Although minute in quantity, each is necessary for the body to function properly.

FAST FACT

If the body becomes contaminated with elements that don't serve a purpose in the body—such as lead or mercury—serious illness or disease may occur. For example, exposure to lead or mercury can lead to heavy-metal poisoning.

That Makes Sense

Each element is represented by a symbol consisting of one or two letters derived from its name. For example, H represents hydrogen, C represents carbon, and He represents helium. Most, but not all, of the symbols are based on their English names. Several are derived from other languages: mostly Latin. For example, the symbol for iron is Fe, which comes from the Latin ferrum; the symbol for potassium is K, which comes from the Latin kalium.

Atoms

Elements consist of particles called **atoms**. Atoms, in turn, consist of even smaller particles called protons, neutrons, and electrons.

ANIMATION

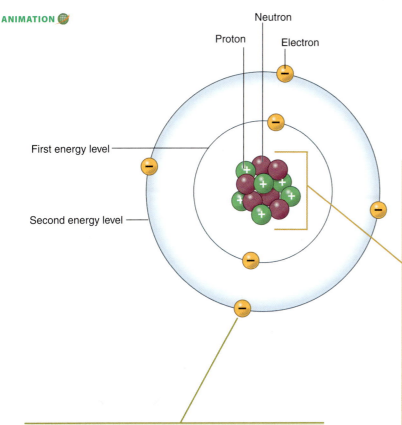

Neutron

Proton   Electron

First energy level

Second energy level

Protons and **neutrons** are packed together in the center of the atom, called the **nucleus**. Protons carry a positive charge, while neutrons are electrically neutral.

- Each element contains a unique number of protons. In other words, the atoms of the 92 elements contain between 1 and 92 protons, with no two elements having the same number of protons.
- The number of protons in the nucleus determines the element's **atomic number**. (For example, hydrogen has one proton, so its atomic number is 1. Oxygen has eight protons, so it has an atomic number of 8.)
- The number of protons and neutrons added together is known as its **atomic weight**. (For example, a carbon atom has six protons and six neutrons; its atomic number is six and its atomic weight is 12. Sodium has 11 protons and 12 neutrons. Its atomic number is 11 and its atomic weight is 23.)

Whirling around the nucleus are one or more concentric clouds of **electrons**: tiny particles with a negative charge.

- The number of electrons equals the number of protons.
- The electron's negative charge cancels out the proton's positive charge, making the atom electrically neutral.
- Each ring, or shell, around the nucleus represents one energy level. The number of shells varies between atoms. For example, hydrogen has only one shell, while potassium has four.
- Each ring can hold a certain maximum number of electrons: the shell closest to the nucleus can hold two electrons; each of the outer shells can hold eight electrons.

FAST FACT

While each element is unique, the protons, neutrons, and electrons that give them form are NOT unique. A proton of lead is the same as a proton of hydrogen. The uniqueness of each atom results from the various combinations of protons, neutrons, and electrons. For example, hydrogen has one proton and one electron, but no neutrons. Adding one proton, one electron, and two neutrons would produce helium.

Isotopes

All of the atoms of the same element contain the same number of protons. Most of them also contain the same number of neutrons. Occasionally, though, an atom of an element will contain a different number of neutrons. This is called an **isotope**.

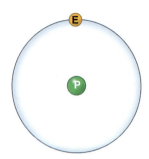

Protium

The most common form of hydrogen, called protium, has one proton and no neutrons. Its atomic number is 1 and its atomic weight is 1.

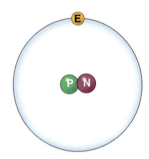

Deuterium

Another, less common form of hydrogen has one proton and one neutron. Called deuterium, it still has an atomic number of 1, but because of the extra neutron, its atomic weight is 2.

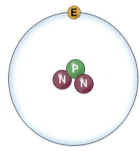

Tritium

Still another form has one proton and two neutrons. This form, called tritium, has an atomic number of 1 and an atomic weight of 3.

Although all of the isotopes of an element have identical chemical properties, some isotopes (such as tritium) are unstable. The nuclei of these isotopes break down, or decay, and, as they do, they emit radiation. These isotopes are called **radioisotopes**, and the process of decay is called **radioactivity**.

FAST FACT

We are continually exposed to low levels of radiation in the environment—including from light and radio waves. This level of radiation exposure is harmless. Higher levels of radiation damage cells and tissues. That's why radiation therapy is used to kill cancer cells. Excessive levels of radiation can cause radiation sickness, a condition that can be mild or, depending upon the level of exposure, fatal.

Life lesson: Radiation therapy

Radioactive isotopes emit particles as they break down. When those particles strike atoms in living cells, they injure or kill the cells. Knowing this, doctors often use radiation to treat patients with cancer. In fact, about half of all cancer patients receive some type of radiation therapy as part of their treatment. While radiation damages healthy cells along with the cancer cells, most healthy cells can recover from the effects of the radiation. The goal of the therapy is to damage as many cancer cells as possible while limiting the damage to nearby healthy tissue.

The type of radiation therapy given depends upon the type and location of the cancer as well as the goal of treatment. Sometimes the goal is to completely destroy the tumor. Other times, the goal is simply to shrink the tumor to help relieve symptoms.

Most often, a machine is used to deliver radiation to the outside of the body. Sometimes radiation may be implanted directly inside the tumor in the form of a tube, wire, capsule, or seeds. Radioactive material also may be administered orally or through an intravenous catheter. A new method of radiation therapy involves injecting tumor-specific antibodies that have been attached to a radioactive substance. Once inside the body, the antibodies seek out cancer cells, which are then destroyed by the radiation.

Chemical Bonds

An atom with a full outer shell is said to be stable. Most atoms are not stable, and they're drawn to other atoms as they attempt to lose, gain, or share the electrons in their outer shells (called **valence electrons**) so as to become stable. For example, an atom with seven electrons in its outer shell will be attracted to an atom with one electron in its outer shell. By joining together, they both end up with eight electrons in their outer shells. This type of interaction results in a **molecule**: a particle composed of two or more atoms united by a **chemical bond**. The three types of chemical bonds are ionic bonds, covalent bonds, and hydrogen bonds.

Ionic Bonds

Ionic bonds are formed when one atom transfers an electron from its outer shell to another atom. Because electrons are negatively charged, when an atom gains or loses an electron, its overall charge changes from neutral to either positive or negative. These electrically charged atoms are called **ions**. Atoms having a positive charge are **cations**; those with a negative charge are **anions**.

Following is an example of a common ionic bond.

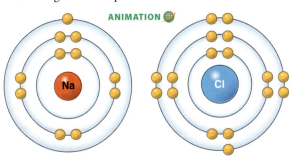

ANIMATION

Sodium has 11 electrons in three electron shells: two in the first shell, eight in the second, and one in the third. If sodium can lose the one electron in its outer shell, the second shell with 8 electrons will become the outer shell, and the atom will be stable.	Chlorine has 17 electrons: two in the first shell, eight in the second, and seven in the third. If it can gain one more electron, its third shell will be full and it, too, will be stable.

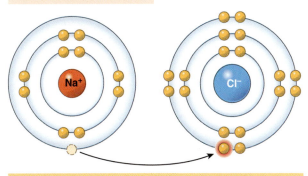

Sodium transfers its one valence electron to chlorine.

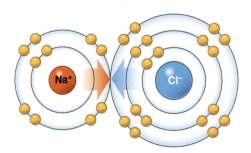

Sodium now has 11 protons in its nucleus and 10 electrons. As a result, it is an ion with a positive charge, symbolized as Na$^+$.	Chlorine has 17 protons and 18 electrons, giving it a negative charge. Called chloride, this ion is symbolized as Cl$^-$.

The positively charged sodium ion (Na$^+$) is attracted to the negatively charged chloride ion (Cl$^-$). The electrostatic force draws the two atoms together, forming an ionic bond, which results in sodium chloride (NaCl): ordinary table salt.

Ionization

When dissolved in water, ionic bonds tend to break, or **dissociate**, creating a solution of positively and negatively charged ions that's capable of conducting electricity. Also called **ionization**, this process can be illustrated by placing salt in water.

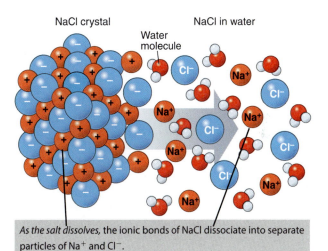

NaCl crystal   NaCl in water

Water molecule

As the salt dissolves, the ionic bonds of NaCl dissociate into separate particles of Na$^+$ and Cl$^-$.

Compounds (such as NaCl) that ionize in water and create a solution capable of conducting electricity are called **electrolytes**. Electrolytes are crucial for heart, nerve, and muscle function; the distribution of water in the body; and the occurrence of chemical reactions. A few of the body's major electrolytes include calcium chloride (CaCl$_2$), magnesium chloride (MgCl$_2$), potassium chloride (KCl), and sodium bicarbonate (NaHCO$_3$).

Maintaining electrolyte balance is a top priority in patient care. Imbalances in electrolytes can cause problems ranging from muscle cramps to cardiac arrest.

That Makes Sense

To remember the difference between cations and anions, think about this: Cations sounds like "cats," and cats have paws; cations are pawsitive. Anions sounds like "onions," and onions make you cry; anions are negative.

*Taking it one step further, **c**ations (which are positive) **c**ontribute electrons, whereas **a**nions (which are negative) **a**ccept electrons.*

Covalent Bonds

Covalent bonds are formed when two atoms *share* one or more pairs of electrons as they attempt to fill their outer shells. The major elements of the body (carbon, oxygen, hydrogen, and nitrogen) almost always share electrons to form covalent bonds. For example,

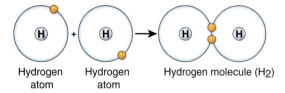

Hydrogen atom · Hydrogen atom · Hydrogen molecule (H₂)

- Hydrogen has one shell with one electron. The inner shell would be full, and the atom stable, if it had two electrons.
- If two atoms of hydrogen share their one electron, a single covalent bond exists and hydrogen gas (H_2) is formed.

Double covalent bonds may also occur, in which atoms are bound together through the sharing of two electrons. Carbon dioxide is one example of a double covalent bond.

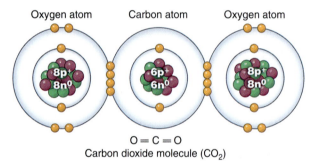

Oxygen atom · Carbon atom · Oxygen atom

$$O = C = O$$
Carbon dioxide molecule (CO_2)

- Oxygen needs two electrons to complete its outer shell. Carbon needs four electrons to complete its outer shell.
- When one carbon atom shares one pair of electrons with *two* oxygen atoms—completing the outer shells for all three atoms—a molecule of carbon dioxide is formed.

The Body AT WORK

Covalent bonds are stronger than ionic bonds, and they're used to create many of the chemical structures found in the body. For example, proteins and carbohydrates are formed through a series of covalent bonds. The fact that covalent bonds don't dissolve in water allows molecules to exist in the fluid environment of the body.

Hydrogen Bonds

Whereas a covalent bond forms a new molecule, a hydrogen bond does not. Rather, a **hydrogen bond** is a weak attraction between a slightly positive hydrogen atom in one molecule and a slightly negative oxygen or nitrogen atom in another. Water is a prime example of how hydrogen bonds function.

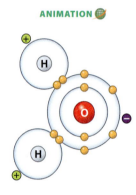

ANIMATION

- Water consists of two hydrogen atoms bonded (with covalent bonds) to an oxygen atom.
- In the bonding process, oxygen shared two of the electrons in its outer shell with hydrogen. Even after bonding, it has four additional electrons in its outer shell. These unpaired electrons give water a partial *negative* (●) charge near the oxygen atom.
- At the same time, the two hydrogen atoms create a slight *positive* (⊕) charge on the other side of the molecule.
- Therefore, although water is electrically neutral, it has an uneven distribution of electrons. This makes it a **polar** molecule.
- The partially positive oxygen side of one water molecule is attracted to the partially negative hydrogen side of another molecule. This attraction results in a weak attachment (hydrogen bond) between water molecules.

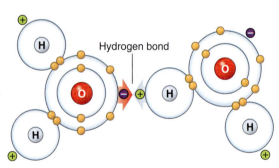

Hydrogen bond

- The ability of water molecules to form hydrogen bonds with other water molecules gives water many unique qualities important for human life. (The properties of water will be discussed in more detail later in this chapter.)

Basic Processes of Life

The microscopic world of atoms and chemical bonds forms the foundation of life. These substances are constantly at work, creating the precise internal environment for survival and providing cells and organs with the energy they need to function.

Energy

Energy is the capacity to do work: to put matter into motion. In the body, this could mean moving a muscle or moving a blood cell. The body works continually—pumping blood, creating new cells, filtering out waste, producing hormones—and therefore needs a constant supply of energy.

In the human body, energy is stored in the bonds of molecules. This is called **potential energy** because it has the potential to do work; it's just not doing work at that moment. Chemical reactions release the energy and make it available for the body to use. Energy in motion is called **kinetic energy**.

Some of the other types of energy include radiant energy (the heat resulting from molecular motion) and electrical energy. Electrical energy can be potential energy (such as when charged particles accumulate on one side of a cell membrane) or kinetic (when the ions move through the cell membrane).

That Makes Sense

For potential energy, think of a bow and arrow pulled taut. The potential for energy to be produced is there, but it's not doing work at the moment. For kinetic energy, think of that same arrow sailing forward, on its way to pierce a target.

Metabolism

The sum of all the chemical reactions in the body is called **metabolism**. (Metabolism will be discussed in more depth in Chapter 21, *Nutrition & Metabolism*.) There are two types of metabolic activity:

1. Catabolism
- This involves breaking down complex compounds (such as large food molecules) into simpler ones.
- The breaking of chemical bonds *releases* energy.
- Some of the energy released is in the form of heat, which helps maintain body temperature.
- Most of it is transferred to a molecule called adenosine triphosphate (ATP), which, in turn, transfers the energy to the cells. (ATP will be discussed in more detail later in this chapter.)

2. Anabolism
- This involves building larger and more complex chemical molecules (such carbohydrates, lipids, proteins, and nucleic acids) from smaller subunits.
- Anabolic chemical reactions *require* energy input.
- The energy needed for anabolic reactions is obtained from ATP molecules.

Chemical Reactions

Chemical reactions involve the formation or breaking of chemical bonds. The course of a chemical reaction is written as a chemical equation, with the *reactants* on the left and an arrow pointing to the *products* of the reaction on the right. Three types of chemical reactions are synthesis reactions, decomposition reactions, and exchange reactions.

Types of Chemical Reactions

Reaction	Description	Formula	Example
Synthesis	• Two or more substances combine to form a different, more complex substance. • Because new bonds are formed, energy is required.	$A + B \rightarrow AB$	Production of collagen-rich scar tissue in a healing wound
Decomposition	• A complex substance breaks down into two or more simpler substances. • Because bonds are broken, energy is released; this energy can be released in the form of heat or stored for future use.	$AB \rightarrow A + B$	Breakdown of a complex nutrient within a cell to release energy for other cellular functions
Exchange	• Two molecules exchange atoms or groups of atoms, which form two new compounds.	$AB + CD \rightarrow AC + BD$	When hydrochloric acid (HCl) and sodium bicarbonate ($NaHCO_3$) meet in the small intestine, the sodium and chlorine atoms exchange, producing salt and bicarbonate: $NaHCO_3 + HCl \rightarrow NaCl + H_2CO_3$

Reversible reactions can go in either direction under different circumstances. Many synthesis, decomposition, and exchange reactions are reversible. These reactions are symbolized by arrows pointed in both directions:

$$A + B \leftrightarrow AB$$

FAST FACT

Reversible reactions always proceed from the side with the greater quantity of reactants to the side with the lesser quantity of reactants.

The Body AT WORK

Molecules—including the molecules in the body— are constantly moving. When mutually reactive molecules collide with each other—in just the right way with the right amount of force— a reaction occurs. Factors that affect reaction rates are:

- *Temperature: Heat speeds up molecular movement, increasing the frequency and force of collisions between molecules.*
- *Concentration: In concentrated solutions, molecules are more densely packed, increasing their rate of collision.*
- *Catalysts: These are chemical substances that speed up the rate of a reaction. Protein catalysts are called **enzymes**. Most metabolic reactions inside cells are controlled by enzymes.*

Compounds of Life

Most of the molecules of the body form organic compounds, which are compounds containing carbon. However, inorganic compounds, which are simple molecules without carbon, are no less important to the maintenance of life.

Inorganic Molecules

Inorganic molecules essential to human life include water, oxygen, and carbon dioxide as well as acids and bases.

Water

Fifty percent or more of an adult's body weight is water: it exists within and around cells and is an essential component of blood. Unlike any other fluid, water has a number of characteristics that make it essential for life.

Characteristics of Water

Characteristic	How It Works in the Body
Water is a solvent—Water dissolves more substances than any other liquid.	Because of its polar nature, water can ionize, or break down, large chemical compounds and then transport them to the body's cells, which need them to function.
Water is a lubricant—Water clings to the body's tissues and forms a lubricating film on membranes.	Water clinging to the pleural and pericardial membranes helps reduce friction as the lungs and heart expand and contract. Also, fluid within the joint cavities prevents friction as the bones move.
Water changes temperature slowly—Water can absorb and release large amounts of heat without changing temperature.	This characteristic allows the body to maintain a stable body temperature. It also allows the body to "cool off" when overheated. Specifically, when water in the form of sweat changes from a liquid to a vapor, it carries with it a large amount of heat.

Body Fluids

The fluids in the body consist of chemicals dissolved or suspended in water. Therefore, the first step in learning about body fluids is to understand the difference between a mixture and a compound.

- **Compound:** When two or more elements *combine* to create a new substance that has its own chemical properties.
  - *Example:* The elements Na and Cl are, by themselves, poisonous; however, when they combine, they create the compound table salt, which is essential for life.
  - *Example:* Water, too, is a molecular compound, resulting from the chemical combination of hydrogen and oxygen.

- **Mixture:** Results when two or more substances *blend* together rather than chemically combine. Each substance retains its own chemical properties, and, because they're not chemically combined, the substances can be separated.
  - *Example:* When you're scrambling eggs and you add salt, you're creating a mixture. The eggs still taste like eggs, and they retain all the properties of an egg; they just have an additional taste of salt.

FAST FACT

Nearly every metabolic reaction in the body depends upon the solvency of water.

Types of Mixtures

Mixtures of substances in water can be solutions, colloids, and suspensions.

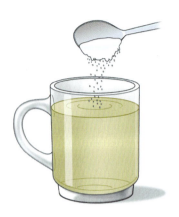

Solution

- A solution consists of particles of matter, called the **solute**, dissolved in a more abundant substance—usually water—called the **solvent**.
- A solution can be gas, solid, or liquid.
- The solvent must be clear—with none of the particles visible—and the particles can't separate out of the solvent when the solution is allowed to stand.
- *Examples:* Sugar in water; glucose in blood

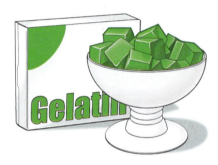

Colloid

- In the human body, these are usually mixtures of protein and water.
- Colloids can change from liquid to a gel.
- The particles are small enough to stay permanently mixed, but large enough so that the mixture is cloudy.
- *Examples:* Gelatin; thyroid hormone (as stored in the thyroid gland)

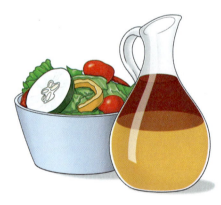

Suspension

- Suspensions contain large particles, making the suspension cloudy or even opaque.
- If allowed to stand, the particles will separate and settle at the bottom of the container.
- *Examples:* Salad dressing; blood cells in plasma

Oxygen and Carbon Dioxide

Oxygen and carbon dioxide are two inorganic substances involved in the process of **cellular respiration**—the production of energy within cells. Cells need oxygen to break down nutrients (such as glucose) to release energy. In turn, the process releases carbon dioxide as a waste product. Although it's a waste product, carbon dioxide plays a crucial role in the maintenance of acid-base balance.

Acids, Bases, and pH

Acids and bases are among the most important chemicals in the body. For the body to function properly, it must maintain a very precise balance between these two chemicals. (For more information on acid-base balance, see Chapter 19, *Fluid, Electrolyte, & Acid-Base Balance.*)

Scientists have long known that acids and bases are chemical opposites: acids taste sour, while bases taste bitter; acids turn litmus paper red, while a base will turn it blue. Acids and bases both dissociate in solution, but when they do, they release different types of ions.

Acids

An **acid** is any substance that releases a hydrogen ion (H^+) when dissolved in water. Because they relinquish an H^+ ion, acids are sometimes called *proton donors*.

ANIMATION

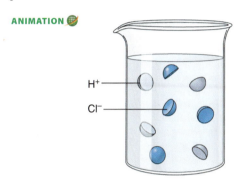

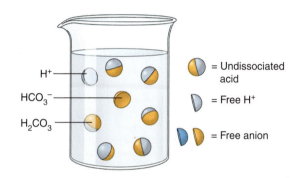

Strong acid

When hydrochloric acid (HCl) is dissolved in water, it dissociates into H^+ and Cl^- ions. A strong acid (like HCl) completely dissociates into H^+ and an ion.

Weak acid

In contrast, carbonic acid (H_2CO_3) dissociates very little and produces few excess H^+ ions in solution. The fact that it produces few H^+ ions makes it a weak acid.

Bases

Bases, or alkaline compounds, are called *proton acceptors*. In general, bases balance out acids by "accepting" excess hydrogen ions.

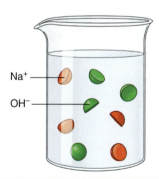

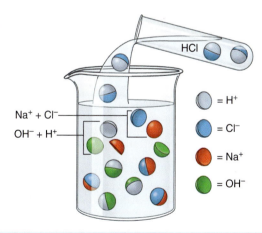

Base

A common base called sodium hydroxide (NaOH) dissociates into Na^+ and OH^- when dissolved in water.

Acid+Base

If an acid like HCl were to be introduced into this solution, the HCl would also dissociate. The solution would then have H^+ ions, Cl^- ions, Na^+ ions, and OH^- ions. The OH^- ions would accept H^+ ions, forming H_2O and reducing the acidity of the solution. The Na^+ and Cl^- ions would also combine, forming NaCl (salt).

The pH Scale

The acidity or alkalinity of a substance is expressed in terms of **pH**. The pH scale ranges from 0 to 14.

FAST FACT

pH is an abbreviation for the phrase "the power of hydrogen."

A solution with a pH less than 7 is **acidic**. The lower the pH value, the more H^+ ions the solution has and the more acidic it is.

A solution with a pH of 7 is neutral, containing equal numbers of H^+ and OH^- ions.

Solutions with a pH greater than 7 are **basic** (alkaline). The higher the pH value, the more OH^- ions the solution has, and the more alkaline it is.

FAST FACT

Each number on the pH scale represents a 10-fold change in H^+ concentration. In other words, a solution with a pH of 3 is 10 times more acidic than a solution with a pH of 4 and 100 times more acidic than one with a pH of 5. Therefore, even slight changes in pH represent significant changes in H^+ concentration.

The Body AT WORK

The normal pH range of human blood is extremely narrow: ranging from 7.35 to 7.45. Even slight deviations of pH can seriously disrupt normal body function. Substances called **buffers** help the body achieve this goal by donating or removing H^+ ions as necessary to keep the pH within the normal range. (For more information on buffers and pH balance, see Chapter 19, Fluid, Electrolyte, & Acid-Base Balance**.**)

0	Hydrochloric acid (0)
1	Gastric acid (0.9–3.0)
2	Lemon juice (2.3)
3	Wine, vinegar (2.4–3.5)
4	Bananas, tomatoes (4.7)
5	Bread, black coffee (5.0)
6	Milk, saliva (6.3–6.6)
	Pure water (7.0)
7	Blood (7.3–7.5)
8	Egg white (8.0)
9	Household bleach (9.5)
10	
	Household ammonia (10.5–11.0)
11	
12	Hair remover (12.5)
13	Oven cleaner, lye (13.4)
14	(NaOH) Sodium hydroxide (14.0)

Organic Compounds

The term *organic* is used to describe the vast array of compounds containing carbon. Carbon serves as the basis for thousands of molecules of varying size and shape. In the human body, the four major groups of organic substances are carbohydrates, lipids, proteins, and nucleic acids.

Carbohydrates

Carbohydrate molecule

Commonly called sugars or starches, **carbohydrates** are the body's main energy source. The body obtains carbohydrates by eating foods that contain them (such as potatoes, vegetables, rice, etc.). Then, through metabolism, the body breaks down carbohydrates to release stored energy.

All carbohydrates consist of carbon, hydrogen, and oxygen; the carbon atoms link with other carbon atoms to form chains of different lengths. The chains consist of units of sugar called saccharide units. Carbohydrates are classified according to the length of their sugar units as being either monosaccharides, disaccharides, or polysaccharides.

Monosaccharides

Contain one sugar unit.

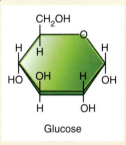

Glucose

There are three primary monosaccharides:

- **Glucose:** the primary source of energy used by most of the body's cells
- **Fructose:** found in fruit; it's converted to glucose in the body
- **Galactose:** found in dairy products; it's also converted to glucose in the body

Disaccharides

Contain two sugar units.

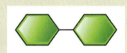

Three important disaccharides are:

- **Sucrose** (table sugar) = glucose + fructose
- **Lactose** (milk sugar) = glucose + galactose
- **Maltose** (found in germinating wheat) = glucose + glucose

Polysaccharides

Consist of many sugar units joined together in straight chains or complex shapes.

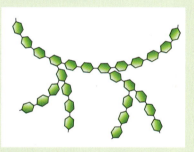

Commonly called complex carbohydrates, polysaccharides include:

- **Glycogen:** the stored form of glucose
  - When glucose levels are high (such as after eating), the liver converts excess glucose into glycogen, which it stores.
  - When glucose levels drop (such as between meals), the liver converts glycogen back into glucose and releases it into the blood to keep blood glucose levels within normal limits and provide cells with a constant supply of energy.
  - The muscles also store glycogen to meet their energy needs.

- **Starch:** the form in which plants store polysaccharides
  - Rice, potatoes, and corn are examples of foods high in starch.
  - When consumed, digestive enzymes split the starch molecule, releasing glucose.

- **Cellulose:** produced by plant cells as part of their cell walls
  - Humans can't digest cellulose and, therefore, don't obtain energy or nutrients from it.
  - Even so, cellulose supplies fiber in the diet, which helps move materials through the intestines.

FAST FACT

Glucose, fructose, and galactose are six-carbon sugars: they contain 6 carbon atoms, 12 hydrogen atoms, and 6 oxygen atoms and have the formula $C_6H_{12}O_6$. Two important monosaccharides—ribose and deoxyribose—have five carbon atoms. These sugars are components of RNA and DNA.

Lipids

Composed mostly of carbon, hydrogen, and oxygen, **lipids** are a large and diverse group. The one characteristic these organic molecules have in common is that they're insoluble in water.

Lipids serve several major roles, including being a reserve supply of energy, providing structure to cell membranes, insulating nerves, serving as vitamins, and acting as a cushion to protect organs. Types of lipids include triglycerides, steroids, and phospholipids.

Triglycerides

Triglycerides—the most abundant lipid—function as a concentrated source of energy in the body. Also called fats, triglycerides result when one molecule of glycerol combines with three fatty acids (hence, the name *tri*glyceride). Fats can be classified as *saturated* or *unsaturated*, depending on their molecular configuration.

Saturated fatty acids

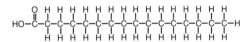

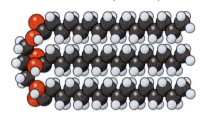

Palmitic acid (saturated)

- Consist of carbon atoms that are *saturated* with hydrogen atoms: each carbon atom in the hydrocarbon chain is bonded to the maximum number of hydrogen atoms by single covalent bonds
- Form a solid mass at room temperature (because the linear structure of the chains allows them to pack closely together)
- Usually derived from animal sources

Unsaturated fatty acids

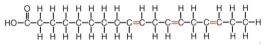

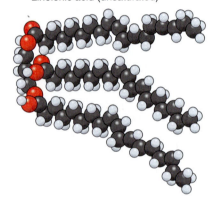

Linolenic acid (unsaturated)

- Consist of carbon atoms that are not saturated with hydrogen atoms: the hydrocarbon chain contains one or more double bonds
- Are liquid at room temperature (because kinks in the chain caused by the double bonds prevent the molecules from packing tightly together)
- Called oils
- Derived mostly from plant sources

Steroids

Steroids are a diverse group of lipids that fulfill a wide variety of roles. The most important steroid—the one from which all other steroids are made—is **cholesterol**. While high cholesterol levels have been implicated in heart disease, it remains an important component of the body. For example, cholesterol:

- is the precursor for other steroids, including the sex hormones (estrogen, progesterone, and testosterone), bile acids (that aid in fat digestion and nutrient absorption), and cortisol
- contributes to the formation of vitamin D
- provides each cell with its three-dimensional structure
- is required for proper nerve function.

About 85% of cholesterol is synthesized in the liver; the remaining 15% is consumed through diet.

Phospholipids

These fat compounds are similar to triglycerides, except that **phospholipids** have a phosphate group in place of one of the fatty acids. Phospholipids help form the structure of cell membranes.

Proteins

Proteins are the most abundant, and most important, organic compounds in the body. The structure of every cell, not to mention most of its metabolic functions, depend on proteins. Here are a few of the body's proteins along with their contributions:

- Keratin gives strength to nails, hair, and skin surface.
- Collagen lends structure to bones, cartilage, and teeth.
- Antibodies defend the body against bacteria.
- Enzymes act as catalysts for crucial chemical reactions.
- Contractile proteins promote muscle contraction.
- Hemoglobin carries oxygen in the blood.
- Hormones, such as insulin, serve as chemical messengers to cells throughout the body.

Proteins are very large molecules consisting of smaller chemical subunits called **amino acids**. All amino acids contain carbon, oxygen, hydrogen, and nitrogen; some are modified by the addition of sulfur, iron, and phosphorus. There are 20 different amino acids; 11 can be manufactured by the body, while nine must be obtained from food. All amino acids have a central carbon atom with an amino group (NH_3) and a carboxyl group (COOH) bonded to it.

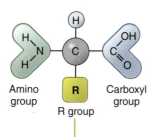

Amino group

R group

Carboxyl group

What differentiates the amino acids from each other is what's called the R group. The R group can be anything, ranging from a single hydrogen atom (as in the amino acid glycine) to a complex configuration of hydrogen and carbon.

The Body AT WORK

*Normal body function depends on proteins. The contraction of muscles, the metabolic reactions that occur inside cells, and the ability of the body to fight off foreign invaders are just a few of the processes that depend on proteins. Each protein consists of various combinations of different amino acids. Although all of these amino acids are essential to the body, the 11 amino acids listed below on the left are called **nonessential amino acids** because they can be manufactured by the body. Those on the right are called **essential amino acids** because it's essential for people to obtain them through food.*

11 Nonessential amino acids	Nine Essential amino acids
Manufactured by body	Obtained through food
Alanine	Histidine
Arginine	Isoleucine
Asparagine	Leucine
Aspartic acid	Lysine
Cysteine	Methionine
Glutamic acid	Phenylalanine
Glutamine	Threonine
Glycine	Tryptophan
Proline	Valine
Serine	
Tyrosine	

Protein Structure

Amino acids link to each other through **peptide bonds.**

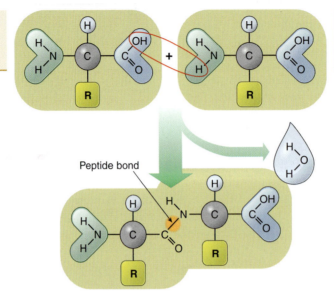

The peptide bond forms when the carboxyl group of one amino acid links to…

…the amino group of another amino acid. In the process, a molecule of water is released.

Peptide bond

A short chain of amino acids linked by peptide bonds is called a polypeptide. A protein may contain anywhere from 50 to several thousand amino acids.

Each protein has a unique three-dimensional shape, and it's this shape that determines the protein's function. Because proteins fulfill roles ranging from the simple to the very complex, it makes sense that the structures of proteins range from the simple (primary structure) to the very complex (quaternary structure).

The *primary structure* consists of a sequence of amino acids in a chain.

Amino acids   Peptide bonds

The *secondary structure* results when the amino acid chain folds or twists.

Folded sheet   Twisted helix

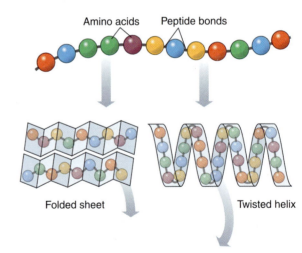

Folded sheet

Helix

The *tertiary structure* occurs when the secondary structure twists or folds a second time, creating a larger, three-dimensional structure.

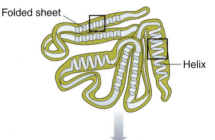

The *quaternary structure* results when two or more separate folded chains join together.

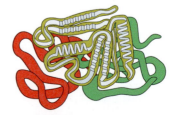

Nucleic Acids

The continuation of any species depends upon two types of **nucleic acids: DNA** (deoxyribonucleic acid) and **RNA** (ribonucleic acid). These nucleic acids consist of thousands and thousands of smaller molecules called **nucleotides**. The nucleotides are made of a five-carbon sugar (pentose sugar), a phosphate group, and one of several nitrogen bases. In DNA nucleotides, the sugar is deoxyribose; in RNA nucleotides, the sugar is ribose.

DNA—the largest molecule in the body—carries the genetic code for every hereditary characteristic ranging from eye color to nose shape. RNA, which is usually a simple strand of nucleotides, copies the genetic code of DNA to direct protein synthesis. (For more information on RNA and DNA, see Chapter 3, *Cells*.)

ATP

Food provides the body with energy. However, even when food is broken down, cells can't use it directly. Instead, cells tap into energy stored within a nucleotide called **ATP (adenosine triphosphate)**. ATP stores the energy released from the breakdown of nutrients and provides it to fuel cellular reactions. Here's how it works:

ANIMATION

ATP consists of a **base**, a **sugar**, and three **phosphate** groups.

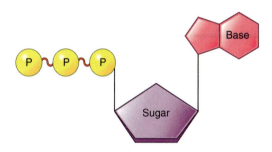

The phosphate groups are connected to each other with high-energy bonds.

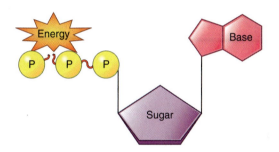

When one of these bonds is broken through a chemical reaction, energy is released that can be used for work (such as muscle movement as well as the body's physiological processes).

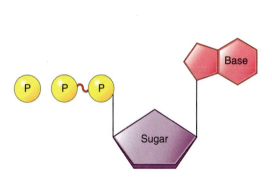

After the bond is broken, adenosine *tri*phosphate becomes adenosine *di*phosphate (ADP) and a single phosphate.

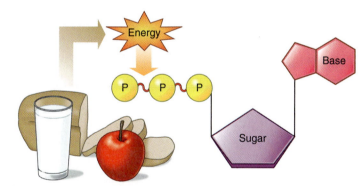

Meanwhile, the cell uses some of the energy released from the breakdown of the nutrients in food to reattach the third phosphate to the ADP, again forming ATP.

FAST FACT

Most ATP is consumed within 60 seconds of being formed. If the synthesis of ATP were to stop suddenly (which is what occurs in cyanide poisoning), death would occur within 1 minute.

Review of Key Terms

Acid: Any substance that releases hydrogen ions in solution

Amino acids: Organic compounds containing an amino (NH_2) group and a carboxyl (COOH) group that are the building blocks of proteins

Anabolism: The constructive phase of metabolism during which cells use nutrients and energy for growth and repair

Anion: An ion with a negative electrical charge

Atom: The smallest part of an element; consists of a nucleus containing protons and neutrons surrounded by electrons

Atomic number: The number of protons in the nucleus of an element

Atomic weight: The number of protons and neutrons added together

Base: Any substance that combines with hydrogen ions

Carbohydrates: Group of organic compounds known as starches or sugars that serves as the body's primary source of energy

Catabolism: Phase of metabolism during which complex substances are converted to simpler ones, resulting in the release of chemical energy

Cations: An ion with a positive electrical charge

Compound: Chemical combination of two or more elements

Covalent bond: Bond formed between two atoms when the atoms share one or more pairs of electrons

Electrolyte: A compound that dissociates in water to create a solution capable of conducting electricity

Electron: Minute particle with a negative electrical charge that revolves around the nucleus of an atom

Element: A substance that cannot be separated into substances different from itself

Enzymes: Substances that change the rate of chemical reactions without being changed themselves

Glucose: Monosaccharide that serves as the primary source of energy for most of the body's cells

Hydrogen bond: A weak attraction between a slightly positive hydrogen atom in one molecule and a slightly negative oxygen or nitrogen atom in another

Ion: Electrically charged atom

Ionic bond: Bond formed when one atom transfers an electron from its outer shell to another atom

Isotope: One of a series of chemical elements that have nearly identical chemical properties but different atomic weights and electrical charges; many are radioactive

Lipid: Group of fats characterized by their insolubility in water

Matter: Anything that has mass and occupies space

Metabolism: The sum of all the chemical reactions in the body

Molecule: A combination of two or more atoms held together by chemical bonds

Neutron: Particle without an electrical charge contained in the nucleus of an atom (along with protons)

pH: A measure of the hydrogen ion concentration of a solution

Proteins: Very large molecules consisting of smaller chemical subunits called amino acids

Proton: Particle with a positive electrical charge contained in the nucleus of an atom (along with neutrons)

Triglyceride: Most abundant lipid that functions as a source of energy in the body

Own the Information

To make the information in this chapter part of your working memory, take some time to reflect on what you've learned. On a separate sheet of paper, write down everything you recall from the chapter. After you're done, log on to the Davis*Plus* website, and check out the Study Group podcast and Study Group Questions for the chapter.

Key Topics for Chapter 2:
- The difference between matter, elements, and compounds
- The main elements in the human body
- The structure of atoms
- Chemical bonds
- Energy, metabolism, and chemical reactions
- Characteristics of water and the roles of water in the body
- The difference between compounds and mixtures
- Acids, bases, and pH
- Types of carbohydrates and their roles in the body
- Types of lipids and their roles in the body
- The structure of protein
- Nucleic acids and ATP

Test Your Knowledge

1. A chemical compound contains at least two:
   a. protons.
   b. ionic bonds.
   c. molecules.
   d. elements.

2. The atomic number of an element is determined by:
   a. the number of electrons it contains.
   b. the number of neutrons in the nucleus.
   c. its atomic weight.
   d. the number of protons in the nucleus.

3. Ionic bonds are formed when:
   a. one atom transfers an electron from its outer shell to another atom.
   b. two atoms share one or more pairs of electrons.
   c. two anions meet.
   d. two elements are dissolved in water.

4. Electrolytes are:
   a. elements that contain an extra neutron.
   b. compounds that dissociate in water.
   c. the building blocks of protein.
   d. atoms joined together by covalent bonds.

5. What is the name of the process used to break down complex compounds into simpler ones to release energy?
   a. Catabolism
   b. Anabolism
   c. Metabolism
   d. Ionization

6. Which is the most abundant inorganic compound in the body?
   a. Carbohydrates
   b. Proteins
   c. Water
   d. Lipids

7. Which type of substance releases a hydrogen ion when dissolved in water?
   a. Base
   b. Salt
   c. Electrolyte
   d. Acid

8. What is the body's main source of energy?
   a. Proteins
   b. Carbohydrates
   c. Lipids
   d. Water

9. The body stores glucose in the form of:
   a. starch.
   b. galactose.
   c. cellulose.
   d. glycogen.

10. How do cells obtain the energy they need?
    a. They receive energy directly from the catabolism of nutrients from food.
    b. They receive energy when ATP is ingested in the diet.
    c. They receive energy when the phosphate bonds of ATP are broken.
    d. Cells don't need an outside supply of energy.

Chapter 2 Answers

1. *Correct answer:* **d.** Protons are particles within an atom. An ionic bond is one type of bond, or force of attraction, that binds a molecule's atoms together. A molecule is a combination of two or more atoms held together by chemical bonds.

2. *Correct answer:* **d.** Atomic weight is determined by adding the number of protons and neutrons together. The number of electrons has nothing to do with an element's atomic number.

3. *Correct answer:* **a.** Covalent bonds are formed when two atoms share one or more electrons. Two anions do not form a bond, nor do they occur when elements are dissolved in water.

4. *Correct answer:* **b.** Compounds that contain an extra neutron are called isotopes. The building blocks of proteins are amino acids. Only ionic bonds dissociate in water.

5. *Correct answer:* **a.** Anabolism involves building larger and more complex chemical molecules (such as carbohydrates, lipids, proteins, and nucleic acids) from smaller subunits. The term *metabolism* is used to describe all the chemical reactions in the body. Ionization is when ionic bonds break or dissociate in water.

6. *Correct answer:* **c.** Carbohydrates, proteins, and lipids are all organic compounds.

7. *Correct answer:* **d.** A base accepts excess hydrogen ions. A salt is a chemical compound resulting from the interaction of an acid and a base. An electrolyte is a compound that dissociates in water.

8. *Correct answer:* **b.** Proteins and lipids can also be used for energy, but neither is the body's main source for energy. Water is necessary for life, but it is not a source of energy.

9. *Correct answer:* **d.** Starch is another name for a complex carbohydrate, or polysaccharide. Galactose and glucose combine to form lactose. Cellulose is a polysaccharide produced by plant cells and is a source of fiber in the diet.

10. *Correct answer:* **c.** Cells use some of the energy released from the breakdown of nutrients in food to reattach the third phosphate to the ADP after it has broken. ATP is not found in the diet. Cells require a constant supply of energy.

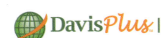

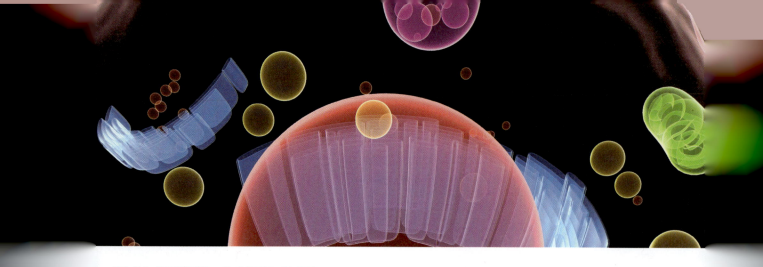

CHAPTER OUTLINE

Cell Variations

Cell Structure

Movement Through Cell Membranes

Cellular Growth and Reproduction

Protein Synthesis

Cell Growth and Reproduction

LEARNING OUTCOMES

1. Explain the reason for the variation in cell shape.

2. Identify the basic structures of a cell.

3. Describe the structure of the plasma membrane.

4. Summarize the role of phospholipids, proteins, and carbohydrates in the plasma membrane.

5. Discuss what is meant by the term "selectively permeable."

6. Describe the structure and function of the nucleus.

7. Identify and explain the functions of the main organelles of a cell, including the endoplasmic reticulum, Golgi apparatus, centrioles, lysosomes, and mitochondria.

8. Recall the structure and function of microvilli, cilia, and flagella.

9. Discuss the mechanisms used to move substances back and forth across a plasma membrane, including diffusion, osmosis, filtration, facilitated diffusion, active transport, and transport by vesicles.

10. Define osmolarity and tonicity, and compare the effects of isotonic, hypertonic, and hypotonic solutions.

11. Describe the structure of DNA, and explain its importance.

12. Describe the structure of RNA, and identify the three key ways it differs from DNA.

13. Discuss the roles of DNA and RNA in protein synthesis.

14. Describe the process of transcription and translation.

15. Describe the events of the cell cycle, including the events of mitosis.

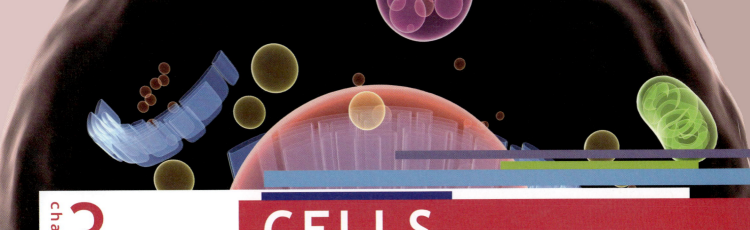

3

CELLS

The adult human body contains over 100 trillion cells. About three billion of those cells die—and most are replaced—every minute.

Cells are the simplest units of all living matter. Some (such as microscopic amoeba and bacteria) exist as independent organisms. Others (such as the cells of the human body) function only when part of a larger organism. These tiny forces of life do more than give the body structure. They also orchestrate all of the processes that make life possible: respiration, movement, reproduction, digestion, and excretion.

The body employs a vast array of cell types to accomplish these varied tasks. In fact, the human body consists of about 200 different types of cells. These cells vary greatly in size and shape, both of which are dictated by the cell's function.

Cell Variations

While human cells vary in size and shape, all are microscopic. Most range in size from 10 to 15 micrometers. (A micrometer is 1/1000 millimeter.) A blood cell measures 7.5 micrometers in diameter, while a human egg, or ovum, is much larger, at about 100 micrometers—or about the size of the period at the end of this sentence. In contrast, a nerve cell may have extensions up to a meter in length. In every instance, though, a cell's function dictates its form.

Types of Cells

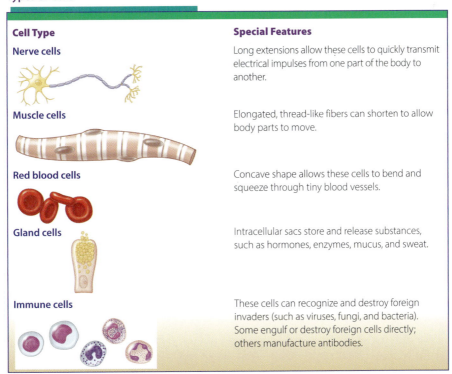

Cell Type	Special Features
Nerve cells	Long extensions allow these cells to quickly transmit electrical impulses from one part of the body to another.
Muscle cells	Elongated, thread-like fibers can shorten to allow body parts to move.
Red blood cells	Concave shape allows these cells to bend and squeeze through tiny blood vessels.
Gland cells	Intracellular sacs store and release substances, such as hormones, enzymes, mucus, and sweat.
Immune cells	These cells can recognize and destroy foreign invaders (such as viruses, fungi, and bacteria). Some engulf or destroy foreign cells directly; others manufacture antibodies.

Cell Structure

The invention of the transmission electron microscope (TEM) has transformed how scientists view cells. For years, scientists thought that a simple mixture of chemicals filled the space between a cell's membrane and its nucleus. They now know, however, that the inner workings of a cell are much more complex and that cells contain a number of highly specialized structures.

The following illustration showcases the most important structures of many different types of cells. Keep in mind that this is a representative rather than an actual cell. No single cell contains all of the specialized components found in the many different cells of the body.

The basic structures of the cell are:

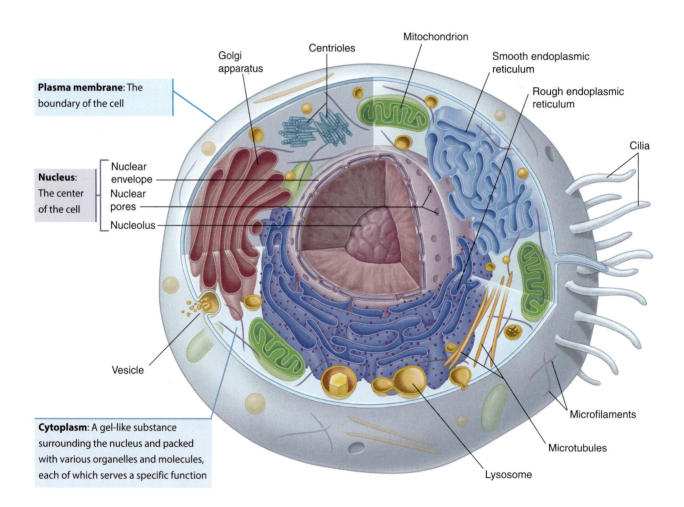

Plasma membrane: The boundary of the cell

Nucleus: The center of the cell
- Nuclear envelope
- Nuclear pores
- Nucleolus

Vesicle

Cytoplasm: A gel-like substance surrounding the nucleus and packed with various organelles and molecules, each of which serves a specific function

Golgi apparatus

Centrioles

Mitochondrion

Smooth endoplasmic reticulum

Rough endoplasmic reticulum

Cilia

Microfilaments

Microtubules

Lysosome

Plasma Membrane

Surrounding the cell is the **plasma membrane**. Besides defining the boundaries of the cell, the plasma membrane regulates the passage of substances into and out of the cell. The plasma membrane consists of phospholipids, cholesterol, and protein.

Phospholipids, which have a head and twin tails, form the bulk of the cell membrane. The heads are "water loving" (hydrophilic), while the tails are "water fearing" (hydrophobic). In an effort to keep their heads facing water, and their tails away from water, the phospholipids position themselves in a double layer (called a bilayer): the heads of some of the phospholipids point toward the fluid-filled cell interior while others point toward the fluid surrounding the cell's exterior. As a result, the tails point toward each other, forming a "hydrophobic" core.

Scattered within the phospholipid molecules are cholesterol molecules. Cholesterol helps stiffen and strengthen the plasma membrane.

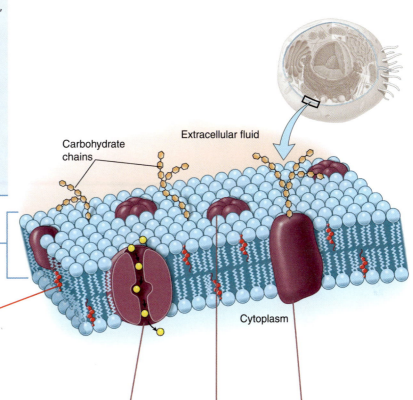

Carbohydrate chains

Extracellular fluid

Cytoplasm

Proteins are embedded in various spots in the membrane and fulfill a number of roles.

Most proteins pass all the way through the membrane and act as channels, allowing solutes to pass in and out of the cell.

Some proteins attach to the surface of the membrane, where they serve as receptors for specific chemicals or hormones.

Many proteins have carbohydrates attached to their outer surface (forming glycoproteins). Glycoproteins act as markers to help the body distinguish its own cells from foreign invaders.

The Body AT WORK

*The phospholipids and proteins forming the membrane are not stationary; they slowly move, which keeps the membrane fluid. The plasma membrane is also like a picket fence as opposed to a wall. This gives the membrane its characteristic of **selective permeability**, meaning that some substances, such as lipid-soluble molecules, pass through easily, while others do not. The various mechanisms the body uses to transport substances into and out of cells will be discussed later in this chapter.*

Nucleus

The central and most important part of the cell is the nucleus. The nucleus is the cell's control center: this microscopic structure contains all of a cell's genetic information. Most cells have only one nucleus, although a few (such as some liver cells and skeletal muscle cells) contain multiple nuclei. Mature red blood cells are the only cells that don't contain a nucleus.

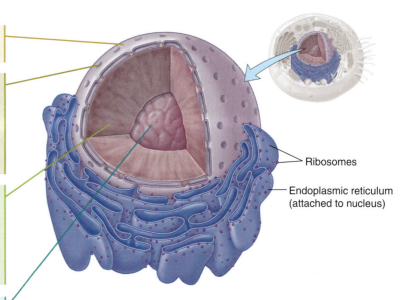

A double-layered membrane called the **nuclear envelope** surrounds the nucleus.

Perforating the nuclear envelope are **nuclear pores**. These pores regulate the passage of molecules into the nucleus (such as those needed for construction of RNA and DNA), as well as out of the nucleus (such as RNA, which leaves the nucleus to perform its work in the cytoplasm).

Extending throughout the nucleoplasm (the substance filling the nucleus) are thread-like structures composed of DNA and protein called **chromatin**. When a cell begins to divide, the chromatin coils tightly into short, rod-like structures called **chromosomes**.

In the center of the nucleus is the **nucleolus**. The nucleolus manufactures components of **ribosomes**, the cell's protein-producing structures.

Ribosomes

Endoplasmic reticulum (attached to nucleus)

FAST FACT

Packed inside the nucleus of every human cell is over 6 feet of DNA. In turn, this large polymer is divided into 46 individual molecules called chromosomes.

Cytoplasm and Organelles

Cytoplasm is the gel-like substance that fills the space between the plasma membrane and the nucleus. Packed into the cytoplasm are hundreds, or even thousands, of "little organs," or **organelles**. Organelles perform specific tasks in cellular metabolism. Following are some of the major cell structures.

Endoplasmic Reticulum

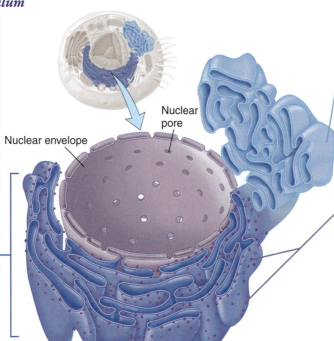

Extending throughout the cytoplasm, from the plasma membrane to the nucleus, is a network of membranous canals and curving sacs called the **endoplasmic reticulum (ER)**. Organelles called ribosomes dot the surface of some of the ER and give the ER a "rough" appearance, earning it the name rough ER. The ribosomes synthesize proteins, which move through the network of canals toward the Golgi apparatus.

Nuclear envelope

Nuclear pore

Smooth ER has no ribosomes. Smooth ER contains enzymes that synthesize certain lipids and carbohydrates.

Ribosomes

Every cell contains thousands of granules of protein and RNA called ribosomes. Some of the ribosomes are attached to the endoplasmic reticulum while others exist alone, scattered throughout the cytoplasm. Ribosomes serve to synthesize protein. Some of the protein produced is used by its host cell; other protein is exported for use elsewhere in the body.

Golgi Apparatus

Made up of flattened membranous sacs stacked one on top of the other, the **Golgi apparatus** receives proteins from the ER and prepares and packages them for export to other parts of the body, as shown in this figure. Keep in mind that the Golgi apparatus processes hundreds of different proteins simultaneously.

1 The ER delivers a protein molecule to the Golgi apparatus.

2 The protein passes through each of the sacs of the Golgi apparatus, undergoing modifications along the way.

3 At the end of the process, the Golgi apparatus envelopes the protein and then pinches off the portion of itself containing the protein, creating a vesicle.

4 Some of the vesicles travel to the surface of the cell, fuse with the plasma membrane, and pop open to release the protein inside. Others become lysosomes; still others become secretory vesicles that store substances like breast milk or digestive enzymes for later secretion.

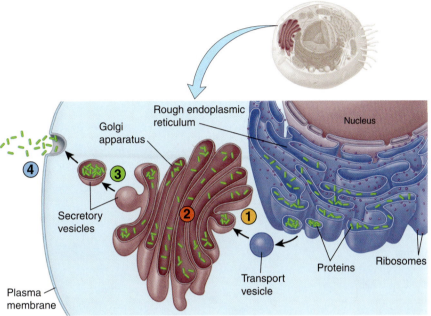

Golgi apparatus
Rough endoplasmic reticulum
Nucleus
Secretory vesicles
Proteins
Ribosomes
Transport vesicle
Plasma membrane

Centrioles

Two **centrioles** lie perpendicular to each other just outside the nucleus. These bundles of microtubules play a role in cell division.

Lysosomes

Lysosomes are membranous vesicles that form from pinched-off pieces of the Golgi apparatus. Inside, they contain various enzymes that help break down protein the cell doesn't need. Besides cleaning out the cell, this allows the cell to "reuse" amino acids. Lysosomal enzymes can also be used to destroy bacteria. These functions have earned lysosomes the nickname "cellular garbage disposals."

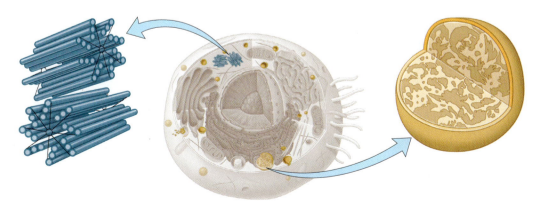

Mitochondria

These sausage-shaped organelles function as the cell's "powerhouses." **Mitochondria** have two membranes: an outer membrane and an inner membrane. The inner membrane folds back and forth across its interior; these folds are called **cristae**. The spaces between the cristae contain enzymes that the organelle uses to convert organic compounds into ATP, which cells use for energy. It makes sense that cells that do a lot of work (such as muscle cells) contain more mitochondria than cells doing less work (such as skin cells).

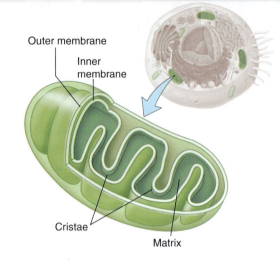

Outer membrane
Inner membrane
Cristae
Matrix

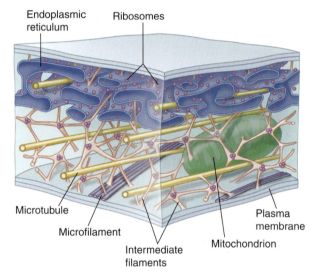

Endoplasmic reticulum
Ribosomes
Microtubule
Microfilament
Intermediate filaments
Mitochondrion
Plasma membrane

Cytoskeleton

The **cytoskeleton** is the supporting framework of the cell. Made of protein filaments and rod-like structures, the cytoskeleton determines the shape of the cell, gives it strength, and also allows the cell to move. It also helps organize the contents of the cell. In some cells, the cytoskeleton forms finger-like processes that extend outward. These processes include microvilli, cilia, and flagella.

Microvilli

Microvilli are folds of the cell membrane that greatly increase the surface area of a cell. Typically found in cells charged with absorbing nutrients—such as the intestines—microvilli can increase a cell's absorptive area as much as 40 times.

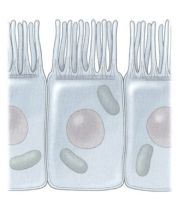

Cilia

Cilia are hair-like processes along the surface of a cell. Unlike microvilli, cilia move. They beat in waves, always in the same direction. They occur primarily in the respiratory tract—where their wave-like motion helps move mucus and foreign particles out of the lungs—and the fallopian tubes—where their motion propels an egg cell or embryo toward the uterus.

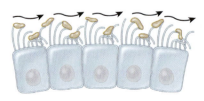

Flagella

Flagella (singular: flagellum) are similar to cilia in that they are also hair-like projections that move. However, flagella are thicker, longer, and fewer in number. Flagella have a whip-like motion that helps move a cell. The only flagellum in humans is the tail of a sperm cell.

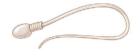

Movement Through Cell Membranes

A cell's survival depends on its ability to move substances such as nutrients and waste products where they're needed. Toward this end, the cell uses a number of transport mechanisms to move substances back and forth across its plasma membrane. These mechanisms fall into one of two categories: passive or active transport.

Passive Transport

Passive transport mechanisms—which include diffusion, osmosis, filtration, and facilitated diffusion—don't require the cells to expend energy.

Diffusion

Diffusion involves the movement of particles from an area of higher concentration to an area of lower concentration. Diffusion occurs in air or water. It can perhaps be best illustrated by placing a dye tablet in water.

ANIMATION

Dye tablet

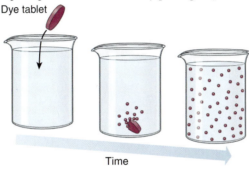

Time

- As the tablet dissolves, the particles move away from the tablet (where concentration is high) to the edges of the container (where the concentration of particles is low).
- Diffusion continues until the particles are evenly distributed. The point at which no further diffusion occurs is called **equilibrium**.

A difference in concentration of a substance from one point to another is called a **concentration gradient**. When the particles move from an area of greater to lesser concentration, as occurs in diffusion, the particles are said to move *down* the concentration gradient. Even when a membrane stands in the way, the particles will still diffuse down the concentration gradient as long as the membrane is permeable to those particles.

Osmosis

A type of diffusion, **osmosis** involves the diffusion of water *down* the concentration gradient through a selectively permeable membrane. In the body, this often happens when a particular substance can't cross the membrane. In that situation, the water—not the particles—moves in an effort to equalize the concentration.

ANIMATION

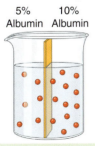

5%   10%
Albumin Albumin

7.5%   7.5%
Albumin Albumin

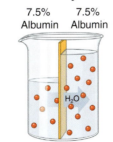

- The membrane in the container above is separating a 5% albumin solution (side A) from a 10% albumin solution (side B). The membrane is permeable to water but not to albumin.
- Side A contains more water molecules in relation to albumin molecules. Therefore, the concentration of water is greater on side A as compared to side B.

- Water molecules move from side A—the side with a higher concentration of water (and lower concentration of albumin)—to side B—the side with the lower concentration of water (and higher concentration of albumin).
- The concentration of the two solutions eventually equalizes. But, in the process, side B ends up with a greater *volume* of water.

The Body AT WORK

*As water diffuses by osmosis into a solution, the volume of that solution increases. As the volume of water on side B increases, it exerts more and more pressure (**hydrostatic pressure**) against the membrane. The greater the volume of water, the greater the hydrostatic pressure. (Think of a water balloon: the more water in the balloon, the more pressure against the sides of the balloon.) Water pressure that develops in a solution as a result of osmosis is called **osmotic pressure**. The more solute there is in a solution, the greater its osmotic pressure.*

Osmolarity and Tonicity

Cells are essentially closed containers. Besides containing fluid, they also contain a variety of solutes, such as salts, sugars, acids, and bases. It's the concentration of these solutes in the fluid that determines whether, and how much, fluid moves into or out of a cell. If a solute can't move through a plasma membrane, and if it's more concentrated on one side of the membrane than on the other, osmosis will occur. The ability of a solution to affect the fluid volume and pressure in a cell through osmosis is called **tonicity**. The three terms used to describe these solutions are isotonic, hypotonic, and hypertonic.

ANIMATION 🌐

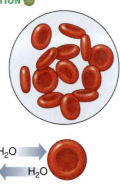

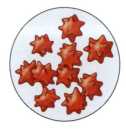

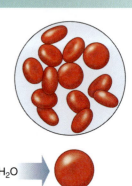

FAST FACT

Understanding tonicity is particularly important when administering intravenous fluids. Most patients receive isotonic fluids (such as normal saline, Ringer's solution, or a mixture of 5% dextrose in water [D_5W]). Isotonic fluids hydrate the body without causing dramatic fluid shifts.

Isotonic	Hypertonic	Hypotonic
An **isotonic** solution is one in which the concentration of solutes is the same as it is in the cell. When a red blood cell is placed in an isotonic solution, water moves into and out of the cell at an equal rate. As a result, the cells remain normal in size and water content.	A **hypertonic** solution contains a higher concentration of solutes compared to the fluid within the cell. If a red blood cell is immersed in a hypertonic solution, such as a concentrated salt solution, water will diffuse out of the cell, causing it to shrivel and perhaps die.	A **hypotonic** solution contains a lower concentration of solutes compared to the fluid within the cell. If a red blood cell is placed in a hypotonic solution (such as distilled water), water will move by osmosis into the cell. This influx of water will cause the cell to swell and, eventually, to burst (called lysis).

Filtration

In contrast to diffusion and osmosis—which occur because of differences in the concentrations of a solute on either side of a selectively permeable membrane—**filtration** occurs because of differences in pressure. In filtration, water and dissolved particles are forced across a membrane from an area of higher to lower hydrostatic pressure. One of the most obvious examples of filtration in the body occurs in capillaries.

ANIMATION 🌐

The hydrostatic pressure of blood inside the capillaries forces water and dissolved materials (such as nutrients) into the surrounding tissue fluid.

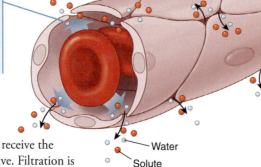

Water

Solute

This is how the body's cells receive the nutrients they need to survive. Filtration is also the method the kidneys use to remove waste products from the blood.

That Makes Sense

A household coffee pot is a perfect example of filtration. The weight of water forces water and dissolved solutes (coffee) through the filter (or membrane) while holding back larger particles (the coffee grounds).

Facilitated Diffusion

Some molecules need other molecules to help, or *facilitate*, their movement across a membrane. This is called **facilitated diffusion**. As with regular diffusion, molecules move down the concentration gradient—from an area of greater to lesser concentration.

ANIMATION

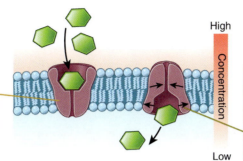

A solute (such as glucose) that can't pass through the membrane enters a channel in a protein molecule that's part of the membrane.

The solute binds to a receptor site on the protein (also called the carrier). The binding process causes the protein to change shape. This alteration in the shape of the carrier protein ejects the solute into the cell's interior.

Active Transport

In **active transport**, solutes move up the concentration gradient—from areas of lesser to greater concentration. Just like swimming upstream, moving against the concentration gradient requires energy, which is provided in the form of ATP. Active transport mechanisms include transport by pumps and transport by vesicles.

Transport by Pumps

By actively pumping, the cell can move ions and other particles to specific areas. For example, for muscle cells to operate properly, they need to maintain a low concentration of calcium whenever they're at rest. So, even though the concentration of calcium in the extracellular fluid is higher than it is inside the cell, special pumps in the cell membrane can force nearly all the intracellular calcium into other compartments.

Perhaps the most important example of active transport in the body is the **sodium-potassium pump.** This crucial pump regulates the volume of fluid within cells, provides the electrical potential necessary for nervous system activity, and helps in heat production.

Normally, the fluid inside the cell contains lower levels of sodium and higher levels of potassium than the fluid outside the cell. Even so, the sodium-potassium pump works to transfer sodium from inside the cell (where sodium levels are low) to outside the cell (where sodium levels are higher), while transferring potassium from the extracellular fluid (where potassium levels are low) to the cell's interior (where potassium levels are higher). Specifically, here's how it works:

FAST FACT

About half the calories you burn each day go to operate the sodium-potassium pump.

ANIMATION

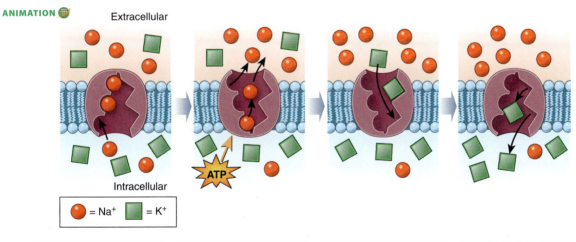

1 Three sodium ions (Na⁺) from inside the cell funnel into receptor sites on a channel protein.

2 Fueled by ATP, the channel protein releases the sodium ions into the extracellular fluid, causing them to move from an area of lower to higher concentration.

3 Meanwhile, two potassium ions (K⁺) from outside the cell enter the same channel protein.

4 The potassium ions are then released inside the cell. This keeps the concentration of potassium higher, and the concentration of sodium lower, within the cell.

Transport by Vesicles

Cells also have the ability to move large particles or numerous molecules at once through the plasma membrane. In this process, which also requires energy, the cell membrane creates a vesicle to transport the matter either into the cell or out of the cell.

Endocytosis

The form of vesicular transport that brings substances *into* the cell is called **endocytosis**. (*Endo* means to "take into.") In brief, the plasma membrane traps a substance that's too large to diffuse through the plasma membrane and brings it into the cell. There are two forms of endocytosis: phagocytosis and pinocytosis.

Phagocytosis (or "cell eating") occurs when the cell engulfs a solid particle and brings it into the cell. A key example is when white blood cells "consume" bacteria.

Pinocytosis (or "cell drinking") occurs when tiny vacuoles bring droplets of extracellular fluid containing dissolved substances into the cell. The cell then uses the engulfed fluid and nutrients.

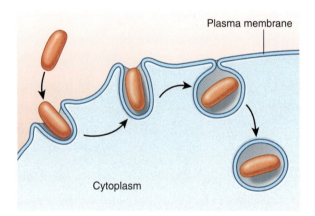

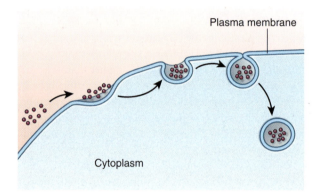

Exocytosis

In contrast to endocytosis, which brings substances into the cell, **exocytosis** uses vesicles to release substances *outside* of the cell. Glands often use this method to release hormones. For example, exocytosis occurs when mammary glands secrete milk as well as when endothelial cells release insulin.

In exocytosis, a vesicle in the cell containing the materials to be released travels to the cell's surface.

The vesicle fuses with the plasma membrane and then releases its contents outside the cell.

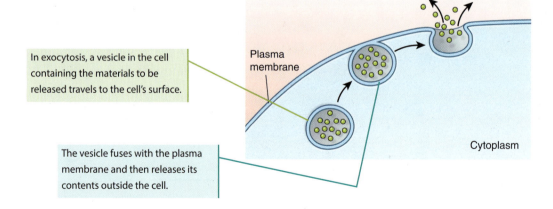

Key Transport Processes

Passive mechanisms

Diffusion
Particles move across a selectively permeable membrane from an area of high to low concentration.

Osmosis
Water diffuses across a selectively permeable membrane from an area of low concentration of solute (and a high concentration of water) to an area of high concentration of solute (and a low concentration of water).

Filtration
Water and solutes move through a selectively permeable membrane as a result of hydrostatic pressure.

Facilitated diffusion
Particles move from an area of high to low concentration with the help of a channel protein that's part of the plasma membrane.

Active mechanisms

Active transport pump
Particles are pumped from an area of low to high concentration by an energy-consuming structure in the plasma membrane.

Phagocytosis
In this form of endocytosis, large particles are trapped in a portion of the plasma membrane and brought into the cell.

Pinocytosis
In this form of endocytosis, fluid and dissolved particles are trapped in a portion of the plasma membrane and brought into the cell.

Exocytosis
Proteins or other cell products move out of a cell when a secretory vesicle containing those products fuses with the plasma membrane.

Cellular Growth and Reproduction

Throughout the nucleus of the cell are numerous thread-like structures composed of DNA and protein. The **DNA (deoxyribonucleic acid)** molecule—a type of **nucleic acid**—is one of the largest and most complex of all molecules. Overriding that is its importance: the DNA molecule stores all of a cell's genetic information—the information it needs to develop, function, and maintain itself.

Nucleic Acids

DNA is a **polymer**, meaning that it's a large molecule made up of many smaller molecules joined together in a sequence that encodes the cell's genetic information. The "building blocks" of DNA are millions of pairs of **nucleotides**. Each nucleotide consists of one sugar, one phosphate group, and one of four possible types of nitrogenous bases. The four types of bases are: **adenine (A)**, **thymine (T)**, **guanine (G)**, and **cytosine (C)**.

The structure of DNA resembles a twisted ladder, called a *double helix*.

The Body AT WORK

A single strand of DNA would stretch about 2 inches (5 cm) if uncoiled. Considering that 46 strands must fit into the microscopic nucleus of a cell, its coiled structure becomes understandable. When the cell isn't dividing, DNA is only loosely coiled. But, when the cell is preparing to divide, DNA forms a dense coil that transforms its appearance into the typical "X" shape of a paired chromosome.

ANIMATION

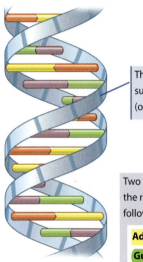

The phosphate group alternates with the sugar **deoxyribose** to form the two sides (or backbone) of the ladder.

Two different bases join together to form the rungs of the ladder. Base combinations follow a specific pattern:

Adenine can pair only with **thymine**
Guanine can pair only with **cytosine**

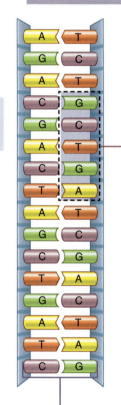

Although the base pair combinations are fixed, their sequence up and down the DNA ladder is not. For example, as you travel up one side of the DNA ladder, the sequence of bases might be A, G, T, C, G, etc. This sequence of bases is the genetic code; this code provides all the necessary information for building and maintaining an organism.

FAST FACT

The sequence of bases determines the genetic code of a strand of DNA, called a chromosome. Because the base *pairings* (such as adenine pairing with thymine, etc.) are predetermined, DNA can unwind and replicate itself exactly.

One of DNA's main functions is to provide information for building proteins. Proteins are the body's main structural molecules; they also contribute to almost every cellular function. However, DNA is too large to leave the nucleus, and protein synthesis takes place in the cytoplasm. Therefore, DNA needs help from another nucleic acid—**ribonucleic acid (RNA)**.

RNA Structure

Similar in structure to DNA, RNA is a long chain of nucleotide units consisting of a sugar, a phosphate group, and a nitrogenous base. The structure of RNA differs from that of DNA, however, in three key ways.

Guanine
Adenine
Cytosine
Uracil

1. RNA is a single strand.
2. RNA contains the sugar ribose instead of deoxyribose.
3. RNA contains the base uracil (U) instead of thymine (T). [Both RNA and DNA contain cytosine (C), guanine (G), and adenine (A).]

RNA exists in three forms: *messenger RNA* (mRNA), *transfer RNA* (tRNA), and *ribosomal RNA* (rRNA), all of which are crucial to protein synthesis.

The Body AT WORK

The bases adenine and guanine are known as purines, while cytosine, thymine, and uracil are known as pyrimidines. Some of the drugs used to fight cancer are purine and pyrimidine analogs. The hope is that, as the replicating cancer cells synthesize protein, they'll latch onto the drug instead of the real base. This will disrupt protein synthesis and kill the cell. Of course, healthy cells aren't immune to the drug, so many of them are also killed.

Protein Synthesis

Manufacture of proteins occurs in two main phases, transcription and translation.

Transcription

1 When the nucleus receives a chemical message to make a new protein, the segment of DNA with the relevant gene unwinds.

2 An RNA enzyme then assembles RNA nucleotides that would be complementary to the exposed bases. The nucleotides attach to the exposed DNA and then bind to each other to form a strand of messenger RNA (mRNA). This strand is an exact copy of the opposite side of the DNA molecule.

Translation

Once in the cytoplasm, the mRNA attaches to a ribosome, which consists of rRNA and enzymes. There, it begins the process of being "translated" into a protein. The ribosome moves along the strand of mRNA reading the codons.

Waiting in the cytoplasm are tRNA molecules. Each tRNA consists of three bases (a triplet called an **anticodon**) that will perfectly complement a specific site (the **codon**) on the mRNA. Attached to the tRNA is the amino acid for that site, according to the genetic "blueprint."

The tRNA finds the three bases that are complementary to its own and deposits the amino acid.

The ribosome then uses enzymes to attach the lengthening chain of amino acids together with peptide bonds.

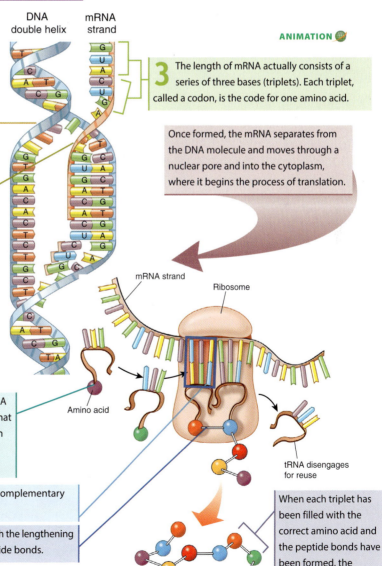

DNA double helix

mRNA strand

ANIMATION

3 The length of mRNA actually consists of a series of three bases (triplets). Each triplet, called a codon, is the code for one amino acid.

Once formed, the mRNA separates from the DNA molecule and moves through a nuclear pore and into the cytoplasm, where it begins the process of translation.

mRNA strand

Ribosome

Amino acid

tRNA disengages for reuse

When each triplet has been filled with the correct amino acid and the peptide bonds have been formed, the protein is complete.

Cell Growth and Reproduction

The survival of all living organisms depends upon the ability of cells to grow and reproduce. These two processes are known as the *cell life cycle*. Besides replacing worn-out cells, the human body must respond to the need for new cells. For example, your body grows new cells following exercise or injury. Also, when you ascend to a higher altitude, your body responds to lower levels of oxygen by producing more red blood cells. The other half of this process—cell reproduction—ensures that genetic information is passed on from one cell to the next, as well as one generation of humans to the next.

While the cell life cycle runs very well, malfunctions can occur. One major disease, cancer, results when cells multiply even though the body doesn't need them. (See "Life lesson: Cancer," later in this chapter.)

The Cell Cycle

Almost all cells periodically divide into two identical daughter cells; this is the key to the continuity of life. The cell life cycle follows the sequence of events illustrated below, starting from the beginning of one division until the beginning of the next. The pattern then repeats itself with the new cells.

1 First gap phase (G₁)
- The cell performs the tasks for which it was created (such as carrying oxygen, secreting digestive enzymes, etc.).
- It accumulates the materials it will need to replicate its DNA.

2 Synthesis phase (S)
The cell makes, or synthesizes, an extra set of DNA.

3 Second gap phase (G₂)
The cell makes final preparations for cell division, including synthesizing necessary enzymes.

4 Mitotic phase (M)
Cell division occurs. (See the following section, "Mitosis," for a detailed discussion of this phase.)

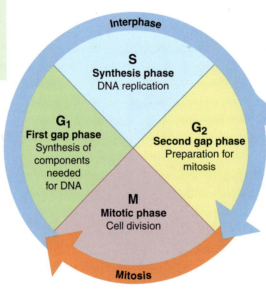

The time between mitotic phases (which includes phases G₁, S, and G₂) is called **interphase**.

Following mitosis, most cells repeat this cycle and divide again. Some cells, however, leave the cycle and enter a period of rest in which they don't divide. This phase, called the **G₀ (G-zero)** phase, can last for days, years, or even decades.

That Makes Sense

The G₁ and G₂ phases are called "gaps" phases because, although the cell is actively working, little is occurring in the nucleus as far as cell replication.

Life lesson: Aging

Scientists still have much to learn about cellular aging, but they have discovered a factor that limits the number of times a cell can divide. Specifically, every time DNA replicates, the ends of chromosomes, called telomeres, shorten. Because the telomeres don't contain important information, the fact that they get "snipped off" is inconsequential until the telomere becomes too short. At that point, essential parts of the DNA can be damaged during replication and the cell stops dividing.

Also, over time, the proteins, lipids, and nucleic acids that make up cells begin to deteriorate. Just like any other "machine," cells begin to wear out. This leads to a decline in cell function, and tissues and organs begin to deteriorate. Skin wrinkles, muscles weaken, and organ systems operate less efficiently.

Mitosis

A key focus of a cell's life cycle is **mitosis**, when the cell splits into two identical daughter cells. The growth of organs and tissues in a developing child, the repair of damaged tissue following an injury, and the replacement of cells that die through the course of everyday living all involve mitosis. The only cells that don't divide through mitosis are sex cells (eggs and sperm). Instead, they use a process called **meiosis**, which will be discussed in Chapter 23, *Reproductive Systems*.

Mitosis consists of the following four phases:

ANIMATION 🌐

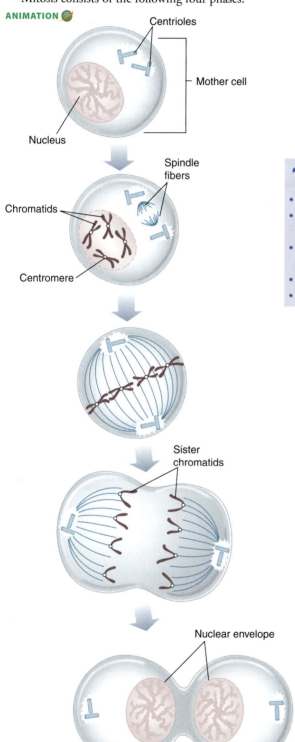

1 Prophase
- Chromatin begins to coil and condense to form chromosomes.
- Each duplicated chromosome consists of two strands (called **chromatids**); each strand contains a single molecule of DNA.
- The two chromatids join together in the middle at a spot called the centromere.
- Centrioles move to opposite poles of the cell.
- The nuclear envelope dissolves, and spindle fibers form in the cytoplasm.

2 Metaphase
- Some of the spindle fibers attach to one side of the chromosomes at the centromere.
- The chromosomes line up along the center of the cell.

3 Anaphase
- The centromeres divide, forming two chromosomes instead of a pair of attached chromatids.
- The spindle fibers pull the newly formed chromosomes to opposite poles of the cell.

4 Telophase
- A new nuclear envelope develops around each set of daughter chromosomes.
- The spindle fibers disappear, and the cytoplasm divides to produce two identical daughter cells.

Life lesson: Cancer

The body normally functions within an orderly system of cell division and cell death. When cells multiply faster than they die, abnormal growths (tumors) result. Tumors are classified as either *benign* or *malignant*. A benign tumor is slow growing and contained within a fibrous capsule that keeps it from spreading to other parts of the body. A *malignant* tumor is cancer.

Cancerous tumors typically grow rapidly. Also, the cells tend to be "slippery" and often break free from the main tumor and migrate to other organs and tissues. This spreading of cancerous cells is called *metastasis* and is the primary cause of death from cancer. Most cancers result from environmental toxins (such as cigarette smoke and chemicals), radiation exposure, and viruses (such as herpes simplex, which may cause some kinds of uterine cancer, and hepatitis C, which can lead to liver cancer).

Chemotherapy is often used to interfere with cell division. Many times patients are treated with cell cycle–specific drugs: drugs that block one or more stages in the cell cycle. For example, some drugs act on cells in the synthesis phase (S), while others target cells in the mitotic phase (M). These types of drugs don't affect cells that are in the resting phase (G_0).

Review of Key Terms

Active transport: Transport process in which solutes move from areas of lesser to greater concentration; requires energy in the form of ATP

Cilia: Hair-like processes on the surface of the cell that propel materials across a surface

Cytoplasm: The gel-like substance surrounding the nucleus and filling the cell

Deoxyribonucleic acid (DNA): Large polymer of a nucleotide that carries the genetic information of a cell

Diffusion: A passive transport mechanism that involves the movement of particles from an area of higher to lower concentration

Endocytosis: Form of vesicular transport that brings substances into the cell

Exocytosis: Form of vesicular transport that releases substances outside the cell

Facilitated diffusion: Transport process involving the diffusion of a substance through a channel protein

Filtration: Transport process in which water and dissolved particles are forced across a membrane from an area of higher to lower pressure

Golgi apparatus: Prepares proteins and packages them for export to other parts of the body

Hydrostatic pressure: Pressure exerted by water

Hypertonic: Pertains to a solution that contains a higher concentration of solutes compared to the fluid within the cell

Hypotonic: Pertains to a solution that contains a lower concentration of solutes compared to the fluid within the cell

Isotonic: Pertains to a solution in which the concentration of solutes in the solution is the same as the concentration of solutes in the cell

Microvilli: Folds of a cell membrane that greatly increase the surface area of a cell to facilitate absorption

Mitochondria: Organelle that converts organic compounds into ATP

Mitosis: Type of cell division in which the "mother" cells splits into two identical daughter cells

Nucleus: The cell's "control center" that contains a complete set of 46 chromosomes

Organelles: The structures within the cell that perform specific tasks in cellular metabolism

Osmosis: A passive transport mechanism involving the diffusion of water from an area of greater concentration of water (and a lesser concentration of solutes) to an area of lesser concentration of water (and a greater concentration of solutes)

Osmotic pressure: Water pressure that develops in a solution as a result of osmosis

Phagocytosis: Process in which large particles are trapped in the plasma membrane and brought into the cell

Pinocytosis: Process in which fluid and dissolved particles are trapped in the plasma membrane and brought into the cell

Plasma membrane: The external boundary of the cell

Polymer: Large molecule consisting of many smaller molecules joined in sequence

Ribonucleic acid (RNA): Nucleotide that assists in protein synthesis

Ribosomes: Granules of protein and RNA scattered throughout the cytoplasm; some are attached to the endoplasmic reticulum

Own the Information

To make the information in this chapter part of your working memory, take some time to reflect on what you've learned. On a separate sheet of paper, write down everything you recall from the chapter. After you're done, log on to the Davis*Plus* website, and check out the Study Group podcast and Study Group Questions for the chapter.

Key Topics for Chapter 3:
- Cell variations
- The basic structures of a cell and the functions of each
- Transport mechanisms for moving substances across the plasma membrane
- Osmolarity and tonicity
- The structure and function of DNA
- The structure and function of RNA
- The process of protein synthesis
- The cell life cycle
- The events of mitosis

Test Your Knowledge

1. The nucleus of the cell is called the control center because it:
   a. controls the function of all the organelles in the cell.
   b. contains all the genetic material for the cell.
   c. regulates the flow of substances into and out of the cell.
   d. resides at the center of the cell.

2. The plasma membrane is made up of:
   a. a rigid layer of protein.
   b. a double layer of protein and cholesterol.
   c. a double layer of phospholipids with cholesterol and proteins embedded at various spots.
   d. a rigid layer of carbohydrate and protein.

3. What is the chief purpose of the Golgi apparatus?
   a. Prepare and package proteins in vesicles for export to other parts of the body
   b. Synthesize proteins
   c. Break down protein the cell doesn't need
   d. Participate in cell division

4. What is the function of the mitochondria?
   a. To destroy bacteria
   b. To burn ATP for energy
   c. To store ATP
   d. To convert organic compounds into ATP

5. The hair-like processes on the surface of a cell that beat in waves to help propel materials across its surface are called:
   a. microvilli.
   b. flagella.
   c. cilia.
   d. centrioles.

6. Which of the following correctly describes diffusion?
   a. It is a form of passive transport in which water moves from an area of higher to lower concentration.
   b. It is a form of active transport in which particles move from an area of higher to lower concentration.
   c. It is a form of passive transport in which particles move from an area of higher to lower concentration.
   d. It is a form of passive transport in which particles pass through channels on the cell membrane to move from an area of higher to lower concentration.

Answers: Chapter 3

1. *Correct answer:* **b.** The nucleus does not control of the function of the various organelles; it also has no control over the flow of substances into and out of the cell. It typically is at the center of the cell; however, that is not why it's called the control center.

2. *Correct answer:* **c.** The plasma membrane does not consist of a rigid layer of protein. It contains cholesterol and protein; however, the cholesterol and protein are scattered throughout the membrane and do not form a layer. It also does not contain carbohydrates.

3. *Correct answer:* **a.** Ribosomes synthesize protein. Lysosomes break down protein the cell doesn't need. Centrioles play a role in cell division.

4. *Correct answer:* **d.** Mitochondria have no role in destroying bacteria. Mitochondria neither burn nor store ATP.

5. *Correct answer:* **c.** Microvilli are folds of the cell membrane that greatly increase the surface area of a cell. Flagella are hair-like projections that serve to propel the cell forward. Centrioles are organelles that serve a role in cell division.

6. *Correct answer:* **c.** The movement of water from an area of higher to lower concentration is osmosis. Diffusion is a passive process that does not require particles to move through channels.

7. *Correct answer:* **d.** Osmosis is driven by the concentration of solutes on either side of a semi-permeable membrane. Hydrostatic pressure is the pressure that drives solutes through capillary walls. Osmotic pressure has no role in venous return.

8. *Correct answer:* **b.** Red blood cells will remain normal in size and water content when immersed in an isotonic solution. A hypotonic solution will cause water to flow into the cell, making it swell and possibly burst. Red blood cells are too large to diffuse through capillary walls.

9. *Correct answer:* **c.** The sodium-potassium pump is an active transport mechanism that consumes, rather than produces, energy. This process pumps sodium and potassium against the concentration gradient: from an area of lower to higher concentration.

10. *Correct answer:* **a.** Endocytosis is a form of vesicular transport that brings substances into the cell. Phagocytosis is when the cell engulfs a solid particle and brings it into the cell. Pinocytosis occurs when vacuoles bring droplets of extracellular fluid containing dissolved substances into the cell.

11. *Correct answer:* **d.** RNA has a single strand, contains the sugar ribose, and contains the base uracil (not thymine).

12. *Correct answer:* **a.** DNA bases have fixed pairings that don't vary. DNA always contains two strands. It's the sequence of bases, not the number, that determines the genetic code.

13. *Correct answer:* **b.** During the first gap phase, the cell accumulates the materials it will need to replicate the DNA; then in the second gap it creates the necessary enzymes. In the mitotic phase, the cell actually divides.

7. Osmotic pressure is the:
   a. force that drives osmosis.
   b. force that drives solutes through the capillary walls.
   c. pressure that aids in venous return.
   d. water pressure that develops as a result of osmosis.

8. If red blood cells are immersed in a hypertonic solution, the cells will:
   a. remain normal in size and water content.
   b. lose fluid and shrivel.
   c. swell and possibly burst.
   d. diffuse through capillary walls.

9. Which statement correctly describes the sodium-potassium pump?
   a. Energy is produced as the cell actively pumps sodium out of the cell and potassium into the cell.
   b. The pump uses energy in the form of ATP to pump sodium into the cell and potassium out of the cell so as to equalize the concentration of these two ions.
   c. The pump uses energy in the form of ATP to transfer sodium from inside the cell (where concentrations of sodium are low) to outside the cell (where concentration of sodium are high) and to transfer potassium from outside the cell (where concentrations of potassium are low) to inside the cell (where concentrations of potassium are high).
   d. The pump uses energy in the form of ATP to transfer sodium from inside the cell (where concentrations of sodium are high) to outside the cell (where concentration of sodium are low) and to transfer potassium from outside the cell (where concentrations of potassium are high) to inside the cell (where concentrations of potassium are low).

10. What is the process by which large molecules can leave the cell even though they are too large to move through the plasma membrane?
    a. Exocytosis
    b. Endocytosis
    c. Phagocytosis
    d. Pinocytosis

11. Which of the following statements about RNA is true?
    a. RNA has a double strand.
    b. RNA contains the sugar deoxyribose.
    c. RNA contains the base thymine.
    d. RNA exists in three forms.

12. What determines the genetic code of a strand of DNA?
    a. The sequence of bases
    b. How the bases are paired
    c. The number of strands
    d. The number of bases

13. In which phase does the cell make an extra set of DNA?
    a. First gap
    b. Synthesis
    c. Second gap
    d. Mitotic

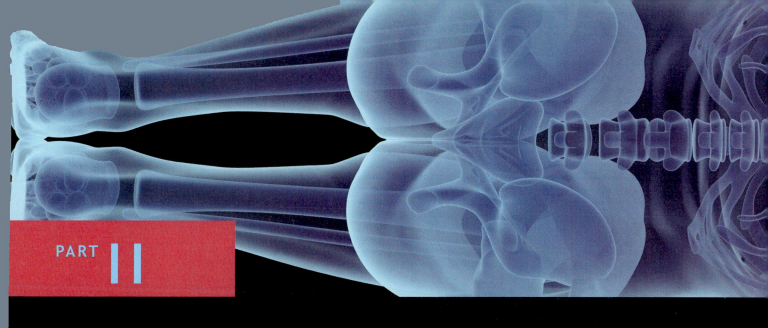

COVERING, SUPPORT, AND MOVEMENT OF THE BODY

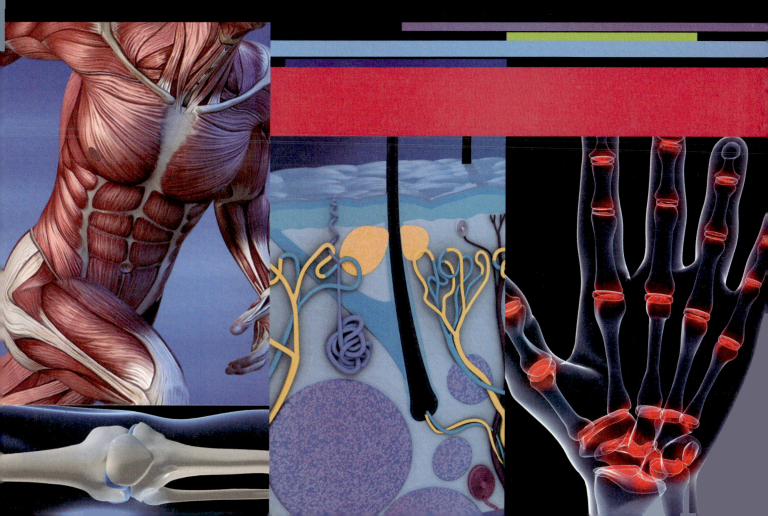

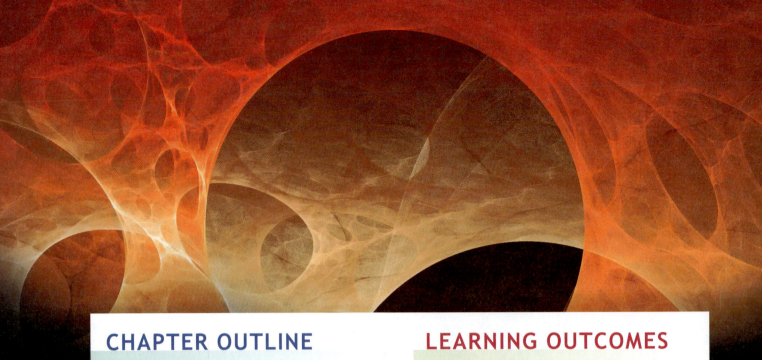

CHAPTER OUTLINE

Tissue Development

Epithelial Tissue

Connective Tissue

Nervous Tissue

Muscle Tissue

Tissue Repair

Membranes

LEARNING OUTCOMES

1. Name the four types of tissue found in the human body.

2. Identify the three germ layers and name the types of tissue arising from each.

3. Define *stem cells,* distinguishing between embryonic and adult stem cells.

4. Discuss the characteristics, functions, and locations of the various types of epithelial tissue.

5. Differentiate between endocrine and exocrine glands.

6. Explain the overriding purpose of connective tissue.

7. Define *extracellular matrix* and identify its components.

8. Name nine types of connective tissue, identify their locations and functions in the body, and describe the matrix and components of each.

9. Explain what makes nervous tissue unique from other tissues.

10. Name the parts of a neuron and describe the function of each.

11. Describe the characteristics and locations in the body of three types of muscle tissue.

12. Discuss the two ways in which tissue can repair itself.

13. Describe the steps in tissue repair.

14. Differentiate between epithelial membranes and connective tissue membranes.

15. Describe the characteristics and locations of mucous, cutaneous, and serous membranes.

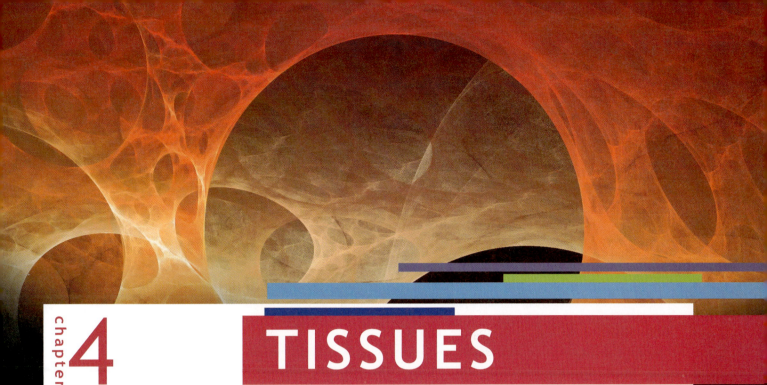

TISSUES

The entire body—including blood and bone—is made of tissue.

Although the human body contains trillions of cells, all of those cells can be categorized as belonging to one of four distinct groups of **tissue**. Tissues are simply groups of similar cells that perform a common function. The four categories of tissue are epithelial, connective, nervous, and muscular.

These four types of tissue exist alone or in combinations to create an amazing array of structures. For example, organs consist of two, three, or even four types of tissue, all working together to fulfill a unique purpose. Tissue is also the connective fabric that holds the body's structures together; it provides the body with its shape and also gives it the ability to move.

Tissue Development

Immediately after an egg and sperm unite to form a single cell, the cells begin to divide rapidly. At first, all the cells are identical. Soon, the cells organize into three layers: the **ectoderm** (outer layer), the **mesoderm** (middle layer), and the **endoderm** (inner layer). The cells of each layer continue to divide, becoming increasingly distinct from the cells of the other layers. Eventually each layer gives rise to the different types of tissue, a process called **differentiation**.

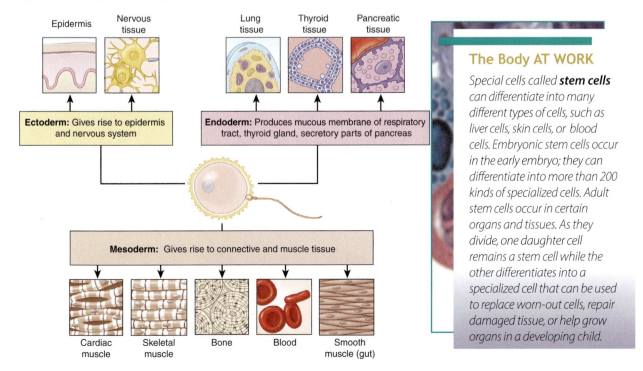

Epidermis | Nervous tissue | Lung tissue | Thyroid tissue | Pancreatic tissue

Ectoderm: Gives rise to epidermis and nervous system

Endoderm: Produces mucous membrane of respiratory tract, thyroid gland, secretory parts of pancreas

Mesoderm: Gives rise to connective and muscle tissue

Cardiac muscle | Skeletal muscle | Bone | Blood | Smooth muscle (gut)

The Body AT WORK

*Special cells called **stem cells** can differentiate into many different types of cells, such as liver cells, skin cells, or blood cells. Embryonic stem cells occur in the early embryo; they can differentiate into more than 200 kinds of specialized cells. Adult stem cells occur in certain organs and tissues. As they divide, one daughter cell remains a stem cell while the other differentiates into a specialized cell that can be used to replace worn-out cells, repair damaged tissue, or help grow organs in a developing child.*

Epithelial Tissue

Also called epithelium (plural: epithelia), **epithelial tissue** is a continuous sheet of tightly packed cells; it covers the body's surface, lines the body cavities and many of the organs, and forms certain glands. The key functions of this tissue involve protection, absorption, filtration, and secretion.

In a sense, the epithelium is a *surface* tissue: its top surface is usually exposed to the environment—such as occurs with the skin or the inside of the mouth—or to an internal body cavity; its bottom surface adheres to underlying connective tissue by means of a **basement membrane**. Epithelial tissue is too thin to contain blood vessels; therefore, it depends on the connective tissue beneath to supply its needs for oxygen and nutrients.

Classification of Epithelial Tissue

Epithelial tissue is classified by the shape of the cells as well as by the number of layers.

Cell Shape

Epithelial cells may assume one of three basic shapes: **squamous**, **cuboidal**, or **columnar**.

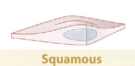

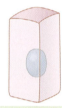

Squamous	**Cuboidal**	**Columnar**
These cells are flat and plate-like. The word *squamous* comes from a Latin word meaning "scaly."	These cells are cube-shaped and contain more cytoplasm than squamous cells.	Higher than they are wide, columnar cells are tall and cylindrical.

Cell Layers

Epithelia may appear as single or multiple layers.

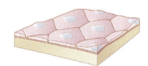
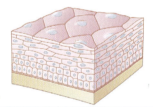

In **simple** epithelia, every cell touches the basement membrane.

In **stratified** epithelia, some cells stack on top of other cells and the upper layers of cells don't touch the basement membrane.

Taking cell shape and number of layers into account, the chart on the next page highlights the various types of epithelial tissue. The epithelium described in that chart is known as membranous epithelium.

Glandular Epithelium

There's another type of epithelium: **glandular epithelium**. A gland is a collection of epithelial cells that specializes in secretion of a particular substance.

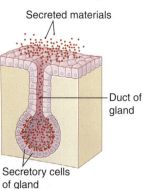

Secreted materials

Duct of gland

Secretory cells of gland

- **Exocrine glands** secrete their products (such as tears, sweat, or gastric juices) into ducts. The ducts then empty onto a body surface or inside a body cavity. For example, sweat glands secrete sweat, which flows through ducts and onto the skin's surface.

- **Endocrine glands** are often called ductless glands. These glands secrete their products, called hormones, directly into the blood. For example, the adrenal glands secrete epinephrine and norepinephrine into the bloodstream. Other examples of endocrine glands include the pituitary, thyroid, and ovaries.

FAST FACT

Goblet cells are modified cells containing secretory vesicles that produce large quantities of mucus.

Types of Membranous Epithelial Tissue

Tissue	Function	Location
One layer		
Simple squamous epithelium:		
• Consists of a single layer of flat, scale-like cells	• Allows for ready diffusion or filtration because of thinness	• Alveoli • Lining of blood and lymphatic vessels
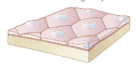 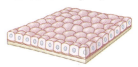		
Simple cuboidal epithelium:		
• Consists of a single layer of cube-like cells	• Secretes and absorbs	• Ducts and tubules of many organs, including the kidneys
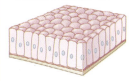		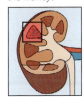
Simple columnar epithelium:		
• Consists of a single layer of columnar cells	• Participates in absorption • Secretes mucus by **goblet cells** (modified columnar cells; see the "Fast Fact" on the previous page)	• Lines the intestines

Pseudostratified columnar epithelium:		
• Consists of a single layer of irregularly shaped columnar cells • Cells of different heights with nuclei at different levels makes it *appear* stratified	• Provides protection • Secretes mucus	• Lines trachea, large bronchi, and nasal mucosa
Several layers		
Stratified squamous epithelium:		
• Contains multiple cell layers (making it stronger than simple epithelia) • The most widespread epithelium in the body	• Resists abrasion and penetration by pathogens • Some contain keratin (such as the epidermis); some do not (such as the mucous membranes)	• Epidermis of the skin • Esophagus • Vagina
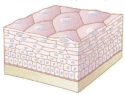		
Transitional epithelium:		
• Consists of multiple cell layers • When stretched, cell layers decrease and cell shape changes from cuboidal to squamous	• Stretches to allow filling of urinary tract	• Urinary tract
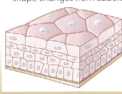		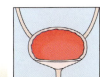

Connective Tissue

The most widespread, and the most varied, of all the tissues is **connective tissue**. Existing in a variety of forms—ranging from tough cords to elastic sheets to fluid—connective tissue performs a variety of tasks. The overriding purposes of this seemingly diverse group of tissues are to connect the body together and to support, bind, or protect organs. This figure shows examples of some of the varied forms of connective tissue.

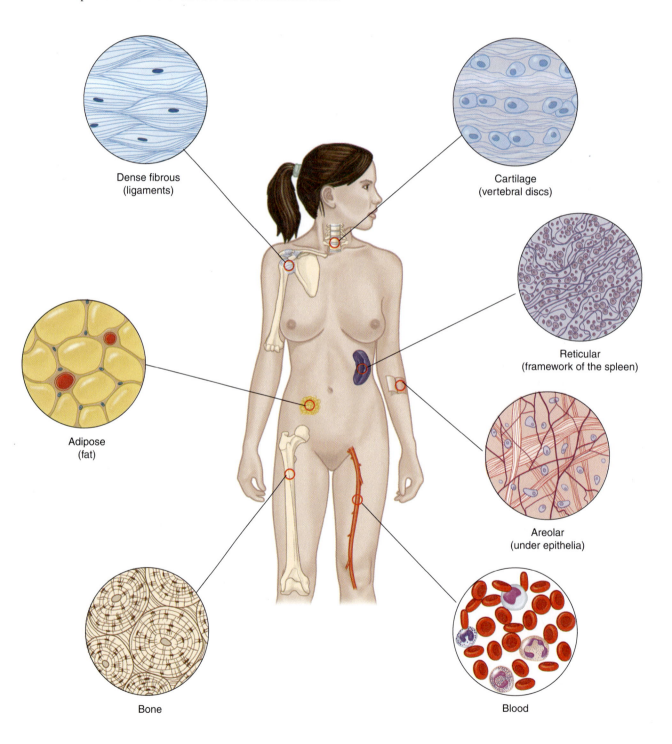

Dense fibrous
(ligaments)

Cartilage
(vertebral discs)

Reticular
(framework of the spleen)

Adipose
(fat)

Areolar
(under epithelia)

Bone

Blood

Components of Connective Tissue

The key component of connective tissue—called **extracellular matrix**—is what allows connective tissues to be so diverse. Extracellular matrix is the framework into which the cells of tissue are embedded. The matrix consists of varying kinds and amounts of protein fibers and fluid; it's the variation in composition that gives tissue its characteristics. For example, the matrix of blood is fluid; it contains many cells but no fibers. In contrast, the matrix of bone contains few cells and many fibers, making it hard and brittle. The matrix may also be gel-like, flexible, tough, or even fragile.

The fibers found in connective tissue may be one of three types:

- **Collagenous fibers:** These are strong and flexible but resist stretching; these are the most abundant fibers.
- **Reticular fibers:** These occur in networks and support small structures such as capillaries and nerve fibers.
- **Elastic fibers:** Made of a protein called *elastin*, these fibers can stretch and recoil like a rubber band.

Types of Connective Tissue

Connective tissues are classified according to their structural characteristics. The basic classifications are fibrous connective tissue, cartilage, bone, and blood. Fibrous connective tissues may be either loose or dense; loose connective tissues are further divided as being areolar tissue, adipose tissue, or reticular tissue.

The Body AT WORK

Collagen is the body's most abundant protein. Besides helping form tendons, ligaments, and the matrix of cartilage and bone, collagen forms the deep layer of the skin. Scientists speculate that many of the skin and body changes associated with aging result because of changes to the molecular structure of collagen. Some people, in an effort to reverse some of these changes, opt to receive collagen injections to fill in wrinkles and plump and smooth the skin.

Fibrous Connective Tissue

An abundance of fiber characterizes fibrous connective tissues. The fibers may be loosely arranged, as in loose connective tissue, or tightly packed, as in dense connective tissue.

Loose Connective Tissue

The most widely distributed of all tissues, loose connective tissue has a stretchable quality. Specific types of loose connective tissue are **areolar**, **adipose**, and **reticular**.

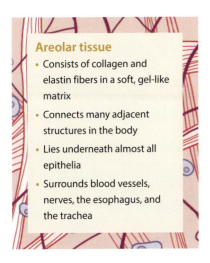

Areolar tissue
- Consists of collagen and elastin fibers in a soft, gel-like matrix
- Connects many adjacent structures in the body
- Lies underneath almost all epithelia
- Surrounds blood vessels, nerves, the esophagus, and the trachea

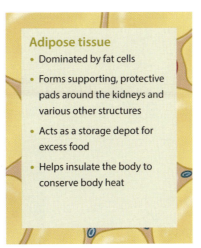

Adipose tissue
- Dominated by fat cells
- Forms supporting, protective pads around the kidneys and various other structures
- Acts as a storage depot for excess food
- Helps insulate the body to conserve body heat

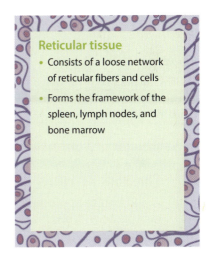

Reticular tissue
- Consists of a loose network of reticular fibers and cells
- Forms the framework of the spleen, lymph nodes, and bone marrow

Dense Connective Tissue

Dense connective tissue consists of closely packed collagen fibers. These dense tissues form **tendons** and **ligaments**, the cord-like structures charged with attaching muscles to bones (tendons) or bones to bones (ligaments). Unlike other connective tissues, which have a rich blood supply, dense connective tissue has few blood vessels. Consequently, injuries to tendons and ligaments heal slowly. Dense connective tissue also forms bands or sheets (called **fascia**) that bind together organs and muscles. This tissue also forms a protective capsule or sheath around the kidneys, spleen, and nerves.

Cartilage

Composed of cells called **chondrocytes,** cartilage has a rubbery, flexible matrix. It contains no blood vessels. Rather, it receives nutrients and oxygen by diffusion from surrounding connective tissue—a slow, inefficient process. Consequently, when cartilage is damaged (such as from a knee injury), it heals very slowly and may not heal at all.

There are three types of cartilage: hyaline, elastic, and fibrocartilage.

Hyaline cartilage

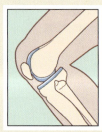

- Found at the ends of movable joints, at the point where the ribs attach to the breastbone, the larynx, and the supportive rings around the trachea
- Forms much of the fetal skeleton (later develops into bone)

Elastic cartilage

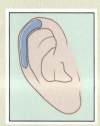

Provides flexible support to the external ear and the epiglottis

Fibrocartilage

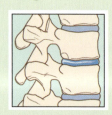

Forms the discs between the vertebrae and in the knee joint because this cartilage resists compression and absorbs shock

Bone

Also called **osseous tissue**, bone is composed of bone cells (called **osteocytes**) embedded in a matrix containing collagen fibers and mineral salt crystals. These mineral crystals are responsible for the hardness of bone.

Bones form the skeleton of the body. They give the body structure, provide support, and offer protection to internal organs, such as the brain. They also offer an attachment point for muscles, making movement possible. The matrix of bone serves as a storage site for calcium, and some bones contain red bone marrow, which produces new blood cells. Bone has a rich blood supply, allowing bone to heal quickly after a fracture. (For more information on bone, see Chapter 6, *Bones & Bone Tissue.*)

Blood

Blood is unique among the connective tissues in that it exists as a fluid. Composed of various types of blood cells surrounded by a liquid matrix (called **plasma**), blood transports cells and dissolved substances from one part of the body to another. Unlike other connective tissues, blood doesn't contain any fibers. (For more information on blood, see Chapter 13, *Blood.*)

The Body AT WORK

Connective tissue performs a number of roles. For example, bones support the body, protect organs, and allow movement. Fat stores energy and generates heat in infants and children. Tendons and ligaments hold organs and muscles in place. Blood transports gases, nutrients, hormones, and wastes. On top of that, connective tissue offers immune protection: connective tissue cells attack foreign invaders while connective tissue fibers provide the location for inflammation.

FAST FACT

Cartilage disorders, whether from injury or osteoarthritis, are the most common cause of knee pain. Researchers are currently exploring various ways to stimulate cartilage regeneration in an attempt to help alleviate these problems.

Types of Connective Tissue

Type	Location	Function
Loose fibrous connective		
• Areolar	Beneath the epithelia; between muscles; surrounding blood vessels and nerves	Connects tissues and organs together (such as skin to muscles)
• Adipose	Beneath the skin, breast, heart's surface; surrounding kidneys and eyes	Provides protective cushion, insulation; stores energy
• Reticular	Spleen; lymph nodes; bone marrow	Provides a supportive framework
Dense fibrous connective	Tendons; ligaments; fascia; dermis of the skin	Provides durable support
Cartilage		
• Hyaline	Ends of bones in joints; connecting point between ribs and sternum; rings in trachea and bronchi; larynx; fetal skeleton	Eases joint movement; firm but flexible support
• Elastic	External ear	Provides flexible support
• Fibrocartilage	Intervertebral discs; knee joint; pelvis	Resists compression and absorbs shock
Bone	Skeleton	Provides support, protection; serves as calcium reservoir
Blood	Inside blood vessels throughout the body	Transports oxygen, nutrients, hormones, wastes from one part of the body to another

Life lesson: Body fat

When an individual consumes more calories than his body burns, the excess calories are stored as fat in adipose tissue. However, men and women tend to store extra fat in different areas. The male sex hormone, testosterone, encourages the accumulation of fat in the abdomen, while the female hormone estrogen encourages fat accumulation in the hips, thighs, and breasts. (After menopause, when estrogen levels decline, fat migrates from the buttocks, hips, and thighs to the waist.)

Increased body fat carries many health risks in general, but the location of the fat may increase risks even further. Specifically, researchers have discovered significantly increased health risks for those who have increased abdominal fat. An increased amount of abdominal fat has been linked to the accumulation of fat around organs, which can interfere with organ function. What's more, increased abdominal fat (called central obesity) has been linked to increased risks for cardiovascular disease, high blood pressure, and diabetes.

A measurement called the waist-hip ratio is used to identify central obesity. In this measurement, the circumference of the waist is divided by that of the hips; a measurement greater than 0.9 for men and 0.85 for women indicates central obesity.

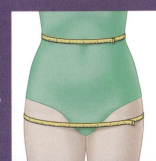

Measure waist at narrowest point

$$\text{Ratio} = \frac{\text{Waist}}{\text{Hips}}$$

Measure hips at widest point

Nervous Tissue

Nervous tissue has a high degree of excitability and conductivity—more so than other tissues. It's these characteristics that allow it to communicate rapidly with other parts of the body. (For more information about the tissue of the nervous system, see Chapter 10, *Nervous System*.)

Found in the brain, spinal cord, and nerves, nerve tissue consists of two types of cells:

- **Neurons**, the units that conduct nervous impulses
- **Neuroglia**, which protect and assist neurons.

FAST FACT

Some axons are quite long; in fact, some extend from the brainstem all the way to the foot.

Each neuron has a large cell body, called a **soma**. The soma contains the nucleus of the nerve cell as well as the organelles.

Extending from the soma are multiple, short processes called **dendrites**. The dendrites receive impulses from other cells, which they then transmit to the soma.

The neuron contains a single, long nerve fiber called the **axon**. The axon transmits signals to other cells.

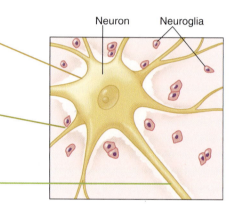

Neuron   Neuroglia

Muscle Tissue

Muscle tissue consists of elongated cells that contract in response to stimulation. The body contains three types of muscle tissue: skeletal, cardiac, and smooth.

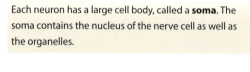

Nucleus
Cylindrical muscle fiber
Striations

Skeletal Muscle

Skeletal muscle consists of long, thin cells called **muscle fibers**. Skeletal muscle may also be called *striated* muscle (because its light and dark bands give it a striped, or striated, appearance) or *voluntary* muscle (because we can move it voluntarily).

Most skeletal muscle is attached to bone. This is the muscle that makes body movements possible. It is also the muscle responsible for breathing, speech, control of urination, and facial expression.

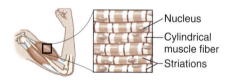

Nucleus
Branched muscle fiber
Striations
Intercalated disc

Cardiac Muscle

Cardiac muscle is found only in the heart. While cardiac muscle also appears striated, it is uniquely different from skeletal muscle. For one thing, cardiac muscle cells are shorter than those of skeletal muscle. In addition, the cells are joined together with junctions called **intercalated discs**. These junctions allow electrical impulses to spread rapidly from cell to cell; this rapid transmission permits almost simultaneous stimulation and contraction. Finally, cardiac muscle is *involuntary* muscle: its contraction is not under voluntary control.

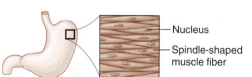

Nucleus
Spindle-shaped muscle fiber

Smooth Muscle

Smooth muscle—which consists of long, spindle-shaped cells—lacks the striped pattern of striated muscle. Stimulated the by autonomic nervous system, smooth muscle is not under voluntary control. This muscle lines the walls of many organs, including those of the digestive, respiratory, and urinary tracts. Smooth muscle controls the diameter of blood vessels, making it important in controlling blood pressure and flow.

Tissue Repair

When damaged, tissue can repair itself in one of two ways:

- **Regeneration** occurs when damaged tissue cells are replaced with the same type of cells, resulting in functional new tissue. Most injuries to the skin, such as cuts and scrapes, heal by regeneration.
- **Fibrosis** occurs when damaged tissue is replaced with scar tissue, which is composed mainly of collagen. Although scar tissue binds the edges of a wound together, it doesn't restore normal function. Severe cuts or burns heal through fibrosis. Also, muscle and nerve tissue have a limited capacity to regenerate; injuries to these tissues heal by fibrosis, causing a loss of at least partial function.

Steps in Tissue Repair

When a cut occurs in the skin, the epithelium regenerates while the underlying tissue heals by fibrosis.

ANIMATION

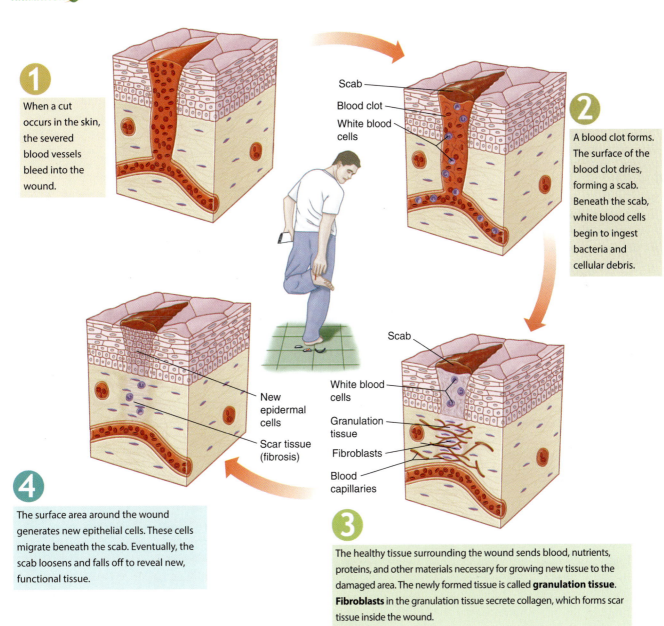

1 When a cut occurs in the skin, the severed blood vessels bleed into the wound.

2 A blood clot forms. The surface of the blood clot dries, forming a scab. Beneath the scab, white blood cells begin to ingest bacteria and cellular debris.

Scab
Blood clot
White blood cells

3 The healthy tissue surrounding the wound sends blood, nutrients, proteins, and other materials necessary for growing new tissue to the damaged area. The newly formed tissue is called **granulation tissue**. **Fibroblasts** in the granulation tissue secrete collagen, which forms scar tissue inside the wound.

Scab
White blood cells
Granulation tissue
Fibroblasts
Blood capillaries

4 The surface area around the wound generates new epithelial cells. These cells migrate beneath the scab. Eventually, the scab loosens and falls off to reveal new, functional tissue.

New epidermal cells
Scar tissue (fibrosis)

Membranes

Thin sheets of tissue, called **membranes**, fulfill many crucial functions in the body. In general, membranes line body cavities, cover body surfaces, and separate organs (or parts of organs) from each other. Some membranes secrete lubricating fluids to reduce friction during movement, such as when the heart beats or a joint bends.

The two categories of membranes are **epithelial membranes** and **connective tissue membranes**.

Epithelial Membranes

The body contains three types of epithelial membranes: mucous membranes, cutaneous membranes, and serous membranes.

1 Mucous membranes

Mucous membranes line body surfaces that open directly to the body's exterior, such as the respiratory, digestive, urinary, and reproductive tracts.

The type of epithelium in each mucous membrane varies according to the location of the membrane and its function. For example, the esophagus contains stratified epithelium, which is tough and resists abrasions, while the stomach is lined with columnar epithelium.

True to the name, mucous membranes secrete **mucus**, a watery secretion that coats and protects the cells of the membrane. Mucus also acts as a lubricant to help propel food through the digestive tract; in the respiratory tract, it traps dust and bacteria.

2 Cutaneous membrane

Known as the skin, this is the body's largest membrane. It consists of a layer of epithelium resting on a layer of connective tissue. (For more information on the skin, see Chapter 5, *Integumentary System*.)

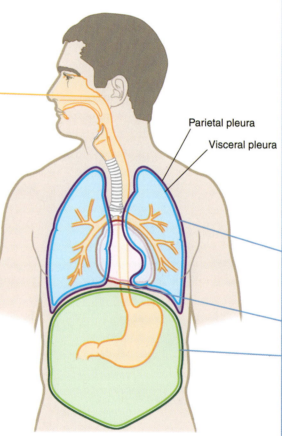

Parietal pleura

Visceral pleura

3 Serous membranes

Composed of simple squamous epithelium resting on a thin layer of areolar connective tissue, serous membranes line some of the closed body cavities and also cover many of the organs in those cavities.

The serous membrane that lines the body cavities is actually one continuous sheet: part of the membrane (called the *parietal membrane*) lines the wall of the cavity; it then folds back and covers the organs. The part of the membrane that covers the organs is called the *visceral membrane*.

There are three serous membranes:

- The pleura , or pleural membrane, surrounds each lung and lines the thoracic cavity.

- The pericardium , or pericardial membrane, surrounds the heart.

- The peritoneum , or peritoneal membrane, lines the abdominal cavity and covers the abdominal organs.

Serous membranes secrete serous fluid, which helps prevent friction as the heart beats and the lungs expand.

Connective Tissue Membranes

Some joints are lined by membranes made of connective tissue. For example, **synovial membranes** line the spaces between bones, where they secrete synovial fluid to prevent friction during movement. (These membranes will be discussed in Chapter 8, *Joints*.)

Review of Key Terms

Adipose tissue: Type of loose connective tissue dominated by fat cells

Areolar tissue: Type of loose connective tissue that lies beneath almost all epithelia

Chondrocytes: Cartilage-forming cells

Columnar epithelium: Epithelial tissue composed of cells having a tall, columnar shape

Connective tissue: The most widespread, and the most varied, of all the tissues; serves to connect the body together and to support, bind, or protect organs

Cuboidal epithelium: Epithelial tissue consisting of cells having a cube-like shape

Endocrine gland: A gland that secretes its product, called a hormone, directly into the bloodstream

Epithelium: The layer of cells forming the epidermis of the skin and the surface layer of mucous and serous membranes

Exocrine gland: A gland that secretes its product into a duct, which then empties onto a body surface or inside a body cavity

Fibroblasts: Cells that secrete collagen, which forms scar tissue inside a wound

Fibrosis: The repair and replacement of damaged tissue with connective tissue, mainly collagen

Glandular epithelium: Type of epithelium consisting of glands that secrete a particular substance

Goblet cell: Modified columnar cell containing secretory vesicles that produce large quantities of mucus

Granulation tissue: Newly formed tissue inside a wound

Mucous membrane: Epithelial membrane that lines body surfaces that open directly to the body's exterior

Muscle tissue: Tissue consisting of contractile cells or fibers that effect movement of an organ or body part

Nervous tissue: Tissue with a high degree of excitability and conductivity that makes up the nervous system

Osseous tissue: Bone tissue

Osteocytes: Bone-forming cells

Reticular tissue: Tissue consisting of a loose network of reticular fibers and cells; forms the framework of the spleen, lymph nodes, and bone marrow.

Serous membrane: Membrane composed of simple squamous epithelium resting on a thin layer of areolar connective tissue; lines some of the closed body cavities and also covers many of the organs in those cavities

Squamous epithelium: Epithelial tissue consisting of thin, flat cells

Stem cell: Specialized cell that can differentiate into many different types of cells

Tissue: Groups of similar cells that perform a common function

Own the Information

To make the information in this chapter part of your working memory, take some time to reflect on what you've learned. On a separate sheet of paper, write down everything you recall from the chapter. After you're done, log on to the Davis*Plus* website, and check out the Study Group podcast and Study Group Questions for the chapter.

Key Topics for Chapter 4:
- How tissues develop
- Classification of epithelial tissue
- Components, types, and characteristics of connective tissue
- Characteristics of nervous tissue
- Types, locations, and characteristics of muscle tissue
- Tissue repair
- Membranes

Test Your Knowledge

Answers: Chapter 4

1. *Correct answer:* **c.** Connective tissue serves to bind the body together and support and protect organs. Muscle tissue consists of elongated cells that contract in response to stimulation. Squamous is a cell shape, not a tissue type.

2. *Correct answer:* **d.** All the other answers are incorrect.

3. *Correct answer:* **a.** In simple epithelia, all cells touch the basement membrane. Cuboidal refers to cells having a cube-like shape. Squamous refers a cells that are flat and plate-like.

4. *Correct answer:* **c.** Endocrine glands secrete their substance directly into the bloodstream. Goblet are a type of cell that contains secretory vesicles that produce mucus. Matrix refers to the key component of connective tissue.

5. *Correct answer:* **d.** Connective tissue is the most widespread tissue in the body and exists in a variety of forms.

6. *Correct answer:* **a.** Reticular tissue forms the framework of the spleen, lymph nodes, and bone marrow. Areolar tissue lies underneath epithelia and serves to connect many adjacent structures in the body. Fascia is dense connective tissue that binds together organs and muscles.

7. *Correct answer:* **b.** Neuroglia is a type of nerve cell that protects and assists neurons. Dendrites receive impulses from other cells and transmit them to the soma. The soma is the neuron's cell body.

1. Which tissue is a continuous sheet of tightly packed cells and covers the body's surface, lines body cavities and many of its organs, and forms certain glands?
   a. Connective tissue
   b. Muscle tissue
   c. Epithelial tissue
   d. Squamous tissue

2. Which of the following statements about epithelial tissue is true?
   a. Epithelial tissue has a rich blood supply, which is why superficial wounds tend to heal quickly.
   b. Epithelial tissue has a poor blood supply, which helps control excess bleeding when it is damaged, such as from a cut or scrape.
   c. Epithelial tissue has an adequate blood supply; however, during tissue repair, when the demand for oxygen and nutrients is high, the connective tissue beneath can furnish it with additional blood.
   d. Epithelial tissue has no blood supply and depends completely on the connective tissue beneath it to supply it with oxygen and nutrients.

3. In what type of epithelia do some cells stack on top of other cells but not touch the basement membrane?
   a. Stratified
   b. Simple
   c. Cuboidal
   d. Squamous

4. Which glands secrete their products into ducts that empty onto a body surface?
   a. Endocrine
   b. Goblet
   c. Exocrine
   d. Matrix

5. Which tissue is the most widespread and varied of all the tissues?
   a. Nervous
   b. Muscular
   c. Epithelial
   d. Connective

6. Which tissue helps to insulate the body to conserve body heat?
   a. Adipose
   b. Reticular
   c. Areolar
   d. Fascia

7. Which part of the neuron transmits impulses to other cells?
   a. Neuroglia
   b. Axon
   c. Dendrite
   d. Soma

8. *Correct answer:* **d.** Fibrosis is when damaged tissue is replaced with scar tissue. Granulation refers to the tissue that fills a damaged area. Ossification is the process of forming bone.

9. *Correct answer:* **b.** Cutaneous membrane is the skin. The serous membrane lines some closed body cavities and covers many organs. Exocrine is a type of gland.

10. *Correct answer:* **d.** Hyaline cartilage exists in the end bones of the joints, the rings of the trachea and bronchi, and the fetal skeleton. Elastic cartilage forms the external ear. There is no such thing as membranous cartilage.

8. The type of healing that occurs when damaged tissue heals and is replaced by new, functional tissue is called:
   a. fibrosis.
   b. granulation.
   c. ossification.
   d. regeneration.

9. Which membranes line body surfaces that open directly to the body's exterior?
   a. Cutaneous
   b. Mucous
   c. Serous
   d. Exocrine

10. Which type of cartilage makes up the discs in the vertebrae?
    a. Hyaline
    b. Elastic
    c. Membranous
    d. Fibrocartilage

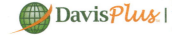

Go to **http://davisplus.fadavis.com** Keyword: Thompson to see all of the resources available with this chapter.

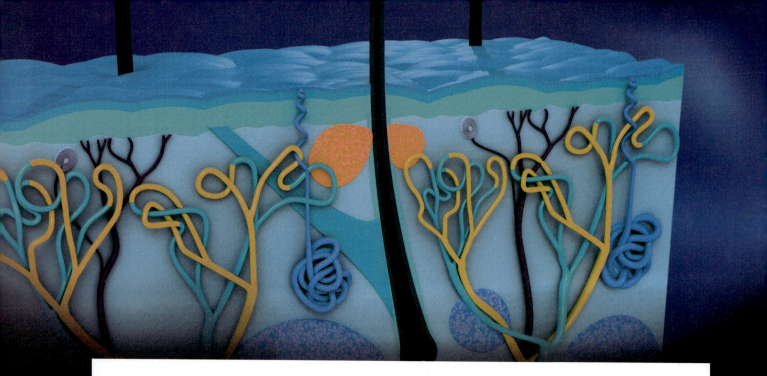

CHAPTER OUTLINE

Structure of the Skin

Skin Color

Functions of the Skin

LEARNING OUTCOMES

1. Name and describe the two layers of the skin.

2. Name and describe the layers of the epidermis.

3. Describe the generation of new cells in the epidermis.

4. Explain the role of melanin in the skin.

5. Discuss potential normal and abnormal skin colors and identify the cause of each.

6. Explain the five functions of skin.

7. Describe the structure and functions of hair.

8. Describe the structure of nails.

9. List some common nail abnormalities and their causes.

10. Name the two types of sweat glands and discuss the structure and functions of each.

11. Differentiate between sebaceous and ceruminous glands, identifying the location, structure, and functions of each.

12. Discuss the three classes of burns, including the complications of each.

13. Describe the three types of skin cancer.

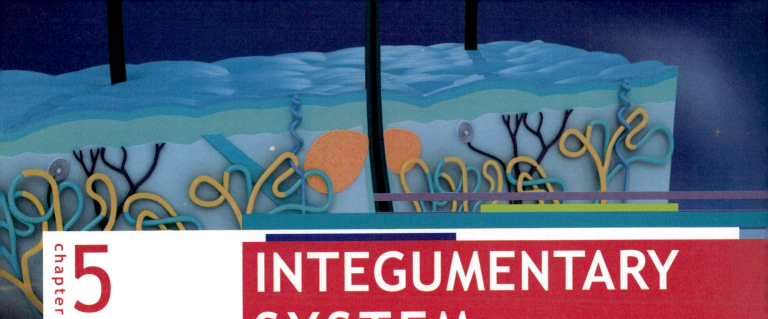

5

INTEGUMENTARY SYSTEM

The skin is the largest organ in the body—covering 17 to 20 square feet (1.5 to 2 square meters). It's also extremely thin, measuring only 0.04 to 0.08 inches (1 to 2 mm) thick in most places.

More than just a covering for the body, skin is crucial for human survival. Perhaps its most obvious task is to define the body's structure: joining forces with the muscular and skeletal systems to build the body's framework. But that's just one small part of the skin's role. This thin, self-regenerating tissue also separates the internal from the external environment, protects the body from invasion by harmful substances, and helps maintain homeostasis. In addition, sensory nerve receptors in the skin gather information about the outside world while its flexibility and ability to stretch permit freedom of movement. Last but not least, changes in the skin can signal diseases or disorders in other body systems. For these reasons and more, the skin and its appendages (hair, nails, and skin glands)—collectively known as the **integumentary system**—deserve close attention.

Structure of the Skin

The skin, also called the **cutaneous membrane**, consists of two layers: the epidermis and the dermis.

The **epidermis**—the outermost layer—consists of stratified squamous epithelial tissue. It contains no blood vessels; instead, it obtains oxygen and nutrients by diffusion from the dermal layer beneath it.

The **dermis**—the inner, deeper layer—is composed of connective tissue. It contains primarily collagen fibers (which strengthen the tissue), but it also contains elastin fibers (which provide elasticity) and reticular fibers (which bind the collagen and elastin fibers together).

The dermis contains an abundance of blood vessels in addition to sweat glands, sebaceous glands, and nerve endings. Hair follicles are also embedded in the dermis. Finger-like projections, called **papillae**, extend upward from the dermis. These projections interlock with downward waves on the bottom of the epidermis, effectively binding the two structures together.

Beneath the skin is a layer of subcutaneous tissue called the **hypodermis**. Made of loose connective (areolar) tissue and adipose tissue, the hypodermis binds the skin to the underlying tissue. Hypodermis that's composed mostly of adipose tissue is called subcutaneous fat. This layer of fat helps insulate the body from outside temperature changes; it also acts as an energy reservoir.

Sweat pores

Hairs

Dermal papilla

Eccrine sweat gland

Sensory nerve fibers
Pressure receptor
Sebaceous gland
Hair follicle
Hair bulb
Apocrine sweat gland
Arrector pili muscle
Motor nerve fibers
Cutaneous blood vessels

Layers of the Epidermis

The epidermis consists of four or five layers, with the extra layer being present in areas receiving a lot of wear and tear, like the soles of the feet. During the course of life, the cells of the outer layer of the epidermis are sloughed off; this means that the skin must continually renew itself by replacing the sloughed off cells with new ones.

Those new cells are created in the lowest level of the epidermis. Once formed, they pass through the layers above, undergoing changes along the way, until they reach the skin's surface. Here's what happens:

FAST FACT

The average person sheds more than 1 pound (0.5 kg) of skin every year. In fact, the outer layer of the epidermis is completely replaced every month.

ANIMATION

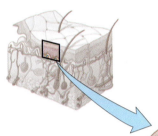

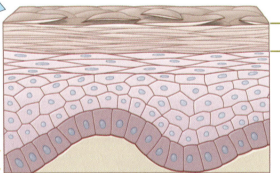

1 The **stratum basale**, or basal layer—also called the **stratum germinativum**—is the innermost layer. It consists of a layer of columnar stem cells. These stem cells continually undergo mitosis, producing new skin cells. As new cells are produced, they push the older cells upward, toward the skin's surface.

2 As the cells are pushed upward, they stop dividing and instead produce **keratin**, a tough, fibrous protein. The keratin replaces the cytoplasm and nucleus in each cell. The cells flatten, and as they move further away from their blood supply, they die.

3 By the time the cells reach the outermost layer—called the **stratum corneum**—all that's left of the dead cells is their keratin. The newly arriving flattened cells—called **keratinocytes**—replace the dead cells that flake away with daily wear.

The stratum corneum actually consists of up to 30 layers of dead, flat keratin-coated cells. This makes the skin's surface durable and resistant to abrasions. It's also an effective barrier, preventing water from entering the body from the outside while still allowing for evaporation.

The Body AT WORK

Skin ranges in thickness: from 0.5 mm on the eyelids to over 5 mm on the back. In most areas, though, skin measures about 1 to 2 mm thick.

Even though skin consists of both dermis and epidermis, it is classified as being thin or thick based on the thickness of the epidermis alone. Most of the body is covered in thin skin, with an epidermis measuring about 0.1 mm thick. Thin skin contains hair follicles, sebaceous glands, and sweat glands. Thick skin doesn't contain any hair follicles and is, therefore, hairless. It covers the palms and soles—areas that receive a lot of friction.

Life lesson:
Subcutaneous and intradermal injections

Subcutaneous tissue has a rich blood supply, making it ideal for absorbing medications. Insulin is a common medication given by *subcutaneous injection*. Ensuring that the medication is deposited in the subcutaneous tissue requires using a relatively short needle and holding the syringe at about a 45° angle. Some medications are given into the skin itself. These injections are called *intradermal injections.*

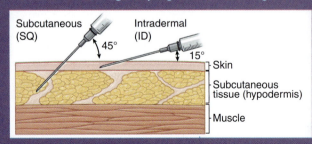

Skin Color

Scattered throughout the basal layer of the epidermis are cells called **melanocytes**. These special cells produce a substance called **melanin**, which accumulates in the cells of the epidermis. There are two types of melanin: a reddish *pheomelanin* and a brown-black *eumelanin*.

A person's skin color is determined by the amount, and type, of melanin—not the number of melanocytes. (In fact, persons of all races have about the same number of melanocytes. The cells in dark-skinned people produce more melanin, and the melanin is broken down more slowly.)

- Melanocytes, which have long projections reaching between cells, release melanin.
- The keratinocytes then bring the melanin into their cells.
- The melanin forms a cap over the top of the cell nucleus to protect it from exposure to the harmful ultraviolet rays of the sun.
- Prolonged exposure to sunlight stimulates the cells to secrete more melanin. This protects the cell's nucleus and also darkens the skin.

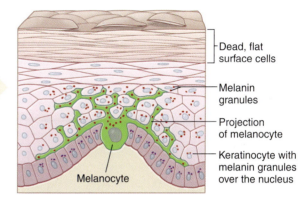

Dead, flat surface cells

Melanin granules

Projection of melanocyte

Keratinocyte with melanin granules over the nucleus

Melanocyte

FAST FACT

When ultraviolet radiation reaches the nucleus of the cell, it damages the cell's DNA and can lead to skin cancer.

The Body AT WORK

Variations in skin tone normally occur. Melanin is not evenly distributed throughout the body: the palms and soles have less melanin than the backs of the hands and the tops of the feet. Melanin can also concentrate in certain areas, such as freckles and moles. A yellow pigment called carotene is also stored in skin tissue. Eating large quantities of foods containing carotene (such as carrots) can give the skin a yellow tint.

Abnormal Changes in Skin Color

Condition	Skin Tone	Cause
Cyanosis	Blue tint	A deficiency of oxygen in circulating blood
Jaundice	Yellow discoloration of skin and the whites of the eyes	Impaired liver function (such as from hepatitis or liver disease) that allows bile to accumulate, which stains the skin
Bronzing	A golden brown skin color	A deficiency of hormones from the adrenal gland, such as occurs with Addison disease
Albinism	Extremely pale skin, white hair, and pink eyes	A genetic lack of melanin
Erythema	Abnormal redness	Increased blood flow in dilated blood vessels close to the skin's surface; may result from heat, exercise, sunburn, or emotions such as embarrassment or anger
Pallor	Pale skin	Decreased blood flow, such as occurs from cold temperatures, fear or emotional stress, low blood pressure, or blood loss
Bruise (hematoma)	Bluish, black, or yellowish mark on the skin	The breakdown of clotted blood under the skin

Functions of the Skin

The skin performs a variety of functions that are crucial to human survival.

Skin Functions	Actions
Protection	• Prevents microorganisms, as well as many harmful chemicals, from invading the body
	• Secretes a residue, or surface film, that helps block toxins and inhibit bacterial and fungal growth
	• Absorbs the force of injuries, protecting delicate underlying structures
Barrier	• Keeps the body from absorbing excess water, such as when swimming or bathing
	• Prevents dehydration by regulating the volume and content of fluid lost from the body
	• Blocks ultraviolet (UV) radiation, keeping it from reaching deeper issue layers
Vitamin D production	• Initiates the production of vitamin D when exposed to ultraviolet light
Sensory perception	• Contains millions of sensory nerve fibers, allowing for perception of temperature, touch, pressure, pain, and vibration
Thermoregulation	• Contains nerves that cause blood vessels in the skin to dilate or constrict to regulate heat loss
	• When chilled, the skin retains heat by constricting blood vessels; this reduces blood flow through the skin and conserves heat
	• When overheated, the blood vessels in the skin dilate; this increases the flow of blood and increases heat loss
	• If the body is still overheated, the brain stimulates sweating; as sweat evaporates, cooling occurs (For more information on thermoregulation, see Chapter 21, *Nutrition & Metabolism*.)

FAST FACT

Scientists have long known that vitamin D helps the body absorb calcium, which is important in the formation and maintenance of strong bones. More recently, research suggests vitamin D may play a role in the function of the immune system. Specifically, vitamin D may help prevent cancer, several autoimmune diseases, and high blood pressure.

The Body AT WORK

While the skin acts as a barrier, it can also absorb many chemicals, making the skin a possible route for medication administration. Called transdermal *administration, a medication in the form of a lotion, gel, or adhesive patch is placed on the skin and allowed to absorb slowly. Some medications administered transdermally include nitroglycerin (to treat certain types of chest pain), hydrocortisone ointment (for inflammation), and nicotine (to treat cigarette addiction).*

The ability to absorb medications means that the skin may absorb toxic chemicals as well. Some of the toxins that can be absorbed through the skin include metals (such as arsenic, mercury, and lead), nail polish remover (acetone), pesticides, and cleaning solvents. Some of these chemicals can cause cancer or brain, kidney, or liver damage, making it important to wear gloves whenever you handle chemicals.

Appendages of the Skin

The appendages of the skin are hair, nails, and glands.

Hair

Hair occurs everywhere on the body except for a few locations: the palms and soles, lips, nipples, and some areas of the genitals. In some locations, hair has a protective role: the eyelashes and eyebrows keep perspiration out of the eyes; hair in the nostrils filters out dust; and the hair on the head provides insulation against heat and cold.

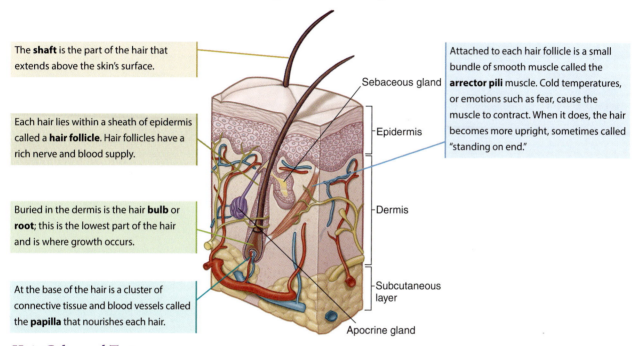

The **shaft** is the part of the hair that extends above the skin's surface.

Each hair lies within a sheath of epidermis called a **hair follicle**. Hair follicles have a rich nerve and blood supply.

Buried in the dermis is the hair **bulb** or **root**; this is the lowest part of the hair and is where growth occurs.

At the base of the hair is a cluster of connective tissue and blood vessels called the **papilla** that nourishes each hair.

Attached to each hair follicle is a small bundle of smooth muscle called the **arrector pili** muscle. Cold temperatures, or emotions such as fear, cause the muscle to contract. When it does, the hair becomes more upright, sometimes called "standing on end."

Sebaceous gland
Epidermis
Dermis
Subcutaneous layer
Apocrine gland

Hair Color and Texture

Hair obtains its color from melanin. The two types of melanin (eumelanin and pheomelanin) give rise to the various shades of hair. Darker hair has a greater concentration of eumelanin. Blond hair contains mostly pheomelanin, while red hair contains a mixture of the two. Gray and white hair result from a lack of melanin.

The shape of the hair shaft determines whether it's straight or curly. A round shaft produces straight hair, while an oval shaft produces curly hair.

Hair Growth and Loss

Hair grows from the base. New cells causing hair growth arise in an area above the papilla. Once formed, these new cells produce keratin and then die. As more cells are formed beneath them, the older cells are pushed toward the surface of the skin; this causes the hair to lengthen. All the cells of the hair—other than the cells just above the papilla—are dead, flattened cells filled with keratin.

Hair has a limited lifespan. Typically, the hair on the head lives between 2 and 6 years. After that it falls out, and after a resting phase, it's replaced by new hair.

Excessive hair loss is called **alopecia**. Alopecia may result from disease, poor nutrition, chemotherapy, or even emotional distress. A common cause of alopecia is aging. Some men exhibit what's known as **male pattern baldness**. This type of hair loss occurs only in individuals who have inherited a specific gene *and* who have high levels of testosterone, which is why it typically occurs in men.

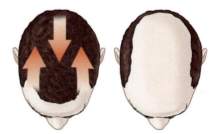

In male pattern baldness, hair recedes in an M shape. Eventually the bald patch on the crown meets the two points of the M, creating a horseshoe shape.

Nails

Nails consist of densely packed, heavily keratinized epithelial cells.

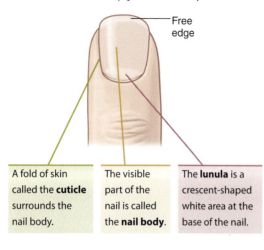

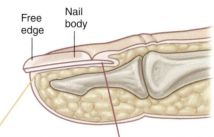

A fold of skin called the **cuticle** surrounds the nail body.	The visible part of the nail is called the **nail body**.

The **lunula** is a crescent-shaped white area at the base of the nail.

The **nail bed** is a layer of epithelium under the nail. It normally appears pink because of the rich blood supply in the area.

The **nail root** is the proximal end of the nail; it's hidden underneath overlying tissue. Nails grow as newly keratinized cells are added to the nail root from the nail matrix. As the new cells are added, the nail is pushed forward. Most fingernails grow about 1/25 inch (1 mm) each week; toenails grow somewhat more slowly.

The shape and color of nails can provide clues about underlying disorders.

Abnormal Nail Changes

Condition	Cause
Clubbing	Long-term oxygen deficiency, usually due to lung disease (This causes the distal ends of the fingers to enlarge, making it look like a drumstick when viewed from above. At the same time the nail bed softens, causing the nail to angle downward, giving it a beaked appearance when viewed from the side.)
Cyanosis	Often is the first sign of oxygen deficiency
Flattened or concave nail beds	May indicate an iron deficiency
Dark lines beneath the nail	May indicate melanoma in lighter-skinned individuals, although such lines may be normal in individuals with dark skin
White nails	May occur in liver diseases such as hepatitis
Yellowish, thickened, slow-growing nails	Often occur in individuals with lung diseases such as emphysema
Pale nail beds	May be a sign of anemia

Life lesson: Changes with aging

The integumentary system may be one of the first body systems to visibly reflect signs of aging. Here are some common results of aging:

- The amount of fat in subcutaneous tissue declines, the dermis thins, the amount of collagen and elastin decreases, and skin cell replacement slows, all leading to wrinkles around the eyes, nose, and mouth.
- Skin cell replacement slows, leading to delayed wound healing and an increased risk for infection.
- The number, and output, of sweat glands declines, making it difficult for elderly individuals to maintain their body temperature.
- Overall melanocyte production slows, increasing sun sensitivity, while the proliferation of melanocytes increases in localized areas, causing brown spots to develop on the skin.
- The pigment in hair decreases, leading to thinning and graying hair.

Glands

The glands associated with the skin include sweat glands, sebaceous glands, and ceruminous glands.

Sweat Glands

These are the most numerous of the skin glands.

The Body AT WORK

*Every day, the body loses about 500 ml of **insensible perspiration**: perspiration that doesn't make the skin feel damp. Perspiration increases dramatically from heat or exercise. In fact, the body can lose as much as a liter of perspiration an hour from intense exercise or extreme heat. If the fluid isn't replaced, dehydration or even circulatory shock may result.*

There are two types of sweat glands: **eccrine glands** and **apocrine glands**.

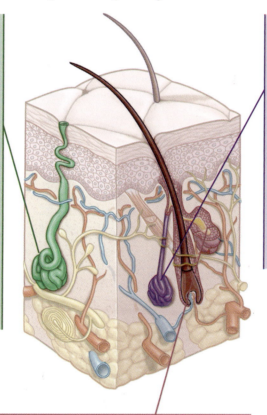

Eccrine glands

- Contain a duct that leads from a secretory portion (consisting of a twisted coil in the dermis), through the dermis and epidermis, and onto the skin's surface
- Are widespread throughout the body, but are especially abundant on the palms, soles, forehead, and upper torso
- Produce a transparent, watery fluid called *sweat*, which contains potassium, ammonia, lactic acid, uric acid, and other wastes
- Sweat plays a chief role in helping the body maintain a constant core temperature and also helps the body eliminate wastes.

Apocrine glands

- Contain a duct that leads to a hair follicle (as opposed to opening onto the skin's surface)
- Are located mainly in the axillary and anogenital (groin) regions
- Are scent glands that respond to stress and sexual stimulation
- Begin to function at puberty
- Sweat produced by these glands does not have a strong odor unless it accumulates on the skin; when this occurs, bacteria begins to degrade substances in the sweat, resulting in body odor.

Sebaceous Glands

Sebaceous glands, which open into a hair follicle, secrete an oily substance called sebum. Sebum helps keep the skin and hair from drying out and becoming brittle. Sebum has a mild antibacterial and antifungal effect. Under the influence of sex hormones, sebum production increases during adolescence. When excess sebum accumulates in the gland ducts, pimples and blackheads can form. (When the accumulated sebum is exposed to air, it darkens, forming a blackhead. A pustule results if the area becomes infected by bacteria.)

Ceruminous Glands

Ceruminous glands, which exist in the external ear canal, secrete a waxy substance called **cerumen**, or ear wax. Cerumen helps keep the ear canal from drying out. However, excess cerumen can accumulate in the ear canal and harden, diminishing hearing.

Life lesson: Burns

Burns can be caused by fire, hot water, steam, electricity, chemicals, and sunlight. Considering the skin's crucial role in protecting against infection, controlling fluid loss, and thermoregulation, it's easy to understand the seriousness of severe or extensive burns. In fact, following a serious burn, a patient may lose as much as 75% of his circulating fluid volume in the first few hours, placing that person at risk for circulatory collapse and cardiac arrest. Another complication of burns is the development of eschar—the dead tissue resulting from a burn. Besides secreting toxins and promoting bacterial growth, eschar can restrict circulation.

Burns are classified according to their depth: in other words, the number of tissue layers affected by the burn.

Burn Classifications

First-degree burn	Second-degree burn	Third-degree burn

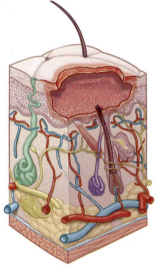
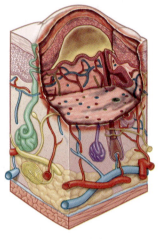
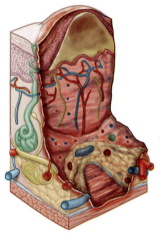

Partial-thickness burn: superficial
- Involves only the epidermis
- Causes redness, slight swelling, and pain
- Often results from sunlight (sunburn)

Partial-thickness burn: deep
- Involves the epidermis as well as part of the dermis
- Results in blisters, severe pain, and swelling
- May result in scarring
- May appear red, white, or tan

Full-thickness burn
- Extends through the epidermis and dermis and into the subcutaneous layer
- May not be painful initially because of the destruction of nerve endings
- May appear white or black and leathery
- Often requires skin grafts

Rule of Nines

Another aspect of burn treatment involves estimating the percentage of body surface area (BSA) affected. A commonly used method, called the Rule of Nines, divides the body into 11 areas of 9%. By adding the corresponding percentages for each body section burned, it's possible to arrive at a quick and accurate estimate of the extent of the burn.

The Rule of Nines isn't accurate in children, however, because a child's BSA differs from that of an adult. For example, a burn to half the head accounts for $9^1/_2$% BSA in a newborn, $6^1/_2$% in a child age 5 years, and $4^1/_2$% in an adult. A table called the Lund–Browder chart—which adjusts the surface area of certain body regions according to age—is used to determine burn size in infants and children.

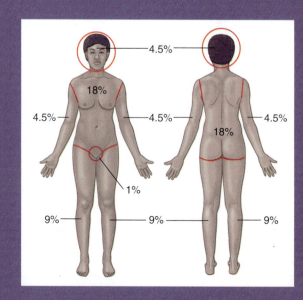

Life lesson: Skin cancer

Skin cancer, which is the most common form of cancer, results from changes in epidermal cells. Each year in the United States, more than 3.5 million cases of basal and squamous cell skin cancer are diagnosed. Melanoma—the most serious of all skin cancers—accounts for another 76,000 cases. The three types of skin cancer are described below:

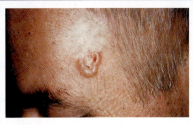

- **Basal cell carcinoma**
  - The most common type
  - Seldom metastasizes, so is the least dangerous
  - Arises from the cells of the stratum basale, typically on the nose or face
  - Lesion first appears as a small, shiny bump; as it enlarges, it often develops a central depression and a beaded, "pearly" edge

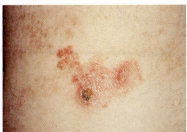

- **Squamous cell carcinoma**
  - Arises in the epidermis and is slow growing
  - Often occurs on the scalp, forehead, backs of the hands, and top of the ears
  - Has a raised, red, scaly appearance
  - Some forms may metastasize

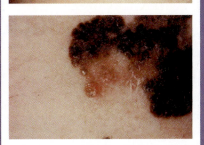

- **Malignant melanoma**
  - Most deadly of all skin cancers
  - Sometimes develops from melanocytes of a preexisting mole
  - Metastasizes quickly and is often fatal when not treated early
  - Risk is greatest in individuals who had severe sunburns as children

Disorders of the Integumentary System

Disorder	Characteristics
Acne	Inflammation of the sebaceous glands, especially during puberty, in which the follicle becomes blocked with keratinocytes and sebum; this results in whiteheads (comedos), while continued inflammation produces pus, causing pimples; oxidation of sebum turns whiteheads into blackheads
Dermatitis	Inflammation of the skin characterized by itching and redness, often the result of exposure to chemicals or toxins (such as poison ivy)
Eczema	Itchy, red rash caused by an allergy; lesions initially weep or ooze serum and may become crusted, thickened, or scaly
Impetigo	Contagious bacterial infection of the skin (usually caused by streptococci or staphylococci), producing yellow to red weeping, crusted, or pustular lesions around the nose, mouth, or cheeks or on the extremities
Psoriasis	A recurring skin disorder characterized by red papules and scaly silvery plaques with sharply defined borders
Tinea	Any fungal infection of the skin; usually occurs in moist areas, such as the groin, axilla, and foot (*athlete's foot*)
Urticaria	Allergic reaction resulting in multiple red patches (wheals) that are intensely itchy

Review of Key Terms

Apocrine glands: Glands located mainly in axillary and anogenital areas that secrete sweat in response to stress and sexual stimulation

Ceruminous gland: Gland in the external ear canal that secretes waxy cerumen

Cutaneous membrane: The skin

Dermis: The layer of the skin lying immediately under the epidermis

Eccrine glands: Glands located throughout the body that secrete sweat directly onto the skin's surface, which helps control body temperature

Epidermis: The outermost layer of the skin

Hair follicle: A sheath of epidermis surrounding each hair

Hypodermis: Subcutaneous tissue composed mostly of fat lying under the dermis

Keratin: A tough, fibrous protein that provides structural strength to the skin, hair, and nails

Melanin: Pigment produced by melanocytes that gives color to the hair and skin

Sebaceous gland: Glands that secrete an oily substance called sebum into each hair follicle

Stratum basale: The innermost layer of the epidermis, where new skin cells are germinated

Stratum corneum: The outermost layer of the epidermis, consisting of dead, flattened cells called keratinocytes

Subcutaneous: Beneath the skin

Own the Information

To make the information in this chapter part of your working memory, take some time to reflect on what you've learned. On a separate sheet of paper, write down everything you recall from the chapter. After you're done, log on to the Davis*Plus* website, and check out the Study Group podcast and Study Group Questions for the chapter.

Key Topics for Chapter 5:
- Structure of the skin
- Layers of the epidermis
- Skin color, both normal and abnormal
- Functions of the skin
- Structure and function of hair
- Structure of nails
- Sweat glands, sebaceous glands, and ceruminous glands
- Burns
- Skin cancer

Test Your Knowledge

1. What is the name of the outermost layer of the skin?
   a. Dermis
   b. Epidermis
   c. Hypodermis
   d. Papillae

2. In which skin layer are new skin cells generated?
   a. Hypodermis
   b. Stratum corneum
   c. Stratum basale
   d. Dermis

3. New skin cells produce which tough, fibrous protein?
   a. Collagen
   b. Elastin
   c. Melanin
   d. Keratin

4. What is the chief purpose of melanin in the skin?
   a. Protect the nucleus of the skin cell against UV radiation
   b. Strengthen the structural integrity of the skin
   c. Prevent excess fluid loss
   d. Aid in thermoregulation

5. The skin initiates the production of which vitamin?
   a. Vitamin C
   b. Vitamin K
   c. Vitamin D
   d. Vitamin A

6. How does the epidermis receive oxygen and nutrients?
   a. It is richly supplied with blood vessels, which provide it with the oxygen and nutrients it needs.
   b. It receives oxygen and nutrients by diffusion from the dermis.
   c. It receives oxygen and nutrients by diffusion from the surrounding environment.
   d. It doesn't need oxygen or nutrients because it is composed only of dead, keratinized cells.

7. Which of the following is a function of the stratum corneum?
   a. Secrete melanin
   b. Generate new skin cells
   c. Act as a barrier
   d. Provide insulation

8. What is the function of the eccrine glands?
   a. They secrete sweat, which plays a role in helping the body maintain a constant core temperature.
   b. They are scent glands that produce sweat in response to stress and sexual stimulation.
   c. They secrete an oily substance that helps keep skin and hair from drying out.
   d. They secrete a waxy substance that helps keep the external ear canal from drying out.

9. The skin helps the body conserve heat by:
   a. dilating blood vessels.
   b. producing sweat.
   c. producing sebum.
   d. constricting blood vessels.

10. Where does hair growth occur?
    a. Hair follicle
    b. Hair bulb
    c. Hair shaft
    d. Papilla

Answers: Chapter 5

1. *Correct answer:* **b.** The dermis is the inner, deeper layer of the skin. The hypodermis is a layer of subcutaneous tissue residing directly beneath the dermis. Papillae are finger-like projections on top of the dermis, which allow it to interlock with the epidermis.

2. *Correct answer:* **c.** The hypodermis and the dermis lie beneath the epidermis and have no role in generating new skin cells. The stratum corneum is the surface layer of the skin, the place to which new cells migrate.

3. *Correct answer:* **d.** Collagen and elastin are connective tissue proteins that help form the dermis. Melanin is a skin pigment.

4. *Correct answer:* **a.** Melanin has no role in strengthening the structural integrity of the skin, preventing fluid loss, or thermoregulation.

5. Correct answer: **c.** The skin has no role in the synthesis of vitamins C, K, or A.

6. *Correct answer:* **b.** The epidermis contains no blood vessels. It does not receive oxygen or nutrients by diffusion from the surrounding environment. The epidermis is living tissue and therefore depends on an adequate supply of oxygen and nutrients.

7. *Correct answer:* **c.** Melanocytes secrete melanin. The stratum basale is where new cells are formed. The hypodermis provides insulation.

8. *Correct answer:* **a.** Apocrine glands are scent glands that produce sweat in response to stress and sexual stimulation. Sebaceous glands secrete sebum, an oily substance that helps keep skin and hair from drying out. Ceruminous glands secrete a waxy substance that helps keep the external ear canal from drying out.

9. *Correct answer:* **d.** Producing sweat and dilating blood vessels are two mechanisms used by the skin to increase heat loss and cool the body. Sebum has no effect on body temperature.

10. *Correct answer:* **b.** The hair follicle is a sheath of epidermis surrounding each hair, and the hair shaft is the portion of the hair that extends above the skin's surface; neither has a role in hair growth. The papilla is a cluster of connective tissue and blood vessels that nourishes each hair, but the growth actually occurs in the hair bulb or root.

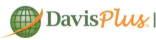 DavisPlus | Go to http://davisplus.fadavis.com Keyword: Thompson to see all of the resources available with this chapter.

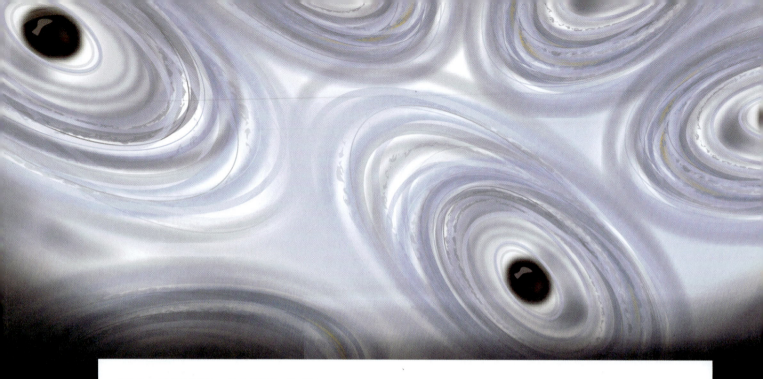

CHAPTER OUTLINE

Bone Functions

Classification of Bones

Bone Tissue

Bone Marrow

Bone Development

Bone Remodeling

Bone Fractures

LEARNING OUTCOMES

1. List the roles of bone in the body.

2. Describe the four types of bone, as classified by shape.

3. Identify the key structures of a long bone.

4. Describe the components of bone, including the specific cells and fibers.

5. Discuss the component that makes bone unique from other connective tissues.

6. Distinguish the unique characteristics of bone.

7. Explain the structure and characteristics of spongy bone and compact bone.

8. Compare the two types of bone marrow, including their functions and locations in the body.

9. Summarize the two processes of bone formation: intramembranous ossification and endochondral ossification.

10. Explain how bone continues to grow throughout the life span.

11. Discuss the process of bone remodeling.

12. Identify five types of bone fractures.

13. Explain the process of fracture repair.

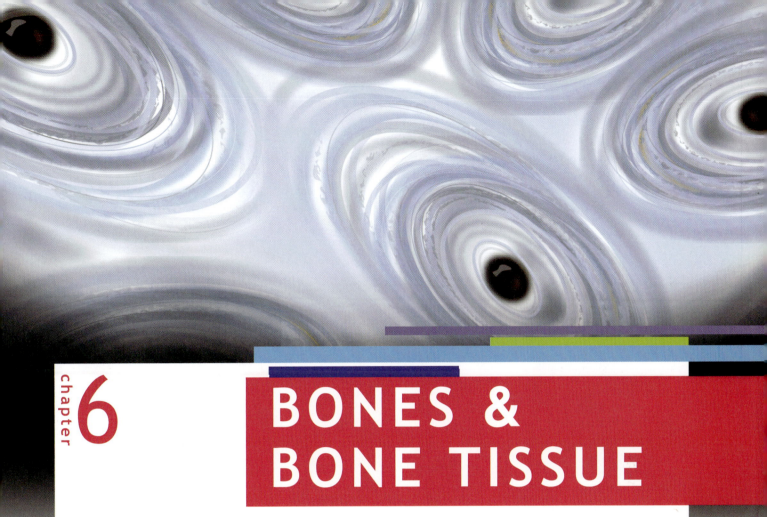

chapter 6

BONES & BONE TISSUE

The strength of bone is similar to that of reinforced concrete. Yet, it is so light it makes up only 14% of an adult's body weight.

The skeleton may appear to be nothing more than a dry, nonliving framework for the body, but it is far from it. The 206 bones in the adult human body are actually dynamic living tissue. Bone constantly breaks down and rebuilds itself, not just during the growth phases of childhood, but throughout the life span. Bone is filled with blood vessels, nerves, and living cells; in addition, its interaction with other body systems is necessary not only for movement, but also for life itself.

Bone Functions

Bone fulfills multiple roles in the body, including:

- **Shape:** Bones give the body its structure.
- **Support:** The bones of the legs, pelvis, and vertebral column support the body and hold it upright.
- **Protection:** Bones protect delicate internal organs, such as the heart, lungs, brain, and spinal cord.
- **Movement:** Movement of the arms and legs as well as the ability to breathe results from the interaction between muscles and bones.
- **Electrolyte balance:** Bones store and release minerals such as calcium and phosphorus—necessary ingredients for a variety of chemical reactions throughout the body.
- **Blood production:** Bones encase bone marrow, a major site of blood cell formation.
- **Acid-base balance:** Bone absorbs and releases alkaline salts to help maintain a stable pH.

FAST FACT

Bone is as strong as steel and as light as aluminum.

Classification of Bones

Bones perform a variety of functions—from supporting the weight of the body (the bones of the legs and pelvis) to performing delicate movements (the fingers). It's those functions that dictate the bone's shape. This variety in the shape of bones lends itself to a classification system.

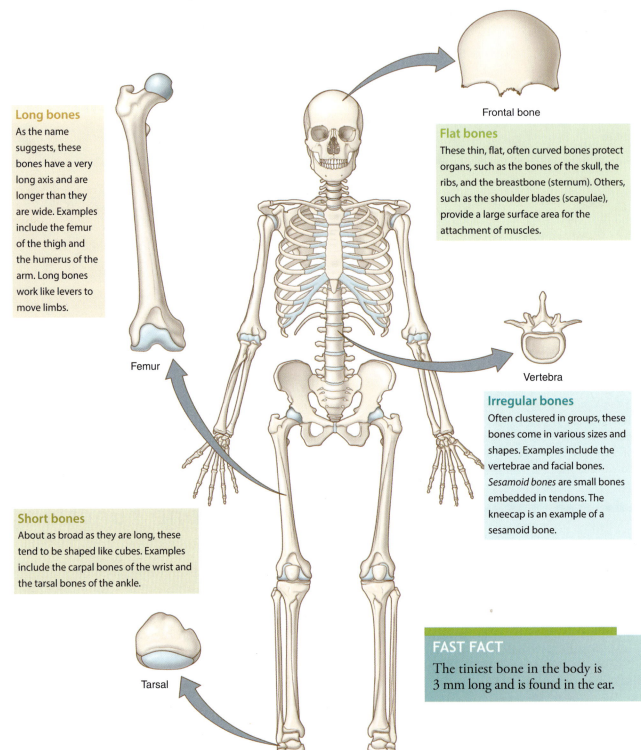

Long bones

As the name suggests, these bones have a very long axis and are longer than they are wide. Examples include the femur of the thigh and the humerus of the arm. Long bones work like levers to move limbs.

Femur

Frontal bone

Flat bones

These thin, flat, often curved bones protect organs, such as the bones of the skull, the ribs, and the breastbone (sternum). Others, such as the shoulder blades (scapulae), provide a large surface area for the attachment of muscles.

Vertebra

Irregular bones

Often clustered in groups, these bones come in various sizes and shapes. Examples include the vertebrae and facial bones. *Sesamoid bones* are small bones embedded in tendons. The kneecap is an example of a sesamoid bone.

Short bones

About as broad as they are long, these tend to be shaped like cubes. Examples include the carpal bones of the wrist and the tarsal bones of the ankle.

Tarsal

FAST FACT

The tiniest bone in the body is 3 mm long and is found in the ear.

Parts of a Long Bone

Long bones consist of several key structures:

The head of each end of a long bone is the **epiphysis**. The bulbous structure of the epiphysis strengthens the joint; it also allows an expanded area for the attachment of tendons and ligaments. The epiphysis is made of porous-looking spongy bone.

Covering the surface of the epiphysis is a thin layer of hyaline cartilage called **articular cartilage**. This cartilage, along with a lubricating fluid secreted between bones, eases the movement of the bone within a joint.

The central hollow portion is called the **medullary cavity**.

- The inside of the medullary cavity is lined with a thin epithelial membrane called the **endosteum**.
- In children, the medullary cavity is filled with blood cell-producing **red bone marrow**. In adults, most of this marrow has turned to **yellow marrow**, which is rich in fat.

The central shaft-like portion of the bone is called the **diaphysis**. Thick, compact bone makes up this hollow cylinder, giving the bone the strength it needs to support a large amount of weight.

A dense fibrous membrane called the **periosteum** covers the diaphysis. Some of the fibers of the periosteum penetrate the bone, ensuring that the membrane stays firmly anchored. Other fibers of the periosteum weave together with the fibers of tendons. (Tendons attach muscle to bone.) This arrangement ensures a strong connection between muscle and bone. The periosteum contains bone-forming cells as well as blood vessels, making its presence crucial for bone survival.

Epiphysis

Articular cartilage

The Body AT WORK

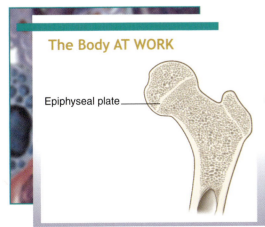

Epiphyseal plate

*In growing children, a layer of cartilage, called the **epiphyseal plate** or **growth plate**, separates the epiphysis from the diaphysis at each end of a long bone. Once growth stops, the plate is replaced by an epiphyseal line. (Bone growth and the epiphyseal plate are discussed in more depth later in this chapter.)*

FAST FACT

Osteomyelitis is an inflammation of bone and marrow, usually the result of a bacterial infection. Bone infections are often difficult to treat and typically require prolonged intravenous antibiotics.

Bone Tissue

Bone, or **osseous tissue**, is a type of connective tissue; like all connective tissues, it consists of cells, fibers, and extracellular material, or matrix. Bone cells include osteoblasts, osteoclasts, and osteocytes.

- **Osteoblasts** help form bone by secreting substances that comprise the bone's matrix.
- **Osteoclasts** dissolve unwanted or unhealthy bone.
- **Osteocytes** are mature osteoblasts that have become entrapped in the hardened bone matrix. Osteocytes have a dual role: some dissolve bone while others deposit new bone. By doing so, they contribute to the maintenance of bone density while also assisting with the regulation of blood levels of calcium and phosphate.

FAST FACT
The study of bone is called *osteology*.

Bone is unique from other connective tissues because of its matrix. Consisting of collagen fibers and crystalline salts (primarily calcium and phosphate), the matrix of bone is hard and calcified. Bone is also incredibly strong; it has a strength rivaling that of steel and reinforced concrete. Bone has significant tensile and compressional strength, but it lacks torsional strength.

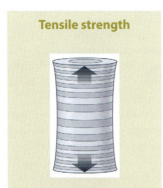

Tensile strength

Collagen fibers in the matrix make bone highly resistant to stretching forces (called **tensile strength**).

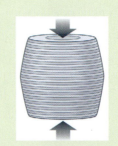

Compressional strength

Calcium salts allow bones to resist strong squeezing forces (called **compressional strength**).

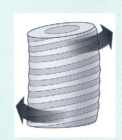

Torsional strength

Bone lacks the ability to endure twisting (called **torsional strength**). In fact, most bone fractures result when torsional forces are exerted on an arm or leg.

The Body AT WORK

Whenever bone experiences an increase in load, osteocytes stimulate the creation of new bone. For example, when an individual participates in weight-bearing exercise, osteocytes trigger the growth of new bone, making bones stronger. This makes any weight-bearing exercise, especially lifting weights, ideal for those at risk for osteoporosis, a disease characterized by a loss of bone density.

Types of Bone Tissue

Not all bone, or osseous tissue, has the same characteristics:

- Some osseous tissue is light and porous; this is spongy, or cancellous, bone. **Spongy bone** is found in the ends of long bones and in the middle of most other bones; it is always surrounded by the more durable compact bone.
- Other osseous tissue—called **compact bone**—is dense and solid. Its density offers strength, which is why it forms the shafts of long bones and the outer surfaces of other bones.

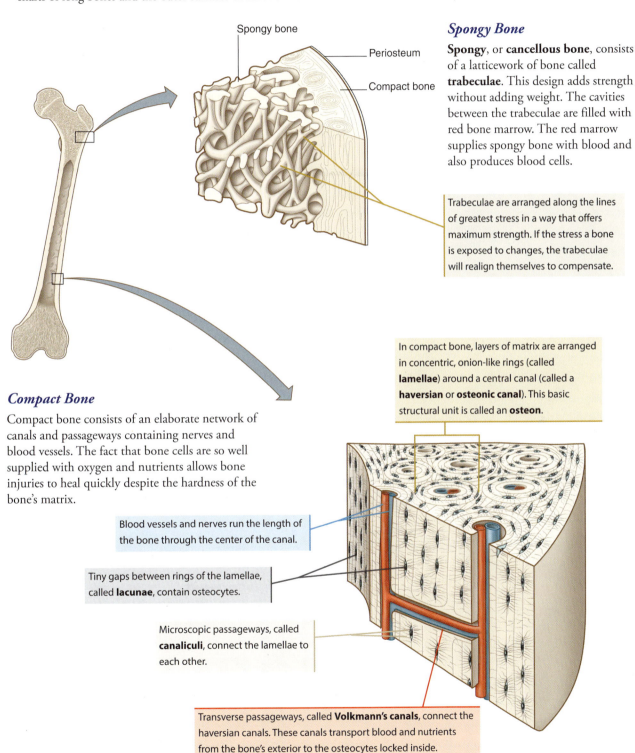

Spongy bone

Periosteum

Compact bone

Spongy Bone

Spongy, or **cancellous bone**, consists of a latticework of bone called **trabeculae**. This design adds strength without adding weight. The cavities between the trabeculae are filled with red bone marrow. The red marrow supplies spongy bone with blood and also produces blood cells.

Trabeculae are arranged along the lines of greatest stress in a way that offers maximum strength. If the stress a bone is exposed to changes, the trabeculae will realign themselves to compensate.

In compact bone, layers of matrix are arranged in concentric, onion-like rings (called **lamellae**) around a central canal (called a **haversian** or **osteonic canal**). This basic structural unit is called an **osteon**.

Compact Bone

Compact bone consists of an elaborate network of canals and passageways containing nerves and blood vessels. The fact that bone cells are so well supplied with oxygen and nutrients allows bone injuries to heal quickly despite the hardness of the bone's matrix.

Blood vessels and nerves run the length of the bone through the center of the canal.

Tiny gaps between rings of the lamellae, called **lacunae**, contain osteocytes.

Microscopic passageways, called **canaliculi**, connect the lamellae to each other.

Transverse passageways, called **Volkmann's canals**, connect the haversian canals. These canals transport blood and nutrients from the bone's exterior to the osteocytes locked inside.

Bone Marrow

Bone marrow is a type of soft tissue that fills the medullary cavity of long bones as well as the spaces of spongy bone. There are two types of bone marrow:

1. **Red bone marrow:** This is the bone marrow charged with producing red blood cells. Nearly all of a child's bones contain red bone marrow.

2. **Yellow bone marrow:** Over time, red marrow is gradually replaced with fatty yellow marrow. Because its marrow cells are saturated with fat, yellow marrow no longer produces blood cells. However, in cases of severe, chronic blood loss or anemia, yellow marrow can change back into red marrow.

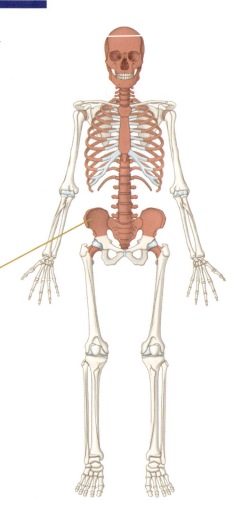

In an adult, red bone marrow can be found only in the ribs, sternum, vertebrae, skull, pelvis, and the upper parts of both the humerus (arm) and femur (thigh). All other bones contain yellow marrow.

Bone Development

The first skeleton in a developing fetus is composed of cartilage and fibrous connective tissue. Through a process called **ossification**, this early skeleton evolves into bone. There are two types of ossification processes: one for fibrous connective tissue and one for cartilage.

Intramembranous Ossification

Some bones, including those of the skull and face, start out as fibrous connective tissue. Called **intramembranous ossification**, this process begins when groups of stem cells in the tissue differentiate into osteoblasts. Clusters of osteoblasts, called *centers for ossification*, deposit matrix material and collagen. Eventually, calcium salts are deposited and the bone is calcified.

The Body AT WORK

*At birth, part of the newborn's skull still consists of fibrous connective tissue. These areas, called **fontanels** or "soft spots," allow for safe compression of the fetus's head while passing through the birth canal. It also allows the skull to expand readily as the brain grows during the months immediately following birth. By age 2, though, the skull is completely ossified.*

Endochondral Ossification

Most bones evolve from cartilage. After about three months' gestation, the fetus has a skeleton composed mostly of cartilage. At that time, the cartilage begins turning into bone. This process, which begins in long bones, is called **endochondral ossification**. The figure below demonstrates how the process occurs.

ANIMATION 🌐

1 Early in the life of a fetus, long bones composed of cartilage can be identified. These cartilaginous bones serve as "models" for bone development.

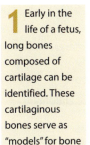

Cartilage model

2 Osteoblasts start to replace the chondrocytes (cartilage cells). The osteoblasts coat the diaphysis in a thin layer of bone, after which they produce a ring of bone that encircles the diaphysis. Soon, the cartilage begins to calcify.

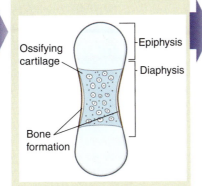

Ossifying cartilage — Epiphysis

Diaphysis

Bone formation

3 Blood vessels then penetrate the cartilage, and a primary ossification center develops in the middle of the diaphysis.

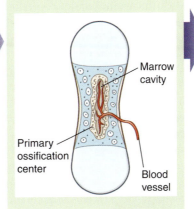

Marrow cavity

Primary ossification center

Blood vessel

4 The bone marrow cavity fills with blood and stem cells. Ossification continues—proceeding from the diaphysis toward each epiphysis—and the bone grows in length. Eventually, secondary ossification centers appear in the epiphyses.

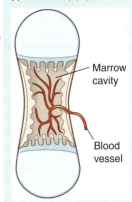

Marrow cavity

Blood vessel

Bone Growth

Bone growth obviously doesn't stop at birth. Bones grow in length, or elongate, for a fixed period. However, bones also widen and thicken throughout the lifespan.

Bone Lengthening

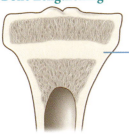

Bone lengthening occurs at the **epiphyseal plate**: a layer of hyaline cartilage at the each end of bone. On the epiphyseal side of the cartilage plate, chondrocytes continue to multiply. As these cells move toward the diaphysis, minerals are deposited and the cartilage becomes calcified. As long as chondrocytes are produced in the epiphyseal plate, the bone continues to elongate.

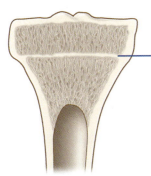

Sometime between the ages of 16 and 25, all of the cartilage of the epiphyseal plate is replaced with spongy bone. When that occurs, bone lengthening stops, and we say that the epiphyses have "closed." What remains is a line of spongy bone called the **epiphyseal line**.

The Body AT WORK

Several hormones, including growth hormone and the sex hormones estrogen and testosterone, influence bone growth. Growth hormone stimulates chondrocytes in the epiphyseal plate to proliferate, causing bones to grow longer. Sex hormones stimulate a growth spurt during puberty; they're also linked to fusion of the epiphyseal plates (which halts growth).

FAST FACT

When overstressed, the epiphyseal plate can separate from the diaphysis or epiphysis, resulting in an **epiphyseal fracture**. When this occurs, future bone growth can be affected.

Bone Widening and Thickening

Unlike bone lengthening, which stops at a certain point, bone widening and thickening continue throughout the lifespan. A bone widens when osteoblasts in the periosteum lay down new layers of bone around the outside of the bone. As this occurs, osteoclasts on the inner bone tissue work to dissolve bone tissue, widening the marrow cavity.

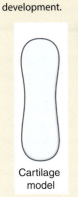

Bone Remodeling

Bone cells work constantly throughout the life span, destroying old bone (**resorption**) and depositing new (**ossification**). In this process, called **remodeling**, osteoclasts remove matrix and reduce the mass of little-used bones. In heavily used bones, osteoblasts deposit new bone tissue on the bone's surface, thickening the bone. Remodeling repairs minor traumas and contributes to homeostasis by releasing calcium into the blood. This same process also leads to the development of projections and bone surface markings as bone is stimulated by the pull of powerful muscles as children grow and begin to walk.

The maintenance of bone density depends upon a balance between the work of osteoclasts (which cause resorption) and osteoblasts (which cause ossification). During early and middle adulthood, ossification and resorption are in balance, with the amount of bone being formed equaling the amount of bone being destroyed. During the growth periods of childhood and adolescence, the creation of bone occurs at a faster rate than resorption. After about age 40, bone loss increases while bone formation slows, causing bones to weaken.

Because bone adapts to withstand physical stress, it's possible to increase bone density through physical exercise. Likewise, a lack of physical exercise causes increased bone loss. This is particularly true in bedridden patients as well as in astronauts experiencing the weightlessness of space.

FAST FACT
Bone remodeling replaces about 10% of the skeleton each year.

The Body AT WORK

A number of factors affect bone growth and maintenance. These include:

- **Heredity:** *Every individual inherits a set of genes that determines his maximum height potential.*
- **Nutrition:** *Children who are malnourished grow very slowly and may not reach their full height, regardless of their genetic potential. Nutrients necessary for proper bone growth include calcium, phosphorus, and vitamins D, C, and A.*
- **Hormones:** *Hormones that contribute to proper bone growth include growth hormone, thyroxine, parathyroid hormone, insulin, and the sex hormones estrogen and testosterone.*
- **Exercise:** *As previously mentioned, without adequate physical stress in the form of weight-bearing exercise (which includes walking), bone destruction will outpace bone creation.*

Life lesson: Osteoporosis

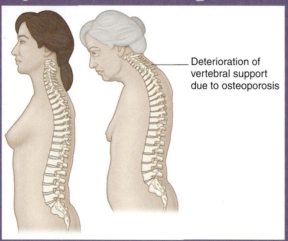

Deterioration of vertebral support due to osteoporosis

Osteoporosis, which means "porous bones," is a condition in which bones lose so much mass that they become extremely brittle. Even minor stresses, such as bending over or coughing, can cause a fracture. Fractures occur most often in the hip, wrist, and vertebral column.

Osteoporosis is the most common bone disease, affecting about 10 million Americans. It's estimated that another 18 million have low bone density. Because women have less bone mass than men, and because they start losing it at an earlier age, women have a higher risk for developing osteoporosis. In particular, postmenopausal white women have the greatest risk. (The drop in estrogen levels that accompanies menopause accelerates bone loss; also, black women tend to have denser bones than white women do.) Other risk factors for osteoporosis include smoking, diabetes mellitus, and diets poor in calcium, protein, and vitamins C and D.

Bone Fractures

A break in a bone is called a **fracture**. There are many different kinds of fractures, as shown below. Typically, broken bones can be manipulated into their original position without surgery. This is called **closed reduction**. Occasionally, surgery is needed to reposition the bones, after which screws, pins, or plates may be used to stabilize the bones. This is called **open reduction**.

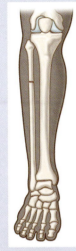

A **simple** fracture is one in which the bone remains aligned and the surrounding tissue is intact.

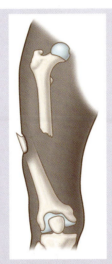

A **compound** fracture is one in which the bone has pierced the skin. Damage to surrounding tissue, nerves, and blood vessels may be extensive. Also, because it has broken through the skin, there is an increased risk for infection.

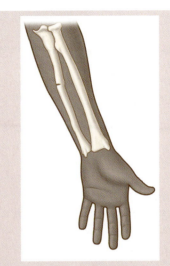

A **greenstick** fracture is one in which the fracture is incomplete, similar to when a green stick breaks. This type of fracture typically occurs in young children, mainly because their bones are softer than adult bones, causing the bone to splinter rather than break completely.

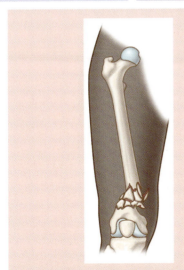

In a **comminuted** fracture, the bone is broken into pieces. This type of fracture is most likely to occur in a car accident.

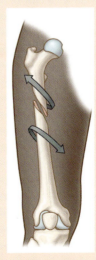

In a **spiral** fracture, the fracture line spirals around the bone, the result of a twisting force. The jagged bone ends often make this type of fracture difficult to reposition.

FAST FACT

Fracture locations typically vary with age: elbow fractures commonly occur in childhood; young persons are more likely to fracture a lower leg bone while playing sports; elderly people are susceptible to hip fractures.

Fracture Repair

Uncomplicated fractures heal in 8 to 12 weeks. Complex fractures, and fractures occurring in bones having a poor blood supply (such as the neck of the femur), take longer. Healing is also slower in elderly people as well as in those who suffer from a poor nutritional state.

In general, healing follows these steps:

ANIMATION 🌐

1 When a fracture occurs, blood vessels in the bone and periosteum are torn, resulting in bleeding and the formation of a clot (hematoma). The hematoma soon transforms into a soft mass of granulation tissue containing inflammatory cells and bone-forming cells that aid in the healing process.

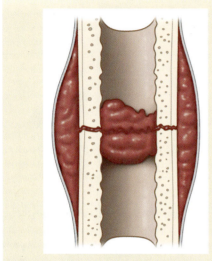

2 Collagen and fibrocartilage are deposited in the granulation tissue, transforming it into a soft callus.

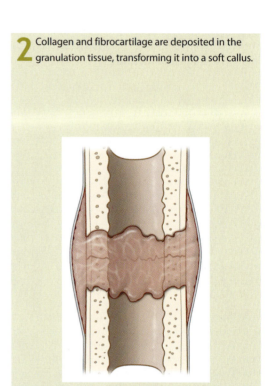

3 Next, bone-forming cells produce a bony, or hard, callus around the fracture. This splints the two bone ends together as healing continues.

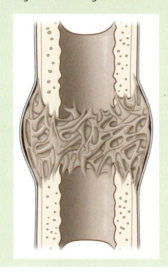

4 Remodeling eventually replaces the callus tissue with bone.

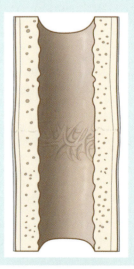

FAST FACT

Orthopedics is the branch of medicine that deals with the prevention or correction of disorders and injuries of bones, joints, and muscles.

Articular cartilage: Thin layer of hyaline cartilage covering the surface of the epiphysis

Canaliculi: Microscopic passageways that connect lamellae to each other

Cancellous bone: Spongy bone found in the ends of long bones and the middle of most other bones

Compact bone: Dense solid bone that forms the shafts of long bones and the outer surfaces of other bones

Diaphysis: The central shaft-like portion of a long bone

Endochondral ossification: Process in the fetus whereby cartilaginous skeleton transforms into bone

Endosteum: Thin epithelial membrane lining the inside of the medullary cavity

Epiphyseal plate: Layer of cartilage separating the epiphysis from the diaphysis at each end of a long bone; the site where bone growth occurs

Epiphysis: The head of each end of a long bone

Haversian canal: A central canal in compact bone containing blood vessels and nerves; surrounded by lamellae

Intramembranous ossification: Process in the fetus whereby fibrous connective tissue evolves into bone

Lacunae: Tiny gaps between rings of lamellae in compact bone

Lamellae: Concentric rings of matrix surrounding haversian canal in compact bone

Medullary cavity: The central hollow portion of a long bone that contains bone marrow

Osseous tissue: Bone tissue

Ossification: The creation of new bone

Osteoblast: Bone-forming cell

Osteoclasts: Bone cells that dissolve old or unhealthy bone

Osteocyte: Mature osteoblast

Osteon: Basic structural unit of compact bone consisting of a haversian canal and surrounding lamellae

Periosteum: Dense fibrous membrane covering the diaphysis

Remodeling: Reshaping or reconstructing part of a bone

Resorption: The destruction of old bone; part of the bone remodeling process

Spongy bone: Also called cancellous bone; found in the ends of long bones and the middle of most other bones

Trabeculae: Latticework of osseous tissue that makes up the structure of spongy or cancellous bone

Own the Information

To make the information in this chapter part of your working memory, take some time to reflect on what you've learned. On a separate sheet of paper, write down everything you recall from the chapter. After you're done, log on to the Davis*Plus* website, and check out the Study Group podcast and Study Group Questions for the chapter.

Key Topics for Chapter 6:
- The roles of bone in the body
- The classification of bones by shape
- The parts of a long bone
- The components of and qualities of bone tissue
- Types of bone tissue
- Types and locations of bone marrow
- Two types of bone development
- Bone growth and remodeling
- Bone fractures and repair

Test Your Knowledge

1. Most fractures occur because bones lack:
   a. tensile strength.
   b. compressional strength.
   c. torsional strength.
   d. both tensile and compressional strength.

2. The head of a long bone is called the:
   a. epiphysis.
   b. endosteum.
   c. diaphysis.
   d. periosteum.

3. The periosteum is crucial to bone survival because it:
   a. helps prevent fractures.
   b. produces bone marrow.
   c. contains blood vessels and bone-forming cells.
   d. secretes immunoglobulin to protect the bone against infection.

4. Which part of bone produces blood cells?
   a. Yellow bone marrow
   b. Red bone marrow
   c. Both red and yellow bone marrow
   d. The medullary cavity

5. The type of bone found in the ends of long bones and in the centers of most other bones is:
   a. compact bone.
   b. cancellous bone.
   c. membranous bone.
   d. endochondral bone.

6. What effect does physical stress have on bone?
   a. It stimulates osteoblasts to break down bone.
   b. It stimulates bone marrow to increase production of red blood cells.
   c. It impairs longitudinal growth.
   d. It stimulates osteocytes to create new bone.

7. A fetus's first skeleton is composed primarily of:
   a. epithelial tissue.
   b. osseous tissue.
   c. cartilage.
   d. fibrous connective tissue.

Answers: Chapter 6

1. *Correct answer:* **c.** Bone is highly resistant to stretching forces (tensile strength) and squeezing forces (compressional strength). It lacks the ability to endure twisting (torsional strength).

2. *Correct answer:* **a.** The endosteum is the membrane lining the inside of the medullary cavity. The diaphysis is the shaft-like portion of the long bone. The periosteum is the fibrous membrane covering the diaphysis.

3. *Correct answer:* **c.** The periosteum has no role in helping prevent fractures; it does not produce bone marrow; it does not secrete immunoglobulin.

4. *Correct answer:* **b.** Yellow bone marrow is mostly fat and does not produce blood cells. The medullary cavity contains bone marrow, but it does not produce blood cells.

5. *Correct answer:* **b.** Compact bone is found in the shafts of long bones and surrounding all other bones. There is no such thing as membranous or endochondral bone.

6. *Correct answer:* **d.** Physical stress stimulates the creation of new bone, not the destruction of bone. Physical stress has no effect on the production of red blood cells or on longitudinal growth.

7. *Correct answer:* **c.** Epithelial tissue is not involved in the formation of bone. Osseous tissue is bone tissue. Parts of the skull start out as fibrous connective tissue; however, most bones evolve from cartilage.

8. *Correct answer:* **a.** Lacunae are the tiny gaps between rings of lamellae that contain osteocytes. Canaliculi are microscopic passageways connecting the lamellae to each other. An osteocyte is a bone cell (not a structural unit).

9. *Correct answer:* **d.** Bone growth and maintenance are affected by a number of factors, including heredity, nutrition, hormones (including the sex hormones estrogen and testosterone), and exercise. However, epinephrine does not affect bone growth or maintenance.

10. *Correct answer:* **b.** A greenstick fracture is an incomplete fracture. A comminuted fracture is one in which the bone is broken into pieces. A spiral fracture is one in which the fracture line spirals around the bone.

8. What is the name of the basic structural unit of bone?
   a. Osteon
   b. Lacunae
   c. Canaliculi
   d. Osteocyte

9. Which of the following does not affect bone growth and maintenance?
   a. Exercise
   b. Sex hormones
   c. Nutrition
   d. Epinephrine

10. What is the name of a fracture in which the bone pierces the skin?
   a. Greenstick
   b. Compound
   c. Comminuted
   d. Spiral

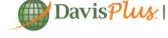

Go to **http://davisplus.fadavis.com** Keyword: Thompson to see all of the resources available with this chapter.

CHAPTER OUTLINE

LEARNING OUTCOMES

1. State the number of bones in an adult's body.

2. Define the common terms related to bone surface markings.

3. Differentiate between the axial and appendicular skeletons.

4. Name the bones of the skull and identify their locations.

5. Describe how an infant's skull differs from the skull of an adult.

6. Name the bones of the face and identify their locations and functions.

7. Discuss the name, location, and function of each of the paranasal sinuses.

8. Discuss the characteristics of the vertebral column, including its structure, function, and the names of its five sections.

9. Identify the characteristics of a typical vertebra.

10. Describe the special features of the atlas and the axis.

11. Describe the structure of the thoracic cage, including the regions of the sternum and how the ribs attach to the vertebral column.

12. Identify and describe the features of the bones of the pectoral girdle.

13. Identify and describe the features of the bones of the upper limb.

14. Name the bones of the hand and identify their features and locations.

15. Name the bones of the pelvic girdle and identify their locations.

16. Explain the difference between the true pelvis, false pelvis, and pelvic outlet.

17. Identify and describe the features of the bones of the lower limb.

18. Name the bones of the foot and ankle and describe their features and locations.

19. Describe the arches of the feet and state their purpose.

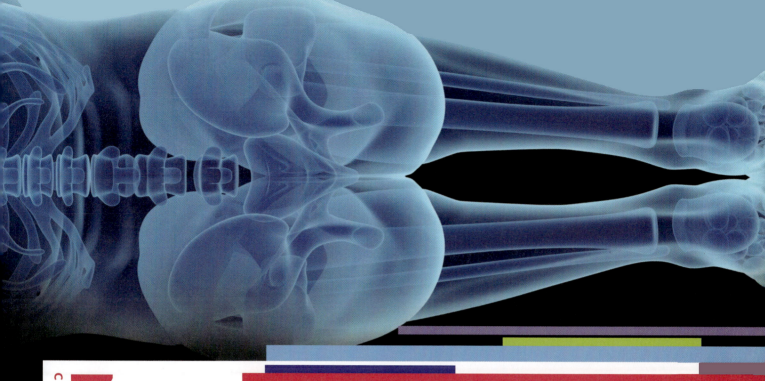

chapter 7

SKELETAL SYSTEM

Newborn babies have 300 or more bones in their bodies. Some of these eventually fuse, leaving the adult with 206 bones.

The skeletal system provides the body's framework as well as its foundation. First of all, the interaction between bones and muscles drives a multitude of movements. Also, many muscles, arteries, veins, and nerves derive their names from nearby bones. Finally, bones provide ready landmarks as clinicians navigate their way around the human body. For all of these reasons, learning the names of the body's major bones is a key part of understanding human anatomy and physiology.

Overview of the Skeletal System

While most adults have 206 bones, there is some variation. Some may have an extra rib, while others have extra bones in the skull. Occasionally, some bones fail to fuse during development, also adding to the total. Of these bones, 80 comprise the upright, central supporting axis of the body, which includes the skull, rib cage, and vertebral column. This is the **axial skeleton**. The other 126 bones make up the bones of the limbs and the pelvic and shoulder area. This is the **appendicular skeleton**.

FAST FACT

The skeleton makes up almost one-fifth of a healthy adult's body weight.

Bone Surface Markings

The surface of bone is not completely smooth. Rather, bones have a number of surface markings, such as flat or rounded areas that allow for joint formation (called **articulations**), projections that allow for muscle attachment, and depressions or passages that provide routes for blood vessels and nerves.

Surface Features of Bones

Articulations	Description
Condyle	Rounded knob; usually fits into a fossa on another bone to form a joint
Facet	A flat surface
Head	The prominent, expanded end of a bone
Projections	
Crest	A moderately raised ridge
Epicondyle	A bump superior to a condyle
Process	A projection or raised area
Spine	A sharp, pointed process
Trochanter	A large process; found only on the femur
Tubercle	A small, rounded process
Tuberosity	A rough, raised bump, usually for muscle attachment
Depressions	
Fossa	A furrow or depression
Fovea	A small pit
Sulcus	Groove or elongated depression
Passages	
Canal	A tunnel through a bone
Fissure	A long slit for blood vessels and nerves
Foramen	A round opening, usually a passageway for vessels and nerves
Meatus	A tube-like opening
Sinus	Cavity within a bone

That Makes Sense

To differentiate between the axial and appendicular skeletons, remember that the axial skeleton relates to the body's axis. *An axis is a straight line around which a body—such as the earth or the human body—revolves. The appendicular skeleton relates to the* appendages *of the body, such as the arms and legs.*

FAST FACT

Each foot consists of 26 bones: that means that $1/4$ of all the body's bones are in the feet.

The Adult Skeleton

The appendicular skeleton is colored turquoise; the other bones are the axial skeleton.

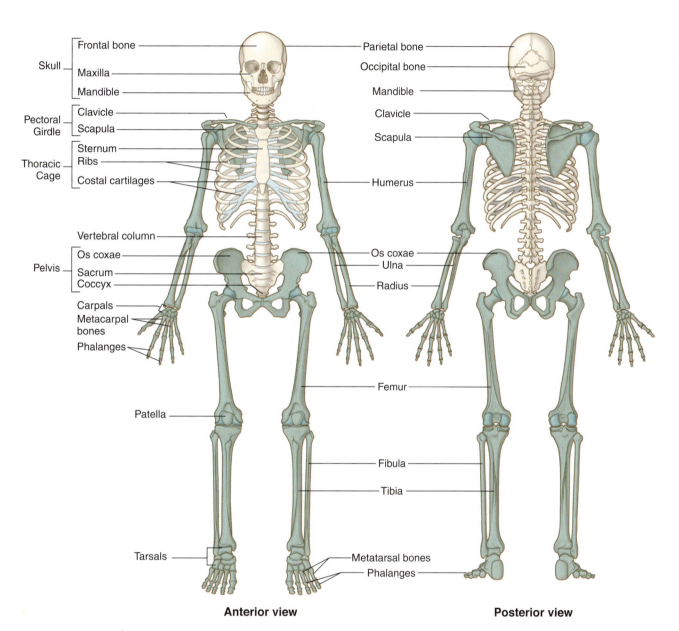

Anterior view   **Posterior view**

Bones of the Skeletal System

The axial skeleton consists of 80 bones, while the appendicular skeleton consists of 126 bones.

Part of the Body	Bones
Axial Skeleton	
Skull (22 bones)	
• Cranium (8 bones)	Frontal (1)
	Parietal (2)
	Temporal (2)
	Occipital (1)
	Sphenoid (1)
	Ethmoid (1)
• Face (14 bones)	Nasal (2)
	Maxillary (2)
	Zygomatic (2)
	Mandible (1)
	Lacrimal (2)
	Palatine (2)
	Inferior nasal conchae (2)
	Vomer (1)
Ear (6 bones)	
	Malleus (2)
	Incus (2)
	Stapes (2)
Hyoid bone (1 bone)	
Vertebral column (26 bones)	
	Cervical vertebrae (7)
	Thoracic vertebrae (12)
	Lumbar vertebrae (5)
	Sacrum (1)
	Coccyx (1)
Thoracic cage (25 bones)	
	Sternum (1)
	Ribs (24)
Appendicular Skeleton	
Pectoral girdle (4 bones)	
	Scapula (2)
	Clavicle (2)
Upper limbs (60 bones)	
	Humerus (2)
	Radius (2)
	Ulna (2)
	Carpals (16)
	Metacarpals (10)
	Phalanges (28)
Pelvic girdle (2 bones)	
	Coxal (2)
Lower limbs (60 bones)	
	Femur (2)
	Patella (2)
	Tibia (2)
	Fibula (2)
	Tarsals (14)
	Metatarsals (10)
	Phalanges (28)

Life lesson: Examining skeletal remains

Detectives know that a great deal of information can be gained by examining a deceased person's bones. Specifically, the scientists who examine skeletal remains are called forensic anthropologists. Some of the information they can obtain include the person's:

- Age (determined by the length of the bones, the extent of fusion of the epiphyseal plates, the status of the teeth, and bone density)
- Gender (through examination of the pubis bone—which has a different shape in women as compared to men—as well as the size of the skull, which is larger in men)
- Stature (through measurement of the femur)

Further examination may reveal the individual's nutritional status, the presence of certain illnesses or diseases, and race. Finally, by isolating the DNA found in bone marrow, the person's identity can be determined.

The Skull

A complex structure, the skull is formed by 22 irregularly shaped bones. These include eight cranial bones and 14 facial bones.

Cranium

The **cranium** is the bony structure housing the brain. It consists of eight **cranial bones:**

Parietal bones (2 bones): Join together at the top of the head to form the top and sides of the cranial cavity

Frontal bone (1 bone): Forms the forehead and the roof of the eye sockets (orbits)

Occipital bone (1 bone): Forms the rear of the skull

Temporal bones (2 bones): Form the sides of the cranium and part of the cranial floor; also contain the structures of the inner and middle ear, including the:
- **External auditory meatus** (an opening into the ear)
- **Mastoid process** (a prominent lump behind the ear)
- **Zygomatic arch** (cheekbone)
- **Styloid process** (an attachment point for several neck muscles)

Sphenoid bone (1 bone): Forms a key part of the cranial floor as well as the floor and side walls of the orbits

Ethmoid bone (1 bone): Contributes to the walls of the orbits, the roof and walls of the nasal cavity, and the nasal septum

The Body AT WORK

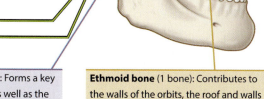

Posterior view

*Viewed posteriorly, the sphenoid bone looks like a giant moth. It lies behind and slightly above the nose and throat. On top of the sphenoid bone is an indented area called the **sella turcica**, which houses the pituitary gland.*

The Body AT WORK

*Just anterior to the sphenoid bone is the **ethmoid bone**. The top of this delicate bone, called the **cribriform plate**, forms part of the roof of the nasal cavity. Tiny perforations in the cribriform plate allow branches of the olfactory nerve to reach the brain. A projection on the cribriform plate provides an attachment for the meninges, the membrane that encloses the brain.*

A sharp, upward blow can drive bone fragments through the cribriform plate and into the brain. If this happens, cerebrospinal fluid will leak out of the nose; it also opens a pathway for infection into the brain. Traumatic injury to this bone can also shear off the olfactory nerves, resulting in a loss of sense of smell.

Suture Lines

The bones of the skull join together at immovable joints called **sutures.**

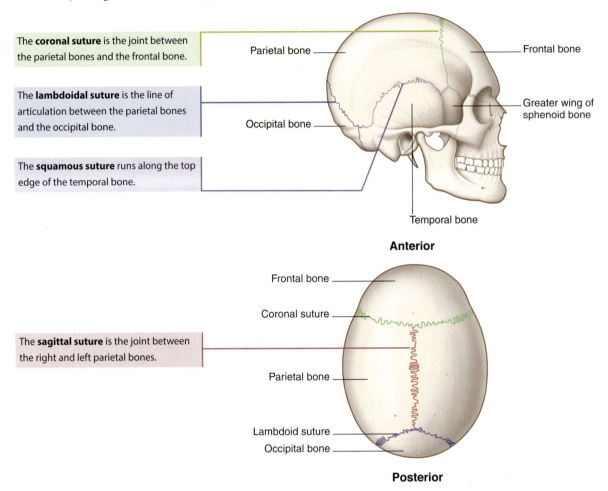

The **coronal suture** is the joint between the parietal bones and the frontal bone.

The **lambdoidal suture** is the line of articulation between the parietal bones and the occipital bone.

The **squamous suture** runs along the top edge of the temporal bone.

Parietal bone — — Frontal bone

Occipital bone — — Greater wing of sphenoid bone

Temporal bone

Anterior

Frontal bone

Coronal suture

The **sagittal suture** is the joint between the right and left parietal bones.

Parietal bone

Lambdoid suture
Occipital bone

Posterior

Foramen Magnum

The skull contains a number of holes called **foramina** that allow for passage of nerves and blood vessels.

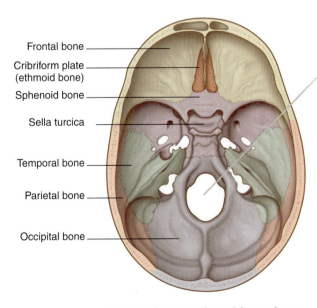

Frontal bone
Cribriform plate (ethmoid bone)
Sphenoid bone
Sella turcica
Temporal bone
Parietal bone
Occipital bone

Cranial floor as viewed from above

A large opening in the base of the skull, called the **foramen magnum**, allows the spinal cord to pass through as it connects to the brainstem.

Life lesson: Brain swelling

Just like any other tissue, when the brain is injured, it swells. However, because the skull can't expand to accommodate the swelling brain, pressure inside the cranium rises as the brain pushes against the sides of the skull. If the swelling becomes severe, the increased pressure will force the brainstem down, through the foramen magnum. The restricted opening of the foramen magnum will constrict the brainstem, resulting in respiratory arrest and, usually, death.

Facial Bones

The 14 bones of the face perform several functions. They support the teeth, provide an attachment point for the muscles used in chewing and for facial expression, form part of the nasal and orbital cavities, and also give each face its unique characteristics.

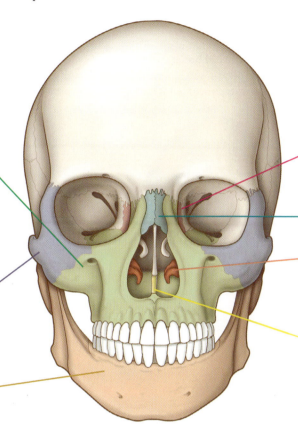

Maxillae (2 bones): These bones meet to form the upper jaw. The maxillae (singular: maxilla) form the foundation of the face; every other facial bone (except for the mandible) articulates with the maxillae. The maxillae form part of the floor of the orbits, part of the roof of the mouth, and part of the floor and walls of the nose.

Zygomatic bones (2 bones): These bones shape the cheeks and form the outer edge of the orbit.

Mandible (1 bone): This is the largest and strongest bone of the face. It articulates with the temporal bone at the **temporomandibular joint (TMJ),** making it the only facial bone that can move.

Lacrimal bones (2 bones): These paper-thin bones form part of the side wall of the orbit.

Nasal bones (2 bones): These rectangular bones form the bridge of the nose; the rest of the nose is shaped by cartilage.

Inferior nasal conchae (2 bones): The conchae bones (singular: concha) contribute to the nasal cavity.

Vomer (1 bone): This small bone forms the inferior half of the nasal septum. (The superior half is formed by the perpendicular plate of the ethmoid bone.)

Palatine bones (2 bones): These bones form the posterior portion of the hard palate, part of the wall of the nasal cavity, and part of the floor of the orbit.

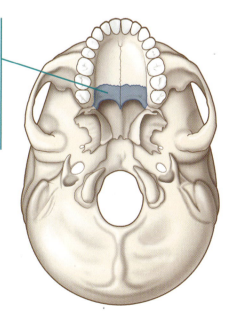

Base of skull as viewed from below

PART II Covering, Support, and Movement of the Body

Bones Associated with the Skull

Several other bones are associated with the skull but not considered a part of the skull. These include the three bones of the middle ear. Called **auditory ossicles**, these bones are named the **malleus** (hammer), **incus** (anvil), and **stapes** (stirrup). (The auditory ossicles are discussed in Chapter 11, *Senses*.)

Hyoid Bone

Another bone associated with the skull is the **hyoid bone**: a U-shaped bone that sits between the chin and the larynx. The hyoid bone—which is the only bone that doesn't articulate with any other bone—serves as an attachment point for muscles that control the tongue, mandible, and larynx.

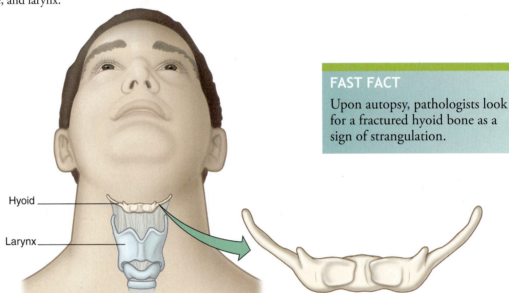

Hyoid

Larynx

FAST FACT

Upon autopsy, pathologists look for a fractured hyoid bone as a sign of strangulation.

Sinuses

The skull contains several cavities, which include the **paranasal sinuses**. The four pairs of sinuses—which are named for the bones in which they reside—open into the internal nose. Filled with air, they lighten the skull and act as resonators for sound production.

The frontal, maxillary, and ethmoid sinuses have well-defined shapes. The sphenoid sinuses are more like sinus cells, having a honeycombed shape.

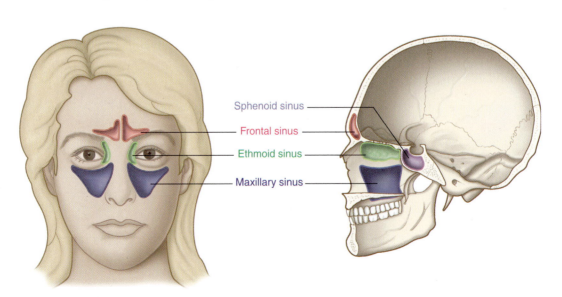

Sphenoid sinus

Frontal sinus

Ethmoid sinus

Maxillary sinus

The Infant Skull

An infant's skull varies from that of an adult in two key ways:

1. **The suture lines in the skull have not yet fused**. Because the suture lines haven't fused, the bones of the skull can shift and overlap, molding the head so the infant can pass through the birth canal. (Consequently, right after birth, a newborn's skull may appear deformed, although it soon assumes a normal shape.) The un-fused suture lines also allow for the rapid brain growth that occurs during infancy.

2. **The infant's skull contains fontanels**. The areas between the un-fused bones, which are covered by fibrous membranes, are called fontanels. Soft to the touch, it's possible to palpate pulsations in these areas. Over time, the fontanels shrink and usually close completely by age two years.

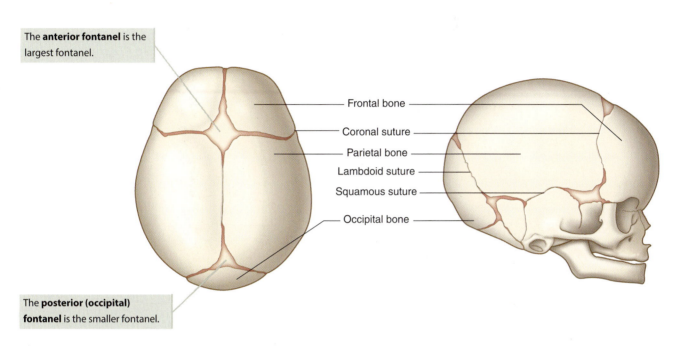

The **anterior fontanel** is the largest fontanel.

Frontal bone
Coronal suture
Parietal bone
Lambdoid suture
Squamous suture
Occipital bone

The **posterior (occipital) fontanel** is the smaller fontanel.

The Body AT WORK

Assessment of the head of a newborn can provide valuable information. For example, suture lines that are abnormally wide suggest hydrocephalus, a condition in which excessive amounts of cerebrospinal fluid accumulate in the brain, causing the cranium to expand. A bulging anterior fontanel signals increased intracranial pressure, such as may occur following a head injury or infection. A sunken fontanel suggests dehydration.

FAST FACT

An infant's skull attains half its adult size by age nine months; it reaches its final size by age eight or nine years. Consequently, the head of an infant or child is larger in proportion to the rest of his body than an adult's head.

The Vertebral Column

The vertebral column—a flexible structure consisting of 33 vertebrae—holds the head and torso upright, serves as an attachment point for the legs, and encases the spinal cord. Its unique structure allows the body to bend forward, backward, and sideways.

After about age three, the vertebral column assumes a slight S shape. This shape centers the head over the body and makes walking possible. (In contrast, newborn infants have a C-shaped spine, mimicking a curled-up fetal position. The normal curves develop as the infant begins to lift his head and, later, as he begins to walk.)

Five Sections of the Vertebral Column

Normal Curvatures of the Spine

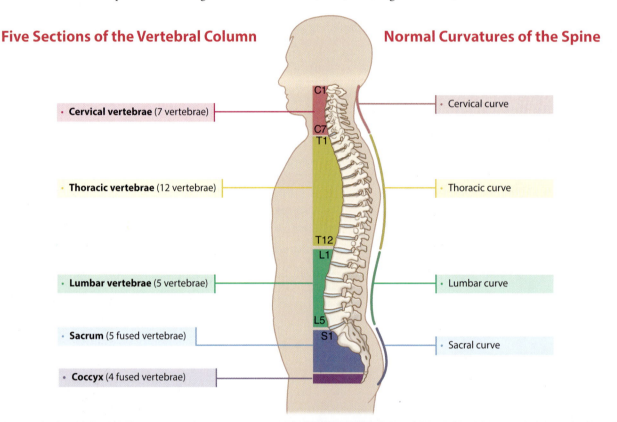

- **Cervical vertebrae** (7 vertebrae)

C1
C7
T1

- **Thoracic vertebrae** (12 vertebrae)

T12
L1

- **Lumbar vertebrae** (5 vertebrae)

L5
S1

- **Sacrum** (5 fused vertebrae)

- **Coccyx** (4 fused vertebrae)

- Cervical curve

- Thoracic curve

- Lumbar curve

- Sacral curve

Life lesson: Abnormal spinal curvatures

Degenerative bone disease, poor posture, and even pregnancy can cause abnormal curvatures in the spine.

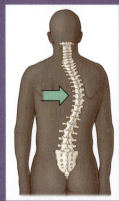

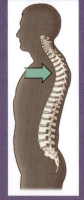

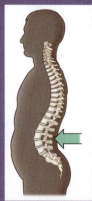

Scoliosis is a lateral curvature of the spine, most often in the thoracic region. It usually occurs in adolescent girls, sometimes the result of the vertebrae failing to develop correctly on one side.

Kyphosis, or "hunchback," is an exaggerated thoracic curvature. While it may result from poor posture, it's also a common finding in individuals with osteoporosis.

Lordosis, or "swayback," is an exaggerated lumbar curvature. It may result from osteoporosis, poor posture, or abdominal weight gain.

Vertebrae Characteristics

Depending upon their location in the vertebral column, the structural characteristics of vertebrae differ slightly from each other. However, all vertebrae have a number of characteristics in common, as illustrated here.

Posterior

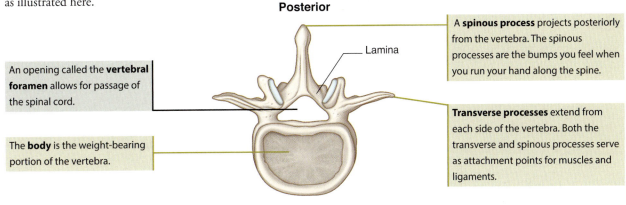

Lamina

A **spinous process** projects posteriorly from the vertebra. The spinous processes are the bumps you feel when you run your hand along the spine.

An opening called the **vertebral foramen** allows for passage of the spinal cord.

Transverse processes extend from each side of the vertebra. Both the transverse and spinous processes serve as attachment points for muscles and ligaments.

The **body** is the weight-bearing portion of the vertebra.

Anterior

Intervertebral Disc

In between each vertebra is an **intervertebral disc**. Designed to support weight and absorb shock, the intervertebral disc consists of two parts:

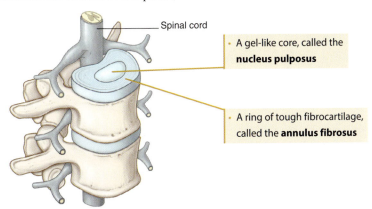

Spinal cord

• A gel-like core, called the **nucleus pulposus**

• A ring of tough fibrocartilage, called the **annulus fibrosus**

Life lesson: Herniated disc

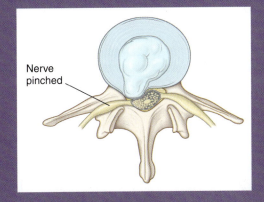

Nerve pinched

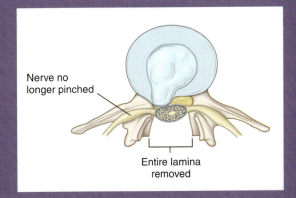

Nerve no longer pinched

Entire lamina removed

Sudden, intense pressure on the intervertebral discs—such as may occur from lifting a heavy object using the back rather than the legs—can cause the annulus of the disc to crack. The nucleus pulposus can then ooze out from the center of the disc and press on the spinal cord or a spinal nerve, causing pain. This is called a **herniated disc**. (Common terms for this condition included *slipped disc* and *ruptured disc*.)

To repair this condition, a procedure called a *laminectomy* may be performed. In this procedure, both laminae and the spinal processes are removed, which relieves pressure on the spinal nerve.

Specialty Vertebrae

The cervical, thoracic, and lumbar vertebrae all differ slightly from each other. However, the most unique of all the vertebrae are the first two cervical vertebrae (C1 and C2), known as the **atlas** and the **axis**, respectively.

Atlas

Named for the Greek god Atlas who carried the world on his shoulders, the role of the first cervical vertebra is to support the skull.

The atlas has no body. Rather, it consists of a delicate ring and a large vertebral foramen.

Depressions on each side of the vertebra articulate with bony projections from the occipital bone of the skull. When the head moves back and forth (such as when nodding "yes"), the projections rock back and forth in these depressions.

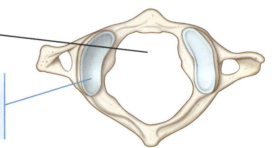

Axis

The C2 vertebra, called the axis, has a projection called the **dens,** or **odontoid process.** The dens projects into the atlas and allows the head to swivel from side to side (such as when saying "no.")

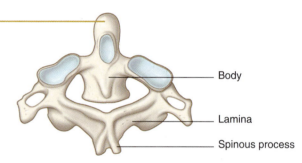

Body

Lamina

Spinous process

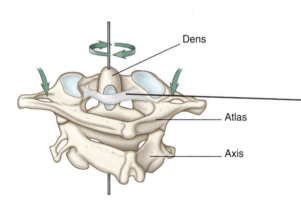

Dens

Atlas

Axis

The **transverse ligament** holds the dens in place. Thus secured, the head can swivel from side to side. In addition, as bony projections from the occipital bone rock back and forth on the depressions of the atlas, the head can move back and forth.

FAST FACT

A hard blow to the top of the head can drive the dens through the foramen magnum and into the brainstem, resulting in sudden death.

The Body AT WORK

While the spinal joints do not offer a wide range of movement, they do allow for significant flexibility. The spine can arch backward, curve forward, and even twist. The structure of the vertebrae allows the spine to bend forward further than it can bend backward. Many different muscles, as well as strong ligaments, stabilize the vertebral column while still allowing flexibility and movement.

The Thoracic Cage

The thoracic cage consists of the thoracic vertebrae, the sternum, and the ribs. These bones form a cone-shaped cage that surrounds and protects the heart and lungs and provides an attachment point for the pectoral girdle (shoulder) and upper limbs. Expansion and contraction of the thoracic cage causes the pressure changes in the lungs that allow breathing to occur.

Sternum

The sternum has three regions.

- **Manubrium**: This is the broadest portion; the **suprasternal notch** (at the top of the manubrium between the two clavicles) is easily palpated.

- **Body**: This is the longest portion; it joins the manubrium at the sternal angle (also called the angle of Louis), which is also the location of the second rib.

- **Xiphoid process**: An important landmark for cardiopulmonary resuscitation (CPR), the xiphoid process provides an attachment point for some abdominal muscles.

Ribs

Twelve pairs of ribs attach to the vertebral column.

Ribs 1 to 7, called **true ribs**, attach to the sternum by a strip of hyaline cartilage called **costal cartilage**.

Ribs 8, 9, and 10 attach to the cartilage of rib 7; these ribs, as well as ribs 11 and 12, are called **false ribs**.

Ribs 11 and 12, called **floating ribs**, do not attach to any part of the anterior thoracic cage.

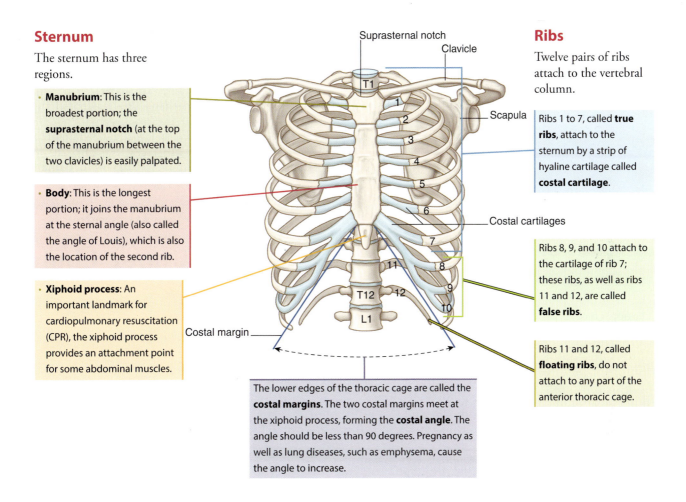

Suprasternal notch
Clavicle
Scapula
Costal cartilages
Costal margin

The lower edges of the thoracic cage are called the **costal margins**. The two costal margins meet at the xiphoid process, forming the **costal angle**. The angle should be less than 90 degrees. Pregnancy as well as lung diseases, such as emphysema, cause the angle to increase.

FAST FACT

Besides protecting the thoracic organs, the ribs also protect the spleen, the liver, and a portion of the kidneys.

Pectoral Girdle

Also called the **shoulder girdle**, the **pectoral girdle** supports the arm. The two pectoral girdles—one on each side of the body—consist of a **clavicle** (collarbone) and a **scapula** (shoulder blade).

A slightly S-shaped bone, the **clavicle** articulates with the sternum and the scapula and helps support the shoulder.

Located on the posterior portion of the thorax, the **scapula** lies over ribs 2 to 7. The lateral portion of this triangle-shaped bone has three main features.

- The **acromion process**: This extension of the scapula articulates with the clavicle; it is the only point where the arm and the scapula attach to the rest of the skeleton.
- The **coracoid process**: This finger-like process provides a point of attachment for some of the muscles of the arm.
- The **glenoid cavity**: This shallow socket articulates with the head of the humerus (upper arm bone).

FAST FACT

The clavicle is the most commonly broken bone in the body.

Upper Limb

The upper limb, or arm, consists of the humerus (upper arm bone), the radius and the ulna (the bones of the lower arm), and the carpals (the bones of the hand).

The **humerus** is the long bone of the upper arm. It contains these features:

- **Head**: The enlarged end of this long bone is covered with articular cartilage; it articulates with the glenoid cavity of the scapula.
- **Olecranon fossa**: This is a depression on the posterior side of the humerus.
- **Olecranon process:** This is the bony point of the elbow; it slides in the olecranon fossa when the arm is extended. (See the pull-out image of the posterior side of the elbow.)

One of the two bones of the lower arm, the **radius**, is located on the same side as the thumb.

- The **proximal head** of the radius is a distinctive disc that rotates on the humerus when the palm is turned forward and back.
- The **radial tuberosity** is where the biceps muscle attaches to the bone.

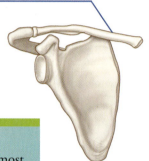

Posterior view of elbow

The **ulna** is the other bone of the lower arm; it is longer than the radius.

The **styloid processes of the radius and ulna** are the bony bumps that can be felt at the wrist.

FAST FACT

When the palm of the hand is facing up (supination), the radius and ulna lie parallel to each other. When the palm is turned down (pronation), the radius and ulna cross.

Anterior view of right arm

Hand

The **hand** consists of the wrist, palm, and fingers.

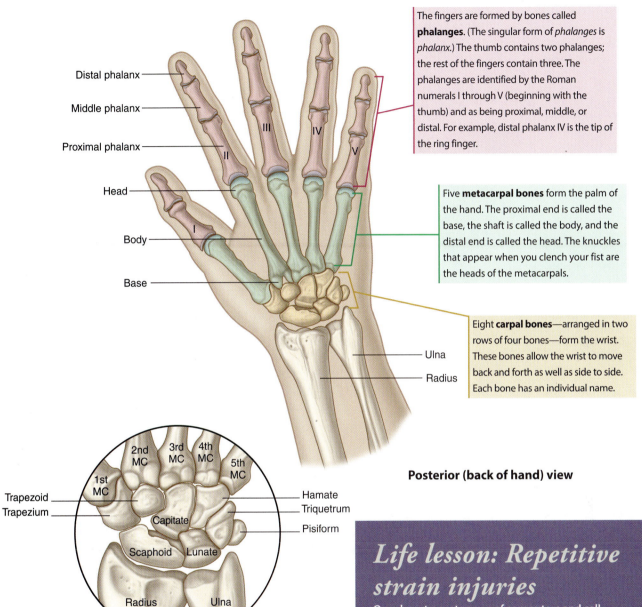

The fingers are formed by bones called **phalanges**. (The singular form of *phalanges* is *phalanx*.) The thumb contains two phalanges; the rest of the fingers contain three. The phalanges are identified by the Roman numerals I through V (beginning with the thumb) and as being proximal, middle, or distal. For example, distal phalanx IV is the tip of the ring finger.

Five **metacarpal bones** form the palm of the hand. The proximal end is called the base, the shaft is called the body, and the distal end is called the head. The knuckles that appear when you clench your fist are the heads of the metacarpals.

Eight **carpal bones**—arranged in two rows of four bones—form the wrist. These bones allow the wrist to move back and forth as well as side to side. Each bone has an individual name.

Posterior (back of hand) view

The carpal bones of the wrist articulate with the five metacarpal (MC) bones. Moving from left to right in two rows, the bones are scaphoid, lunate, triquetrum, pisiform, trapezium, trapezoid, capitate, and hamate. (To help you remember, use the mnemonic "Stop Letting Those People Touch the Cadaver's Hand.")

Life lesson: Repetitive strain injuries

Our almost nonstop use of computers and cell phones is taking a toll on the hands and wrists of millions of people. The resultant injuries are known as *repetitive strain injuries*. When someone performs the same motion over and over—even typing on a keyboard—without rest, the muscles in the wrists become fatigued and, eventually, the joint becomes inflamed. The resulting pain can be debilitating.

Doctors have dubbed an inflammation of the tendons of the wrist as "Guitar Hero syndrome," because it has been occurring in those who have spent many hours strumming to the video game. Another high-tech injury is "BlackBerry thumb": a painful inflammation in the thumb as a result of frequent texting.

Pelvic Girdle

Each of the two large bones of the hip is called an **os coxae**; it may also be called a **coxal bone** or **innominate bone**. Together they form what's known as the **pelvic girdle**: the foundation of the pelvis. The os coxae is not a single bone; rather, it consists of three bones fused together, as shown here.

Ilium: A large, flaring section you can feel under the skin

Ischium: The lower posterior portion

Pubis: The most anterior portion that joins with the other pubis at the symphysis pubis, a disc of cartilage that separates the two pubic bones.

Sacrum

Symphysis pubis

Posteriorly, each os coxae articulates with the sacrum at the **sacroiliac joint**.

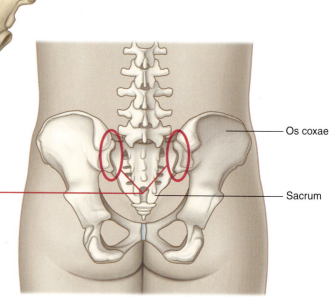

Os coxae

Sacrum

The os coxae contains a number of features that serve as landmarks. Some of these are best viewed laterally, as shown here:

Iliac crest: The upper, outer edge of the ilium

Greater sciatic notch: Point through which the sciatic nerve passes on its path to the back of the thigh

Acetabulum: A depression that houses the head of the femur to form the "hip socket"

Ischial spine: Projection into the pelvic cavity

Lesser sciatic notch

Ischial tuberosity: Supports your body when you're sitting

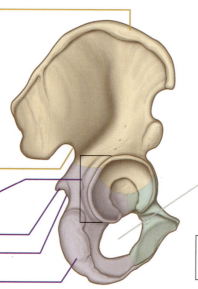

Lateral view of right os coxae

Obturator foramen: Large hole below the acetabulum that's closed by a ligament

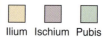

Ilium   Ischium   Pubis

FAST FACT

Because the marrow contained in the ilium produces blood cells, it is a common site for bone marrow biopsies.

Pelvis

The combination of the os coxae and the sacrum is known as the **pelvis**. The pelvis supports the trunk, provides an attachment point for the legs, and also protects the organs of the pelvis (including the lower colon, reproductive organs, and urinary bladder). The pelvis is divided into a **true (lesser) pelvis** and a **false (greater) pelvis**.

The **true pelvis** extends between what's known as the **pelvic brim**.

The **pelvic outlet** is the lower edge of the true pelvis. The diameter of the pelvic outlet is measured as the distance between the two ischial bones. The pelvic outlet is the passageway through which an infant enters the world; therefore, the distance between the two ischial bones must be wide enough to allow his head to pass.

The **false pelvis** extends between the outer, flaring edges of the iliac bones.

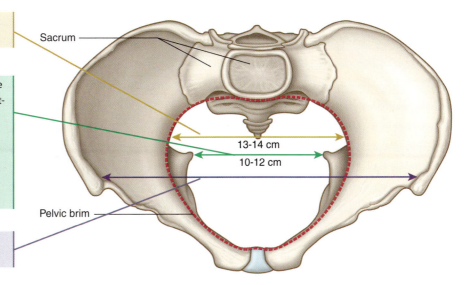

Sacrum

13-14 cm

10-12 cm

Pelvic brim

Pelvis as viewed from above

The Body AT WORK

The male and female pelvises have a number of differences, mainly because the female pelvis is adapted for pregnancy and childbirth.

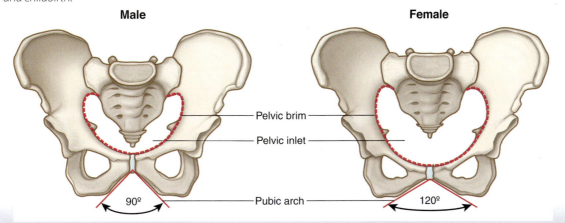

Male   Female

Pelvic brim

Pelvic inlet

90°   Pubic arch   120°

In general, the true pelvis is wide and shallow in females and narrow and deep in males. Also, females have a larger pelvic outlet and wider pubic arch than males do. The female symphysis pubis softens before delivery, which allows the pelvic outlet to expand as the newborn's head passes through the birth canal.

Lower Limb

The bones of the lower limb—which consist of the femur (thigh bone), patella (kneecap), tibia and fibula (bones of the lower leg), and foot—join with the pelvis to give the body a stable base. More importantly, the bones of the lower limb are articulated in such a way as to allow the body to move.

Femur

The longest and strongest bone in the body, the femur articulates with the acetabulum of the pelvis to form a ball-and-socket joint.

The **head** of the femur fits into the rounded contour of the acetabulum.

The **neck** of the femur is a frequent site for fractures in elderly persons.

Greater trochanter

Lesser trochanter

These two bony projections provide attachment points for hip muscles.

Shaft

Medial epicondyle

Lateral epicondyle

The **medial** and **lateral epicondyle** are the widest points of the femur at the knee.

Patella

Commonly known as the kneecap, the **patella** is a triangular sesamoid bone embedded in the tendon of the knee. At birth, the patella is composed of cartilage. It ossifies between the ages of three and six years.

Fibula

The long and slender **fibula** resides alongside the tibia and helps stabilize the ankle. It does not bear any weight.

- The head of the fibula articulates with the tibia.

- The distal end of the fibula forms the **lateral malleolus** of the ankle.

Tibia

Of the two bones in the lower leg, the **tibia** is the only one that bears weight. Commonly called the shinbone, the tibia articulates with the femur.

- The **tibial tuberosity** (which can be palpated just below the patella) serves as the attachment point for thigh muscles.

- The bony knob you can palpate on your inner ankle is the **medial malleolus**.

Foot and Ankle

The bones of the foot and ankle are arranged similarly to those of the hand. However, because the foot and ankle bear the weight of the body, the size of the bones, as well as how they're arranged, differs.

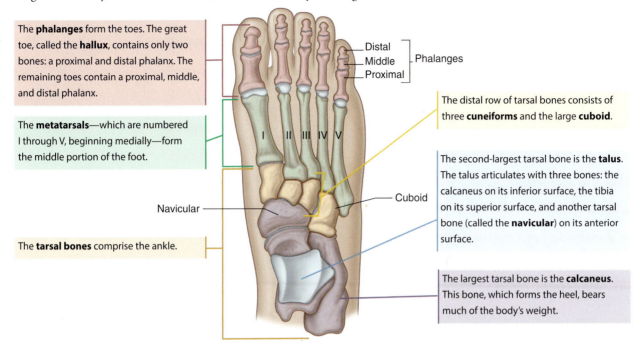

The **phalanges** form the toes. The great toe, called the **hallux**, contains only two bones: a proximal and distal phalanx. The remaining toes contain a proximal, middle, and distal phalanx.

The **metatarsals**—which are numbered I through V, beginning medially—form the middle portion of the foot.

The **tarsal bones** comprise the ankle.

Distal
Middle
Proximal
} Phalanges

The distal row of tarsal bones consists of three **cuneiforms** and the large **cuboid**.

The second-largest tarsal bone is the **talus**. The talus articulates with three bones: the calcaneus on its inferior surface, the tibia on its superior surface, and another tarsal bone (called the **navicular**) on its anterior surface.

Navicular

Cuboid

The largest tarsal bone is the **calcaneus**. This bone, which forms the heel, bears much of the body's weight.

Arches of the Foot

Strong ligaments hold the foot bones together in a way that forms arches in the foot. Just as arches add supporting strength to a building, foot arches give the foot more strength to support the weight of the body.

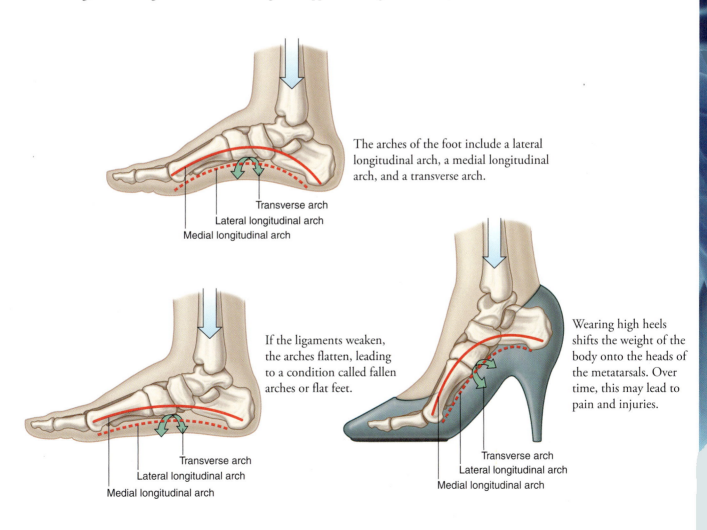

The arches of the foot include a lateral longitudinal arch, a medial longitudinal arch, and a transverse arch.

Transverse arch
Lateral longitudinal arch
Medial longitudinal arch

If the ligaments weaken, the arches flatten, leading to a condition called fallen arches or flat feet.

Transverse arch
Lateral longitudinal arch
Medial longitudinal arch

Wearing high heels shifts the weight of the body onto the heads of the metatarsals. Over time, this may lead to pain and injuries.

Transverse arch
Lateral longitudinal arch
Medial longitudinal arch

Review of Key Terms

Appendicular skeleton: Bones making up the limbs, pelvis, and shoulder areas

Articulation: The site of close approximation of two or more bones

Axial skeleton: The skeleton that forms the central supporting axis of the body

Carpal bones: Small bones of the wrist

Condyle: Rounded knob; usually fits into a fossa on another bone to form a joint

Crest: A moderately raised ridge

Epicondyle: A bump superior to a condyle

Facet: A flat surface

False pelvis: Portion of the pelvis that extends between the edges of the iliac bones

Fontanel: Un-fused area of an infant's skull

Fossa: A furrow or depression

Foramen: A round opening in a bone, usually a passageway for vessels and nerves

Head: The prominent, expanded end of a bone

Kyphosis: An exaggerated thoracic curvature

Meatus: A tube-like opening

Process: A projection or raised area

Scoliosis: A lateral curvature of the spine

Sinus: Cavity in the skull filled with air

Sulcus: Groove or elongated depression

Sutures: Immovable joints of the skull

Trochanter: A large process; found only on the femur

True pelvis: Portion of the pelvis that extends between the pelvic brim

Tubercle: A small, rounded process

Tuberosity: A rough, raised bump, usually for muscle attachment

Own the Information

To make the information in this chapter part of your working memory, take some time to reflect on what you've learned. On a separate sheet of paper, write down everything you recall from the chapter. After you're done, log on to the Davis*Plus* website, and check out the Study Group podcast and Study Group Questions for the chapter.

Key Topics for Chapter 7:
- Bone surface markings
- Bones of the axial and appendicular skeleton
- Bones of the skull and face
- Sinuses
- The vertebral column
- Characteristics of vertebrae
- The thoracic cage
- Bones of the upper limb and hand
- Bones of the pelvic girdle
- Bones of the lower limb and foot

Test Your Knowledge

1. Which bone is a facial bone?
   a. Sphenoid
   b. Ethmoid
   c. Mastoid
   d. Vomer

2. Which bones form the upper jaw?
   a. Maxillae
   b. Mandible
   c. Zygomatic bones
   d. Lacrimal bones

3. The bumps you feel when you run your hand along the spine in the back are:
   a. transverse processes.
   b. spinous processes.
   c. intervertebral discs.
   d. vertebral foramen.

4. Why are ribs 8 through 12 called false ribs?
   a. These ribs are made of cartilage instead of bone.
   b. These ribs do not attach to the thoracic vertebrae.
   c. These ribs do not attach to the anterior thoracic cage.
   d. These ribs attach to the manubrium.

5. What are the bony processes that can be felt at the wrist?
   a. The styloid processes of the radius and ulna
   b. The radial tuberosity
   c. The carpal bones
   d. The acromion process

6. Which part of the os coxae supports your body weight when sitting?
   a. Obturator foramen
   b. Ischial tuberosity
   c. Sacroiliac joint
   d. Acetabulum

7. Which bone does not support any body weight?
   a. Tibia
   b. Fibula
   c. Medial malleolus
   d. Lateral malleolus

8. The bone that forms the heel is the:
   a. talus.
   b. calcaneus.
   c. metatarsal.
   d. navicular.

9. To form the hip joint, the head of the femur rests in the:
   a. ilium.
   b. ischium.
   c. obturator foramen.
   d. acetabulum.

10. The pituitary gland rests in an indented area in which cranial bone?
   a. Frontal
   b. Sphenoid
   c. Ethmoid
   d. Temporal

Answers: Chapter 7

1. *Correct answer:* **d.** All of the other bones are cranial bones.

2. *Correct answer:* **a.** The mandible is the lower jaw. The zygomatic bones shape the cheeks. The lacrimal bones form part of the side wall of the orbit.

3. *Correct answer:* **b.** Transverse processes extend from each side of the vertebra. Intervertebral discs sit in between each vertebra. Vertebral foramen are openings that allow for passage of the spinal cord. None of these structures can be palpated.

4. *Correct answer:* **c.** All of the ribs attach to the vertebral column. Ribs 1 through 7 (the true ribs) attach to the sternum. Ribs 8 through 12 are called false ribs; ribs 8, 9, and 10 attach to the cartilage of rib 7 while ribs 11 and 12 (called floating ribs) do not attach to any part of the anterior thoracic cage.

5. *Correct answer:* **a.** The radial tuberosity is where the biceps muscle attaches to the bone. The carpal bones are the small bones of the wrist. The acromion process is an extension of the scapula that articulates with the clavicle.

6. *Correct answer:* **b.** The obturator foramen is a large hole below the acetabulum. The sacroiliac joint is the joint where the os coxae articulates with the sacrum. The acetabulum is a depression that houses the head of the femur.

7. *Correct answer:* **b.** The fibula articulates with the tibia but does not support any weight. The tibia is the primary bone of the lower leg that supports weight. The medial and lateral malleolus are projections from the tibia and fibula, respectively, that form the bony knob of the ankle.

8. *Correct answer:* **b.** The talus and navicular bones are both tarsal bones, but the calcaneus is the largest tarsal bone and it is the one that forms the heel. The metatarsals are bones that make up the middle portion of the foot.

9. *Correct answer:* **d.** The ilium is the large, flaring portion of the os coxae. The ischium forms the lower posterior portion of the os coxae. The obturator foramen is a hole below the acetabulum.

10. *Correct answer:* **b.** The frontal bone forms the forehead and roof of the eye sockets. The ethmoid bone lies anterior to the sphenoid bone and forms part of the roof of the nasal cavity. The temporal bones form the sides of the cranium and part of the cranial floor.

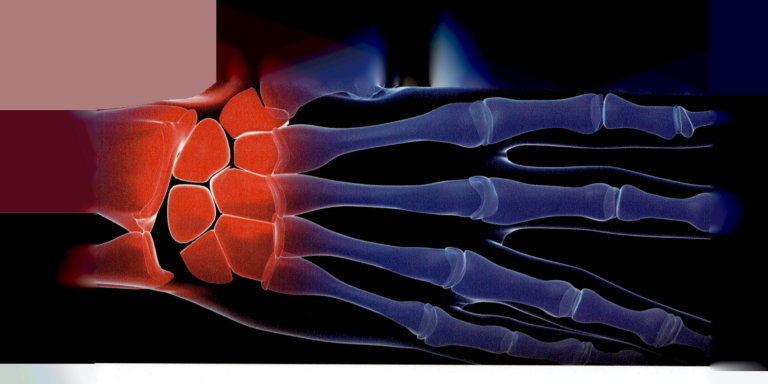

CHAPTER OUTLINE

Classifications of Joints

LEARNING OUTCOMES

1. Explain what joints are and the functions they serve.

2. Identify and describe the four classifications for joints.

3. Describe the structures found in all synovial joints.

4. Name and describe the five types of synovial joints.

5. Name and describe the range of movements of synovial joints.

6. Identify the major anatomical features of the shoulder, elbow, knee, and hip.

JOINTS

*The body contains over 300 joints. In fact, the only bone **without** a joint is the hyoid bone in the neck.*

Joints—also called **articulations**—are points where bones meet. Some joints are completely immovable; others allow only limited movement. Most joints, however, permit considerable movement. Through the interaction of multiple interconnecting parts, these incredible structures allow the body to walk, run, dance, throw a ball, and even type on a computer.

Classifications of Joints

Joints may be classified according to how movable they are: fixed, semi-movable, or freely movable. They may also be classified according to the material that binds them together. For example, fixed joints are bound by fibers and are called fibrous joints; semi-movable joints are joined by cartilage and are called cartilaginous joints; freely movable joints contain a fluid-filled joint capsule and are called synovial joints.

> **FAST FACT**
>
> The branch of science that studies joint structure, function, and dysfunction is called **arthrology**.

Fibrous Joints

Fibrous joints—also called **synarthroses**—result when collagen fibers from one bone penetrate the adjacent bone, anchoring the bones in place.

The adult skull's suture joints are fibrous joints: once growth is complete, the bones of the skull knit together securely, offering protection to the brain.

Cartilaginous Joints

In **cartilaginous joints**, two bones are joined by cartilage. These joints—called **amphiarthroses**—are slightly movable.

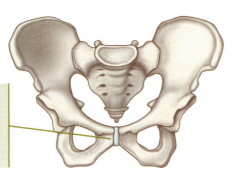

The two pubic portions of the os coxae are joined by a pad of cartilage called a **symphysis**, thus forming the joint known as the symphysis pubis.

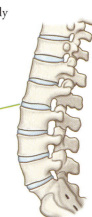

Fibrocartilaginous pads (called intervertebral discs) reside between each vertebrae, making the vertebrae of the spine cartilaginous joints. These pads of cartilage absorb shock and allow for limited movement.

Synovial Joints

Synovial joints—also called **diarthroses**—are freely movable. They're also the most numerous and versatile of all the body's joints. Every synovial joint contains the following structures:

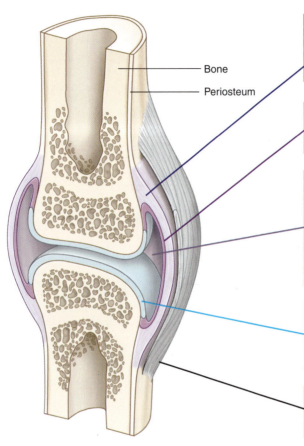

Bone

Periosteum

Joint capsule: Extending from the periosteum of each of the articulating bones is a sheet of connective tissue that encloses the joint cavity.

Synovial membrane: This moist, slippery membrane lines the inside of the joint capsule, where it secretes synovial fluid.

Joint cavity: This small space between the bones allows for freedom of movement. It also contains **synovial fluid**, a slippery, viscous fluid that has the consistency of an egg white. Synovial fluid lubricates the joint, nourishes the cartilage, and contains phagocytes to remove debris.

Articular cartilage: A thin layer of hyaline cartilage covers the bone surfaces. In combination with synovial fluid, the articular cartilage permits friction-free movement.

Ligaments: Tough cords of connective tissue help bind the bones more firmly together.

Bursae in Synovial Joints

Some joints—such as the knee, shoulder, and elbow—contain small sacs filled with synovial fluid called **bursa** (plural: **bursae**). Residing in areas where muscles and tendons pass over bony prominences, the bursae facilitate movement and ease friction.

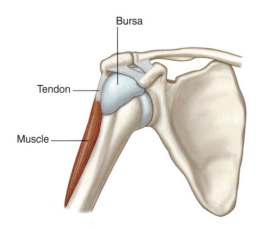

Bursa

Tendon

Muscle

The Body AT WORK

*Joints are typically named for the bones involved. For example, the **humeroscapular joint** is the articulation of the humerus and the scapula. The **temporomandibular joint** is the articulation between the mandible and the temporal bone in the skull. The **sacroiliac joint** is the point where the sacrum and the ilium meet.*

Types of Synovial Joints

Not all synovial joints are configured the same. In fact, the body contains six types of synovial joints, with each joint type offering a specific movement.

Ball-and-Socket Joint

The ball-shaped head of one bone fits into a cup-like socket of another bone to form this joint to offer the widest range of motion of all joints. The shoulder and hip joints are both ball-and-socket joints.

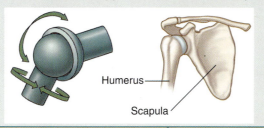

Humerus

Scapula

Pivot Joint

In this joint, a projection from one bone articulates with a ring-shaped socket of another bone, allowing the bones to rotate, or pivot. For example, the dens of the second cervical vertebra turns within a ring-shaped portion of the first vertebra, allowing the head to rotate. Another example is the radioulnar joint, in which the head of the radius rotates within a groove of the ulna.

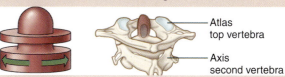

Atlas
top vertebra

Axis
second vertebra

Hinge Joint

Just like the hinge on a door, these joints allow only back-and-forth movements (flexion and extension). To form a hinge joint, the convex surface of one bone (such as the humerus) fits into a concave depression on another bone (such as the ulna). Besides the elbow, other examples of hinge joints include the knee and the interphalangeal joints of the fingers and toes.

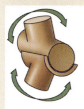

Humerus
Radius
Ulna

Saddle Joint

The surfaces of both bones in this joint are shaped like the surface of a saddle: concave in one direction (like the front to rear curvature of a horse's saddle) and convex in the other (like the right to left curvature of a saddle). When perched on top of each other, this shape allows the bones to move back and forth and from side to side, although the side-to-side motion is limited. Found only in the thumbs, this joint's unique shape allows the thumb to move over to touch the tips of the fingers, which gives us the ability to grasp small objects.

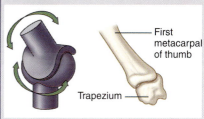

First
metacarpal
of thumb

Trapezium

Condyloid Joint

Here, an oval convex surface on one bone fits into a similarly shaped depression on another. Examples include the articulation of the distal end of the radius with the carpal bones of the wrist as well as the joints at the base of the fingers. Condyloid joints allow flexion and extension as well as side-to-side movement.

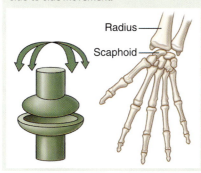

Radius

Scaphoid

Gliding Joint

In this joint, the two bone surfaces—which are relatively flat—slide over each other. Surrounding ligaments limit the amount of movement, making these the least mobile of all the synovial joints. Examples of these joints include the tarsal bones of the ankle, the carpal bones of the wrist, and the articular processes of the vertebrae.

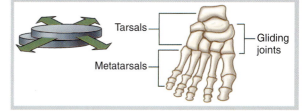

Tarsals

Gliding
joints

Metatarsals

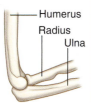

Movements of Synovial Joints

The movements a joint can make depend upon the shape of the joint (as previously discussed) as well as the involvement of nearby muscles, tendons, and ligaments. The terms used to describe the movements are shown here.

Flexion and Extension
ANIMATION 🌐

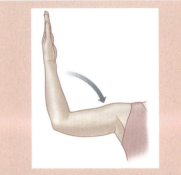

Flexion involves bending a joint so as to decrease the angle of the joint.

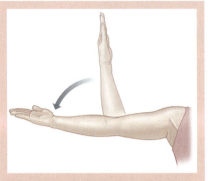

Extension involves straightening a joint, increasing the angle between the bones.

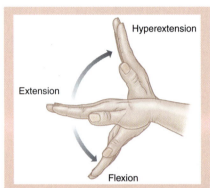

Hyperextension

Extension

Flexion

Hyperextension is the extreme extension of a joint beyond its normally straight position.

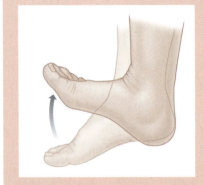

Dorsiflexion involves moving the toes or foot upward.

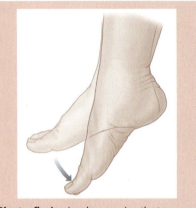

Plantar flexion involves moving the toes or foot downward (toward the plantar surface).

Abduction and Adduction
ANIMATION 🌐

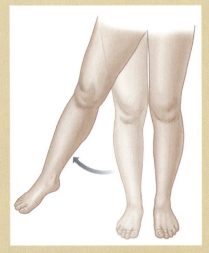

Abduction is the movement of a body part *away* from the midline of the body.

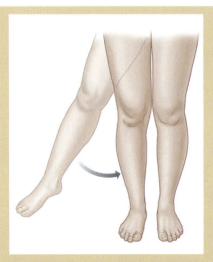

Adduction is the movement of a body part *toward* the midline of the body.

Circumduction
ANIMATION 🌐

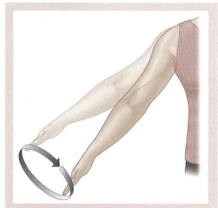

In circumduction, the distal end of an appendage, such as the arm or leg, moves in a circle.

Rotation

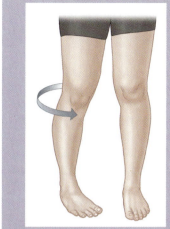 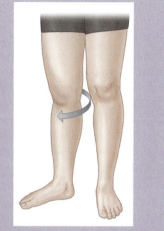

Internal rotation occurs when a bone spins *toward* the body's midline. (For example, the femur undergoes internal rotation when you turn your foot toward the body's midline.)

External rotation occurs when a bone spins *away* from the body's midline. (For example, the femur undergoes external rotation when your turn foot away from the midline of the body.)

Supination and Pronation

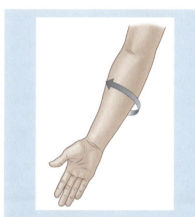

Supination is a movement that turns the palm *upward*.

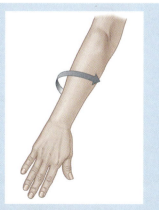

Pronation is a movement that turns the palm *downward*.

Inversion and Eversion
ANIMATION 🌐

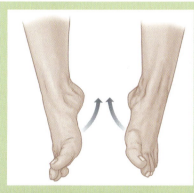

Inversion is a foot movement that turns the sole medially, toward the other foot.

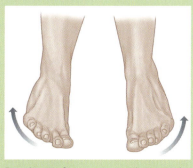

Eversion is a foot movement that turns the sole laterally, away from the other foot.

Protraction and Retraction

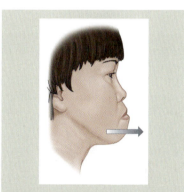

Protraction moves a part forward.

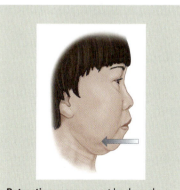

Retraction moves a part backward.

Key Synovial Joints

The joints that most often require medical attention include the shoulder, elbow, knee, and hip.

Shoulder

The shoulder is called the **humeroscapular joint** (denoting the articulation of the humerus with the scapula) or the **glenohumeral joint** (denoting the articulation of the head of the humerus with the glenoid cavity of the scapula). The ball-and-socket joint of the shoulder has the greatest range of motion of any joint in the body.

Because the shoulder is more mobile than it is stable, it is supported by a number of muscles, tendons, ligaments, and bursae. Specifically, the joint is supported by five principal ligaments and four bursae. In addition, the tendons of several surrounding muscles form the rotator cuff, which helps hold the head of the humerus in the shallow glenoid cavity.

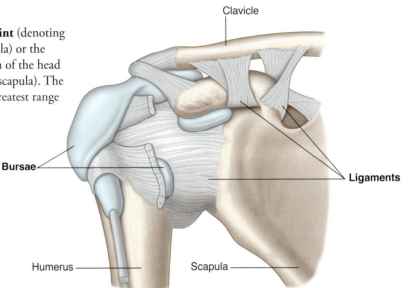

Anterior view

Life lesson: Shoulder dislocation

Of all the joints in the body, the shoulder is the one most likely to suffer a dislocation. When it does dislocate, it usually does so inferiorly, a result of a downward-driving force. That's because the rotator cuff protects the joint in every area *except* inferiorly; the top of the joint also has additional protection from the clavicle and coracoid and acromion processes. Most dislocations occur when an outstretched arm receives a blow from above.

Children are especially prone to shoulder dislocations because their shoulders aren't fully ossified. Their injuries usually result from being jerked off the ground by one arm or from a forceful tug on the arm.

Elbow

The elbow is a hinge joint consisting of two articulations: one between the humerus and the ulna (the **humeroulnar joint**) and the second between the humerus and the head of the radius (the **humeroradial joint**). A single joint capsule encases both articulations. Ligaments on either side help stabilize the joint.

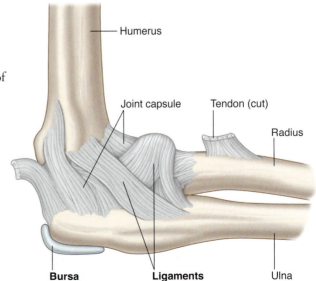

Knee

The knee, or **tibiofemoral joint**, is the largest joint in the body: it's also the most complex. Besides the structures shown here, the knee also contains 13 bursae, which serve as pads around the knee joint.

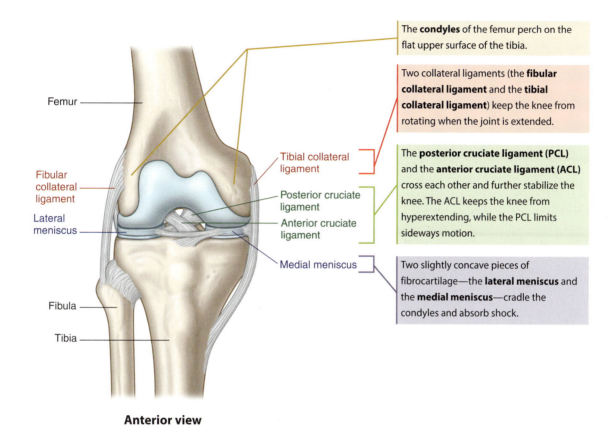

The **condyles** of the femur perch on the flat upper surface of the tibia.

Two collateral ligaments (the **fibular collateral ligament** and the **tibial collateral ligament**) keep the knee from rotating when the joint is extended.

The **posterior cruciate ligament (PCL)** and the **anterior cruciate ligament (ACL)** cross each other and further stabilize the knee. The ACL keeps the knee from hyperextending, while the PCL limits sideways motion.

Two slightly concave pieces of fibrocartilage—the **lateral meniscus** and the **medial meniscus**—cradle the condyles and absorb shock.

Femur

Fibular collateral ligament

Lateral meniscus

Fibula

Tibia

Tibial collateral ligament

Posterior cruciate ligament

Anterior cruciate ligament

Medial meniscus

Anterior view

Life lesson: Knee injuries

Because the knee has few surrounding muscles, it's injured more often than the hip. It's particularly susceptible to blows or sudden stops or turns, making knee injuries one of the most common athletic injuries. In particular, the meniscus and the anterior cruciate ligament (ACL) are most frequently injured. Because cartilage has no blood supply, and ligaments have a minimal blood supply, these types of injuries heal slowly, or not at all. Consequently, surgical repair is often necessary, usually by *arthroscopy*. In this procedure, the joint is viewed and repaired through the use of a pencil-thin, tube-like instrument called an *arthroscope*.

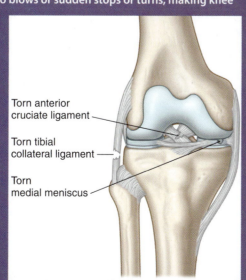

Torn anterior cruciate ligament

Torn tibial collateral ligament

Torn medial meniscus

Life lesson: Joint replacement

Arthroplasty is a surgical procedure that replaces a diseased joint with an artificial device, or *prosthesis*. Joint replacements are most commonly performed on the hip and the knee, although they can also be done on fingers, the elbow, and the shoulder. In fact, more than 1 million Americans have a hip or knee replacement each year. The procedure is most often done to replace joints that have been damaged by osteoarthritis. (See *Life lesson: Arthritis* on the next page.)

In a joint replacement, the heads of long bones are replaced with a prosthesis made of a metal alloy, while the joint socket is made of high-density polyethylene. In the past, prostheses were cemented in place. Newer prostheses, however, allow bone to grow into the artificial material, thus increasing stability.

Hip

The hip is a ball-and-socket joint, just like the shoulder. However, the hip is more stable than the shoulder, mainly due to the fact that the hip socket—the depression into which the head of the femur sits—is much deeper than the socket of the shoulder joint.

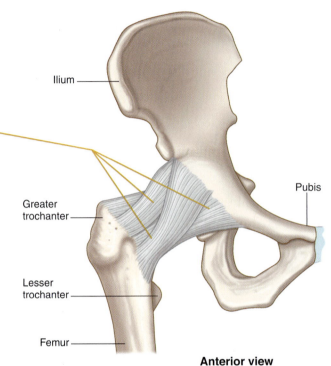

Several ligaments help hold the femur in place. When you stand, the ligaments twist, pulling the head of the femur into the acetabulum.

Ilium

Pubis

Greater trochanter

Lesser trochanter

Femur

Anterior view

Life lesson: Arthritis

Arthritis refers to inflammation of a joint. While there are over 100 types of arthritis and related conditions, the most common form is *osteoarthritis*. Referred to as "wear-and-tear" arthritis, the disorder is a common effect of aging. In fact, osteoarthritis affects 85% of people over age 70. With age, articular cartilage softens and degenerates, sometimes to the point that bone is exposed to bone, resulting in pain. Osteoarthritis most often affects the hips, knees, intervertebral joints, and fingers.

In contrast, *rheumatoid arthritis* is an autoimmune disease in which the body's antibodies attack the synovial membranes, leading to degeneration of the articular cartilage and thickening of the synovial membrane. Over time, the disease may destroy the synovial membrane and calcify the joint. This severe form of arthritis causes pain and joint deformity along with systemic symptoms such as fatigue, fever, and anemia. While there is no cure, drug and physical therapy can help control symptoms.

The Body AT WORK

Regular exercise may help protect articular cartilage from "wear and tear." Here's why: Cartilage depends on synovial fluid for oxygen and nutrients. During exercise, joint compression squeezes fluid and metabolic wastes out of the cartilage. Then, when the weight is removed, the cartilage sucks up synovial fluid like a sponge. The periods of compression and relaxation accompanying exercise cause the synovial fluid, along with its supply of oxygen, nutrients, and phagocytes, to cycle through the cartilage. Without exercise, articular cartilage deteriorates more rapidly because of a lack of nutrition, oxygenation, and waste removal.

Warming up before vigorous exercise also helps protect articular cartilage. Once warm, the synovial fluid is less viscous, which allows the cartilage to soak it up more easily. This causes the cartilage to swell, making it a more effective cushion against compression.

Abduction: Movement away from the body

Adduction: Movement toward the body

Arthrology: The branch of science that studies the structure, function, and dysfunction of joints

Articulation: The point at which bones meet to form a joint

Ball-and-socket joint: Joint in which the ball-shaped head of one bone fits into a cup-like socket of another

Bursae: Small sacs filled with synovial fluid that ease friction in areas where muscles and tendons pass over bony prominences

Cartilaginous joints: Semi-movable joints joined by cartilage

Condyloid joint: Joint (such as occurs at the base of the fingers) in which an oval convex surface on one bone fits into a similarly shaped depression on another bone

Eversion: Foot movement that turns sole laterally, away from the other foot

Fibrous joints: Fixed joints bound by collagen fibers

Gliding joint: Joint (such as occurs in the tarsal bones of the ankle) in which two bone surfaces slide over each other

Hinge joint: Joint that allows only back-and-forth movement

Inversion: Foot movement that turns the sole medially

Pivot joint: Joint (such as occurs between the first and second cervical vertebrae) in which a projection from one bone articulates with the ring-shaped socket of another bone, allowing the bones to pivot

Pronation: Movement that turns the palms downward

Saddle joint: Joint (such as occurs in the thumbs) in which the surfaces of both bones are concave in one direction and convex in the other, allowing the bones to move back and forth and from side to side

Supination: Movement that turns the palms upward

Synovial joints: Freely movable joints that contain a fluid-filled joint capsule

Own the Information

To make the information in this chapter part of your working memory, take some time to reflect on what you've learned. On a separate sheet of paper, write down everything you recall from the chapter. After you're done, log on to the Davis*Plus* website, and check out the Study Group podcast and Study Group Questions for the chapter.

Key Topics for Chapter 8:

- Classifications of joints
- Characteristics of fibrous joints
- Characteristics of cartilaginous joints
- Characteristics of synovial joints
- Types of synovial joints
- Movements of synovial joints
- Characteristics of the shoulder, elbow, knee, and hip

Test Your Knowledge

PART II Covering, Support, and Movement of the Body

Answers: Chapter 8

1. *Correct answer:* **a.** Cartilaginous joints are slightly movable while synovial joints are freely movable. A pivot joint is a type of joint that allows rotation.

2. *Correct answer:* **b.** Synovial joints outnumber fibrous and cartilaginous joints. Synarthroses are another name for fibrous joints.

3. *Correct answer:* **d.** The joint capsule is a sheet of connective tissue enclosing the joint cavity, and the synovial membrane secretes synovial fluid. Both contribute to joint function but aren't the key structures that allow friction-free movement. Ligaments help stabilize the joint and do not contribute to friction-free movement.

4. *Correct answer:* **b.** A gliding joint allows a limited sliding movement in the bones of the wrist and ankle; the saddle joint is found in the thumb and permits both a back-and-forth and side-to-side motion; a hinge joint allows back-and-forth movement.

5. *Correct answer:* **d.** A hinge joint allows only back-and-forth movement, a gliding joint allows limited sliding movement, and a condyloid joint allows flexion and extension as well as side-to-side movement. In contrast, a ball-and-socket joint offers a full range of motion.

6. *Correct answer:* **d.** Abduction is movement away from the midline of the body. Pronation is a movement that turns palms downward. Inversion is a foot movement that turns the sole medially, toward the other foot.

7. *Correct answer:* **a.** The hip is more stable than the shoulder because it has a deep socket. Neither the elbow nor the knee is prone to dislocation.

1. The least movable joint is a:
   a. fibrous joint.
   b. cartilaginous joint
   c. pivot joint.
   d. synovial joint.

2. Most of the joints in the body are:
   a. fibrous joints.
   b. synovial joints.
   c. cartilaginous joints.
   d. synarthroses.

3. Along with synovial fluid, this structure permits friction-free movement in synovial joints.
   a. Joint capsule
   b. Ligaments
   c. Synovial membrane
   d. Articular cartilage

4. Which type of joint allows the head to rotate (such as when shaking the head "no")?
   a. Gliding joint
   b. Pivot joint
   c. Saddle joint
   d. Hinge joint

5. The joint offering the widest range of motion is the:
   a. hinge joint.
   b. gliding joint.
   c. condyloid joint.
   d. ball-and-socket joint.

6. An extreme extension of a joint beyond its normally straight position is called:
   a. abduction.
   b. pronation.
   c. inversion.
   d. hyperextension.

7. Which joint is most likely to be dislocated?
   a. Shoulder
   b. Hip
   c. Knee
   d. Elbow

8. *Correct answer:* **c.** Only the knee contains a medial and lateral meniscus.

9. *Correct answer:* **c.** All the other choices pertain to osteoarthritis.

10. *Correct answer:* **b.** Only the shoulder has a rotator cuff.

8. Which joint has a medial and lateral meniscus?
   a. Hip
   b. Elbow
   c. Knee
   d. Shoulder

9. Which statement about rheumatoid arthritis is true?
   a. It is known as "wear-and-tear" arthritis.
   b. It affects 85% of people over age 70.
   c. It is an autoimmune disease.
   d. It often affects the knees, hips, intervertebral joints, and fingers.

10. The rotator cuff is found in which joint?
    a. Knee
    b. Shoulder
    c. Hip
    d. Elbow

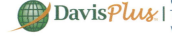 Go to **http://davisplus.fadavis.com** Keyword: Thompson to see all of the resources available with this chapter.

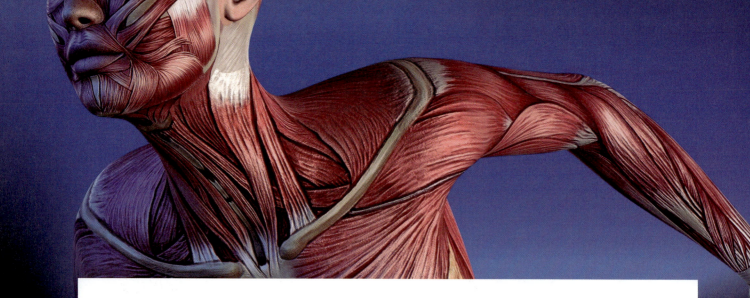

CHAPTER OUTLINE

Types of Muscle

Skeletal Muscle Structure

Muscle Contraction and Relaxation

Muscle Function

Superficial Muscles

How Muscles Are Named

Major Muscles of the Body

LEARNING OUTCOMES

1. Identify three types of muscle and the general characteristics of each.

2. Discuss the structure of skeletal muscle.

3. Explain the two ways skeletal muscle attaches to bone.

4. Describe the components of a muscle fiber.

5. Identify the two proteins found within a muscle fiber and the function of each.

6. Describe the structure of a sarcomere.

7. Discuss the sliding filament model of contraction.

8. Summarize the process of muscle contraction and relaxation.

9. Explain the role of calcium and ATP in muscle contraction.

10. Discuss how the length of muscle fibers affects the strength of a contraction.

11. Summarize how the stimulus of a muscle fiber stimulates contraction.

12. Define *muscle twitch*.

13. Explain the two key ways used by the nervous system to control the strength of a contraction.

14. Explain the difference between isometric and isotonic contractions.

15. Describe how muscles meet their demands for energy at rest and during exercise.

16. Describe how muscles work in groups to create movement.

17. State how muscles are named.

18. Identify the major muscles of the body.

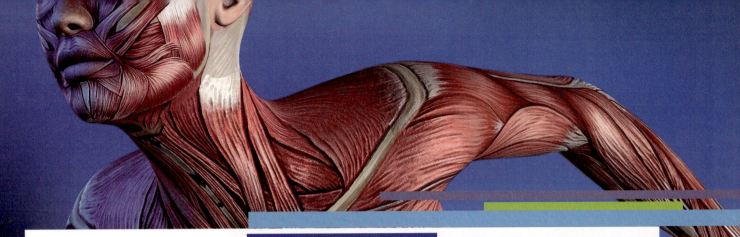

chapter 9

MUSCULAR SYSTEM

The body contains over 600 muscles, which comprise about 40% of an adult's body weight.

Muscles are a unique form of tissue that transform energy into motion. Everything your mind conceives is transmitted to your muscles to perform. The words you speak, the expression on your face, the motion of your fingers as you write or play an instrument are possible only because of muscular movement. Even more, muscles operate behind the scenes to propel blood through blood vessels, drive the flow of air into and out of the lungs, digest food, and produce body heat. Indeed, this sophisticated tissue helps sustain life.

Types of Muscle

The body contains three types of muscle: cardiac muscle, smooth muscle, and skeletal muscle.

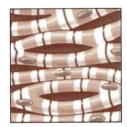

Cardiac Muscle

- Found only in the heart
- Consists of short, branching fibers that fit together at **intercalated discs**
- Appears striped, or **striated**, when viewed under a microscope
- Is a type of **involuntary** muscle because it contracts automatically

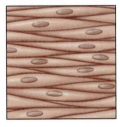

Smooth Muscle

- Found in the digestive tract, blood vessels, bladder, airways, and uterus
- Does not appear striped when viewed under a microscope, so is called **nonstriated**
- Known as involuntary muscle, because it contracts automatically (such as when the digestive tract processes food)

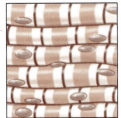

Skeletal Muscle

- Attached to bone and causes movement of the body
- Known as **voluntary** muscle because it can be contracted at will
- Appears markedly striated when examined with a microscope

The remainder of this chapter will focus on skeletal muscle.

Skeletal Muscle Structure

Skeletal muscle consists of bundles of tiny fibers that run the length of the muscle. Most fibers are about $1\,^{1}/_{5}$ inches (3 cm) long and 1/500 inch (0.05 mm) wide.

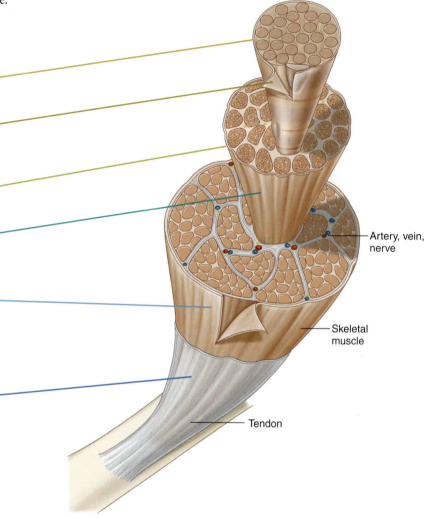

A skeletal muscle cell is called a **muscle fiber**.

A delicate connective tissue called **endomysium** covers each muscle fiber.

Muscle fibers are grouped in bundles called **fascicles**.

A sheath of tougher connective tissue called the **perimysium** encases the fascicles.

Still another layer of connective tissue, called the **epimysium**, surrounds the muscle as a whole and binds all the muscle fibers together.

Connective tissue called **fascia** surrounds the muscle outside the epimysium. **Deep fascia** lies between muscles, while **superficial fascia** (hypodermis) resides just under the skin.

Artery, vein, nerve

Skeletal muscle

Tendon

FAST FACT

Tendons and aponeuroses are so strong that they rarely break, even by forces strong enough to break a bone or tear a muscle. They can, however, be pulled away from a bone.

The Body AT WORK

Skeletal muscle may attach to a bone in one of two ways: direct attachment or indirect attachment.

- *In **direct attachment**, muscle fibers merge with the periosteum of the bone, forming a strong attachment.*
- *In **indirect attachment**, the epimysium extends past the muscle as a **tendon** (a strong, fibrous cord). The tendon then merges with the periosteum.*

*Occasionally, instead of attaching to bone, a muscle attaches to another muscle. In these instances, the epimysium extends past the muscle as a flat, broad tendon called an **aponeurosis**. The aponeurosis then fuses with the covering of the other muscle. Occasionally, aponeuroses also attach to bone.*

Structure of Muscle Fibers

Because of their long, thread-like appearance, muscle cells are called muscle fibers. Unlike other cells, muscle fibers have multiple nuclei pressed against the side of the plasma membrane. Furthermore, even though muscle fibers are extremely thin, they contain a complex interior—just like other human cells.

The plasma membrane surrounding each fiber is called a **sarcolemma**, while the cytoplasm of the cell is called **sarcoplasm**.

Long protein bundles called **myofibrils** fill the sarcoplasm. Myofibrils store glycogen (which is used for energy) as well as oxygen.

Sarcoplasmic reticulum (SR)—the smooth endoplasmic reticulum of a muscle fiber—surrounds each myofibril. This is where calcium ions are stored.

Myofibrils consist of even finer fibers, called **myofilaments**. There are two types of myofilaments: thick and thin. Thick myofilaments are made of a protein called **myosin**, while thin myofilaments consist of a protein called **actin**. The arrangement of actin and myosin gives skeletal muscle its striated appearance.

A system of tubules, called **transverse (T) tubules**, extend across the sarcoplasm. Formed from inward projections of the sarcolemma, the T tubules allow electrical impulses to travel deep into the cell.

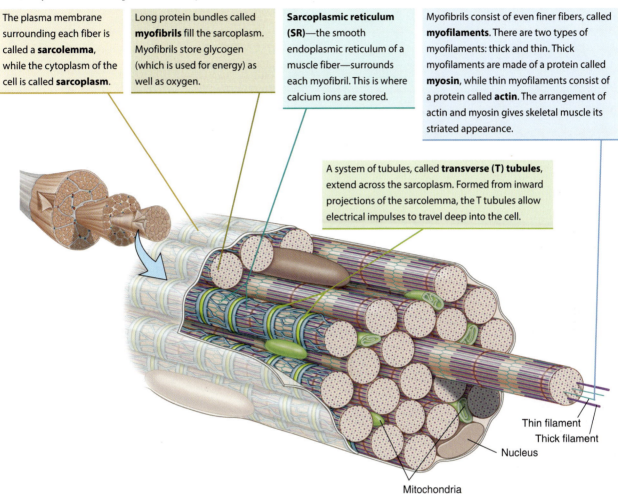

Thin filament
Thick filament
Nucleus
Mitochondria

Thick Filaments

Each thick myofilament consists of hundreds of myosin molecules stacked together, with the myosin heads facing outward.

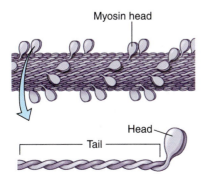

Myosin head

Head
Tail

The myosin molecule, which makes up thick myofilaments, is shaped like a golf club with a globular head and shaft-like tail.

Thin Filaments

Consisting of two chains of the contractile protein **actin**, thin myofilaments look like a string of beads. Entwined with the actin are two other proteins: **tropomyosin** and **troponin**.

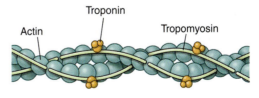

Troponin
Actin
Tropomyosin

Structure of Myofibril

The thin and thick myofilaments stack together, one alternating with the other, to form myofibrils. They do not completely overlap. Instead, they're arranged in a type of latticework to form units called **sarcomeres.**

ANIMATION

A plate or disc called a **Z-disc**, or **Z-line**, serves as an anchor point for thin myofilaments.

The section between the Z-discs is called a **sarcomere**. This is where muscle contraction occurs.

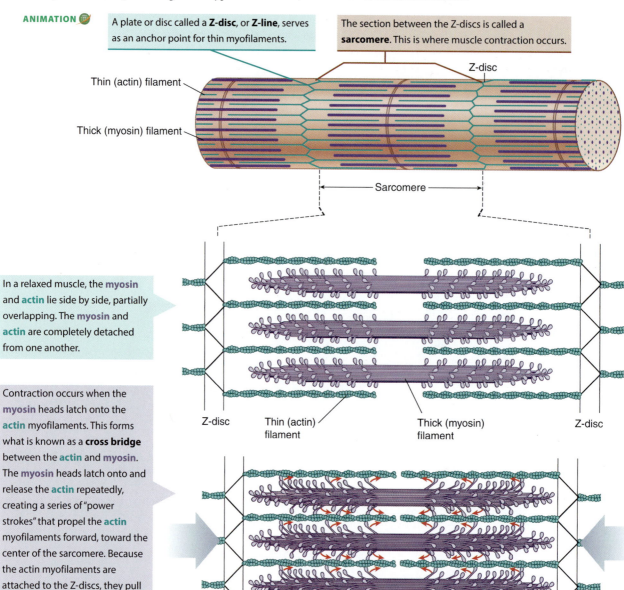

Thin (actin) filament

Thick (myosin) filament

Z-disc

Sarcomere

In a relaxed muscle, the **myosin** and **actin** lie side by side, partially overlapping. The **myosin** and **actin** are completely detached from one another.

Z-disc

Thin (actin) filament

Thick (myosin) filament

Z-disc

Contraction occurs when the **myosin** heads latch onto the **actin** myofilaments. This forms what is known as a **cross bridge** between the **actin** and **myosin**. The **myosin** heads latch onto and release the **actin** repeatedly, creating a series of "power strokes" that propel the **actin** myofilaments forward, toward the center of the sarcomere. Because the actin myofilaments are attached to the Z-discs, they pull the Z-discs closer together, shortening the sarcomere. As the sarcomere shortens, so does the myofibril and the entire muscle. This is known as the **sliding-filament model** of contraction.

FAST FACT

Keep in mind that the myofilaments don't shorten; they stay the same length. The sarcomere shortens because the filaments slide over the top of one another.

The Body AT WORK

Muscle contraction requires energy in the form of adenosine triphosphate (ATP). In fact, ATP allows the myosin heads to release their grip on the actin filament. The myosin then splits the ATP, giving it fuel to form a new cross bridge. This cycle of gripping and releasing causes a series of "power strokes" that moves the actin smoothly forward.

Besides ATP, contraction requires calcium. That's because, when calcium is absent, tropomyosin and troponin—the two protein molecules entwined with the actin filament—block the sites where the myosin heads would attach. With the sites blocked, a cross bridge can't form, and contraction can't occur. When calcium is present, it binds with the troponin to expose the myosin attachment points, allowing contraction to occur.

Muscle Contraction and Relaxation

To contract, a skeletal muscle must be stimulated by a nerve, specifically a **motor neuron**. The cell bodies of motor neurons reside in the brainstem and spinal cord. Extensions from the cell bodies, called **axons**, carry impulses to skeletal muscles. Each axon branches numerous times, with each branch stimulating a different muscle fiber.

The connection between a motor neuron and a muscle fiber is called a **neuromuscular junction**. Between the end of the motor nerve and the muscle fiber is a narrow space called the **synaptic cleft**.

How Muscle Fibers Contract

1. When an impulse reaches the end of a motor neuron, it causes small vesicles to fuse with the cell membrane and release a **neurotransmitter** (a chemical messenger) called **acetylcholine (ACh)** into the synaptic cleft.
2. The ACh quickly diffuses across the synaptic cleft, where it stimulates receptors in the sarcolemma (the membrane surrounding the muscle fiber).
3. In turn, this sends an electrical impulse over the sarcolemma and inward along the T tubules. The impulse in the T tubules causes the sacs in the sarcoplasmic reticulum to release calcium.
4. The calcium binds with the troponin on the actin filament to expose attachment points. In response, the myosin heads of the thick filaments grab onto the thin filaments, and muscle contraction occurs.

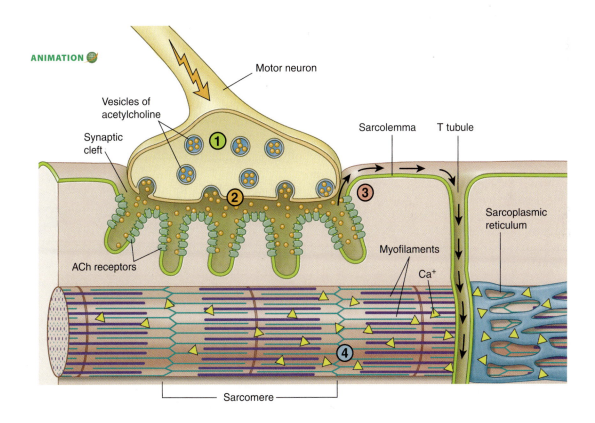

ANIMATION

Motor neuron

Vesicles of acetylcholine

Synaptic cleft

Sarcolemma   T tubule

Sarcoplasmic reticulum

ACh receptors

Myofilaments

Ca^+

Sarcomere

How Muscle Fibers Relax

When nerve impulses stop arriving at the neuromuscular junction, ACh is no longer released. The enzyme **acetylcholinesterase** breaks down any remaining ACh while calcium ions are pumped back into the sarcoplasmic reticulum. With the calcium removed, troponin and tropomyosin again prevent the myosin heads from grasping the thin filament, and the muscle fiber relaxes.

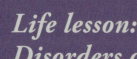

Life lesson:
Disorders of the neuromuscular junction

Interference with any of the steps necessary for skeletal muscle contraction will result in muscle weakness or paralysis. A number of toxins and diseases target the neuromuscular junction. Following are just a few:

- *Botulism:* This is a form of food poisoning usually acquired from eating improperly canned foods. The bacteria *Clostridium botulinum* blocks release of ACh, inhibiting nerve transmission so muscles can't contract. Death results from paralysis of respiratory muscles.

- *Myasthenia gravis:* In this disease, the body produces antibodies against receptors for ACh. As a result, not all ACh can find a receptor. Nerve transmission is poor, and profound muscular weakness results.

- *Tetanus ("lockjaw"):* This disease results from the bacterium *Clostridium tetani,* which causes motor neurons to fire excessively. This leads to overstimulation of muscles, resulting in severe muscle spasms and sustained contractions. Jaw muscles are typically affected first, hence the name lockjaw.

- *Curare:* Once used to poison arrows, curare is now used in anesthesia to relax skeletal muscles. Curare binds to ACh receptor sites, stopping nerve transmission and causing paralysis. Because the diaphragm is paralyzed, patients receiving curare must be mechanically ventilated.

Muscle Tone

The strength of a contraction depends upon the length of the fibers before the contraction begins. This is called the **length-tension relationship**.

1. In overly contracted fibers, the sarcomeres are shortened. As a result, even after stimulation, the fiber can't contract very far before the thick filaments bump into the Z-discs. Therefore, contraction is weak.

2. In overly stretched fibers, the thick and thin filaments have little overlap. Only a small portion of the thin filament is accessible for the myosin heads to grab onto when stimulation occurs. Again, the contraction is weak.

3. The strongest contraction occurs when the thin and thick filaments are partially overlapped. In this situation, the Z-discs are far enough apart to allow for movement during contraction; also, the thin and thick filaments overlap enough to allow the myosin heads to get a firm grip on the thin actin filaments.

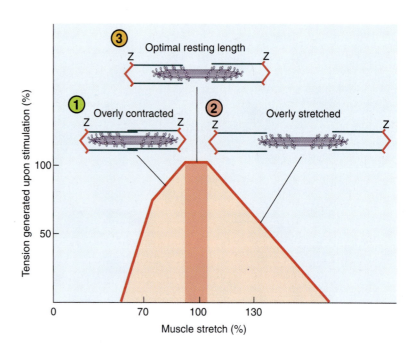

The nervous system constantly monitors skeletal muscles, stimulating muscle fibers just enough to achieve their *optimal resting length.* This continuous state of partial contraction is called **muscle tone**. Muscle tone is what allows you to stand, hold up your head, and maintain your posture. Having your muscles in a partial state of contraction also allows you to react quickly to a dangerous situation, such as righting your balance when you slip or jumping out of the way of an approaching car.

Contraction of an Entire Muscle

Now that we've discussed how individual muscle fibers contract, we need to apply that knowledge to the muscle as a whole. To begin, recall that one motor neuron stimulates a group of muscle fibers. The neuron and all the fibers it stimulates are called a **motor unit**. A single motor unit can consist of a few fibers…or a few hundred. These fibers are scattered throughout the muscle rather than bunched together, allowing the contraction to be spread over a wide area.

To contract, muscle fibers must receive an electrical stimulus. The stimulus needs to be of a certain strength, or voltage. If the stimulus is too weak, the muscle fiber won't respond.

The minimum voltage needed to cause a muscle fiber to contract is called the **threshold**. When a fiber receives a stimulus at or above threshold, it responds after a brief lag by quickly contracting and then relaxing. This single, brief contraction is called a **twitch**.

Obviously, one twitch can't aid a muscle in performing a task. For a muscle to perform any kind of work, many fibers must contract at the same time. In addition, the muscle needs to stay contracted for longer than a split second.

Also, muscles are often called upon to contract at different *strengths*. For example, lifting a pencil requires an entirely different amount of contraction than does, say, lifting a sofa. The force of contraction is affected by a number of things, including the size of the muscle, the degree of stretch, and the number of muscle fibers contracting.

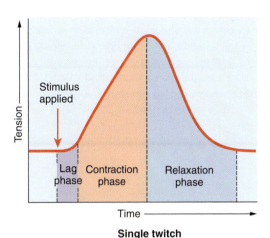

Single twitch

The Body AT WORK

Typically, smaller motor units are found in muscles that perform precise movements, such as the muscles of the eyeball or the fingers. In contrast, larger motor units are found in muscles that don't perform precise movements, such as the muscles of the back.

FAST FACT

Muscles typically become rigid (a condition called rigor mortis) when someone dies. That's because, at the time of death, the production of ATP stops. Without ATP, the myosin heads remain locked onto the actin filaments. No sliding occurs, and muscles become rigid. Rigor mortis peaks about 12 hours after death and then fades over the next 48 hours.

Life lesson: Sports and muscle fibers

Not all muscle fibers are alike, and not all muscle fibers are suited for the same task. Some muscle fibers, called slow-twitch, or type I, fibers, respond slowly to stimuli. These fibers contain abundant mitochondria and a rich blood supply, making them efficient at using oxygen to generate ATP for energy. Although these fibers respond slowly to stimuli, they can fire for a long time before becoming fatigued. Endurance athletes, such as marathon runners, tend to have a preponderance of slow-twitch fibers.

Other fibers, called fast-twitch, or type II, fibers, are better at generating short bursts of speed or strength. Although these fibers do not contain as many mitochondria and have a poorer supply of blood, they can absorb and release calcium quickly. This allows them to fire rapidly, although they fatigue more quickly than slow-twitch fibers do. Athletes such as sprinters tend to have an abundance of fast-twitch fibers.

Controlling the Strength of a Contraction

The nervous system responds to the various demands placed on muscles in two key ways: altering the *frequency* of the stimulus and altering the *intensity* of the stimulus.

Stimulus Frequency

The frequency of stimuli—even if the strength of the stimulus remains the same—can alter contraction strength.

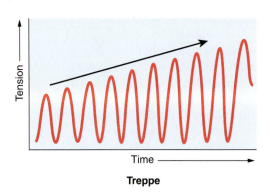

Treppe

When a muscle contracts several times in a row, the last contraction will be stronger than the first contraction. Here's what happens: When stimuli come quickly, the sarcoplasmic reticulum doesn't have time to completely reabsorb all of the calcium ions that were previously released. The increased concentration of calcium leads to a more forceful contraction. This phenomenon, in which each successive twitch contracts more forcefully than the previous one, is called **treppe**, or the staircase phenomenon.

When impulses reach muscle fibers even faster, the fibers don't have a chance to relax completely before the next impulse arrives. As a result, the force of a subsequent contraction builds on the force of the previous contraction. This condition of rapid contraction with only partial relaxation is called **incomplete tetanus**.

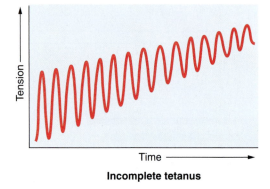

Incomplete tetanus

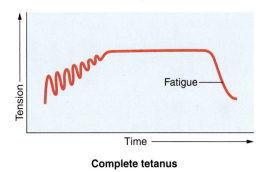

Complete tetanus

If the impulses arrive so fast that the muscle can't relax at all between stimuli, the twitches merge into one prolonged contraction called **complete tetanus**. (Don't confuse the use of the term *tetanus* with the disease tetanus, which is discussed in the "Life Lesson" on page 136.) The state of complete tetanus rarely occurs in the body.

The Body AT WORK

Most skeletal muscles normally remain in a state of incomplete tetanus—mostly due to rapid-fire stimulation of nerve fibers. At some point, though, the fibers become fatigued and have to relax. To allow for this without the muscle falling limp, the motor units of a muscle fire in an asynchronous, overlapping pattern, so that one group of fibers is contracting while another group is relaxing.

Stimulus Intensity

In general, a stronger stimulus elicits a stronger contraction. Specifically, a stronger stimulus excites more nerve fibers in a motor nerve, which then stimulates more motor units.

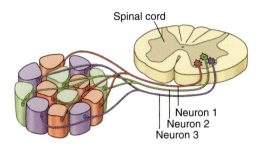

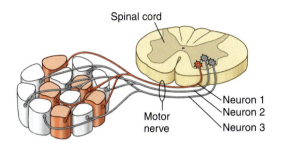

Strong Stimulus

A strong stimulus may stimulate all the fibers in a motor nerve. In turn, the nerve fibers call on all their accompanying muscle fibers to contract. The more fibers contracting at once, the stronger the contraction. (The process by which an increasing number of motor units are called into action is called **recruitment**.)

Weak Stimulus

In contrast, a weak stimulus stimulates just a few nerve fibers. As shown here, a weak stimulus may stimulate just one nerve fiber and the muscle fibers connected to it. The fewer fibers contracted at once, the weaker the response.

Isotonic and Isometric Contraction

While muscle contraction often shortens the muscle (called isotonic contractions), sometimes muscles contract by increasing tension while the length stays the same. These are called isometric contractions.

Isometric Contractions

In isometric contractions, the tension within a muscle increases while its length remains the same. For example, if you pull on a cable fastened to a stationary object, the muscle in your upper arm will tighten, but its length will remain the same.

Isotonic Contractions

In isotonic contractions, the muscle changes length and moves a load, while the tension within the muscle remains the same. For example, when you lift a barbell, the muscle in your upper arm shortens; as you lower the weight, the muscle lengthens.

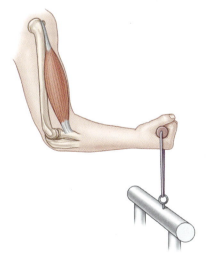

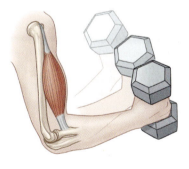

That Makes Sense!

The prefix iso- *means "equal"; the suffix* -tonic *means "tension." Therefore,* isotonic *means "equal tension." The suffix* -metric *means "measurement"; therefore,* isometric *means "same measurement."*

Energy Source for Contraction

All muscle contraction requires energy in the form of ATP. However, muscles store only very small amounts of ATP. In fact, just a few seconds of activity will completely deplete the ATP within a muscle fiber. Consequently, the constant synthesis of ATP is a necessity. Depending upon activity level, muscles obtain their energy supply in several ways.

At rest, muscles obtain most of their energy by metabolizing fatty acids. Because oxygen is plentiful, it uses the process of **aerobic respiration** to break down fatty acids for energy. (The term *aerobic* means "with oxygen.")

When beginning to exercise, the demand for oxygen suddenly increases. The heart and lungs work harder to meet this demand, but, in the short term, the supply of oxygen drops. When this happens, muscles quickly restock their waning supply of ATP by breaking down a compound called **creatine phosphate (CP)**, which is stored in muscle. This high-energy compound can furnish the muscle with fuel for about 20 seconds of high-energy activity or a minute of more moderate activity.

If exercise continues, the supply of CP is exhausted before the supply of oxygen has reached an acceptable level. At this point, muscles switch to **anaerobic** (meaning "without oxygen") **respiration** of glucose. Muscles receive much of their glucose through the bloodstream; however, some is stored within muscle in the form of glycogen. Anaerobic respiration can generate energy quickly; therefore, it's useful for intense bursts of activity. However, it also produces a byproduct called **lactic acid**, which, as it accumulates in muscle, leads to muscle fatigue.

After about 10 minutes of more moderate activity, the heart and lungs have had a chance to increase the supply of oxygen to the muscles. This allows muscles to shift back to aerobic respiration. Aerobic respiration produces more ATP than anaerobic respiration. Also, its byproducts are carbon dioxide and water, which, unlike lactic acid, aren't toxic to muscle.

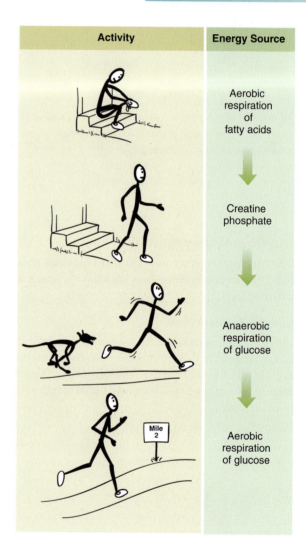

Activity	Energy Source
	Aerobic respiration of fatty acids
	Creatine phosphate
	Anaerobic respiration of glucose
	Aerobic respiration of glucose

The Body AT WORK

Following strenuous exercise, some of the lactic acid produced during anaerobic respiration travels to the liver, where it is converted back into glucose. However, the conversion process consumes a lot of oxygen, which is why you continue to breathe heavily for several minutes following a hard workout. The extra oxygen that's needed to process lactic acid is called an oxygen debt.

Muscle Function

The role of a muscle is to move a body part. Each end of most skeletal muscles adheres to a different bone. The contraction of the muscle causes one bone to move while the other remains relatively still.

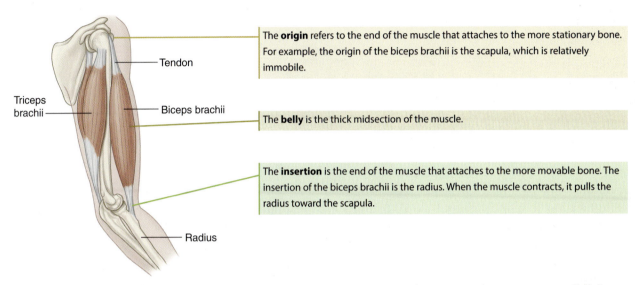

Triceps brachii

Tendon

Biceps brachii

Radius

The **origin** refers to the end of the muscle that attaches to the more stationary bone. For example, the origin of the biceps brachii is the scapula, which is relatively immobile.

The **belly** is the thick midsection of the muscle.

The **insertion** is the end of the muscle that attaches to the more movable bone. The insertion of the biceps brachii is the radius. When the muscle contracts, it pulls the radius toward the scapula.

Skeletal muscles typically work in groups to create movement. The main muscle triggering the movement is called the **prime mover;** the muscles that assist are called **synergists.** Muscles balancing these movements are called **antagonists.** Antagonists **oppose** the action of the prime mover. When the prime mover contracts, the antagonist must relax and give the prime mover control. Typically, the antagonist works to moderate the speed or range of movement, helping to prevent joint injury. The prime mover for one movement is the antagonist for the opposite movement.

The biceps brachii and brachialis muscles work together to flex the elbow, with the brachialis being the prime mover and the biceps brachii being the synergist. The triceps brachii is the antagonist.

When extending the arm, the triceps brachii is the prime mover and the brachialis is the antagonist.

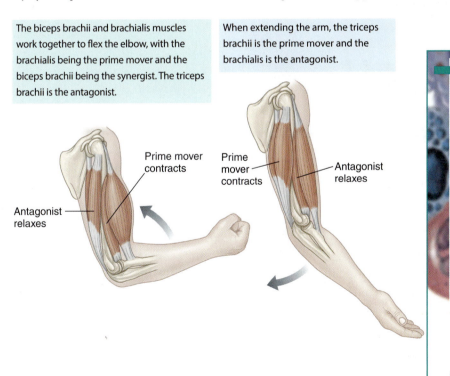

Prime mover contracts

Antagonist relaxes

Prime mover contracts

Antagonist relaxes

The Body AT WORK

*Exercise, or a lack of exercise, causes physiological changes in skeletal muscles. Strength training, such as lifting weights, causes a muscle to enlarge. This is called **hypertrophy.** Specifically, intense exercise, such as from resistance training, slightly injures muscle fibers. As the body repairs the damage, the fibers enlarge, and consequently so does the muscle. In contrast, a lack of use causes the muscle fibers, and therefore the entire muscle, to shrink, or **atrophy.***

Endurance (aerobic) exercise stimulates the growth of blood vessels in the muscle. This allows for an increased supply of oxygen and glucose—two necessary ingredients for ATP production.

Superficial Muscles

The following two figures display some of the major muscles of the body. Keep in mind, though, that the body contains over 600 muscles, all of which can't be shown here. These figures show the major superficial muscles, the ones you are most likely to be able to palpate. Underneath these muscles are many more muscles.

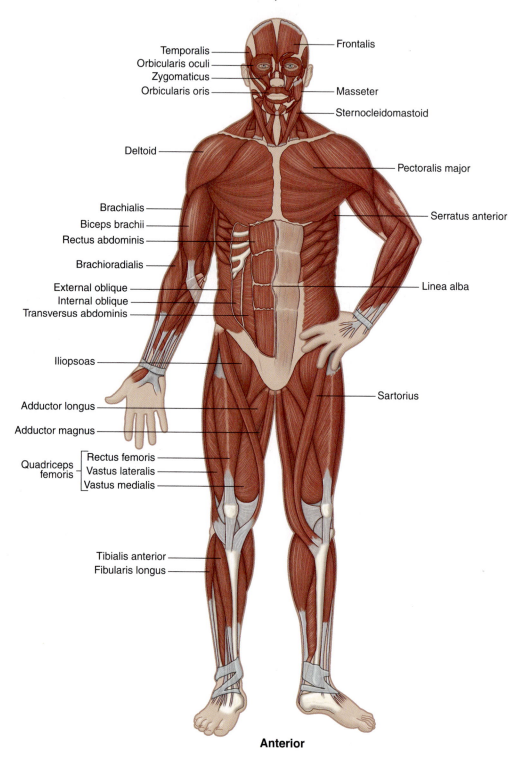

Temporalis
Orbicularis oculi
Zygomaticus
Orbicularis oris

Frontalis

Masseter

Sternocleidomastoid

Deltoid

Pectoralis major

Brachialis
Biceps brachii
Rectus abdominis

Serratus anterior

Brachioradialis

External oblique
Internal oblique
Transversus abdominis

Linea alba

Iliopsoas

Adductor longus

Adductor magnus

Sartorius

Quadriceps femoris
Rectus femoris
Vastus lateralis
Vastus medialis

Tibialis anterior
Fibularis longus

Anterior

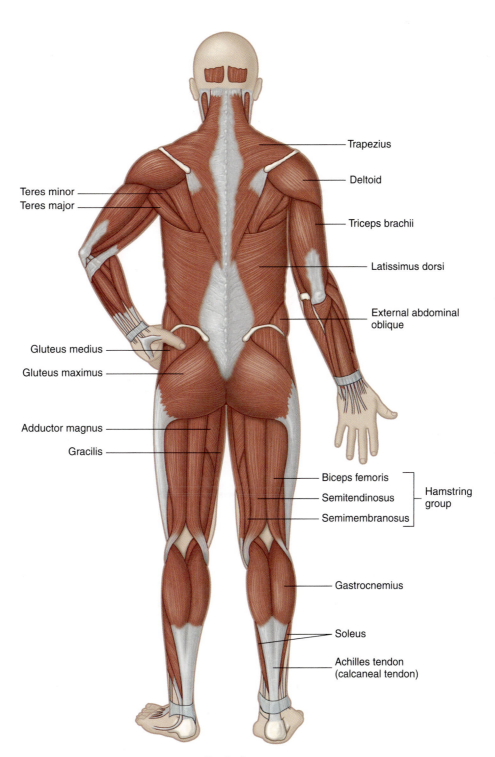

Trapezius

Deltoid

Teres minor

Teres major

Triceps brachii

Latissimus dorsi

External abdominal oblique

Gluteus medius

Gluteus maximus

Adductor magnus

Gracilis

Biceps femoris

Semitendinosus

Semimembranosus

Hamstring group

Gastrocnemius

Soleus

Achilles tendon (calcaneal tendon)

Posterior

How Muscles Are Named

Muscles are named according to their size, shape, location, number of origins, the direction of muscle fibers, or their action. Learning key terms, such as the ones listed in the chart below, can help you figure out the location and function of many muscles. When studying these terms, keep in mind that Latin roots form the basis of many of these words.

Characteristic	Term	Meaning	Example
Size	Maximus	Largest	Gluteus maximus
	Minimus	Smallest	Gluteus minimus
	Major	Large	Pectoralis major
	Minor	Small	Pectoralis minor
	Longus	Longest	Peroneus longus
	Brevis	Shortest	Peroneus brevis
Shape	Deltoid	Triangular	Deltoid
	Rhomboid	Diamond-shaped	Rhomboideus major
	Serratus	Sawtoothed (like a serrated knife)	Serratus anterior
	Trapezius	Trapezoidal	Trapezius
Location	Pectoralis	Chest	Pectoralis major
	Brachio-	Upper arm	Brachioradialis
	Radialis	Radius	Brachioradialis
	Gluteus	Buttock	Gluteus maximus
	Femoris	Femur	Quadriceps femoris
	Sterno-	Sternum	Sternocleidomastoid
	Cleido-	Clavicle	Sternocleidomastoid
	Mastoid	Mastoid process	Sternocleidomastoid
	Digiti	Finger or toe	Extensor digiti minimi
	Pollicis	Thumb	Opponens pollicis
Number of origins	Biceps	Two origins	Biceps femoris
	Triceps	Three origins	Triceps brachii
	Quadriceps	Four origins	Quadriceps femoris
Direction	Rectus	Straight	Rectus abdominis
	Transverse	Across	Transversus abdominis
	Oblique	Diagonal	External oblique
Action	Adductor	Adducts	Adductor magnus
	Abductor	Abducts	Abductor pollicis
	Flexor	Flexes	Flexor carpi radialis
	Extensor	Extends	Extensor digitorum
	Levator	Elevates	Levator scapula

Muscles of the Head and Neck

Muscles in this region are typically grouped according to their function: muscles of facial expression, muscles of chewing (called mastication) and swallowing, and muscles that move the head. Of all the muscles of the face, the area around the mouth is the most complex. This makes sense considering that the mouth is the most expressive part of the face; the movement of the lips is also pivotal in the formation of words.

Muscles of Facial Expression

Frontalis: Raises the eyebrows when glancing upward or when showing surprise

Orbicularis oculi: A sphincter muscle that closes the eye when blinking or squinting

Zygomaticus: Draws the mouth upward when laughing

Orbicularis oris: Closes the mouth and purses the lips, such as when kissing

Buccinator (shown on the other side of the face): Assists in smiling and blowing (such as when playing a trumpet or whistling) as well as chewing

Muscles of Chewing

Temporalis: Aids in closing the jaw

Masseter: Closes the jaw

Muscles That Move the Head

Sternocleidomastoid: Flexes the head (so is sometimes called the praying muscle); rotates the head to the opposite side when only one muscle contracts

Trapezius: Extends the head (such as when looking upward) and flexes the head to one side; also elevates the shoulder

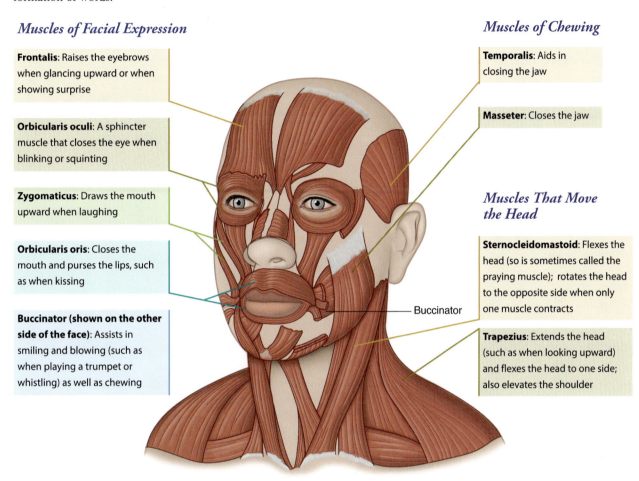

Buccinator

FAST FACT
The face contains over 30 muscles, which allow us to express a variety of emotions.

FAST FACT
The human face is considerably more expressive than the faces of other mammals: all due to the wide variety of facial muscles.

The Body AT WORK

Besides contributing to facial expression, the muscles of the face allow us to speak, chew, and perform other oral functions. Almost every muscle of the face is innervated by the facial nerve (cranial nerve VII). Consequently, an injury or disorder of the facial nerve can cause paralysis on one side of the face. For example, a viral infection of the facial nerve, called Bell's palsy, results in paralysis of the muscles on the affected side. The muscles on that side of the face droop, and those afflicted have trouble eating, drinking, blinking, or forming any facial expression (such as smiling, grimacing, or raising eyebrows).

Muscles of the Trunk

Some of the muscles of the truck participate in respiration and form the abdominal wall. Additional muscles support and allow movement in the vertebral column, while several other muscles lie on top of each other to form the pelvic floor.

Muscles Involved in Breathing

Muscles are the driving force behind our ability to breathe. (For more information on the muscles of respiration, see Chapter 17, *Respiratory System.*)

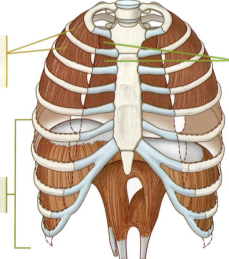

External intercostals: Lie superficially between ribs; elevate the ribs during inspiration

Internal intercostals: Lie deeper than the external intercostals; depress the ribs during forced exhalation

Diaphragm: Enlarges the thorax to trigger inspiration

Muscles Forming the Abdominal Wall

While the trunk receives support from the skeleton, the abdominal wall derives its strength from alternating layers of muscle. The muscle fibers in each of the three layers forming the abdominal wall run in different directions: downward and anterior (as in the external oblique muscle: the most superficial layer), upward and anterior (as in the internal oblique muscle: the next layer), and horizontal (as in the transverse abdominal muscle: the deepest layer).

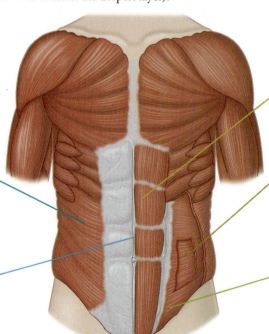

Rectus abdominis: Flexes the lumbar region of the spinal column to cause bending forward at the waist; extends from the sternum to the pubic bone

Transversus abdominis: Compresses the contents of the abdomen

External oblique: Compresses the abdominal organs, which aids in forceful expiration, vomiting, and defecation; also allows flexion of the vertebral column and rotation and lateral bending of the trunk

The aponeuroses of the muscles forming the abdominal wall meet in the midline of the abdomen, where they form a tough band of connective tissue called the **linea alba** (white line).

Internal oblique: Stabilizes the spine and maintains posture, just like the external oblique muscles; also permits rotation of the waist

Muscles of the Shoulder and Upper Arm

The shoulder and upper arm perform a wide variety of movements. Some movements—such as throwing a ball or swimming—require power and a full range of motion. Others, such as writing, depend upon more subtle movements. To make these motions possible, the shoulder draws on a complex variety of muscles. A few of those muscles are illustrated in the figure below.

Deltoid: Abducts, flexes, and rotates the arm; involved in swinging the arm (walking or bowling); also raises the arm to perform tasks, such as writing on an elevated surface

Pectoralis major: Flexes and adducts the upper arm, such as when climbing or hugging

Serratus anterior: Drives all forward-reaching and pushing movements; pulls the shoulder down and forward

Anterior

Trapezius: Raises and lowers the shoulders; stabilizes the scapula during arm movements

Latissimus dorsi: Adducts the humerus; extends the upper arm backward (such as when rowing or swimming); when grasping an object overhead, such as when climbing, serves to pull the body upward

Rotator cuff: The tendons of four muscles (attached to the scapula) form the rotator cuff. They are the:

- **supraspinatus**
- **infraspinatus**
- **teres minor** and
- **subscapularis** (on the anterior scapula)

Nicknamed the "SITS" muscles (derived from the first letter of names for each of the muscles), the tendons of these muscles fuse with the joint capsule and form a "cuff" around the shoulder joint, helping to hold the head of the humerus in place.

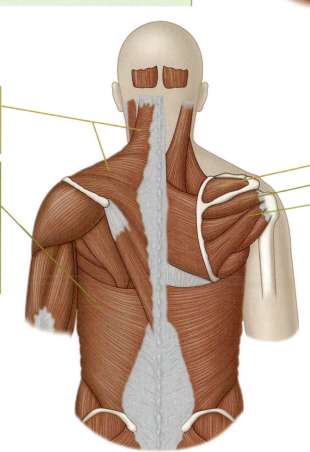

Posterior

Life lesson: Rotator cuff injury

The shoulder is the body's most mobile joint. Along with this great mobility, however, comes a tendency toward injury. In particular, a fall or hard blow to the shoulder, or repetitive use of the arm in an overhead motion (such as by baseball pitchers, tennis players, weight lifters, and swimmers), can injure the muscles forming the rotator cuff. Overuse can also cause one or more of the tendons to become inflamed, resulting in pain. If the inflammation happens repeatedly, the tendon can degenerate and eventually rupture.

Muscles That Move the Forearm

The muscles that flex and extend the forearm are located on the humerus.

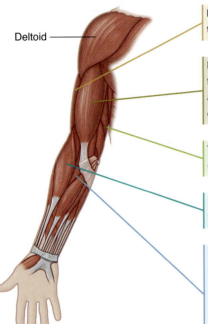

Deltoid

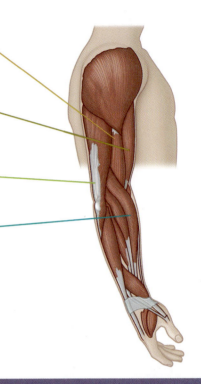

Brachialis: The prime mover when flexing the forearm

Biceps brachii: Assists the brachialis when flexing the forearm; also flexes the elbow and supinates the forearm (such as when opening a bottle with a corkscrew)

Triceps brachii: The prime mover when extending the forearm

Brachioradialis: Helps the brachialis and the biceps brachii flex the forearm

Pronator muscles allow the arm to pronate (palms down). A **supinator muscle**—not visible here—lies deep in the forearm near the elbow; it joins forces with the biceps brachii to allow supination (palms up).

Muscles of the Wrist and Hand

Some of the muscles that move the wrist, hand, and fingers are in the hand itself; others are located in the forearm.

Muscles that flex the wrist—called **flexors**—are located on the anterior of the forearm. (Examine the above illustration to locate the flexors.) Similar muscles, called **extensors**, are found on the posterior of the forearm; these act to extend the wrist. (This makes sense: *Flexing* your wrist pulls your hand back toward the anterior surface of the forearm, which is where the *flexors* are located. *Extending* your wrist bends your hand toward the posterior surface of your forearm: the location of the *extensors*.) The muscles in the hands also work with the flexors and extensors to help the fingers make delicate, precise movements.

FAST FACT

A bulging biceps brachii symbolizes upper arm strength. Even so, the brachialis, which lies underneath the biceps brachii, is the prime mover for flexing the elbow.

Life lesson: Carpal tunnel syndrome

On the palm side of the wrist, near the thumb, is a narrow passageway surrounded by bones and ligaments called the *carpal tunnel*. Tendons that allow finger flexion as well as a key nerve of the hand (the median nerve) pass through this channel. Difficulties arise when repetitive flexion and extension of the wrist triggers inflammation and swelling in the sheath surrounding the tendons. Because the carpal tunnel can't expand, the swelling presses on the median nerve, which produces tingling, weakness, and pain in the thumb, index finger, middle finger, and middle side of the ring finger. Called *carpal tunnel syndrome*, the disorder commonly afflicts those who spend long hours at computer keyboards, although any repetitive wrist motion may trigger the condition.

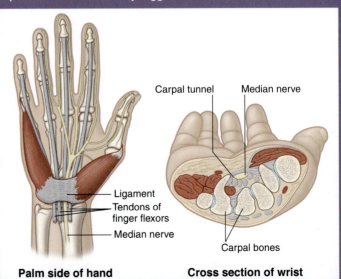

Carpal tunnel

Median nerve

Ligament

Tendons of finger flexors

Median nerve

Carpal bones

Palm side of hand

Cross section of wrist

Muscles Acting on the Hip and Thigh

Unlike the arms, which are geared for free movement and precise maneuvers, the legs are built for stability and power. The muscles of the hip and thigh enable the body to stand, walk, and maintain balance. Consequently, this area contains some of the body's largest, and most powerful, muscles.

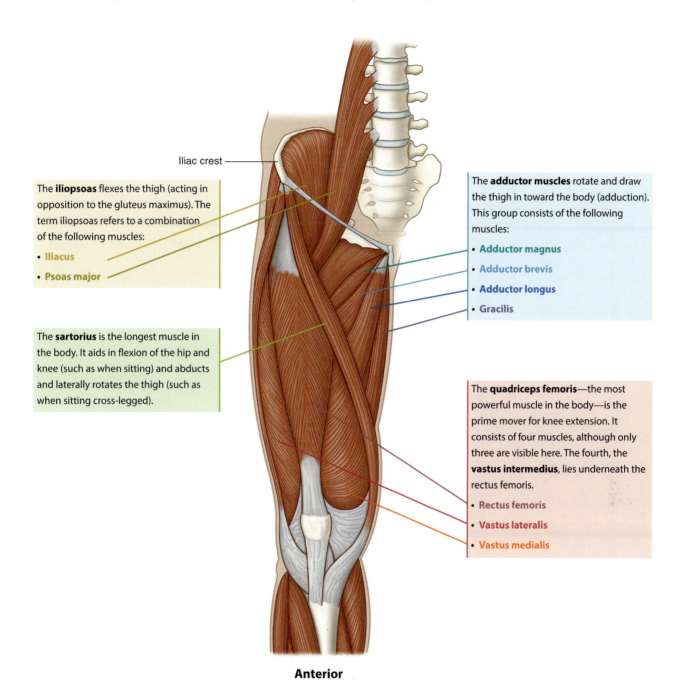

Iliac crest

The **iliopsoas** flexes the thigh (acting in opposition to the gluteus maximus). The term iliopsoas refers to a combination of the following muscles:

- Iliacus
- Psoas major

The **sartorius** is the longest muscle in the body. It aids in flexion of the hip and knee (such as when sitting) and abducts and laterally rotates the thigh (such as when sitting cross-legged).

The **adductor muscles** rotate and draw the thigh in toward the body (adduction). This group consists of the following muscles:

- Adductor magnus
- Adductor brevis
- Adductor longus
- Gracilis

The **quadriceps femoris**—the most powerful muscle in the body—is the prime mover for knee extension. It consists of four muscles, although only three are visible here. The fourth, the **vastus intermedius**, lies underneath the rectus femoris.

- Rectus femoris
- Vastus lateralis
- Vastus medialis

Anterior

FAST FACT

The sartorius muscle has the nickname "tailor's muscle," supposedly because tailors sat cross-legged while sewing, supporting their work on their knee.

The gluteal muscles consist of the following three muscles:

Gluteus medius: Abducts and rotates the thigh outward

Gluteus maximus: The bulkiest muscle in the body; it produces the backswing of the leg when walking and provides most of the power for climbing stairs

Gluteus minimus: This muscle lies beneath the other two gluteal muscles

Adductor magnus

Gracilis

The **hamstrings** are a group of muscles consisting of the following three muscles, all of which work to extend the thigh at the hip, flex the knee, and rotate the leg. You can easily feel the tendons of these muscles as the prominent cords on either side of the back of the knee.

Biceps femoris

Semitendinosus

Semimembranosus

Posterior

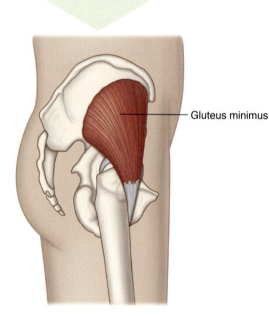

Gluteus minimus

FAST FACT

Severing the hamstrings makes someone immediately immobile, which is why ancient knights would use their swords to slice the back of an opponent's thighs.

FAST FACT

The gluteus medius is a common site for intramuscular injections, particularly if the amount of medication to be administered is more than 2 to 3 ml. If 2 ml or less is to be injected, the deltoid muscle is often used.

Muscles Acting on the Foot

Muscles in the lower leg are primarily responsible for moving the foot and ankle.

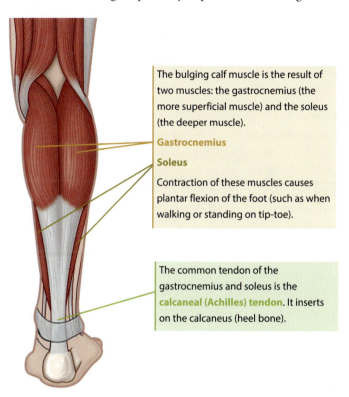

The bulging calf muscle is the result of two muscles: the gastrocnemius (the more superficial muscle) and the soleus (the deeper muscle).

Gastrocnemius

Soleus

Contraction of these muscles causes plantar flexion of the foot (such as when walking or standing on tip-toe).

FAST FACT

The calcaneal, or Achilles, tendon is the strongest tendon in the body. Even so, it's a frequent site of athletic injuries. It's particularly vulnerable to sudden stress, such as sprinting.

The common tendon of the gastrocnemius and soleus is the **calcaneal (Achilles) tendon**. It inserts on the calcaneus (heel bone).

Muscles on the anterior of the lower leg also participate in moving the foot and ankle.

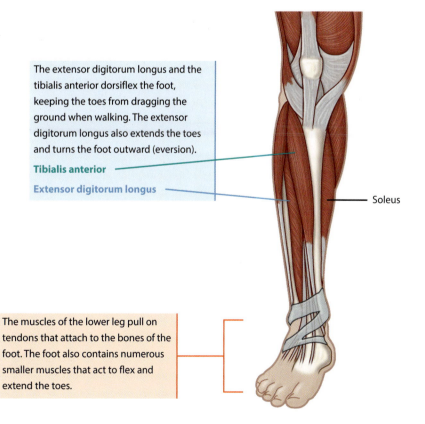

The extensor digitorum longus and the tibialis anterior dorsiflex the foot, keeping the toes from dragging the ground when walking. The extensor digitorum longus also extends the toes and turns the foot outward (eversion).

Tibialis anterior

Extensor digitorum longus

Soleus

The muscles of the lower leg pull on tendons that attach to the bones of the foot. The foot also contains numerous smaller muscles that act to flex and extend the toes.

Major Muscles of the Body

Muscle	Origin	Insertion	Function
Muscles of the head and neck			
Muscles of facial expression			
Frontalis	Occipital bone	Tissues of eyebrows	Raises eyebrows; expressions of surprise
Orbicularis oculi	Encircles eyelid		Closes eye
Zygomaticus	Zygomatic bone	Angle of mouth	Laughing
Orbicularis oris	Encircles mouth		Draws lips together
Buccinator	Maxillae	Skin of cheeks and lips	Smiling; blowing (playing a trumpet)
Muscles of chewing			
Temporalis	Temporal bone	Mandible	Closes jaw
Masseter	Zygomatic arch	Mandible	Closes jaw
Muscles that move the head			
Sternocleidomastoid	Sternum; clavicle	Mastoid process of temporal bone	Flexes head; "prayer muscle"
Trapezius	Occipital bone; vertebrae	Clavicle; scapula	Extends head (looking up); flexes head to one side; elevates shoulder
Muscles of the trunk			
Muscles involved in breathing			
External intercostals	Rib	Rib	Elevate ribs
Internal intercostals	Rib	Rib	Depress ribs
Diaphragm	Lower edge of ribcage; xiphoid process; lumbar vertebrae	Central tendon of diaphragm	Enlarges thorax to trigger inspiration
Muscles forming the abdominal wall			
Rectus abdominis	Pubic bone	Xiphoid process of sternum	Flexes lumbar region to allow bending forward
Transverse abdominal	Ribs; pelvis	Pubic bone; linea alba	Compresses contents of abdomen
Internal oblique	Pelvis	Ribs	Stabilizes spine to maintain posture; permits rotation at waist
External oblique	Ribs	Pelvis	Stabilizes spine
Muscles of the shoulder and upper arm			
Deltoid	Clavicle; scapula	Humerus	Abducts, flexes, and rotates arm
Pectoralis major	Clavicle; sternum	Humerus	Flexes and adducts upper arm
Serratus anterior	Ribs	Scapula	Pulls shoulder down and forward
Trapezius	Occipital bone; vertebrae	Clavicle; scapula	Raises or lowers shoulders
Latissimus dorsi	Vertebrae	Humerus	Adducts and extends the arm backward
Rotator cuff:	Scapula	Humerus	Rotates and adducts arm
• Supraspinatus			
• Infraspinatus			
• Teres minor			
• Subscapularis			

Muscle	Origin	Insertion	Function
Muscles that move the forearm			
Brachialis	Humerus	Ulna	Flexes the forearm
Biceps brachii	Scapula	Radius	Flexes the forearm
Triceps brachii	Scapula; humerus	Ulna	Extends the forearm
Brachioradialis	Humerus	Radius	Helps flex the forearm
Pronator muscles	Humerus; ulna	Radius	Pronates the forearm
Supinator	Humerus; ulna	Radius	Supinates the forearm
Muscles acting on the hip and thigh			
Iliacus	Ilium	Femur	Flexes the thigh
Psoas major	Ilium	Femur	Flexes the thigh
Sartorius	Iliac spine	Tibia	Adducts and flexes the leg; permits sitting "cross-legged"
Adductor muscles: • Adductor magnus • Adductor brevis • Adductor longus • Gracilis	Pubic bone	Femur	Adduct the thigh
Quadriceps femoris: • Rectus femoris • Vastus lateralis • Vastus medialis • Vastus intermedius	Ilium; femur	Tibia	Flexes the thigh; extends the leg
Gluteus medius	Ilium	Femur	Abducts and rotates the thigh outward
Gluteus maximus	Ilium	Femur	Extends and rotates the thigh outward
Gluteus minimus	Ilium	Femur	Abducts and rotates the thigh
Hamstring group: • Biceps femoris • Semitendinosus • Semimembranosus	Ischium; femur	Fibula; tibia	Extends the thigh
Muscles acting on the foot			
Gastrocnemius	Femur	Calcaneus	Plantar flexion of the foot
Soleus	Tibia; fibula	Calcaneus	Plantar flexion of the foot
Tibialis anterior	Tibia	Tarsal bone	Dorsiflexion of the foot
Extensor digitorum longus	Tibia; fibula	Phalanges	Dorsiflexion of the foot

Life lesson: Exercise and muscle conditioning

Endurance (aerobic) exercise, such as jogging, cycling, or swimming, trains muscles to resist fatigue. This primarily occurs because exercise stimulates slow-twitch fibers to produce more mitochondria and glycogen; the blood supply to these fibers also improves. Exercise affects more than muscle fibers: it strengthens bones, improves the oxygen-carrying capacity of the blood by increasing the number of red blood cells, and enhances the function of the cardiovascular, respiratory, and nervous systems.

Endurance exercise does not significantly increase muscle strength, however. Increased muscle strength requires *resistance exercise,* such as weight lifting, that involves the contraction of muscles against a load that resists movement. This action stimulates muscle fibers to synthesize more myofilaments and the myofibrils grow thicker and increase in number. As a result, muscles become both larger and stronger. A few minutes a day, several times a week, is enough to stimulate muscle growth.

Because endurance and resistance exercise produces different results, an optimal exercise program should include both types of training.

Review of Key Terms

Acetylcholine: Chemical messenger released from the end of a motor neuron

Actin: Protein of which the thin myofilaments are composed

Aerobic respiration: Process that breaks down fatty acids for energy when oxygen is present

Anaerobic respiration: Process that breaks down glucose for energy when oxygen is not plentiful

Antagonist: Muscles that oppose the action of a prime mover

Aponeurosis: Flat, broad tendon that attaches a muscle to another muscle or to bone

ATP: Adenosine triphosphate; used for energy in cells to perform various functions, including muscle contraction

Atrophy: Decrease in the size of a muscle

Belly: The thick midsection of the muscle

Complete tetanus: Condition in which impulses arrive so fast the muscle cannot relax between stimuli and twitches merge into one prolonged contraction

Creatine phosphate: Compound stored in muscle that is used for short bursts of high-energy activity

Endomysium: Delicate connective tissue covering each muscle fiber

Epimysium: Connective tissue covering that surrounds muscles as a whole and binds all muscle fibers together

Fascia: Connective tissue surrounding the muscle

Fascicles: Bundles of muscle fibers

Hypertrophy: Enlargement of a muscle

Incomplete tetanus: Condition of rapid muscle contraction with only partial relaxation

Insertion: The end of a muscle that attaches to the more mobile bone

Isometric contraction: Contraction in which the tension within a muscle increases while its length remains the same

Isotonic contraction: Contraction in which the muscle changes length to move a load

Motor unit: A neuron and all the muscle fibers it stimulates

Muscle fiber: A skeletal muscle cell

Muscle tone: Continuous state of partial muscle contraction that allows for the maintenance of posture

Myofibrils: Long protein bundles that fill the sarcoplasm of a muscle fiber

Myofilaments: Fine protein fibers that make up a myofibril

Myosin: Protein of which the thick myofilaments are composed

Neuromuscular junction: Connection between a motor neuron and a muscle fiber

Origin: The end of a muscle that attaches to the more stationary bone

Perimysium: Sheath of connective tissue encasing fascicles

Prime mover: The main muscle triggering a movement

Sarcomere: The unit of contraction of the myofibrils of a muscle

Sarcoplasm: The cytoplasm of a muscle fiber

Synaptic cleft: Narrow space between the end of a motor nerve and the muscle fiber

Synergists: Muscles that assist in the movement of a bone

Tendon: Strong, fibrous cord through which a muscle attaches to a bone

Transverse (T) tubules: Tubules that extend across the sarcoplasm and allow electrical impulses to travel deep into the cell

Treppe: Phenomenon in which each successive twitch contracts more forcefully than the previous one

Twitch: Single, brief contraction

Own the Information

To make the information in this chapter part of your working memory, take some time to reflect on what you've learned. On a separate sheet of paper, write down everything you recall from the chapter. After you're done, log on to the Davis*Plus* website, and check out the Study Group podcast and Study Group Questions for the chapter.

Key Topics for Chapter 9:
- Types of muscle
- Skeletal muscle structure
- How skeletal muscles contract and relax
- Controlling the strength of a contraction
- Types of muscle contractions
- Energy sources for contractions
- How muscles function
- Names and actions of the body's major muscles

Test Your Knowledge

1. A single muscle cell is called a:
   a. myofilament.
   b. muscle fiber.
   c. myofibril.
   d. fascicle.

2. Which statement correctly describes what occurs when a skeletal muscle contracts?
   a. Myosin and actin myofilaments form cross bridges, and the actin pulls the myosin myofilament toward the center of the sarcomere.
   b. The myosin and actin myofilaments shorten, pulling the Z-discs closer.
   c. After forming cross bridges with the actin myofilament, the myosin myofilament propels the actin myofilament toward the center of the sarcomere.
   d. The sarcomere shortens, pulling the actin and myosin myofilaments toward the center, which pulls the Z-discs closer together.

3. A continuous state of partial muscle contraction in which muscles are at their optimal resting length is called:
   a. muscle tone.
   b. incomplete tetanus.
   c. complete tetanus.
   d. twitch.

4. At rest, muscles obtain most of their energy by metabolizing:
   a. glucose.
   b. lactic acid.
   c. creatine phosphate.
   d. fatty acids.

5. The end of a muscle that's attached to the more mobile bone is called the:
   a. belly.
   b. prime mover.
   c. origin.
   d. insertion.

6. The prefix *bi-* in a muscle name, such as in biceps brachii, refers to the fact that the muscle:
   a. exists in two locations (such as both arms).
   b. has two different actions.
   c. has two directions.
   d. has two origins.

7. A tendon is an extension of what muscle component?
   a. Endomysium
   b. Epimysium
   c. Perimysium
   d. Sarcolemma

8. During the process of muscle contraction, the sarcoplasmic reticulum is stimulated to release which substance?
   a. Calcium
   b. Acetylcholine
   c. ATP
   d. Acetylcholinesterase

9. Which muscle is often called the "praying muscle" because of its role in flexing the head?
   a. Trapezius
   b. Temporalis
   c. Sternocleidomastoid
   d. Buccinator

10. The prime mover for knee extension is the:
    a. gluteus maximus.
    b. quadriceps femoris.
    c. iliacus.
    d. sartorius.

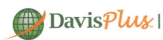 **DavisPlus** | Go to **http://davisplus.fadavis.com** Keyword: Thompson to see all of the resources available with this chapter.

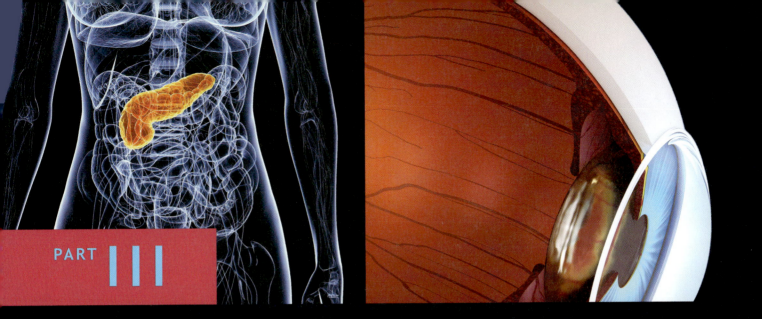

REGULATION AND
INTEGRATION OF THE BODY

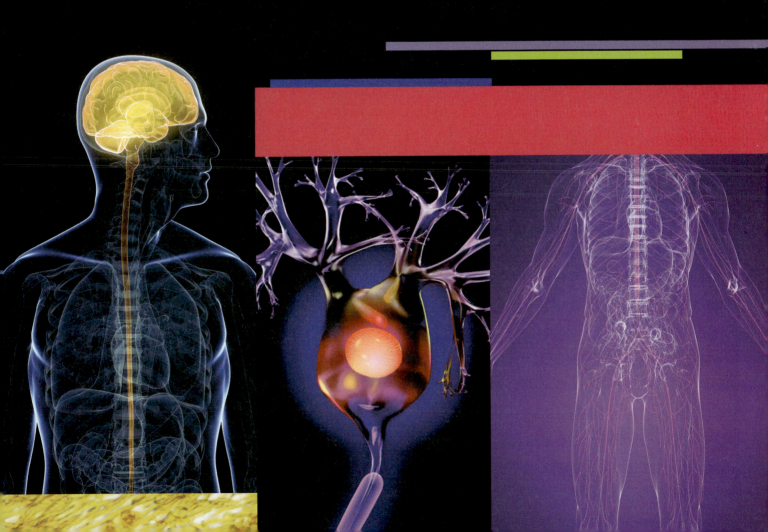

CHAPTER OUTLINE

Overview of the Nervous System

Divisions of the Nervous System

Nervous System Cells

Repair of Nerve Fibers

Impulse Conduction

Synapses

Structure of the Spinal Cord

Spinal Nerves

Somatic Reflexes

General Structures of the Brain

Divisions of the Brain

Functions of the Cerebral Cortex

Cranial Nerves

Visceral Reflexes

Structure of the Autonomic Nervous System

Divisions of the Autonomic Nervous System

Effects of the ANS on Target Organs

LEARNING OUTCOMES

Overview of the Nervous System

1. Describe the two divisions of the nervous system.

2. Name the two types of cells that make up the nervous system and describe the function of each.

3. List the basic parts of a neuron.

4. Recall the structure and function of the myelin sheath.

5. Explain the process of impulse conduction in both myelinated and unmyelinated nerve fibers.

6. Discuss how a nerve impulse is transmitted from one neuron to another.

7. Describe the anatomy of the spinal cord.

8. Define the structure and general function of spinal nerves.

9. Identify the categories of spinal nerves.

10. Recall the four components of a reflex arc.

The Brain and Cranial Nerves

11. Describe the major subdivisions of the brain and the functions of each.

12. Identify the location of gray and white matter in the brain.

13. Name the layers of the meninges and relate its function.

14. Summarize the production and circulation of cerebrospinal fluid.

15. Summarize the function of the reticular activating system.

16. List the 12 cranial nerve, using name and number and identify the functions of each.

Autonomic Nervous System

17. Describe how visceral reflexes differ from somatic reflexes.

18. Compare the structure and function of the autonomic and somatic nervous system.

19. Identify the differences in structure and function between the sympathetic and parasympathetic divisions of the autonomic nervous system.

10

NERVOUS SYSTEM

There are more nerve cells in the human body than there are stars in the Milky Way.

To remain in balance (homeostasis), the various organ systems of the body must work together. Even an act as simple as eating lunch requires input from multiple body systems, including the endocrine system (which senses a drop in blood glucose levels and triggers the sensation of hunger), the muscular system (which allows you to chew your food), and the digestive system (which processes the food and eliminates the waste). The nervous system coordinates these systems so each knows exactly what to do and when to do it.

The **nervous system**—consisting of the brain, spinal cord, and nerves—constantly receives signals about changes within the body as well the external environment. It then processes the information, decides what action needs to occur, and sends electrical and chemical signals to the cells, telling them how to respond. The nervous system also powers our ability to learn, feel, create, and experience emotion. Of all the body's systems, the nervous system is the most complex.

Overview of the Nervous System

The body has two organ systems dedicated to coordinating the activities of the trillions of cells making up the human form. One of those systems—the **endocrine system**—employs chemical messengers called hormones to communicate with cells. In contrast, the **nervous system** uses electrical signals to transmit messages at lightning speed.

The nervous system has three essential roles:

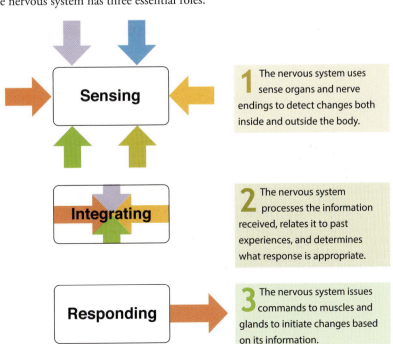

Sensing

Integrating

Responding

1 The nervous system uses sense organs and nerve endings to detect changes both inside and outside the body.

2 The nervous system processes the information received, relates it to past experiences, and determines what response is appropriate.

3 The nervous system issues commands to muscles and glands to initiate changes based on its information.

FAST FACT

During fetal development, neurons grow at a rate of about 250,000 neurons per minute.

Divisions of the Nervous System

The nervous system contains two main divisions: the **central nervous system** (CNS) and the **peripheral nervous system** (PNS).

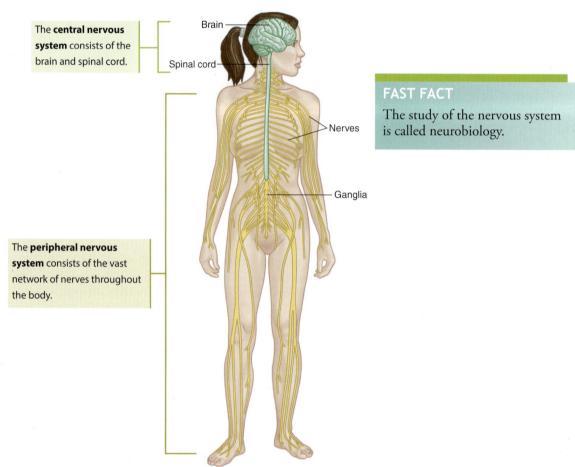

The **central nervous system** consists of the brain and spinal cord.

Brain

Spinal cord

Nerves

Ganglia

FAST FACT
The study of the nervous system is called neurobiology.

The **peripheral nervous system** consists of the vast network of nerves throughout the body.

In brief, the peripheral nervous system consists of everything outside of the brain and spinal cord. However, because the nervous system performs so many different functions, it's helpful to further subdivide the peripheral nervous system, as shown in the flowchart below.

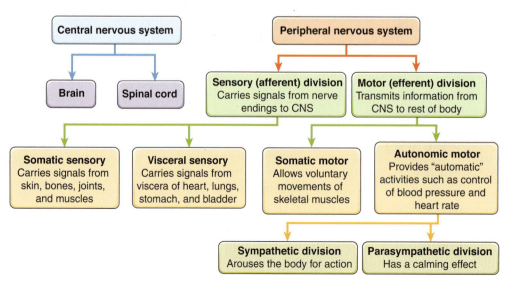

Central nervous system

- **Brain**
- **Spinal cord**

Peripheral nervous system

- **Sensory (afferent) division**
  Carries signals from nerve endings to CNS
  - **Somatic sensory**
    Carries signals from skin, bones, joints, and muscles
  - **Visceral sensory**
    Carries signals from viscera of heart, lungs, stomach, and bladder
- **Motor (efferent) division**
  Transmits information from CNS to rest of body
  - **Somatic motor**
    Allows voluntary movements of skeletal muscles
  - **Autonomic motor**
    Provides "automatic" activities such as control of blood pressure and heart rate
    - **Sympathetic division**
      Arouses the body for action
    - **Parasympathetic division**
      Has a calming effect

Nervous System Cells

Two types of cells make up the nervous system: **neurons** and **neuroglia**. Neurons are the excitable, impulse-conducting cells that perform the work of the nervous system, while neuroglia protect the neurons.

Neuroglia

Also called **glial cells,** neuroglia are the supportive cells of the nervous system. (The word *glia* means "glue," and neuroglia do just that: they bind neurons together.) They also perform various functions that enhance the performance of the nervous system. Underscoring the importance of neuroglia is the fact that the nervous system contains about 50 glial cells for each neuron.

The nervous system contains five major types of glia. Diverse in shape as well as function, the following table summarizes each type. Schwann cells are found in the peripheral nervous system; all the rest reside in the central nervous system.

Types of Glial Cells

Cell Type	Function
Neuroglia of CNS	
Oligodendrocytes	Form myelin sheath in the brain and spinal cord; speed signal conduction
Ependymal cells	Line spinal cord and cavities of the brain; some secrete cerebrospinal fluid, whereas others have cilia that aid fluid circulation
Microglia	Perform phagocytosis, engulfing microorganisms and cellular debris
Astrocytes	Extend through brain tissue; nourish neurons; help form blood-brain barrier; attach neurons to blood vessels; provide structural support
Neuroglia of PNS	
Schwann cells	Form myelin sheath around nerves in PNS; form neurilemma

The Body AT WORK

Star-shaped astrocytes—the most numerous of all glial cells—are pervasive throughout the brain. A tiny "foot" exists at the end of each of the astrocyte's star-like projections. Some of the feet latch onto a capillary while others connect with a neuron. This arrangement allows the astrocyte to funnel glucose from the bloodstream to the neuron for nourishment. What's more, the feet of the astrocytes join with the endothelial cells lining the walls of capillaries to create a semi-permeable membrane called the **blood-brain barrier (BBB)**. *The BBB, which exists throughout the brain, allows small molecules (like oxygen, carbon dioxide, and water) to diffuse across to the brain but blocks larger molecules. This helps protect the brain from foreign substances. However, it also prevents most medications from reaching brain tissue, making treating disorders of the brain challenging.*

Life lesson: Brain tumors

Unlike neurons, which don't undergo mitosis, glial cells retain the ability to divide throughout life. While this allows them to replace worn-out or damaged cells, it also makes them susceptible to tumor formation. In fact, most adult brain tumors consist of glial cells. These types of tumors—called *gliomas*—are highly malignant and grow rapidly. Because of the blood-brain barrier (see "The Body at Work" on this page), most medications aren't effective in treating these tumors, which is why surgery and radiation continue to be treatment mainstays. Certain techniques that may help augment drug delivery to the tumor include administering a concentrated sugar solution to make the BBB permeable, injecting drugs directly into spinal fluid, or implanting a chemotherapy wafer within the brain tissue.

Neurons

Nerve cells called **neurons** handle the nervous system's role of communication. There are three classes of neurons: sensory (afferent) neurons, interneurons, and motor (efferent) neurons. Each neuron type fulfills one of the three general functions of the nervous system.

Sensory neurons

Sensory (afferent) neurons detect stimuli—such as touch, pressure, heat, cold, or chemicals—and then transmit information about the stimuli to the CNS.

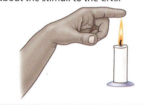

Interneurons

Interneurons, which are found only in the CNS, connect the incoming sensory pathways with the outgoing motor pathways. Besides receiving, processing, and storing information, the connections made by these neurons make each of us unique in how we think, feel, and act.

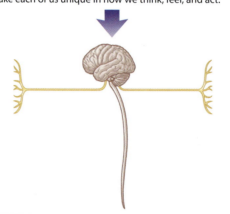

Motor neurons

Motor (efferent) neurons relay messages from the brain (which the brain emits in response to stimuli) to the muscle or gland cells.

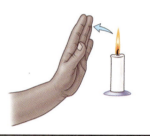

Types of Neurons

Neurons vary greatly in both size and shape. They also vary according to the type, number, and length of projections.

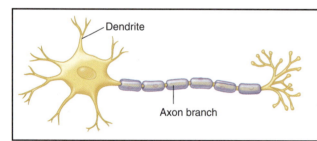

Dendrite

Axon branch

Multipolar neurons

Multipolar neurons have one axon and multiple dendrites. This is the most common type of neuron and includes most neurons of the brain and spinal cord.

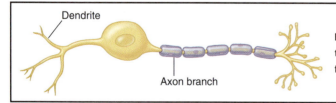

Dendrite

Axon branch

Bipolar neurons

Bipolar neurons have two processes: an axon and a dendrite with the cell body in between the two processes. These neurons can be found in the retina of the eye and olfactory nerve in the nose.

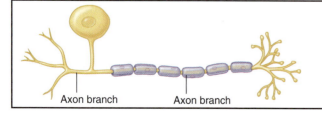

Axon branch

Axon branch

Unipolar neurons

Unipolar neurons have one process—an axon—that extends from the cell body before branching in a T shape. These neurons mostly reside in the sensory nerves of the peripheral nervous system.

FAST FACT

About 90% of the body's neurons are interneurons.

Neuron Structure

Neurons are perhaps the most diverse of all body cells, assuming a variety of shapes and sizes. In general, though, neurons have three basic parts: a cell body and two extensions called an **axon** and a **dendrite**.

The **cell body** (also called the **soma**) is the control center of the neuron and contains the nucleus.

Dendrites, which look like the bare branches of a tree, receive signals from other neurons and conduct the information to the cell body. Some neurons have only one dendrite; others have thousands.

The **axon**, which carries nerve signals away from the cell body, is longer than the dendrites and contains few branches. Nerve cells have only one axon; however, the length of the fiber can range from a few millimeters to as much as a meter.

The axons of many (but not all) neurons are encased in a **myelin sheath**. Consisting mostly of lipid, myelin acts to insulate the axon. In the peripheral nervous system, Schwann cells form the myelin sheath. In the CNS, oligodendrocytes assume this role. (For more information, see "Myelin" on the next page.)

Gaps in the myelin sheath, called **nodes of Ranvier**, occur at evenly spaced intervals.

The end of the axon branches extensively, with each axon terminal ending in a **synaptic knob**. Within the synaptic knobs are vesicles containing a neurotransmitter.

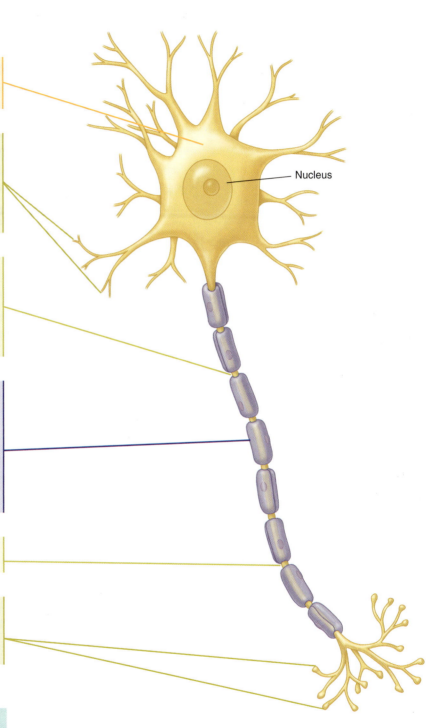

Nucleus

FAST FACT

The sciatic nerve contains the longest axon in the body; it extends from the base of the spine to the big toe in each foot.

Myelin

Not all nerve fibers are myelinated. However, because myelin helps speed impulse conduction, unmyelinated fibers conduct nerve impulses more slowly. Typically, unmyelinated nerve fibers perform functions in which speed isn't essential, such as stimulating the secretion of stomach acid. In contrast, nerve fibers stimulating skeletal muscles, where speed is more important, are myelinated.

In the peripheral nervous system, the myelin sheath is formed when Schwann cells wrap themselves around the axon, laying down multiple layers of cell membrane. It's these inside layers that form the myelin sheath. The nucleus and most of the cytoplasm of the Schwann cell are located in the outermost layer. This outer layer, called the **neurilemma**, is essential for an injured nerve to regenerate.

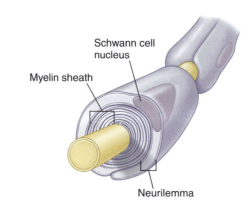

Schwann cell nucleus

Myelin sheath

Neurilemma

In the CNS, the myelin sheath is formed by oligodendrocytes. Unlike Schwann cells—which wrap themselves completely around one axon—one oligodendrocyte forms the myelin sheath for several axons. Specifically, the nucleus of the cell is located away from the myelin sheath and outward projections from the cell wrap around the axons of nearby nerves. As a result, there is no neurilemma, which prevents injured CNS neurons from regenerating. This explains why paralysis resulting from a severed spinal cord is currently permanent, although researchers continue to explore possible solutions.

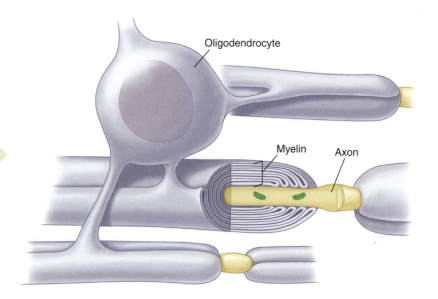

Oligodendrocyte

Myelin

Axon

The Body AT WORK

Although myelination begins during the fourteenth week of fetal development, it is not complete until late adolescence. In fact, at birth, very few of the neurons in a newborn's brain are myelinated. During infancy and childhood, however, myelination proceeds rapidly. For this to occur properly, children need an adequate supply of dietary fat. (Remember: Myelin is mostly fat.) That's why children younger than age two should never be placed on a low-fat diet.

Repair of Nerve Fibers

When nerves are injured (such as from a cut, crushing injury, or some other type of trauma), their ability to repair themselves depends upon the extent of the injury as well as their location. Nerves in the peripheral nervous system can regenerate as long as the soma and neurilemma are intact. Because nerves in the central nervous system lack a neurilemma, they cannot regenerate. Therefore, most injuries to the brain and spinal cord cause permanent damage. The following figures illustrate the repair process in a somatic motor neuron.

1 When a nerve fiber is cut, the distal portion of the axon is separated from its source of nutrition. Consequently, it begins to degenerate along with the myelin sheath and Schwann cells. Macrophages move in to clean up the resulting debris.

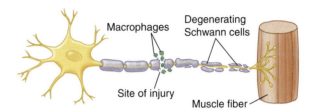

Macrophages   Degenerating Schwann cells

Site of injury   Muscle fiber

2 Because the muscle fibers normally innervated by the nerve are deprived of nervous input, they begin to atrophy, or shrink. Meanwhile, the severed portion of the axon sprouts new growth processes. At the same time, the neurilemma forms a tunnel near the site of the injury; new Schwann cells grow within the tunnel.

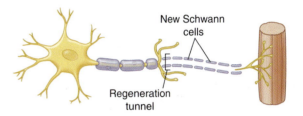

New Schwann cells

Regeneration tunnel

3 When one of the new growth processes finds its way into the tunnel, it begins to grow rapidly (3 to 5 mm/day). At that point, the other growth processes begin to retract.

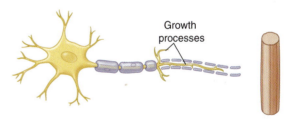

Growth processes

4 The new fiber continues to grow, guided by the tunnel, until it reestablishes contact with the muscle. After that occurs, the reinnervated muscle fibers regrow.

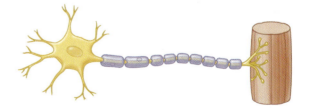

Life lesson: Nerve injuries

When a peripheral nerve is severed, neurosurgeons may try to realign the nerve ends surgically. If the severed ends aren't adjacent to one another, the surgeon may use a nerve or vein graft to bridge the gap. Success with these techniques is variable, however. Another method currently being researched is the use of synthetic guidance channels to help direct newly growing axons. The channels may be implanted empty, or they may be filled with growth factors or neural cells.

Impulse Conduction

To relay messages to organs and tissues throughout the body, nerves must initiate and then transmit signals from one neuron to the next neuron at lightning speed. Signal transmission occurs through an electrical current, which, like all electrical currents, results from the flow of charged particles from one point to another.

In the body, whenever ions with opposite electrical charges are separated by a membrane, the potential exists for them to move toward one another (depending, of course, upon the permeability of the membrane). This is called **membrane potential**. A membrane that exhibits membrane potential—an excess of positive ions on one side of the membrane and an excess of negative ions on the other side—is said to be **polarized**.

ANIMATION

1 Resting potential

- Inside of cell has negative charge; outside has positive charge
- Exterior rich in Na$^+$; interior rich in K$^+$

When a neuron is not conducting an electrical signal, its interior has a negative electrical charge, while the charge on the outside is positive. The outside of the cell is rich with sodium ions (Na$^+$) while the inside contains an abundance of potassium ions (K$^+$). The interior of the cell contains other ions as well, particularly large, negatively charged proteins and nucleic acids. These additional particles give the cell's interior its overall negative charge. Because of the membrane's permeability, a certain amount of sodium and potassium ions leak across the membrane. However, the sodium-potassium pump constantly works to restore the ions to the appropriate side. (For more information on the sodium-potassium pump, see Chapter 3, *Cells*.) This state of being inactive and polarized is called **resting potential**. The neuron is resting, but it has the potential to react if a stimulus comes along.

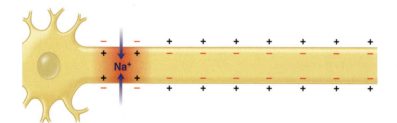

2 Depolarization

- Stimulus causes Na$^+$ to enter cell
- Region of interior changes from negative to positive

When a stimulus (such as chemicals, heat, or mechanical pressure) comes along, channels on the resting neuron's membrane open and the Na$^+$ from outside the membrane rushes into the cell. The addition of all these positively charged ions changes the charge of a region of the cell's interior from negative to positive. As the membrane becomes more positive, it is said to **depolarize**.

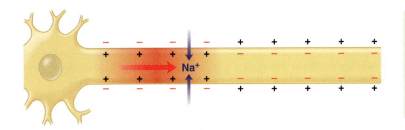

3 Action potential
- Channels in adjacent areas open and more Na⁺ enters the cell
- Nerve impulse continues down the length of the axon

If the depolarization is strong enough—in other words, if the stimulus goes above what's known as the threshold level—adjacent channels also open, allowing even more Na⁺ to flood the cell's interior. This creates an **action potential**, meaning that the neuron has become active as it conducts an impulse along the axon. Another term for action potential is *nerve impulse*. The action potential continues down the axon as one segment stimulates the segment next to it.

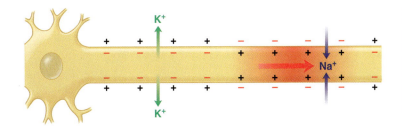

4 Repolarization
- K⁺ flows out of cell
- Electrical balance restored: interior has negative charge and exterior has positive charge

Meanwhile, the sudden influx of Na⁺ triggers the opening of other channels to allow K⁺ to flow out of the cell. Soon after K⁺ begins to exit, the Na⁺ channels shut to prevent any more Na⁺ from flowing into the cell. This **repolarizes** the cell; however, Na⁺ and K⁺ are now flip-flopped, with the outside containing more K⁺ and the inside containing more Na⁺.

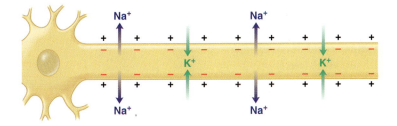

5 Refractory period
- Membrane is polarized, but Na⁺ and K⁺ are on wrong sides of membrane
- Sodium-potassium pump works to restore ions to rightful sides

Although the membrane is polarized, the neuron won't respond to a new stimulus as long as the Na⁺ and K⁺ are on the wrong sides of the membrane. This is known as the **refractory period.** The sodium-potassium pump works to return Na⁺ to the outside and K⁺ to the inside. When this is completed, the nerve is again polarized and in resting potential until it receives another stimulus.

The Body AT WORK

Action potential is an "all or nothing" event. When a stimulus reaches a threshold and depolarizes the neuron, the neuron fires at its maximum voltage. If the stimulus doesn't reach the threshold, the neuron doesn't fire at all. What's more, a stronger stimulus doesn't produce a stronger response. In this way, as each neuron segment triggers firing in the segment next to it, the nerve impulse continues at the same strength all the way to the synaptic knobs.

Impulse Conduction in Myelinated Fibers

Nerve impulses move through unmyelinated fibers as previously described. In myelinated fibers, however, the thick layer of myelin encasing the axons of most nerve fibers blocks the free movement of ions across the cell membrane. The only place ion exchange can occur is at the nodes of Ranvier: the evenly spaced gaps in myelin. The following illustration shows how a nerve impulse travels down a myelinated fiber.

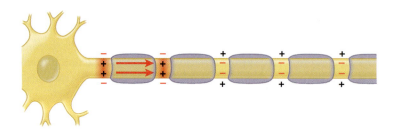

Electrical changes occur at the nodes of Ranvier, creating an action potential. The current flows under the myelin sheath to the next node, where it triggers another action potential.

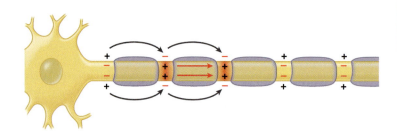

This process continues as the signal moves down the axon. Because the action potentials occur only at the nodes, the impulse seems to "leap" from node to node. This type of signal conduction is called **saltatory conduction**. (The word *saltatory* comes from the Latin word *saltare*, which means "to leap.")

> **FAST FACT**
> Neurons can transmit impulses amazingly fast: up to 120 meters per second (268 miles per hour).

Life lesson: Multiple sclerosis

Multiple sclerosis (MS) is a disease in which the myelin sheaths surrounding the nerves of the CNS deteriorate and are replaced by hard scar tissue (called plaques). These changes disrupt nerve conduction and cause symptoms that vary, depending upon which nerves are affected. Common symptoms include visual disturbances (such as blindness or double vision), weakness, loss of coordination, and speech disturbances. The disease progresses over many years; symptoms typically improve and then worsen in unpredictable cycles. MS tends to strike women between the ages of 20 and 40 years. Although the exact cause is unknown, experts speculate that a virus may trigger an autoimmune reaction in which the patient's immune system attacks the myelin of the CNS. There is no known cure.

Synapses

Nerve impulses usually travel through several different neurons before reaching their target organ or tissue. For this to happen, the impulse must have some way of transferring from one neuron to the next. The area where this occurs is called a **synapse**. Chapter 9 discussed the synapses that occur between nerves and muscles; now we'll examine the synapses that occur between two neurons.

Some synapses (such as those between cardiac muscle cells and certain types of smooth tissue cells) are electrical. In these instances, adjacent neurons touch, which allows an action potential to pass smoothly from one neuron to the next. More commonly, synapses are chemical. In these instances, the two neurons don't touch. Instead, a chemical called a neurotransmitter bridges a very narrow gap (the synaptic cleft) to carry the message from the first neuron (the **presynaptic neuron**) to the next (the **postsynaptic neuron**). Although greatly simplified, here's what basically happens:

ANIMATION

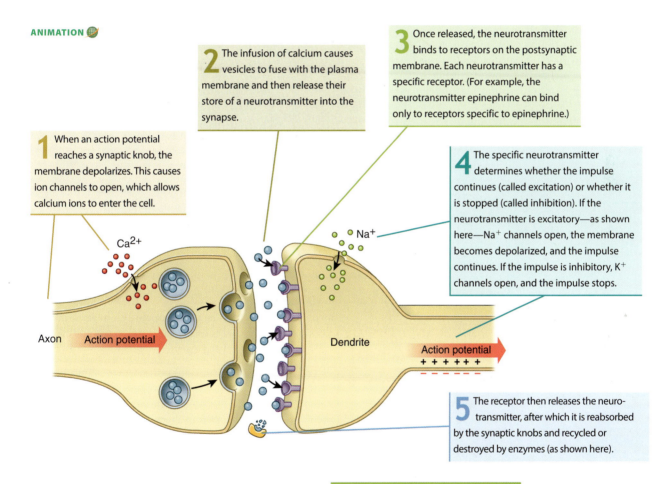

2 The infusion of calcium causes vesicles to fuse with the plasma membrane and then release their store of a neurotransmitter into the synapse.

3 Once released, the neurotransmitter binds to receptors on the postsynaptic membrane. Each neurotransmitter has a specific receptor. (For example, the neurotransmitter epinephrine can bind only to receptors specific to epinephrine.)

1 When an action potential reaches a synaptic knob, the membrane depolarizes. This causes ion channels to open, which allows calcium ions to enter the cell.

4 The specific neurotransmitter determines whether the impulse continues (called excitation) or whether it is stopped (called inhibition). If the neurotransmitter is excitatory—as shown here—Na^+ channels open, the membrane becomes depolarized, and the impulse continues. If the impulse is inhibitory, K^+ channels open, and the impulse stops.

Ca^{2+}

Na^+

Axon   Action potential

Dendrite   Action potential
+ + + + + +

5 The receptor then releases the neurotransmitter, after which it is reabsorbed by the synaptic knobs and recycled or destroyed by enzymes (as shown here).

FAST FACT

Scientists have discovered more than 100 different neurotransmitters in the human body. Some common neurotransmitters include acetylcholine, epinephrine, norepinephrine, serotonin, dopamine, and histamine.

FAST FACT

One neuron can have multiple synapses. In fact, in a particular portion of the brain, one neuron can have up to 100,000 synapses.

SPINAL CORD AND SOMATIC REFLEXES

The spinal cord is the information passageway that relays messages from the brain to the rest of the body. Thirty-one pairs of spinal nerves branch out from the spinal cord, linking it to the far reaches of the body. Although the spinal cord is part of the central nervous system and the peripheral nerves are part of the peripheral nervous system, the two are inseparable.

FAST FACT
The spinal cord is as wide as your finger and extends for about 17" (43 cm).

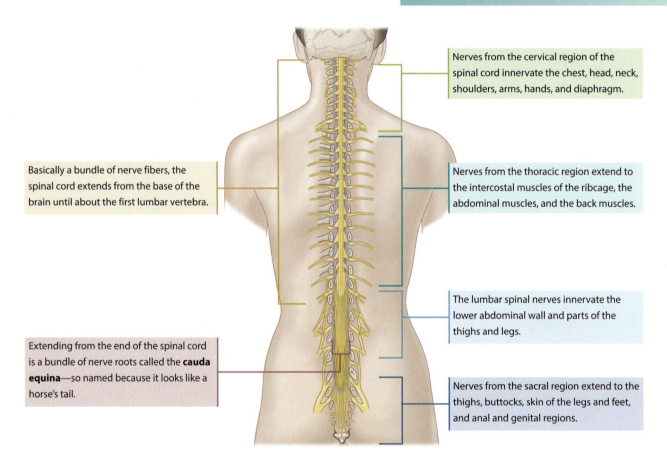

Nerves from the cervical region of the spinal cord innervate the chest, head, neck, shoulders, arms, hands, and diaphragm.

Basically a bundle of nerve fibers, the spinal cord extends from the base of the brain until about the first lumbar vertebra.

Nerves from the thoracic region extend to the intercostal muscles of the ribcage, the abdominal muscles, and the back muscles.

The lumbar spinal nerves innervate the lower abdominal wall and parts of the thighs and legs.

Extending from the end of the spinal cord is a bundle of nerve roots called the **cauda equina**—so named because it looks like a horse's tail.

Nerves from the sacral region extend to the thighs, buttocks, skin of the legs and feet, and anal and genital regions.

The Body AT WORK

Early in fetal development, the spinal cord extends all the way down the vertebral column. However, the vertebral column grows faster than the spinal cord and, by the time a baby is born, the spinal cord ends at about the level of L3. By adulthood, the spinal cord extends only as far as L1. This explains why lumbar punctures (procedures in which a needle is inserted into spinal canal to withdraw cerebrospinal fluid for analysis) are performed between L3 and L4. At that location, there's no danger of nicking the spinal cord with the needle.

Structure of the Spinal Cord

The spinal cord sits inside a protective, bony tunnel created by the stacked vertebrae. A cross section clearly shows the two types of nervous tissue (white matter and gray matter) that make up the spinal cord.

Gray matter—which appears gray because of its lack of myelin—contains mostly the cells bodies of motor neurons and interneurons. This H-shaped mass is divided into two sets of horns: the **posterior (dorsal) horns** and the **ventral (anterior) horns**.

A small space—called the **epidural space**—lies between the outer covering of the spinal cord and the vertebrae; it contains a cushioning layer of fat as well as blood vessels and connective tissue.

White matter appears white because of its abundance of myelin. It contains bundles of axons (called **tracts**) that carry impulses from one part of the nervous system to another.

A minute opening called the **central canal** carries cerebrospinal fluid through the spinal cord.

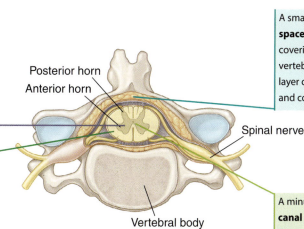

Posterior horn
Anterior horn
Spinal nerve
Vertebral body

Attachment of Spinal Nerves

Spinal nerves travel through gaps between the vertebrae (which are held apart by intervertebral discs) and attach to the spinal cord by way of two roots: the dorsal and the ventral roots.

The **dorsal (posterior) nerve root** contains fibers that carry sensory information into the spinal cord. It enters the dorsal horn of the spinal cord.

Cell bodies of the dorsal neurons are clustered in a knot-like structure called a **ganglion**.

A **spinal nerve** is a single nerve resulting from the fusion of the dorsal and ventral nerve roots. Because the nerve contains both sensory and motor fibers—meaning it can transmit impulses in two directions—it's called a **mixed nerve**.

Fibers in the **ventral (anterior) nerve roots** exit from the ventral horn to carry motor information out of the spinal cord.

Meninges of the Spinal Cord

In addition to the bony protection offered by the vertebrae, the spinal cord is further protected by three layers of fibrous connective tissue, called the meninges. (The meninges also covers the brain.) The three layers of the meninges, from the inside out, are the pia mater, the arachnoid mater, and the dura mater.

The **pia mater** is the innermost layer. This transparent membrane clings to the outer surface of the brain and spinal cord. It also contains blood vessels.

The **subarachnoid space** lies between the arachnoid mater and the pia mater. It is filled with cerebrospinal fluid.

The **arachnoid mater**—a delicate layer resembling a cobweb—lies between the dura mater and the pia mater.

The **dura mater** is the tough outer layer.

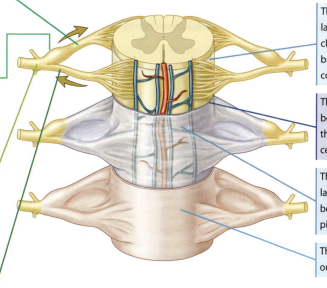

Spinal Tracts

Within the white matter of the spinal cord are bundles of axons called **tracts** that serve as the routes of communication to and from the brain. All the nerve fibers of a single tract have a similar origination, destination, and function. As an example, the fibers of the spinothalamic tract originate in the spinal cord (*spino-*) and end in the thalamus (*thalamic*). In addition, they all convey sensations of pain, touch, and temperature to the thalamus in the brain.

Some of the most important tracts are highlighted in the figure below. *Note:* All tracts exist on both sides of the spinal cord, but, in this illustration, the ascending tracts are highlighted on the left and the descending tracts on the right.

 Ascending tracts convey *sensory* signals (such as pain) *up* the spinal cord to the brain.

Descending tracts conduct motor impulses down the spinal cord to skeletal muscles.

The **dorsal column** relays sensations of deep pressure and vibration as well as those needed to create awareness of the body's position (proprioception).

The **corticospinal tracts** (also called the **pyramidal tracts**) are responsible for fine movements of hands, fingers, feet, and toes on the opposite side of the body.

The **spinocerebellar tract** is responsible for proprioception.

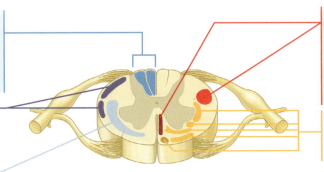

The **extrapyramidal tracts** are a group of tracts associated with balance and muscle tone.

The **spinothalamic tract** relays sensations of temperature, pressure, pain, and touch.

The Body AT WORK

*Most of the spinal cord tracts cross from one side of the body to the other in the brainstem. This is called **decussation**. For example, sensory signals from the right side of the body are sent to the left side of the brain. Also, motor signals being sent to the right side of the body originate on the left side of the brain. This is why someone who suffers a stroke affecting motor centers in the left side of the brain will have weakness or paralysis on the right side of the body and vice versa.*

That Makes Sense

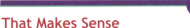

*To remember the difference between ascending and descending tracts, think about this: When you step on a nail, the **sensation** of pain **ascends** to your brain. (Ascending: sensory.) In response, your brain issues an impulse that travels **down** to your foot, telling you to **move**. (Descending: motor.)*

FAST FACT
All the axons in a given tract serve one general function.

Life lesson: Spinal cord injury

Over 10,000 people in the United States suffer from spinal cord injuries each year. Males between the ages of 16 and 30 have the greatest risk, mainly because of their tendency for high-risk behaviors. Most injuries result from car and motorcycle accidents.

If the spinal cord is severed—often because of a vertebral fracture—it causes a loss of movement and sensation below the level of the injury. For example, a spinal cord injury between the levels of T1 and L1 causes paralysis in the legs (*paraplegia*); an injury above the C5 vertebra causes paralysis in all the limbs (*quadriplegia*). An injury above C4 is especially serious because this is where the phrenic nerve exits the spinal cord. Because the phrenic nerve innervates the diaphragm, an injury here can cause respiratory failure.

Spinal Nerves

Spinal nerves (part of the peripheral nervous system) relay information from the spinal cord to the rest of the body.

A **nerve** consists of many nerve fibers (axons) encased by connective tissue. The number of nerve fibers contained in a single nerve varies from a few to as many as a million. (Remember: A neuron is a nerve cell; a nerve contains many neurons.)

Nerve fibers are gathered together in bundles called **fascicles**; in turn, several fascicles are grouped together—along with blood vessels—and wrapped in a dense connective tissue.

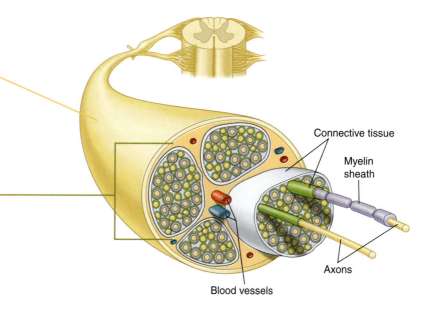

Connective tissue

Myelin sheath

Axons

Blood vessels

Most nerves contain both sensory and motor fibers and are called **mixed nerves**. These nerves can transmit signals in two directions. A few nerves (such as the optic nerves) are **sensory nerves** and contain only sensory (afferent) fibers. They carry sensations toward the spinal cord. Others are **motor nerves** and contain only motor (efferent) fibers and carry messages to muscles and glands.

That Makes Sense

To make sense of the terms used for nerves and nerve tracts, think about this: Sensation always travels toward the CNS. Sensory nerves transmit impulses toward the spinal cord; once there, they travel up the spinal cord (ascend) along the ascending tract. As a further hint, remember that **a**fferent *(sensory) nerves link to the* **a**scending *tract. Motor nerves carry messages about movement; therefore, those impulses leave (or* **e**xit*) the spinal cord along* **e**fferent *(motor) nerves.*

Categories of Spinal Nerves

Thirty-one pairs of spinal nerves connect to the spinal cord. They include:

- 8 cervical nerves (C1-C8)
- 12 thoracic nerves (T1-T12)
- 5 lumbar nerves (L1-L5)
- 5 sacral nerves (S1-S5)
- 1 coccygeal nerve (Co)

The first cervical nerve exits the spinal cord between the skull and the axis. The other nerves pass through holes in the vertebra (intervertebral foramina).

Once outside the spinal column, each spinal nerve forms several large branches. Some of these branches subdivide further to form nerve networks called plexuses. The four major plexuses are the cervical plexus, the brachial plexus, the lumbar plexus, and the sacral plexus.

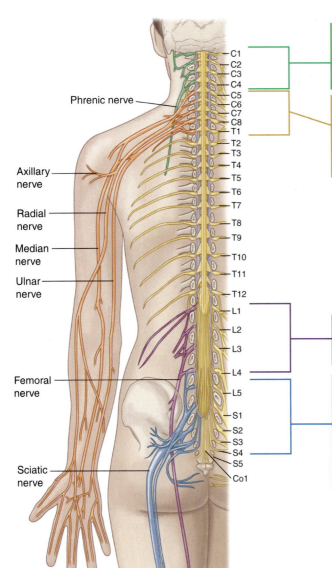

The **cervical plexus** contains nerves that supply the muscles and skin of the neck, tops of the shoulders, and part of the head. The **phrenic nerve**, which stimulates the diaphragm for breathing, is located here.

The **brachial plexus** innervates the lower part of the shoulder and the arm. Key nerves traveling into the arm from this region include the **axillary nerve** (which passes close to the armpit, making it susceptible to damage from the use of crutches), the **radial nerve**, the **ulnar nerve**, and the **median nerve**.

The **lumbar plexus**—derived from the fibers of the first four lumbar vertebrae—supplies the thigh and leg. A key nerve in this region is the large **femoral nerve**.

The **sacral plexus** is formed from fibers from nerves L4, L5, and S1 through S4. (Because of the co-mingling of fibers of the sacral plexus with those of the lumbar plexus, these two plexuses are often referred to as the *lumbosacral plexus*.) The **sciatic nerve**, the largest nerve in the body, arises here and runs down the back of the thigh. Irritation of this nerve causes severe pain down the back of the leg, a condition called *sciatica*.

Dermatomes

Each spinal nerve (except for C1) innervates a specific area of the skin. These areas are called **dermatomes**. Clinicians use this information to identify the location of a nerve abnormality by testing a patient's response to pinpricks in the different areas.

The Body AT WORK

Your ability to stand, walk, and correct your balance can all be attributed to reflexes. Specifically, skeletal muscles contain sensory receptors that send messages to the brain about the amount of stretch in a muscle as well as the movement of body parts. This allows the brain to emit signals to correct muscle tone and control movement; it also allows it to trigger a reflex to correct posture. For example, keeping your balance can be attributed to the reflexive contracting and relaxing of various muscles—all without your awareness.

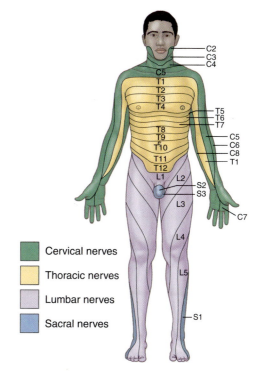

Cervical nerves

Thoracic nerves

Lumbar nerves

Sacral nerves

Somatic Reflexes

Reflexes are a quick, involuntary, predictable response to a stimulus. Reflexes employ a neural circuit called a **reflex arc**, which bypasses regions of the brain where conscious decisions are made. That's why someone becomes aware of a reflex only after it's occurred. Some reflexes—called autonomic (visceral) reflexes—involve secretion from glands or the contraction of smooth muscle (such as dilation of the pupil). These reflexes are governed by autonomic neurons, which will be discussed later in this chapter.

Somatic reflexes involve the contraction of a skeletal muscle after being stimulated by a somatic motor neuron. Somatic reflexes often help protect the body against harm—such as causing you to withdraw your hand from a hot stove. Other reflexes help you maintain your posture. (See "The Body at Work" on this page.) Several reflexes (such as the patellar reflex, described below) are commonly tested during physical exams to identify certain diseases.

ANIMATION

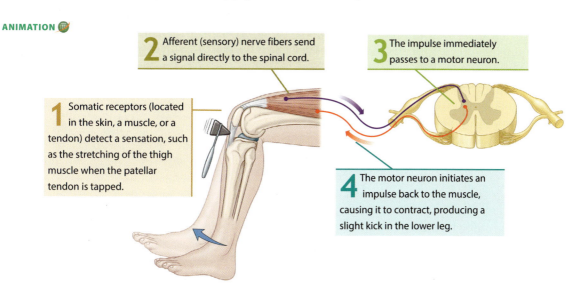

2 Afferent (sensory) nerve fibers send a signal directly to the spinal cord.

3 The impulse immediately passes to a motor neuron.

1 Somatic receptors (located in the skin, a muscle, or a tendon) detect a sensation, such as the stretching of the thigh muscle when the patellar tendon is tapped.

4 The motor neuron initiates an impulse back to the muscle, causing it to contract, producing a slight kick in the lower leg.

THE BRAIN AND CRANIAL NERVES

The brain is the site for thought, learning, reasoning, memory, and creativity. Indeed, the brain performs numerous amazing functions, many of which remain beyond our grasp.

General Structures of the Brain

The brain is divided into four major regions: the cerebrum, the diencephalon, the cerebellum, and the brainstem.

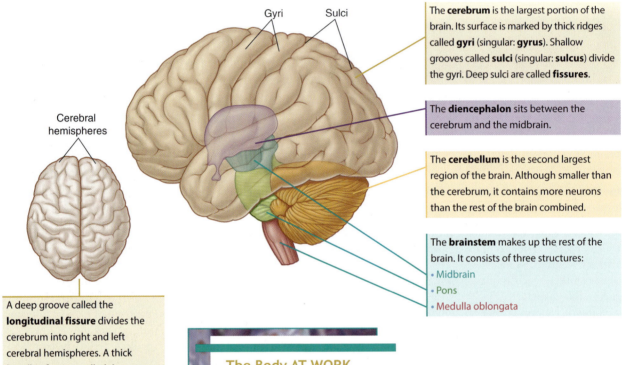

Gyri

Sulci

The **cerebrum** is the largest portion of the brain. Its surface is marked by thick ridges called **gyri** (singular: **gyrus**). Shallow grooves called **sulci** (singular: **sulcus**) divide the gyri. Deep sulci are called **fissures**.

Cerebral hemispheres

The **diencephalon** sits between the cerebrum and the midbrain.

The **cerebellum** is the second largest region of the brain. Although smaller than the cerebrum, it contains more neurons than the rest of the brain combined.

The **brainstem** makes up the rest of the brain. It consists of three structures:
• Midbrain
• Pons
• Medulla oblongata

A deep groove called the **longitudinal fissure** divides the cerebrum into right and left cerebral hemispheres. A thick bundle of nerves called the **corpus callosum** runs along the bottom of the fissure and serves to connect the two hemispheres.

The Body AT WORK

Because the brain's gray matter (the part charged with thought, learning, and reasoning) is located at its surface, the folds allow more gray matter to be packed into the small area of the skull. (As an analogy, think of fitting a large piece of paper into a small space: it becomes possible if you crunch it into a ball.) Scientists have long thought that the brain's folds explain why humans are more intelligent than species with smoother brains. Recent discoveries have revealed that the folding pattern varies with each individual, making a person's brain folds as unique as his fingerprints. What's more, scientists have discovered abnormal folding patterns in those suffering from a variety of mental and neurodevelopment disorders, ranging from depression to autism.

Gray and White Matter

Like the spinal cord, the brain contains both gray and white matter. Unlike the spinal cord (in which gray matter forms the interior), in the brain, gray matter forms the surface. Specifically, gray matter (consisting of cell bodies and interneurons) covers the cerebrum and cerebellum in a layer called the **cortex**. Underneath the cortex is white matter, although gray matter exists in patches called **nuclei** throughout the white matter. The white matter contains bundles of axons that connect one part of the brain to another.

Meninges of the Brain

Like the spinal cord, meninges covers the outside surface of the brain, offering protection. Nearby bone also helps protect the brain from trauma.

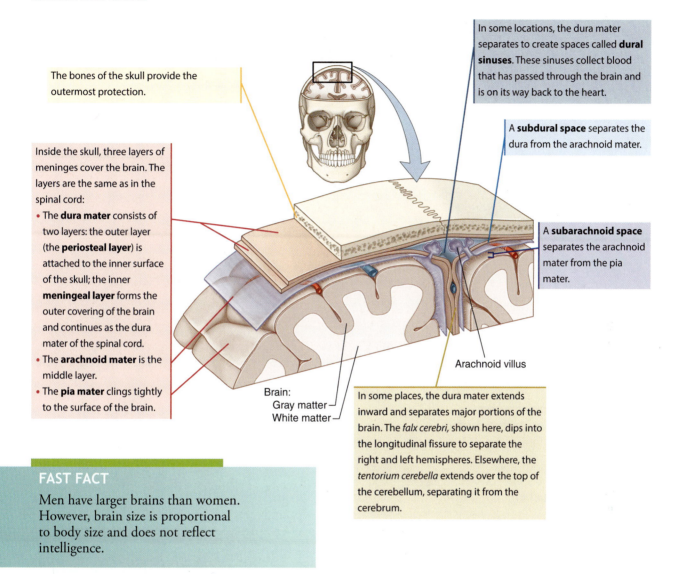

In some locations, the dura mater separates to create spaces called **dural sinuses**. These sinuses collect blood that has passed through the brain and is on its way back to the heart.

A **subdural space** separates the dura from the arachnoid mater.

The bones of the skull provide the outermost protection.

A **subarachnoid space** separates the arachnoid mater from the pia mater.

Inside the skull, three layers of meninges cover the brain. The layers are the same as in the spinal cord:

- The **dura mater** consists of two layers: the outer layer (the **periosteal layer**) is attached to the inner surface of the skull; the inner **meningeal layer** forms the outer covering of the brain and continues as the dura mater of the spinal cord.
- The **arachnoid mater** is the middle layer.
- The **pia mater** clings tightly to the surface of the brain.

Brain:
Gray matter
White matter

Arachnoid villus

In some places, the dura mater extends inward and separates major portions of the brain. The *falx cerebri*, shown here, dips into the longitudinal fissure to separate the right and left hemispheres. Elsewhere, the *tentorium cerebella* extends over the top of the cerebellum, separating it from the cerebrum.

FAST FACT

Men have larger brains than women. However, brain size is proportional to body size and does not reflect intelligence.

Life lesson: Meningitis

Infection or inflammation of the meninges is called *meningitis*. Infection may be caused by several different bacteria or viruses that gain entry to the central nervous system by spreading from other locations in the body, such as from an ear or sinus infection. Bacterial meningitis occurs less frequently than viral meningitis, but it can be life-threatening without immediate treatment.

Symptoms of meningitis include fever, stiff neck, irritability, headache, drowsiness, and seizures. Infants with meningitis may have different symptoms, including poor feeding, bulging fontanelles, and a high-pitched cry. Viral meningitis usually causes milder symptoms, such as those similar to a cold or the flu. In fact, viral meningitis often goes undiagnosed because the symptoms are so mild.

To diagnose meningitis, a sample of cerebrospinal fluid is obtained through a lumbar puncture. The fluid is then examined for bacteria and white blood cells, a sign of inflammation. Viral meningitis usually resolves on its own in 7 to 10 days, while bacterial meningitis requires hospitalization and treatment with intravenous antibiotics.

Ventricles

The brain contains four chambers, called ventricles.

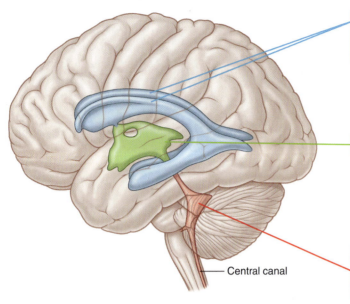

Two **lateral ventricles** arch through the cerebral hemispheres: one in the right hemisphere and one in the left.

Each of the lateral ventricles connects to a **third ventricle**.

Central canal

A canal then leads to the **fourth ventricle**. This space narrows to form the central canal, which extends through the spinal cord.

Cerebrospinal Fluid

A clear, colorless fluid called **cerebrospinal fluid (CSF)** fills the ventricles and central canal; it also bathes the outside of the brain and spinal cord. CSF is formed from blood by the **choroid plexus** (a network of blood vessels lining the floor or wall of each ventricle).

The Body AT WORK

The brain produces about 500 ml of CSF each day; however, much of that is reabsorbed. At any one time, an adult brain contains about 140 ml of CSF. CSF is not stagnant; rather, it constantly flows through the central nervous system, providing nourishment in the form of glucose and protein and helping to remove metabolic wastes.

CSF plays other roles as well. For example, CSF helps protect the brain against minor trauma: When the head is jolted, CSF acts as a cushion to keep the brain from striking the inside of the skull. In addition, CSF plays a role in the maintenance of homeostasis. Specifically, the brain monitors the level of CO_2 in CSF and triggers responses as needed to help the body regain equilibrium.

FAST FACT

Although the brain constitutes only 2% of an adult's body weight, it receives 15% of the blood and consumes 20% of the body's oxygen and glucose.

Life lesson: Hydrocephalus

If the flow of CSF becomes blocked anywhere on its route, the fluid accumulates in the brain's ventricles. This condition is called *hydrocephalus*, or, more commonly, "water on the brain." The accumulating CSF causes the ventricles to expand. In an infant whose cranial bones haven't fused, the entire head expands. An adult, however, has no such "release valve." In this situation, the expanding ventricles compress the brain tissue against the sides of the skull and intracranial pressure rises. Untreated, the condition can prove fatal. It can, however, be successfully treated by inserting a tube, or shunt, to drain fluid from the ventricles into a vein in the neck.

Formation and Flow of CSF

ANIMATION 🌐

1 The choroid plexus in each lateral ventricle secretes CSF.

2 The CSF flows into the third ventricle, where another choroid plexus adds more fluid.

3 It then flows into the fourth ventricle, where still more CSF is added by the choroid plexus in that ventricle.

4 Some of the CSF moves into the central canal of the spinal cord. Most flows through two tiny openings (foramina) into a space leading to the subarachnoid space.

5 The CSF then flows through the subarachnoid space, up the back of the brain, down around the spinal cord, and up the front of the brain.

6 The CSF is reabsorbed into the venous bloodstream by projections of the arachnoid mater into the dural sinuses (called **arachnoid villi**).

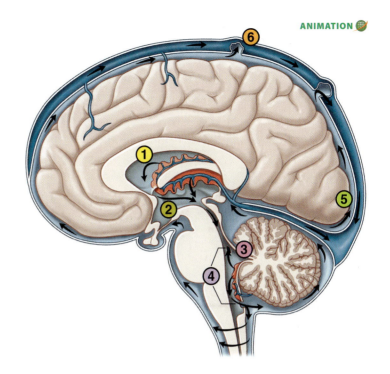

Blood-Brain Barrier

The brain demands a high volume of blood to function properly. However, blood also contains substances such as antibodies and macrophages that would harm the brain. As a means of protection, a **blood-brain barrier** serves to restrict what substances can pass from the bloodstream into the tissue fluid of the brain. This barrier consists mainly of capillaries formed by tightly joined endothelial cells (as opposed to the loosely overlapping cells that form the capillaries in general circulation). A thick basement membrane adds to the barrier, as do the feet of astrocytes, which reach out and surround the endothelial cells. This arrangement creates a semi-permeable membrane throughout the brain. As discussed previously, the membrane allows small molecules (like oxygen, carbon dioxide, and water) to diffuse across to the brain but blocks larger molecules. Other substances that can diffuse across the barrier include alcohol, nicotine, caffeine, and anesthetics. Trauma or inflammation can damage the blood-brain barrier and allow pathogens to enter. (For more information, see "The Body at Work" under the section on neuroglia on page 161.)

FAST FACT

The circulation of CSF is aided by pulsations in the choroid plexus and by the motion of the cilia of ependymal cells.

FAST FACT

An interruption in the flow of blood to the brain for as little as 10 seconds causes unconsciousness; an interruption for 4 minutes produces irreparable brain damage.

Divisions of the Brain

The divisions of the brain, starting at the bottom, are the brainstem, cerebellum, diencephalon, and cerebrum.

Brainstem

The brainstem consists of the midbrain, pons, and medulla oblongata.

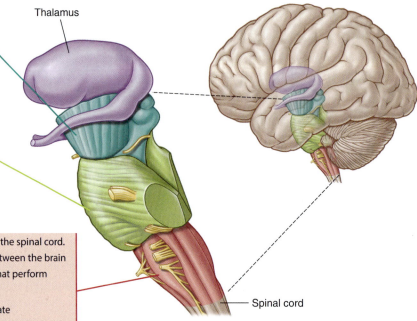

Thalamus

The **midbrain** contains tracts that relay sensory and motor impulses. It also contains centers for auditory and visual reflexes as well as clusters of neurons integral to muscle control.

The **pons** contains tracts that convey signals to and from different parts of the brain. Several cranial nerves arise from this area; they include cranial nerves V (trigeminal), VI (abducens), VII (facial), and VIII (vestibulocochlear). (The cranial nerves will be discussed later in this chapter.)

The **medulla oblongata** attaches the brain to the spinal cord. Besides relaying sensory and motor signals between the brain and spinal cord, the medulla contains nuclei that perform functions vital to human life. These include:

- The **cardiac center**, which regulates heart rate
- The **vasomotor center**, which controls blood vessel diameter, which, in turn, affects blood pressure
- Two **respiratory centers**, which regulate breathing

The medulla also houses reflex centers for coughing, sneezing, swallowing, and vomiting. Several cranial nerves (cranial nerve IX [glossopharyngeal], X [vagus], XI [accessory], and XII [hypoglossal]) either begin or end in the medulla.

Spinal cord

FAST FACT

Because the medulla contains centers that regulate heart rate, blood pressure, and breathing, an injury here—such as from a blow to the base of the skull—can prove fatal.

Cerebellum

About the size of a fist, the cerebellum houses more neurons than the rest of the brain combined. Connected to the cerebral cortex by approximately 40 million neurons, the cerebellum receives, and processes, messages from all over the brain. Long known to play a key role in motor functions, recent discoveries show that the cerebellum assumes a powerful role in sensory, cognitive, and even emotional functions as well. In brief, the cerebellum:

- Joins forces with the cerebral cortex to monitor body movements and send messages crucial for balance, coordination, and posture
- Stores the information necessary for muscle groups to work together to perform smooth, efficient, and coordinated movements
- Evaluates sensory input, such as touch, spatial perception, and sound

People with cerebellar dysfunction (such as from a tumor, hemorrhage, or trauma) have a spastic gait, poor balance, jerky movements, and tremors. They also tend to have poor impulse control and overreact emotionally.

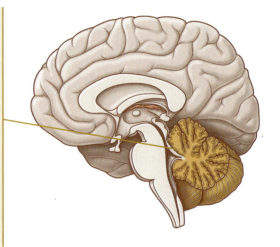

Diencephalon

The diencephalon is a region deep inside the brain consisting of several structures, with the chief ones being the thalamus and the hypothalamus.

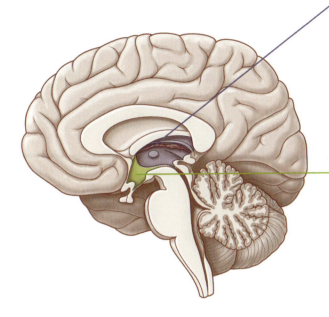

Thalamus

Shaped like two eggs sitting side by side, the **thalamus** resides on the top of the brainstem. It acts as a gateway for nearly every sensory impulse (including smell, sight, taste, pain, pressure, heat, cold, and touch) travelling to the cerebral cortex. The thalamus processes and filters these impulses, transmitting some, but not all, to the cerebral cortex.

The thalamus plays other roles as well. For example, it relays messages regarding certain complex movements; it also is involved in memory and emotion.

Hypothalamus

The **hypothalamus'** small size belies its crucial function. In fact, this tiny area of the brain extends its influence to nearly every organ of the body. The hypothalamus plays a key role in numerous functions. For example, it:

- Controls the autonomic nervous system (which is responsible for such vital functions as heart rate and blood pressure)

- Contains centers responsible for hunger, thirst, and temperature regulation

- Controls the pituitary gland—often called the "master gland" because of its influence on most endocrine glands (such as the thyroid, testes, ovaries, and adrenal glands)

- Is involved in multiple emotional responses, including fear, anger, pleasure, and aggression

The Body AT WORK

*Scattered throughout the brainstem is a set of interconnected nuclei called the **reticular formation**. Fibers extend from there to many parts of the cerebrum, the cerebellum, and the spinal cord. One component of the reticular formation is the **reticular activating system (RAS).** Charged with maintaining a state of wakefulness and alertness, the RAS receives sensory input from the eyes and ears. After filtering out insignificant signals (such as routine noise), it sends impulses to the cerebral cortex so the mind remains conscious and alert. Drugs that depress the reticular activating system induce sleep.*

The reticular formation also has tracts extending into the spinal cord that are involved in posture and equilibrium. Other components of the reticular formation include the cardiac and vasomotor centers of the medulla oblongata, which are responsible for heart rate and blood pressure.

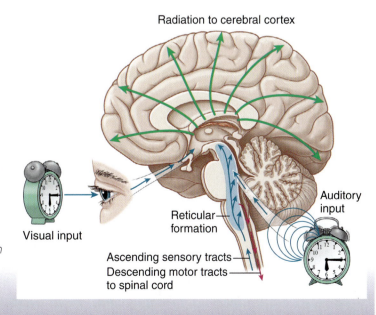

Radiation to cerebral cortex

Visual input

Auditory input

Reticular formation

Ascending sensory tracts

Descending motor tracts to spinal cord

Cerebrum

The largest, and most obvious, portion of the brain is the **cerebrum**. Your ability to think, remember, feel, use judgment, and move can be credited to the cerebrum.

Some of the more obvious sulci (grooves) divide the cerebrum into five distinct lobes. Each lobe is named for the bones of the skull that lie directly over them.

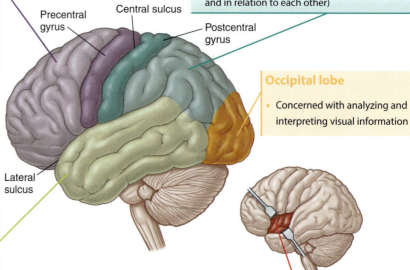

Frontal lobe
- Central sulcus forms the posterior boundary
- Governs voluntary movements, memory, emotion, social judgment, decision making, reasoning, and aggression; is also the site for certain aspects of one's personality

Parietal lobe
- Central sulcus forms the anterior boundary
- Concerned with receiving and interpreting bodily sensations (such as touch, temperature, pressure, and pain); also governs proprioception (the awareness of one's body and body parts in space and in relation to each other)

Occipital lobe
- Concerned with analyzing and interpreting visual information

Temporal lobe
- Separated from the parietal lobe by the lateral sulcus
- Governs hearing, smell, learning, memory, emotional behavior, and visual recognition

Insula
- Hidden behind the lateral sulcus
- Plays a role in many different functions, including perception, motor control, self-awareness, and cognitive functioning

Precentral gyrus · Central sulcus · Postcentral gyrus · Lateral sulcus

FAST FACT

If the brain's surface were flattened, it would measure about 465 square inches (3000 cm^2), or about the size of an opened newspaper.

Life lesson: Brain lesions

The symptoms resulting from injuries to key areas of the brain have been a primary source of information about the role those areas play. Following are some examples of symptoms that may occur following trauma or stroke to specific brain regions.

- *Parietal lobe lesion:* Dysfunction in this part of the brain causes people to ignore objects on the opposite side of the body—even their own arm and leg. Patients may dress only half their body and even deny that the opposite arm or leg belongs to them.
- *Temporal lobe lesion:* An injury here can impair the ability to identify familiar objects. Some may not even recognize their own face. In other instances, the person may lose the ability to differentiate between sounds, causing him to lose any appreciation of music.
- *Frontal lobe lesion:* A lesion or injury here can result in severe personality disorders and cause socially inappropriate behavior.

Inside the Cerebrum

The bulk of the cerebrum is **white matter**, which consists of bundles of myelinated nerve fibers, called tracts. Tracts carry impulses from one part of the cerebrum to the other, or from the cerebrum to other parts of the brain or spinal cord.

Most of the tracts that pass from one hemisphere to the other travel through a large "bridge" called the **corpus callosum**. This arrangement allows the brain's two hemispheres to communicate with each other.

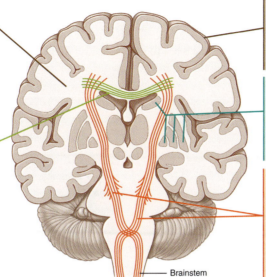

The surface of the cerebrum, called the **cerebral cortex**, consists of a thin layer of gray matter. (Even though the layer is thin, gray matter actually makes up about 40% of the brain's mass.)

Masses of gray matter—called **basal nuclei**, or, sometimes, **basal ganglia**—lie deep within the cerebrum. These structures play a role in the control of movement.

Other tracts carry information back and forth between the brain and the spinal cord. These tracts are extensions of the ascending (sensory) spinothalamic tracts and the descending (motor) corticospinal tracts. Note how the tracts cross in the brainstem, with the right side of the brain sending impulses to the left side of the body (and vice versa).

Brainstem

The Limbic System

Sometimes called the "emotional brain," the limbic system is the seat of emotion and learning. It's formed by a complex set of structures that encircle the corpus callosum and thalamus. In brief, it links areas of the lower brainstem (which control automatic functions) with areas in the cerebral cortex associated with higher mental functions. Two key structures of the limbic system include the hippocampus and amygdala.

Feelings of anger, fear, sexual feelings, sorrow, and pleasure only result because of a functioning limbic system. However, to ensure that those feelings are expressed in socially acceptable ways, other parts of the cerebral cortex must also be engaged. Limbic system activity, without the moderating influence of other parts of the cerebrum, leads to attacks of uncontrollable rage.

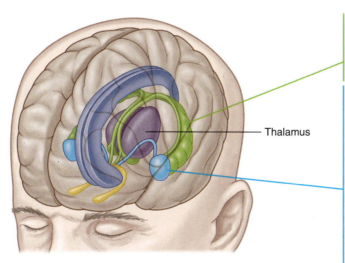

Thalamus

Hippocampus: Charged with converting short-term memory into long-term memory, making it crucial for memory and learning.

Amygdala: Two almond-shaped masses of neurons on either side of the thalamus; concerned with emotions such as anger, jealousy, and fear; it also stores, and can recall, emotions from past events. This explains why a current event can trigger emotions from a previous experience, such as feeling pleasure when viewing a picture of a favorite vacation spot or crying in grief on the anniversary of a loved one's death.

Functions of the Cerebral Cortex

Even though specific areas of the brain focus on certain functions, these areas are not absolute and can vary among individuals. They can also shift within an individual to compensate for an injury, a characteristic known as *plasticity*. Keep in mind that no area of the brain acts alone. Normal brain function requires multiple structures of the central nervous system to work together. Many of the brain's roles require the integration of both sensation and movement.

Motor Functions of the Cerebral Cortex

The primary somatic motor area is the precentral gyrus.

Movement begins with the intention to move. Neurons in the **motor association area** determine which movements are required to perform a specific task. It then sends the appropriate signals to the precentral gyrus.

In response, neurons in the **precentral gyrus** send impulses through the motor tracts in the brainstem and spinal cord. The impulses travel to the skeletal muscles, and movement occurs.

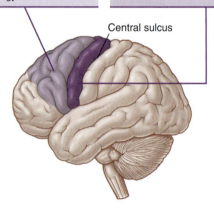

Central sulcus

Sensory Functions of the Cerebral Cortex

Sensory nerve fibers transmit signals up the spinal cord to the thalamus, which forwards them to the postcentral gyrus.

The **postcentral gyrus** is the **primary somatic sensory area** of the brain. It receives impulses of heat, cold, and touch from receptors all over the body. (Because of decussation, the right postcentral gyrus receives signals from the left side of the body and the left gyrus receives signals from the right.)

Adjacent to the postcentral gyrus is the **somatic sensory association area**. This area allows us to pinpoint the location of pain, identify a texture, and be aware of how our limbs are positioned.

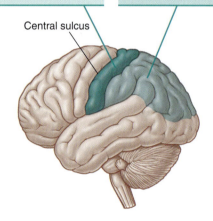

Central sulcus

The Body AT WORK

The illustration shown here, called a **homunculus**, *maps the parts of the cerebral cortex dedicated to specific regions of the body. The size of the body parts in the illustration reflects the amount of cortical tissue dedicated to sending signals to, and processing information from, those areas. For example, the hands perform many intricate movements and can detect a variety of sensations. Therefore, they demand a large amount of brain tissue. In contrast, the back performs few movements and has limited sensitivity; consequently, it commands a much smaller area of the cortex.*

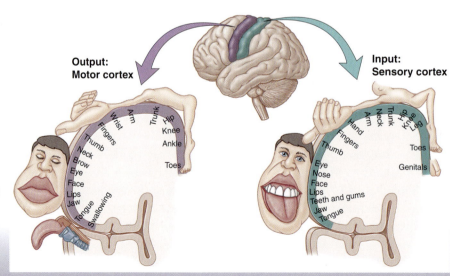

Output:
Motor cortex

Input:
Sensory cortex

Language

Each aspect of language—which includes the ability to read, write, speak, and understand—is handled by a different region of the cerebral cortex.

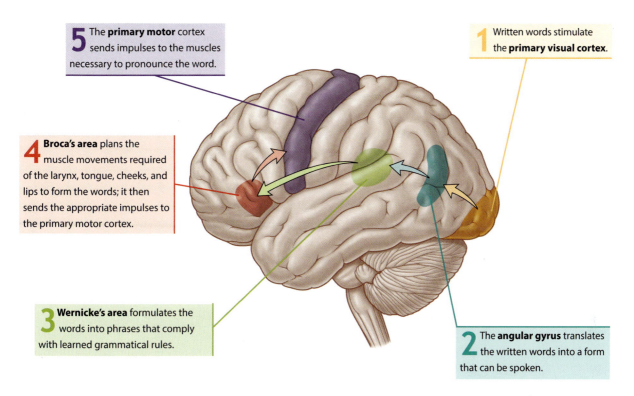

5 The **primary motor** cortex sends impulses to the muscles necessary to pronounce the word.

4 **Broca's area** plans the muscle movements required of the larynx, tongue, cheeks, and lips to form the words; it then sends the appropriate impulses to the primary motor cortex.

3 **Wernicke's area** formulates the words into phrases that comply with learned grammatical rules.

1 Written words stimulate the **primary visual cortex**.

2 The **angular gyrus** translates the written words into a form that can be spoken.

FAST FACT

Only about 4% of brain cells are active at any given time.

The Body AT WORK

Because Wernicke's area (located in the left temporal lobe) is responsible for language comprehension, patients suffering an injury to this part of the brain have difficulty comprehending what others are saying. They will also have difficulty forming their own sentences, to the extent that they may make no sense. This condition is called Wernicke's aphasia.

Because Broca's area (located in the left frontal lobe) controls the muscle movements required for speech, those suffering an injury to this area will understand what's being said, but they'll find it difficult, or even impossible, to speak. This condition is called Broca's aphasia.

Special Senses

The primary senses of taste, smell, vision, and hearing are handled by specialized regions of the brain, as shown below. (For more information on the senses, see Chapter 11, *Sense Organs*.)

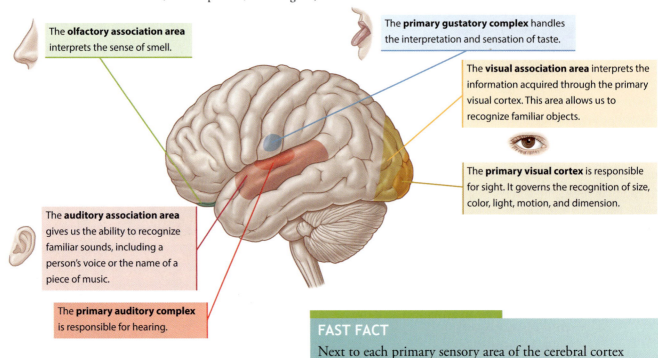

The **olfactory association area** interprets the sense of smell.

The **primary gustatory complex** handles the interpretation and sensation of taste.

The **visual association area** interprets the information acquired through the primary visual cortex. This area allows us to recognize familiar objects.

The **primary visual cortex** is responsible for sight. It governs the recognition of size, color, light, motion, and dimension.

The **auditory association area** gives us the ability to recognize familiar sounds, including a person's voice or the name of a piece of music.

The **primary auditory complex** is responsible for hearing.

FAST FACT

Next to each primary sensory area of the cerebral cortex is an association area that identifies and interprets sensory information so that it meaningful and useful.

Sleep

The body, as well as the brain, requires periods of sleep, and even dreaming, to function optimally. However, scientists still have much to learn about both sleep and dreaming. What is known, however, is that sleep occurs in repetitive phases called stages.

Stages of Sleep

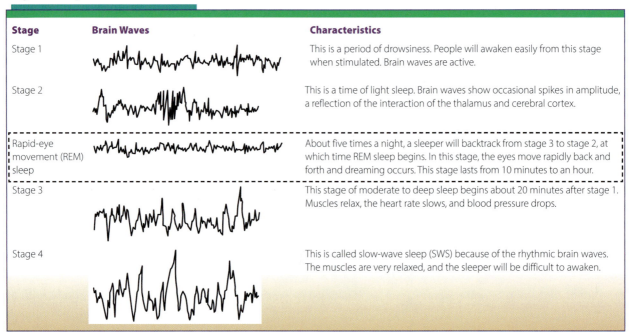

Stage	Brain Waves	Characteristics
Stage 1		This is a period of drowsiness. People will awaken easily from this stage when stimulated. Brain waves are active.
Stage 2		This is a time of light sleep. Brain waves show occasional spikes in amplitude, a reflection of the interaction of the thalamus and cerebral cortex.
Rapid-eye movement (REM) sleep		About five times a night, a sleeper will backtrack from stage 3 to stage 2, at which time REM sleep begins. In this stage, the eyes move rapidly back and forth and dreaming occurs. This stage lasts from 10 minutes to an hour.
Stage 3		This stage of moderate to deep sleep begins about 20 minutes after stage 1. Muscles relax, the heart rate slows, and blood pressure drops.
Stage 4		This is called slow-wave sleep (SWS) because of the rhythmic brain waves. The muscles are very relaxed, and the sleeper will be difficult to awaken.

Memory

The ability to store and retrieve information is one of the brain's key functions. The cerebral cortex handles two types of memory: *short-term memory*—in which information is stored briefly and then forgotten—and *long-term memory*—in which information is stored for days or years. Many parts of the cerebral cortex participate in creating memory. Memory most likely results when repeated stimulation permanently changes the synapses of a specific circuit of neurons. Although still poorly understood, experts think the synaptic changes facilitate impulse transmission.

Experts also know that the limbic system as a whole, and the hippocampus in particular, plays a role in memory. If the hippocampus is damaged, the ability to form new memories is impaired. In fact, the hippocampus is one of the first regions to suffer damage in Alzheimer's disease, although it can also be damaged due to hypoxia, encephalitis, or temporal lobe epilepsy.

Cerebral Lateralization

While the two hemispheres of the brain may look identical, they handle different functions. In brief, the left hemisphere is the more analytical side; it focuses on language and the types of reasoning used in math and science. The right hemisphere is more concerned with creativity and spatial ability.

In a normal brain, the two hemispheres communicate with each other via the corpus callosum, allowing for the smooth integration of information. While neither hemisphere is "dominant," the left hemisphere is usually considered the *categorical* hemisphere, although this varies somewhat with hand dominance. For example, the left hemisphere is dominant for speech in 95% of those who are right-handed, while the right hemisphere is dominant for speech in only 4% of right-handers. In contrast, among left-handers, the right hemisphere is dominant for speech in about 15%; the left hemisphere, in 70%; and neither, in 15%.

The following illustration highlights some of the specializations of each hemisphere.

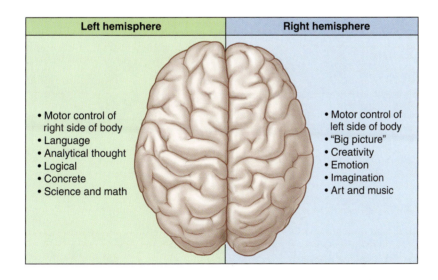

Left hemisphere	Right hemisphere
• Motor control of right side of body • Language • Analytical thought • Logical • Concrete • Science and math	• Motor control of left side of body • "Big picture" • Creativity • Emotion • Imagination • Art and music

FAST FACT

Cerebral lateralization, or dominance, seems to be stronger in men than in women. In fact, when the left hemisphere is damaged, men are three times as likely to suffer aphasia. Although the reason for this isn't completely clear, scientists speculate that women have more communication between their right and left hemispheres.

Cranial Nerves

The brain has 12 pairs of **cranial nerves** to relay messages to the rest of the body. While still part of the peripheral nervous system, these nerves—unlike the spinal nerves—arise directly from the brain.

Each cranial nerve is identified by a name (suggestive of its function) as well as a number. Designated by a Roman numeral, the nerves are numbered I to XII according to their order, beginning in the anterior portion of the brain. Some cranial nerves contain only sensory fibers, some contain primarily motor fibers, while others contain both.

I Olfactory nerve (I, sensory)

- Governs sense of smell
- Terminates in olfactory bulbs in the cribriform plate, just above the nasal cavity
- Impairment results in an impaired sense of smell (which may be linked to a loss of taste)
- *To test:* Ask person to smell substances such as vanilla or coffee

VII Facial nerve (VII, mixed)

- Sensory portion concerned with taste; motor portion controls facial expression and secretion of tears and saliva
- Damage causes sagging facial muscles and a distorted sense of taste
- *To test:* Check sense of taste on anterior two-thirds of tongue; test ability to smile, frown, whistle, and raise eyebrows

VIII Vestibulocochlear nerve (VIII, sensory)

- Concerned with hearing and balance
- Damage results in deafness, dizziness, nausea, and loss of balance
- *To test:* Test hearing, balance, and ability to walk a straight line

X Vagus nerve (X, mixed)

- Longest and most widely distributed cranial nerve
- Supplies organs in the head and neck as well as those in the thoracic and abdominal cavities
- Plays key role in many heart, lung, digestive, and urinary functions
- Damage causes hoarseness or loss of voice and impaired swallowing; damage to both vagus nerves can be fatal
- *To test:* Perform same tests as those for cranial nerve IX

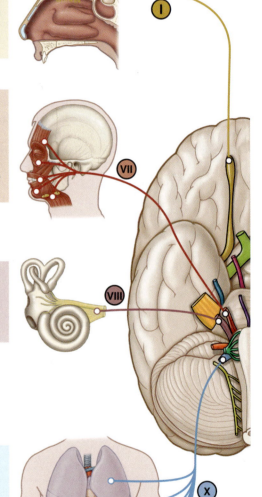

Optic nerve (II, sensory)

- Concerned with vision
- Links the retina to the brain's visual cortex
- Damage causes blindness in part or all of a visual field
- *To test:* Check visual acuity and peripheral vision

Oculomotor, trochlear, and abducens nerves (III, IV, VI, mainly motor)

- Regulate voluntary movements of the eyelid and eyeball; oculomotor also controls pupil constriction
- Damage can cause drooping eyelid, dilated pupil (oculomotor only), inability to move eye in some directions, double vision
- *To test:* Inspect size, shape, and reaction of pupils; check eye movements and ability to follow moving object

Trigeminal nerve (V, two sensory and one mixed branch)

- Sensory branches (ophthalmic and maxillary) sense touch, temperature, and pain on the eye, face, and teeth; mixed branch (mandibular) controls chewing and detects sensations in the lower jaw
- Ophthalmic branch triggers the corneal reflex: blinking in response to a light touch on the eyeball
- Damage to the sensory branches causes loss of sensation in upper face; damage to mixed branch results in impaired chewing and loss of sensation in jaw
- *To test:* Lightly touch eyeball with cotton swab to check corneal reflex; evaluate sense of touch, pain, and temperature with pin as well as hot and cold objects; evaluate ability to open mouth and move jaw side to side

Glossopharyngeal nerve (IX, mixed)

- Motor fibers govern tongue movements, swallowing, and gagging
- Sensory fibers handle taste, touch, and temperature from the tongue; also concerned with regulation of blood pressure
- Damage causes impaired swallowing, choking, and bitter or sour taste
- *To test:* Test gag reflex, swallowing, and coughing; check taste on posterior one-third of tongue

Hypoglossal nerve (XII, mainly motor)

- Controls tongue movements
- Damage causes impaired speech and swallowing; deviation of tongue toward injured side
- *To test:* Check for tongue deviation when tongue is protruded

Spinal accessory nerve (XI, mainly motor)

- Controls movement in the head, neck, and shoulders
- Damage impairs movement of the head, neck, and shoulders
- *To test:* Check ability to rotate head and shrug shoulders against resistance.

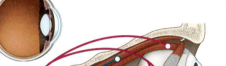
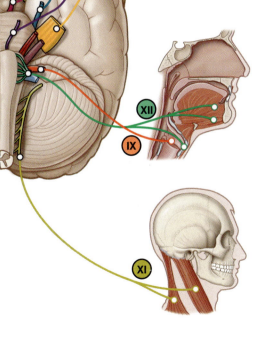

That Makes Sense

A number of different mnemonic devices have evolved over the years to aid in the memorization of the cranial nerves. Here's a common one, in which the first letter of each word represents the name of a cranial nerve, in order:

Cranial Nerve Mnemonic

Mnemonic	Nerves
On	• **O**lfactory (I)
Old	• **O**ptic (II)
Olympus'	• **O**culomotor (III)
Towering	• **T**rochlear (IV)
Top,	• **T**rigeminal (V)
A	• **A**bducens (VI)
Friendly	• **F**acial (VII)
Viking	• **V**estibulocochlear (VIII)
Grew	• **G**lossopharyngeal (IX)
Vines	• **V**agus (X)
And	• **A**ccessory (XI)
Hops.	• **H**ypoglossal (XII)

FAST FACT

Brain swelling from an injury or tumor can cause pressure on the oculomotor nerve. This will interfere with the ability of the pupils to respond to light, which is why a patient's pupils are checked following a head injury.

FAST FACT

Most cranial nerves transmit impulses to receptors on the same side of the body. Consequently, a lesion on one side of the brainstem will produce sensory or motor symptoms on the same side of the body. (Exceptions are the optic and trochlear nerves.)

Life lesson: Cranial nerve disorders

Inflammation of the trigeminal nerve can cause *trigeminal neuralgia*, or tic douloureux. In this disorder, such things as eating, drinking, tooth brushing, shaving—or even changes in temperature—can trigger brief episodes of intense pain. Although the pain lasts only a few seconds, it strikes frequently at unpredictable times. Severe cases may require surgery to sever the trigeminal nerve. This stops the attacks of pain, but it also leads to numbness of the face, scalp, teeth, and conjunctiva on the afflicted side.

In *Bell's palsy*, dysfunction of the facial nerve causes paralysis of the facial muscles on one side. Consequently, the muscles on one side of the face sag, the eyelid droops, and that side of the face shows no expression. The cause of Bell's palsy is often unclear, although infection by a virus is suspected. Other possible causes include Lyme disease or a middle ear infection. The condition usually resolves in 3 to 5 weeks.

AUTONOMIC NERVOUS SYSTEM

The **autonomic nervous system (ANS)** is a subdivision of the nervous system responsible for regulating the activities that maintain homeostasis. These activities include such things as the secretion of digestive enzymes, the constriction and dilation of blood vessels for the maintenance of blood pressure, and the secretion of hormones. Most of these activities occur without your awareness or control; in other words, they happen independently, or *autonomously*, which is how the ANS received its name.

The ANS sends motor impulses to cardiac muscle, glands, and smooth muscle (as opposed to skeletal muscle, which is innervated by the peripheral nervous system). Because the ANS targets organs, it's sometimes called the **visceral motor system**.

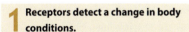

Visceral Reflexes

The ANS asserts control through **visceral reflexes**—similar to somatic reflexes discussed earlier, but, instead of affecting a skeletal muscle, these reflexes affect an organ. While the following illustration shows the visceral reflex arc responsible for the regulation of blood pressure, all visceral reflexes follow similar steps.

ANIMATION

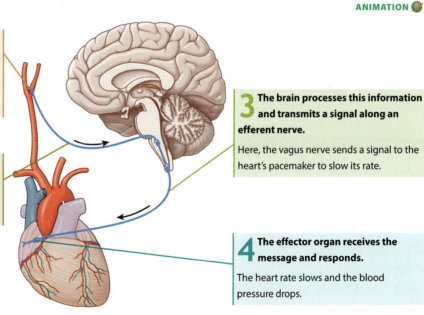

1 Receptors detect a change in body conditions.

In this instance, pressure receptors in the carotid artery, called baroreceptors, detect a rise in blood pressure.

2 Afferent neurons transmit information about this change to the CNS.

The glossopharyngeal nerve relays this information to the medulla oblongata.

3 The brain processes this information and transmits a signal along an efferent nerve.

Here, the vagus nerve sends a signal to the heart's pacemaker to slow its rate.

4 The effector organ receives the message and responds.

The heart rate slows and the blood pressure drops.

Structure of the Autonomic Nervous System

Autonomic motor pathways (both sympathetic and parasympathetic) differ from the somatic motor pathways discussed earlier. As previously learned, somatic pathways are structured as follows:

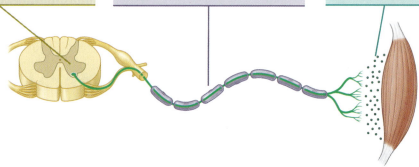

The neuron's cell body lies within the CNS (either the brain or spinal cord).

A single myelinated axon extends from the brainstem or spinal cord to a skeletal muscle.

At the target muscle, the neurotransmitter acetylcholine (ACh) is released to cause muscle contraction.

In contrast, autonomic pathways employ *two* neurons to reach a target organ.

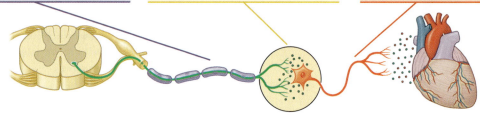

A myelinated **preganglionic neuron** extends from the brainstem or spinal cord to a ganglion.

In the ganglion, it synapses with a **postganglionic neuron**; here, the neurotransmitter ACh is released.

The axon of the unmyelinated postganglionic neuron extends to the target organ. Here, the neurotransmitter released varies: parasympathetic fibers release ACh while sympathetic fibers release norepinephrine (NE).

Comparison of Somatic and Autonomic Nervous Systems

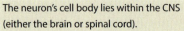

Somatic	Autonomic
• Innervates skeletal muscle	• Innervates glands, smooth muscle, and cardiac muscle
• Consists of one nerve fiber leading from CNS to target (no ganglia)	• Consists of two nerve fibers that synapse at a ganglion before reaching target
• Secretes neurotransmitter acetylcholine	• Secretes both acetylcholine and norepinephrine as neurotransmitters
• Has an excitatory effect on target cells	• May excite or inhibit target cells
• Operates under voluntary control	• Operates involuntarily

Divisions of the Autonomic Nervous System

The ANS consists of two divisions: the **sympathetic** division and the **parasympathetic** division. These two divisions have separate neural pathways and perform different functions; however, they often both innervate the same organ.

The sympathetic division prepares the body for physical activity. It's also the system that's called into play during times of extreme stress, anger, or fear. Because this division prepares someone to fight or flee from danger, its effects are called the "fight or flight" reaction. In contrast, the parasympathetic division has a calming effect on body functions. The following chart contrasts some of the effects of these two systems.

Sympathetic Division	Parasympathetic Division
• Increases alertness	• Has a calming effect
• Increases heart rate	• Decreases heart rate
• Dilates bronchial tubes to increase air flow in the lungs	• Constricts bronchial tubes to decrease air flow in lungs
• Dilates blood vessels of skeletal muscles to increase blood flow	• Has no effect on blood vessels of skeletal muscles
• Inhibits intestinal motility	• Stimulates intestinal motility and secretion to promote digestion
• Stimulates secretion of thick salivary mucus	• Stimulates secretion of thin salivary mucus
• Stimulates sweat glands	• Has no effect on sweat glands
• Stimulates adrenal medulla to secrete epinephrine	• Has no effect on adrenal medulla
• Has no effect on the urinary bladder or internal sphincter	• Stimulates the bladder wall to contract and the internal sphincter to relax to cause urination
• Causes "fight or flight" response	• Causes the "resting and digesting" state

That Makes Sense

To remember the effects of the sympathetic division of the ANS, think about a time when you were really angry or scared. How did you feel? Most likely your heart pounded; you took deep, rapid breaths; your palms sweated; your pupils dilated; your mouth felt dry. These symptoms illustrate the "fight or flight" response of the sympathetic division, all of which are designed to promote energy use by the skeletal muscles.

The Body AT WORK

*Both the sympathetic and parasympathetic divisions of the ANS work at the same time, providing a background level of activity called **autonomic tone**. The balance between sympathetic and parasympathetic activity constantly changes depending on the body's needs: during times of activity or stress, the sympathetic division dominates; at rest, parasympathetic activity takes center stage.*

However, neither the sympathetic nor parasympathetic divisions ever stops working completely. For example, during a time of rest, the parasympathetic division is primarily active. However, even then, the sympathetic division constantly stimulates the blood vessels, keeping them partially constricted so as to maintain blood pressure. If sympathetic stimulation were to stop, blood pressure would drop drastically and the person would go into shock.

The Sympathetic Division

The sympathetic division is also called the **thoracolumbar division** because it arises from the thoracic and lumbar regions of the spinal cord.

ANIMATION

Sympathetic preganglionic neurons begin within the spinal cord.

From the cell bodies, myelinated fibers reach to sympathetic ganglia, most of which exist in chains along both sides of the spinal cord (even though the illustration here depicts the ganglia only along one side). Because the ganglia lie close to the spinal cord, the preganglionic neurons are short.

Not all preganglionic neurons synapse in the first ganglion they encounter. Some travel up or down the chain to synapse with other ganglia at different levels. Others pass through the first ganglion to synapse with another ganglion a short distance away.

Unmyelinated postganglionic fibers leave the ganglia and extend to the target organs. Postganglionic fibers tend to be long.

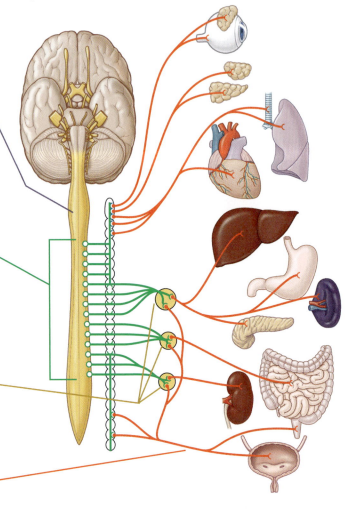

The Body AT WORK

Rather than synapsing with a single postganglionic neuron, each preganglionic neuron of the sympathetic division branches and synapses with multiple postganglionic neurons. This arrangement allows one preganglionic neuron to excite multiple postganglionic neurons simultaneously. That's why the sympathetic division can ignite such an immediate, widespread response, such as what occurs during "fight or flight."

The Adrenal Glands

The adrenal glands—triangular-shaped glands perched on the tops of each kidney—play a role in the function of the sympathetic nervous system. Sympathetic preganglionic fibers pass through the outer cortex of the adrenal gland and terminate in the center, which is called the **adrenal medulla**. When stimulated, the adrenal medulla secretes the hormone *epinephrine* (along with small amounts of *norepinephrine*) into the bloodstream. Epinephrine, as well as norepinephrine, can bind to the receptors of sympathetic effectors, which helps prolong the sympathetic response.

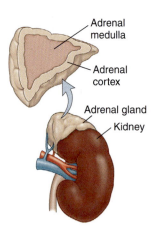

Adrenal medulla

Adrenal cortex

Adrenal gland

Kidney

The Parasympathetic Division

The neurons of the parasympathetic division arise from the brain and the sacral region of the spinal cord—which is why this division of the ANS is also called the **craniosacral division**.

Parasympathetic fibers leave the brainstem by joining one of the following cranial nerves:

- **Oculomotor nerve (III):** Parasympathetic fibers carried in this nerve innervate the ciliary muscle, which thickens the lens of the eye, and the pupillary constrictor, which constricts the pupil.

- **Facial nerve (VII):** These parasympathetic fibers regulate the tear glands, salivary glands, and nasal glands.

- **Glossopharyngeal nerve (IX):** The parasympathetic fibers carried in this nerve trigger salivation.

- **Vagus nerve (X):** This nerve carries about 90% of all parasympathetic preganglionic fibers. It travels from the brain to organs in the thoracic cavity (including the heart, lungs, and esophagus) and the abdominal cavity (such as the stomach, liver, kidneys, pancreas, and intestines).

Parasympathetic fibers leave the sacral region by way of pelvic nerves and travel to portions of the colon and bladder.

Unlike the ganglia of the sympathetic division, the ganglia of the parasympathetic division reside in or near the target organ. As a result, the preganglionic fibers of the parasympathetic division are long while the postganglionic fibers are short.

Because the ganglia are more widely dispersed, the parasympathetic division produces a more localized response than that of the sympathetic division.

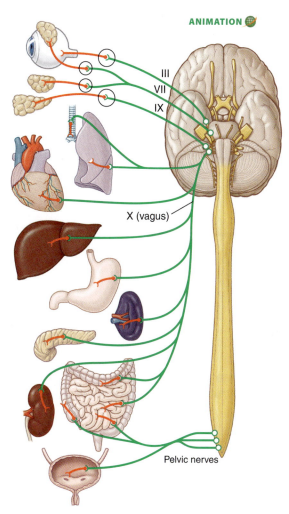

ANIMATION

III
VII
IX

X (vagus)

Pelvic nerves

Comparison of Sympathetic and Parasympathetic Divisions

Sympathetic	Parasympathetic
• Originates in thoracolumbar region	• Originates in craniosacral region
• Ganglia lie in chain alongside spinal cord	• Ganglia lie in or near target organs
• Has short preganglionic and long postganglionic fiber	• Has long preganglionic and short postganglionic fiber
• Employs mostly norepinephrine as a neurotransmitter (occasionally uses acetylcholine)	• Employs acetylcholine as a neurotransmitter
• Produces widespread, generalized effects	• Produces local effects

Effects of the ANS on Target Organs

The two divisions of the ANS tend to exert opposite effects. For example, the sympathetic division increases the heart rate while the parasympathetic division slows it down. However, that's not always the case. For example, the sympathetic division triggers dilation of blood vessels leading to skeletal muscles, but it also constricts blood vessels leading to most organs.

Two factors determine the effect of each division: the neurotransmitter released and the type of receptor on the target cells.

Neurotransmitters

The ANS employs two different neurotransmitters: acetylcholine (ACh) and norepinephrine (NE). Fibers that secrete acetyl*choline* are called **cholinergic fibers**. Fibers that secrete NE (sometimes called nor*adrenaline*) are called **adrenergic fibers**.

Cholinergic Fibers

- Include the preganglionic fibers of both the sympathetic and parasympathetic divisions
- Include the postganglionic fibers of the parasympathetic division
- Secrete acetylcholine

Adrenergic Fibers

- Include most (but not all) of the postganglionic fibers of the sympathetic division
- Secrete norepinephrine

The Body AT WORK

The effects of the parasympathetic division tend to be short lived, while the effects of the sympathetic division last much longer. The difference in the length of these responses is linked to the speed with which the neurotransmitter is broken down after its release.

For example, once ACh is released into the synaptic cleft, it's quickly broken down by the enzyme acetylcholinesterase (AChE). As a result, the parasympathetic division exerts only short-term effects.

In contrast, NE—the neurotransmitter released only by postganglionic sympathetic fibers—may be disposed of by one of three methods, none of which are as rapid as the breakdown of ACh. Some NE is reabsorbed by the nerve fiber (where it is either reused or broken down by the enzyme monoamine oxidase [MAO]); some of it is also absorbed by the surrounding tissue (where it is broken down by another enzyme). In addition, some of the NE may be absorbed by the bloodstream and carried throughout the body, further prolonging the effects of the sympathetic division.

That Makes Sense

Remember: In all pathways, preganglionic fibers are cholinergic and secrete acetylcholine. Most sympathetic postganglionic fibers are adrenergic. (See the diagram at the end of the chapter for a clear example of this complex process.)

FAST FACT

Recent research has shown that neurotransmitters other than norepinephrine and acetylcholine can bind to autonomic receptors—thus opening the door for the development of new medications.

Receptors

After being released, the neurotransmitters bind to receptors on the effector cells of the target organs. In brief, ACh binds to cholinergic receptors and NE binds to adrenergic receptors. However, within these two categories of receptors are several subtypes of receptors; it's these different types of receptors that determine the effect produced by a neurotransmitter.

To illustrate the importance of the type of receptor, consider the fact that the sympathetic division secretes NE to constrict the blood vessels of the skin and also to dilate the blood vessels of skeletal muscles. Likewise, the parasympathetic division secretes ACh to contract the bladder wall and also to relax the internal urethral sphincter. These opposite effects occur then, not because of the neurotransmitter, but because of the receptor.

Cholinergic Receptors

Acetylcholine may bind to one of two different types of receptors:

Nicotinic Receptors

- These receptors occur within the ganglia of the ANS, in the adrenal medulla, and in the neuromuscular junction.
- All cells with nicotinic receptors are excited by ACh.

Muscarinic Receptors

- These receptors occur on the glands, smooth muscle, and cardiac muscle cells of the organs innervated by cholinergic fibers.
- Cells with muscarinic receptors exhibit a variable response to ACh: some are excited while others are inhibited. (This variable response occurs because several subtypes of muscarinic receptors exist.)
- This variable response allows ACh to stimulate intestinal smooth muscle while inhibiting cardiac muscle.

Adrenergic Receptors

There are also two basic types of adrenergic receptors: **alpha-(α-)adrenergic receptors** and **beta-(β-)adrenergic receptors.** The following principles are true most of the time:

- Cells with *α-adrenergic receptors* are *excited* by NE.
- Cells with *β-adrenergic receptors* are *inhibited* by NE.

To illustrate, the binding of NE to α-adrenergic receptors in blood vessels causes the blood vessels to constrict. Arteries that supply blood to the heart and skeletal muscles contain β-adrenergic receptors. The binding of NE to these receptors causes the vessels to dilate.

(Be aware, however, that both alpha and beta receptors contain subtypes—alpha-1 [α_1], alpha-2 [α_2], beta-1 [β_1], and beta-2 [β_2]—which can cause exceptions to these principles.)

FAST FACT

A group of drugs called beta blockers bind to beta receptors, effectively "blocking" norepinephrine and epinephrine from binding to those same receptors. (Remember that the sympathetic nervous system stimulates the adrenal medulla to secrete epinephrine, a hormone that prolongs the sympathetic response.) Blocking these hormones effectively lessens the sympathetic response, making the drugs useful for treating such disorders as high blood pressure and irregular heartbeats.

Neurotransmitters and Receptors

The following diagrams summarize the different neurotransmitters and receptors of the two divisions of the autonomic nervous system.

Sympathetic Division

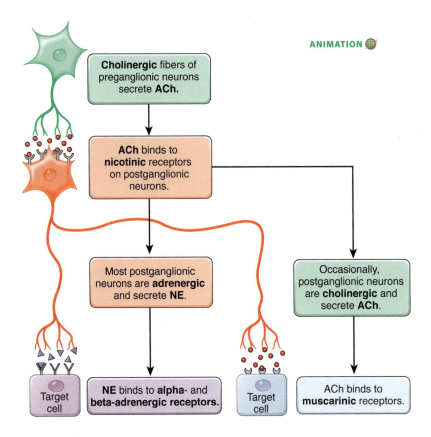

ANIMATION

Cholinergic fibers of preganglionic neurons secrete **ACh.**

ACh binds to **nicotinic** receptors on postganglionic neurons.

Most postganglionic neurons are **adrenergic** and secrete **NE.**

Occasionally, postganglionic neurons are **cholinergic** and secrete **ACh.**

Target cell

NE binds to **alpha-** and **beta-adrenergic receptors.**

Target cell

ACh binds to **muscarinic** receptors.

Parasympathetic Division

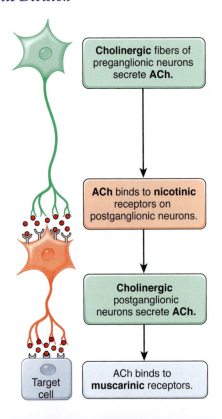

Cholinergic fibers of preganglionic neurons secrete **ACh.**

ACh binds to **nicotinic** receptors on postganglionic neurons.

Cholinergic postganglionic neurons secrete **ACh.**

Target cell

ACh binds to **muscarinic** receptors.

The Body AT WORK

*Most organs receive nerve fibers from both the sympathetic and parasympathetic divisions. This is called **dual innervation**. Typically, the effects of the two divisions oppose one other. For example, the sympathetic division increases heart rate, while the parasympathetic division slows it down; also, the sympathetic division dilates pupils, while the parasympathetic division constricts them.*

Sometimes, though, the effects of the two divisions complement each other to produce a desired effect. For example, parasympathetic division stimulates salivary glands to produce a thin secretion containing enzymes while the sympathetic division stimulates the production of thick mucus; both of these substances are needed to make saliva.

FAST FACT

Sympathetic fibers cause both blood vessel constriction and dilation. They do this by altering their frequency of firing. An increase in firing causes blood vessels to constrict; a decrease in firing results in dilation. This allows the sympathetic division to regulate blood pressure and blood flow without any help from parasympathetic fibers.

Life lesson: Medications and the nervous system

A number of drugs work by enhancing or inhibiting the effects of neurotransmitters. Following are some of the major classifications of these types of drugs:

- *Sympathomimetics:* These drugs enhance sympathetic action by either promoting the release of epinephrine or stimulating adrenergic receptors. A common example is phenylephrine, a drug found in many cold remedies. This drug stimulates α_1 receptors, which dilates the bronchial tubes (to ease breathing) and constricts blood vessels in the nose (to ease nasal congestion).
- *Sympatholytics:* These drugs block the effects of epinephrine and norepinephrine, primarily by inhibiting adrenergic receptors. This class of drug is often used to treat high blood pressure: blocking α-adrenergic receptors causes the blood vessels to dilate and blood pressure to fall.
- *Parasympathomimetics:* These drugs—also called cholinergics—stimulate or mimic the parasympathetic division. They do this by either stimulating the nicotinic or muscarinic receptors or by inhibiting acetylcholinesterase (the enzyme that breaks down ACh). One such drug is physostigmine, which is used to treat glaucoma (increased pressure in the eye) and delayed gastric emptying.
- *Parasympatholytics:* Also called anticholinergics, these drugs inhibit ACh release or block its receptors to reduce the activity of the parasympathetic division. Because one of its effects is to dilate the bronchiole tubes in the lungs, this class of drug may be used to treat asthma.

Life lesson: Changes with aging

The type and degree of age-related changes in the brain and nervous system varies from one individual to the next. Some experience significant nerve degeneration while others have few changes. In general, most people experience slight slowing of thought and memory as the speed of nerve conduction slows. Other possible changes include reduced reflexes or sensation, leading to problems with safety.

Dementia and severe memory loss are not a normal part of aging. When they occur, they often signal underlying disease. Illnesses not related to the brain, however, can cause changes in thinking and behavior. For example, an infection or unregulated blood glucose levels can cause severe confusion.

Some evidence suggests that both physical and mental exercise (such as reading, doing crossword puzzles, and engaging in stimulating conversations) can help keep thinking sharp.

Review of Key Terms

Action potential: Nerve impulse

Adrenergic fibers: Nerve fibers that secrete norepinephrine

Afferent neuron: Sensory nerve that carries impulses toward the central nervous system

Alpha-adrenergic receptors: Receptors to norepinephrine that generally produce an excitatory response

Autonomic nervous system: Subdivision of the nervous system responsible for regulating activities that maintain homeostasis; also called visceral motor system

Axon: Fiber extending from a neuron's cell body that conducts impulses

Beta-adrenergic receptors: Receptors to norepinephrine that generally produce an inhibitory response

Brainstem: Stem-like portion of the brain that connects the cerebral hemispheres to the spinal cord; consists of the midbrain, pons, and medulla oblongata

Central nervous system: Portion of the nervous system consisting of the brain and spinal cord

Cerebellum: Portion of the brain responsible for coordination of voluntary movement and balance

Cerebral cortex: The surface of the cerebrum consisting of a thin layer of gray matter

Cerebrospinal fluid: Clear, colorless fluid that fills the brain's ventricles and central canal and also bathes the outside of the brain and spinal cord

Cerebrum: Largest portion of the brain

Cholinergic fibers: Nerve fibers that secrete acetylcholine

Cranial nerves: Nerves of the peripheral nervous system that arise directly from the brain (instead of from the spinal cord)

Dermatome: A specific area of the skin innervated by a spinal nerve

Efferent neuron: Motor nerve that carries impulses away from the central nervous system

Epidural space: Small space between the outer covering of the spinal cord and the vertebrae

Frontal lobe: Portion of the cerebrum responsible for decision making, reasoning, memory, and voluntary movements

Gray matter: Nervous tissue containing mostly cell bodies of motor neurons and interneurons

Hypothalamus: The bottom half of the diencephalon of the brain, which is responsible for many vital body functions

Limbic system: Complex set of structures in the brain responsible for emotion and learning

Medulla oblongata: Attaches brain to spinal cord; contains centers that govern heart rate, blood pressure, and breathing

Meninges: Layer of fibrous connective tissue covering the brain and spinal cord

Mixed nerve: Nerve that contains both sensory and motor fibers

Muscarinic receptors: Receptors to acetylcholine on target cells that exhibit a variable response

Myelin: Fatty sheath encasing the axons of many neurons; formed by Schwann cells in the peripheral nervous system and oligodendrocytes in the central nervous system

Nerve: A bundle of neurons that transmits impulses between the brain and spinal cord and the rest of the body

Neuroglia: Cells in the nervous system that support neurons but do not conduct impulses

Neurons: Nervous system cells that conduct impulses

Nicotinic receptors: Receptors to acetylcholine on target cells that produce an excitatory response

Occipital lobe: Portion of the cerebrum responsible for analyzing and interpreting visual information

Parasympathetic division: Division of the autonomic nervous system that primarily has a calming effect; also called craniosacral division

Parietal lobe: Portion of the cerebrum concerned with bodily sensations and proprioception

Peripheral nervous system: Portion of the nervous system consisting of the network of nerves throughout the body

Plexus: A network of nerves

Polarization: The electrical state of a cell membrane that has an excess of positive ions on one side of the membrane and an excess of negative ions on the other

Reflex arc: A neural circuit that bypasses regions of the brain where conscious decisions are made

Somatic reflex: Reflex involving contraction of a skeletal muscle after being stimulated by a somatic motor neuron

Sympathetic division: Division of the autonomic nervous system responsible for "fight or flight" response; also called thoracolumbar division

Synapse: Space between the junction of two neurons in a neural pathway

Temporal lobe: Portion of the brain responsible for hearing, smell, and visual recognition

Tracts: Bundles of axons in the spinal cord that serve as routes of communication to and from the brain

Visceral reflexes: Reflex of the autonomic nervous system affecting organs

White matter: Nervous tissue containing bundles of axons that carry impulses from one part of the nervous system to another

Own the Information

To make the information in this chapter part of your working memory, take some time to reflect on what you've learned. On a separate sheet of paper, write down everything you recall from the chapter. After you're done, log on to the Davis*Plus* website, and check out the Study Group podcast and Study Group Questions for the chapter.

Key Topics for Chapter 10:
- Divisions of the nervous system
- Types of cells found in the nervous system
- Neuron structure
- The repair of nerve fibers
- Impulse conduction in both myelinated and unmyelinated nerve fibers
- Synapse structure and function
- The structure of the spinal cord
- Spinal tracts
- Spinal nerves
- Somatic reflexes
- Divisions of the brain
- Structure and function of the meninges
- Creation and circulation of cerebrospinal fluid
- Divisions of the brain, including the brainstem, cerebellum, diencephalon, and cerebrum
- The limbic system
- Sensory and motor functions of the cerebral cortex
- Regions of the brain responsible for language and special senses
- Types of brain waves as related to different stages of sleep
- Brain regions involved in memory
- The relationship between the right and left hemispheres
- Cranial nerves
- Visceral reflexes
- The structure and function of the autonomic nervous system
- The structure and function of the sympathetic and parasympathetic divisions of the autonomic nervous system
- The neurotransmitters and receptors employed by the autonomic nervous system
- The effects of the sympathetic and parasympathetic nervous systems on target organs

Test Your Knowledge

Answers: Chapter 10

1. *Correct answer:* **b.** Neuroglia are nervous system cells that protect neurons. Microglia are a type of neuroglia that perform phagocytosis and engulf microorganisms and debris. Ependymal cells line the spinal cord and cavities in the brain and secrete cerebrospinal fluid.

2. *Correct answer:* **c.** The brain requires a large supply of blood to function. The blood supply to the brain is not separate from the blood supplied to the rest of the body. Cerebrospinal fluid follows its own circulatory route and is eventually reabsorbed into the venous system; it has nothing to do with the blood-brain barrier.

3. *Correct answer:* **c.** Efferent neurons are motor neurons; these relay messages from the brain to muscles and gland cells. Interneurons are found only in the CNS; they connect incoming sensory pathways with outgoing motor pathways. Schwann cells wrap around the axons of many peripheral nerves to form the myelin sheath.

4. *Correct answer:* **d.** Resting potential is the phase in which the neuron is resting but has the potential to react. Action potential is when the neuron becomes active and conducts an impulse along an axon. Repolarization is when the nerve cell restores its electrical balance in preparation for a new stimulus. While a neuron won't necessarily react to an impulse during action potential and repolarization, the most correct answer is the refractory period, because, although the membrane is polarized, the cell won't react to a new impulse until sodium and potassium have been restored to their rightful sides of the membrane.

5. *Correct answer:* **a.** Spinal nerves carry both sensory and motor fibers, making them capable of transmitting impulses both to and from the CNS. Spinal nerves regulate voluntary function, not autonomic function; they are not part of the autonomic nervous system.

6. *Correct answer:* **c.** The phrenic nerve is part of the cervical plexus and innervates the diaphragm. The axillary nerve is part of the brachial plexus and leads into the arm. The femoral nerve is derived from the lumbar plexus and supplies the thigh and leg.

7. *Correct answer:* **c.** CSF nourishes the brain by providing glucose and protein and removing metabolic wastes. An adult brain contains about 140 ml of CSF; the brain monitors levels of carbon dioxide; CSF continually circulates through the central nervous system.

8. *Correct answer:* **b.** The pons contains tracts that convey signals to and from different parts of the brain; it's also the site where several cranial nerves originate. The midbrain contains centers for auditory and visual reflexes as well as neurons essential for motor control. The cerebellum plays a key role in motor functions as well as in sensory and emotional functions.

9. *Correct answer:* **d.** The thalamus is the gateway for nearly all sensory impulses. The limbic system is the seat of emotion and learning. The cerebral cortex is the gray matter covering the surface of the brain; it handles the cerebrum's functions, which include thought, reasoning, judgment, and memory.

---

1. The impulse-conducting cells of the nervous system are called:
   a. neuroglia.
   b. neurons.
   c. microglia.
   d. ependymal cells.

2. What is the blood-brain barrier?
   a. It's a membrane surrounding the brain that keeps blood from penetrating brain tissue.
   b. It's a membrane surrounding the brain that keeps the blood in the brain separate from the blood in the rest of the body.
   c. It's a semi-permeable membrane that permits small molecules like oxygen and carbon dioxide to diffuse across to the brain but blocks larger molecules.
   d. It's a semi-permeable membrane that prevents cerebrospinal fluid from leaving the brain and entering the bloodstream.

3. Which neurons detect sensations such as touch or heat and then relay information about the stimuli to the central nervous system?
   a. Efferent neurons
   b. Interneurons
   c. Afferent neurons
   d. Schwann cells

4. A nerve cell in which phase cannot respond to a new stimulus?
   a. Resting potential
   b. Action potential
   c. Repolarization
   d. Refractory period

5. Which statement regarding spinal nerves is true?
   a. Spinal nerves are mixed nerves, containing both sensory and motor fibers, making it capable of transmitting impulses in two directions.
   b. Spinal nerves are primarily motor nerves, responsible for transmitting impulses to skeletal muscles.
   c. Spinal nerves are primarily sensory nerves, responsible for transmitting sensations from the muscles to the brain and spinal cord.
   d. Spinal nerves are a chief component of the autonomic nervous system and are responsible for controlling autonomic functions.

6. Which key nerve is part of the sacral plexus?
   a. Phrenic nerve
   b. Axillary nerve
   c. Sciatic nerve
   d. Femoral nerve

7. Which statement about cerebrospinal fluid (CSF) is true?
   a. An adult's brain contains about 500 ml of CSF.
   b. The brain monitors the level of oxygen in CSF.
   c. CSF furnishes the brain with glucose and protein.
   d. CSF remains relatively stagnant within the cerebral cavity.

8. Which portion of the brain contains centers responsible for such vital functions as heart rate, breathing, and blood pressure?
   a. Pons
   b. Medulla oblongata
   c. Midbrain
   d. Cerebellum

9. Which brain structure influences nearly every organ and exerts control over the autonomic nervous system and pituitary gland?
   a. Thalamus
   b. Limbic system
   c. Cerebral cortex
   d. Hypothalamus

10. *Correct answer:* **a.** The parietal lobe handles the awareness of one's body parts; an injury here may cause someone to ignore objects on one side of the body, even his own arm or leg. The temporal lobe governs hearing and memory; an injury here may impair the ability to identify familiar objects. The occipital lobe is concerned with analyzing and interpreting visual information; an injury here would affect the ability to see.

11. *Correct answer:* **d.** Neurons in the precentral gyrus send impulses through the motor tracts in the brainstem and spinal cord to skeletal muscles. Wernicke's area (in the left temporal lobe) and Broca's area (in the left frontal lobe) are both concerned with language: Wernicke's area formulates the words into phrases that comply with learned grammatical rules; Broca's area plans the muscle movements required to form the words and sends the appropriate impulses to the primary motor cortex.

12. *Correct answer:* **c.** The glossopharyngeal nerve governs tongue movements, swallowing, and gagging. The hypoglossal nerve controls tongue movements. The vestibulocochlear nerve is concerned with hearing and balance.

13. *Correct answer:* **a.** The olfactory nerve governs the sense of smell. The optic nerve is concerned with vision (not pupillary response). The facial nerve is concerned with taste as well as facial expression.

14. *Correct answer:* **d.** All the other statements are characteristics of the autonomic nervous system.

15. *Correct answer:* **b.** All of the other actions listed can be attributed to the sympathetic division.

16. *Correct answer:* **c.** Adrenergic fibers secrete norepinephrine. Cholinergic fibers include the preganglionic fibers of both the sympathetic and parasympathetic divisions as well as the postganglionic fibers of the parasympathetic division.

17. *Correct answer:* **c.** The amount of neurotransmitter would influence the strength of a response, but not the type of response. The effect produced does vary according to the type of neurotransmitter; however, the same neurotransmitter bound to a different receptor will have a different response. Therefore, it's the receptor, not the neurotransmitter, that ultimately determines the response. If the receptors are blocked (thus decreasing the number available), then the strength of the response would be diminished.

10. An injury to which part of the brain may result in a severe personality disorder and cause socially inappropriate behavior?
 a. Frontal lobe
 b. Parietal lobe
 c. Temporal lobe
 d. Occipital lobe

11. Which area of the brain receives impulses of heat, cold, and touch from receptors all over the body and is, therefore, known as the primary somatic sensory area?
 a. Precentral gyrus
 b. Wernicke's area
 c. Broca's area
 d. Postcentral gyrus

12. Which cranial nerve supplies most of the organs in the thoracic and abdominal cavities as well as those in the head and neck?
 a. Glossopharyngeal
 b. Hypoglossal
 c. Vagus
 d. Vestibulocochlear

13. Brain swelling from a head injury can compress this nerve and interfere with the ability of the pupils to react to light.
 a. Oculomotor
 b. Olfactory
 c. Optic
 d. Facial

14. Which of the following is a characteristic of the somatic nervous system?
 a. It innervates glands, smooth muscle, and cardiac muscle.
 b. It consists of two nerve fibers that synapse at a ganglion before reaching a target organ.
 c. It secretes both acetylcholine and norepinephrine.
 d. It operates under voluntary control.

15. Which of the following is one of the actions of the parasympathetic division of the autonomic nervous system?
 a. Increases heart rate
 b. Constricts bronchial tubes
 c. Stimulates sweat glands
 d. Inhibits intestinal motility

16. Which of the following statements correctly describes cholinergic fibers?
 a. Cholinergic fibers secrete norepinephrine.
 b. Cholinergic fibers include the postganglionic fibers of the sympathetic and parasympathetic divisions.
 c. Cholinergic fibers secrete acetylcholine.
 d. Cholinergic fibers include the preganglionic fibers of the parasympathetic division only.

17. The effect produced by a neurotransmitter (such as whether it constricts or dilates blood vessels) is ultimately determined by:
 a. the amount of neurotransmitter released.
 b. the type of neurotransmitter released.
 c. the type of receptor.
 d. the number of receptors.

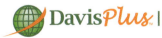

Go to **http://davisplus.fadavis.com** Keyword: Thompson to see all of the resources available with this chapter.

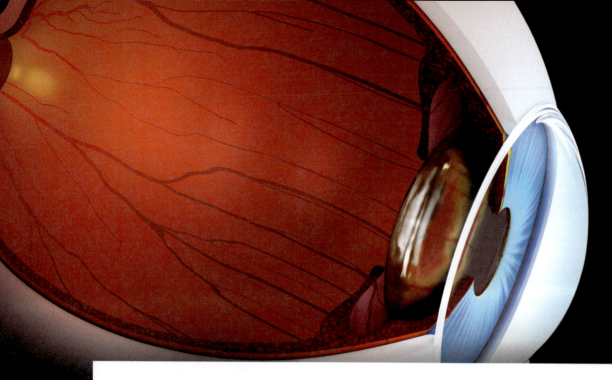

LEARNING OUTCOMES

1. Distinguish between sensory receptors and sense organs.

2. List three kinds of information obtained by sensory receptors.

3. Name five classifications of sensory receptors.

4. Identify two categories of pain receptors.

5. Summarize the main pain pathway.

6. Name the five special senses.

7. Specify the location of taste receptors and describe how the sensation of taste occurs.

8. Identify the location of smell receptors and describe how the sensation of smell occurs.

9. Describe the anatomy of the inner, middle, and outer ear.

10. Explain how hearing occurs.

11. Discuss how the vestibule and semicircular canals allow the brain to interpret body movement and position.

12. Describe the anatomy of the eye and its accessory structures.

13. Describe the structure and function of the retina.

14. Discuss how vision occurs.

15. Explain how the size of the pupil and curvature of the lens affect vision.

16. Describe the location and purpose of rods and cones.

11

SENSE ORGANS

Although human sense organs detect a vast array of sensations, the environment is full of physical and chemical energy beyond our comprehension.

Sense organs allow us to taste our food, see a beautiful sunset, hear music, and feel the touch of another person. But senses do more than contribute to our enjoyment of life. For one thing, our senses protect us from danger: being able to see or hear danger, and to feel pain, allows us to avoid injury. Even more importantly, experiencing sensation is vital to our mental well-being. In fact, in experiments in which subjects were placed in isolation tanks that deprived them of all sensation, the subjects soon experienced hallucinations, extreme anxiety, delusions, and panic.

The five main senses are sight, hearing, taste, smell, and touch; however, the body's sensory experiences involve more than those few. In fact, many of the body's sensory processes take place without our awareness. For example, the sensory system is integral in maintaining such vital functions as blood pressure, body temperature, and balance.

Sensory Receptors

Scattered throughout the body are millions of sensory **receptors**. Some of these receptors combine with muscle and tissue to form sense organs (such as the eyes, ears, and nose). Most, though, are specialized nerve cells or nerve endings that detect physical or chemical events outside the cell membrane.

| A sensation begins when a receptor detects a stimulus. | If the stimulus is strong enough, the receptor causes a sensory neuron to send an impulse to the brain and spinal cord. | When the impulse arrives at the brain, we may experience a sensation, such as a sight or sound. |

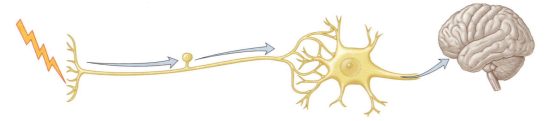

The Body AT WORK

Normally, the brain filters out most of the stimuli detected by receptors, keeping them below our level of awareness. That's because many of the stimuli relate to body processes that operate subconsciously. Also, the filtering process protects us from being overwhelmed by an overabundance of stimuli.

FAST FACT

One type of energy beyond the scope of human senses is electric fields. However, some fish, such as sharks, have electroreceptive organs that allow them to detect weak electrical impulses emitted by the gills of their prey.

Sensory receptors transmit information about the type, the location, and the intensity of each sensation.

- **Type:** Each sensory receptor responds to a different stimulus; for example, cold receptors respond only to cold while light receptors respond only to light. This allows the nervous system to differentiate between the various sensations.

- **Location:** Each sensory neuron responds to stimuli in a certain area, called a *receptive field*. Therefore, when a particular neuron carries a stimulus to the brain, the brain knows where the stimulus originated. This is known as **sensory projection**. Sensitive areas of the body, such as the tips of the fingers, contain a dense population of receptors. Because each neuron covers a tiny territory, the brain can pinpoint the location of a stimulus. In less sensitive areas, such as the back, a single neuron covers a much larger territory. Consequently, the brain can only identify that a stimulus occurred in that area; it can't pinpoint the spot with accuracy.

- **Intensity:** The stronger a particular stimulus, the more nerve fibers fire. This allows the brain to interpret the intensity of a sensation.

Classification of Receptors

Receptors are classified according to the type of stimuli they detect.

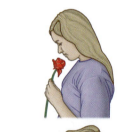

Chemoreceptors

These receptors react to various chemicals, including odors and tastes, as well as the concentration of various chemicals (such as glucose or carbon dioxide) in the body.

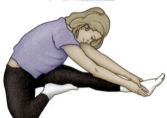

Mechanoreceptors

These receptors respond to factors—such as pressure, stretch, or vibration—that change the position of a receptor.

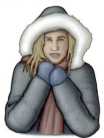

Thermoreceptors

These receptors are activated by a change in temperature.

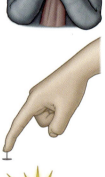

Nociceptors

These are pain receptors that respond to tissue damage from trauma as well as from heat, chemicals, pressure, or a lack of oxygen.

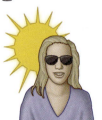

Photoreceptors

Found only in the eyes, these receptors respond to light.

The Body AT WORK

When a stimulus is continuous, the firing frequency of the nerve begins to slow, causing the sensation to diminish. This is known as **adaptation**. As an example, think of entering a cold body of water. When you first step in, the water may seem very cold. After a few minutes, your senses adapt and it doesn't feel as cold.

The Body AT WORK

Another type of specialized receptor is the **proprioceptor**. Found in skeletal muscle, joints, and tendons, proprioceptors provide information about body movement, muscle stretch, and the general orientation of the body. For example, proprioceptors allow you to orient your body in space and to know the position of your body parts (such as your arm or leg) without looking.

The General Senses

The general senses include pain as well as the sensations of pressure, touch, stretch, and temperature. Receptors for the general senses are widely distributed in the skin, muscles, tendons, joints, and viscera.

Pain

Nociceptors, or pain receptors, consist of free nerve endings that carry pain impulses to the brain. They're especially abundant in the skin and mucous membranes and also found in almost every organ. (They're not, however, found in the brain.) They fall into one of two categories:

- **Fast pain fibers:** Abundant in the skin and mucous membranes, these fibers produce a sharp, localized, stabbing-type pain at the time of injury. This is the type of pain you experience when you stub your toe or slam your finger in a door.
- **Slow pain fibers:** These fibers are congregated on deep body organs and structures and produce a dull, aching pain. For example, pain sensations from a bowel obstruction or appendicitis would be carried along these fibers.

Pain can travel by a number of different routes (making the true source of pain often difficult to identify). The following illustration portrays the main pain pathway for most areas of the body.

> **FAST FACT**
> While nociceptors don't occur in the brain, they do occur in the meninges. Headaches, therefore, don't result from pain in the brain but from the surrounding tissues.

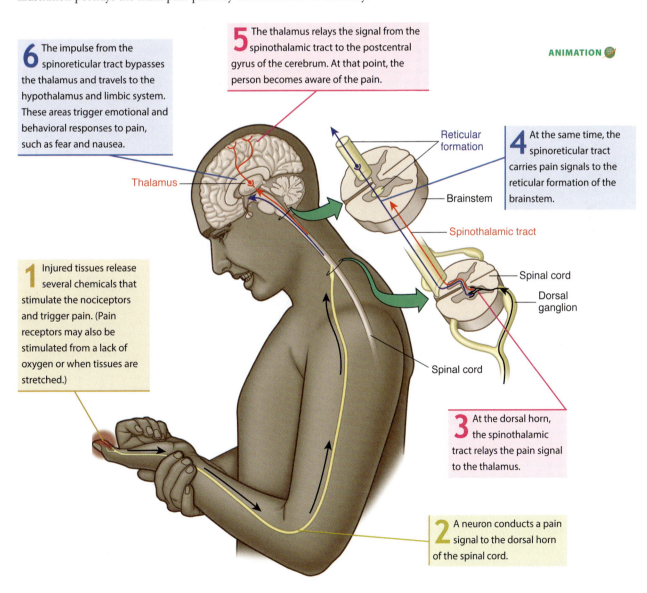

6 The impulse from the spinoreticular tract bypasses the thalamus and travels to the hypothalamus and limbic system. These areas trigger emotional and behavioral responses to pain, such as fear and nausea.

5 The thalamus relays the signal from the spinothalamic tract to the postcentral gyrus of the cerebrum. At that point, the person becomes aware of the pain.

ANIMATION 🌐

4 At the same time, the spinoreticular tract carries pain signals to the reticular formation of the brainstem.

Reticular formation

Thalamus

Brainstem

Spinothalamic tract

Spinal cord

Dorsal ganglion

1 Injured tissues release several chemicals that stimulate the nociceptors and trigger pain. (Pain receptors may also be stimulated from a lack of oxygen or when tissues are stretched.)

Spinal cord

3 At the dorsal horn, the spinothalamic tract relays the pain signal to the thalamus.

2 A neuron conducts a pain signal to the dorsal horn of the spinal cord.

Referred Pain

Pain originating in a deep organ may be sensed as if it's originating from the body's surface—sometimes at a totally different part of the body. Called **referred pain**, this occurs because sensory fibers from an organ and those from an area of skin converge in a single pathway. The illustration shown here identifies common sites of referred pain.

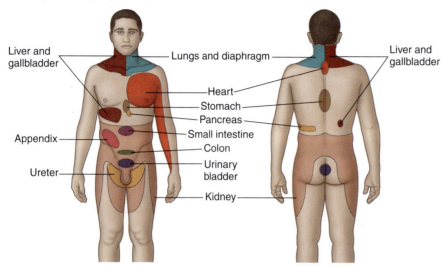

Liver and gallbladder

Lungs and diaphragm

Heart

Stomach

Pancreas

Small intestine

Appendix

Colon

Urinary bladder

Ureter

Kidney

Liver and gallbladder

An example of referred pain includes one of the classic symptoms of myocardial infarction: pain in the left arm or over the left chest. Those symptoms occur because pain fibers from the heart and pain fibers from the skin over the left side of the chest and left arm enter the spinal cord at the same level. Sensory impulses from both these areas travel to the brain over the same pathway, which may cause the brain to misidentify pain from the heart as coming from the chest or arm.

FAST FACT

Drugs used to relieve pain are called **analgesics**.

The Body AT WORK

No one likes to be in pain; however, pain is one of the body's chief protective mechanisms. Pain alerts us to danger—such as letting us know that a stove is hot—and warns us about internal injury or disease. Those with an impaired perception of pain have an increased risk for injury because they can't sense the warning signs that pain provides. For example, a common complication of diabetes is nerve damage (neuropathy) in the feet. Because the neuropathy impairs the sensation of pain, someone with diabetic neuropathy may overlook a seemingly minor injury that can later become infected.

Temperature

Free nerve endings called **thermoreceptors** mediate sensations of heat and cold.

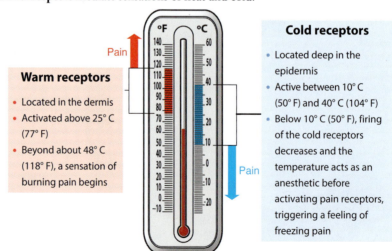

Pain

Warm receptors

- Located in the dermis
- Activated above 25° C (77° F)
- Beyond about 48° C (118° F), a sensation of burning pain begins

Cold receptors

- Located deep in the epidermis
- Active between 10° C (50° F) and 40° C (104° F)
- Below 10° C (50° F), firing of the cold receptors decreases and the temperature acts as an anesthetic before activating pain receptors, triggering a feeling of freezing pain

Pain

Touch

Specialized nerve endings, most of which are mechanoreceptors, provide for the senses of touch, pressure, and stretch. Some receptors are enveloped in connective tissue while others are uncovered. These receptors, which are located on sensitive, hairless areas of the skin such as the fingertips, palms, eyelids, lips, nipples, and genitals, have different sizes and shapes. This broad variety allows us to feel the difference between a wide range of textures, such as being able to differentiate between smooth silk and rough burlap.

The Special Senses

The special senses—which include taste, smell, hearing, equilibrium, and vision—involve receptors that are either grouped together or clustered in specialized organs.

Taste

The sense of taste, or **gustation**, results when chemicals come in contact with taste buds. Most taste buds are located around protrusions on the tongue called **papillae**, although a few reside in the lining of the mouth and soft palate. The tongue contains four types of papillae:

- **Vallate papillae** are large papillae found at the rear of the tongue; although few in number, they contain up to half of all taste buds.

- **Foliate papillae** form ridges at the sides of the tongue.

- **Filiform papillae** are thread-like papillae that contain no taste buds; they play a role in helping us distinguish the texture of food.

- **Fungiform papillae** are especially concentrated at the tip and sides of the tongue.

Epiglottis

Lingual tonsil

Papillae

Taste buds reside along and between the papillae.

Taste buds look similar to an orange, with each segment containing 25 to 50 chemoreceptors called **gustatory cells** or **taste cells**.

Tongue epithelium

Supporting cell
Gustatory cell

A hair-like tip projects into an opening called the taste pore, which is bathed in saliva. Chemicals dissolved in saliva stimulate the gustatory cells, which, in turn, stimulate certain cranial nerves.

Taste buds send gustatory impulses directly to the brain by one of three cranial nerves (the facial nerve [VII], the glossopharyngeal nerve [IX], and the vagus nerve [X]). The cranial nerve used depends on the location of the taste bud stimulated.

FAST FACT

A child has about 10,000 taste buds. The number declines with age, and elderly people may have fewer than 5000 taste buds.

The Body AT WORK

The four primary tastes are salty, sweet, sour, and bitter. Researchers have suggested a new primary taste called umami. *A Japanese slang word meaning "delicious," umami refers to a "meaty" taste resulting from amino acids.*

Despite previously held views, the tongue is not divided into different regions according to taste. All tastes can be detected in all areas of the tongue that contain taste buds; however, some areas are more sensitive to certain tastes. For example, the tip of the tongue is most sensitive to sweet tastes while the taste buds at the rear of the tongue are most sensitive to bitter tastes.

Smell

Lining the roof of the nasal cavity is a small area of epithelium that contains receptor cells for **olfaction** (the sense of smell). The receptor cells—which are essentially neurons—leave the nasal cavity through pores in the ethmoid bone; they then gather together to form cranial nerve I (the olfactory nerve).

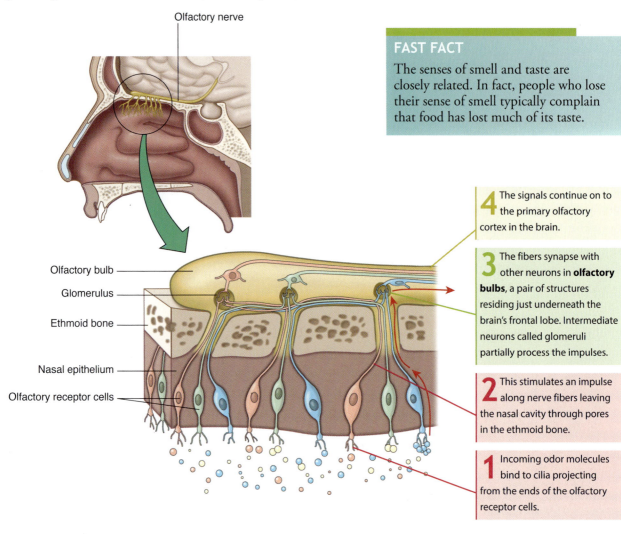

Olfactory nerve

Olfactory bulb

Glomerulus

Ethmoid bone

Nasal epithelium

Olfactory receptor cells

4 The signals continue on to the primary olfactory cortex in the brain.

3 The fibers synapse with other neurons in **olfactory bulbs**, a pair of structures residing just underneath the brain's frontal lobe. Intermediate neurons called glomeruli partially process the impulses.

2 This stimulates an impulse along nerve fibers leaving the nasal cavity through pores in the ethmoid bone.

1 Incoming odor molecules bind to cilia projecting from the ends of the olfactory receptor cells.

FAST FACT

The senses of smell and taste are closely related. In fact, people who lose their sense of smell typically complain that food has lost much of its taste.

FAST FACT

Olfactory receptors are quickly fatigued; they will stop sensing even the strongest smells after a short time.

The Body AT WORK

After a stimulus reaches the primary olfactory cortex, it may continue on to a number of other locations in the cerebrum and brainstem—including the hippocampus and amygdala. This explains why certain odors can evoke a memory, an emotional response, or even a physical response—such as vomiting.

Also noteworthy is that certain odors (such as those produced by the chemicals ammonia, chlorine, and menthol) stimulate nociceptors on the trigeminal nerve instead of olfactory cells. The strong, unpleasant response that results from smelling these chemicals is what makes "smelling salts" effective in reviving someone who is unconscious.

Hearing

The ears provide the sense of hearing; they're also essential for balance (equilibrium). The ear has three sections: the outer ear, the middle ear, and the inner ear.

Outer Ear

The outer, or external, ear consists of the auricle (or pinna) and the auditory canal.

The **auricle (pinna)** is the visible part of the ear. Shaped by cartilage, this part of the ear funnels sound into the auditory canal.

The **auditory canal** leads through the temporal bone to the eardrum. (The opening of the auditory canal to the outside of the body is called the **external acoustic meatus.**) Glands lining the canal produce secretions that mix with dead skin cells to form cerumen (ear wax). Cerumen waterproofs the canal and also traps dirt and bacteria. The cerumen usually dries and then, propelled by jaw movements during eating and talking, works its way out of the ear.

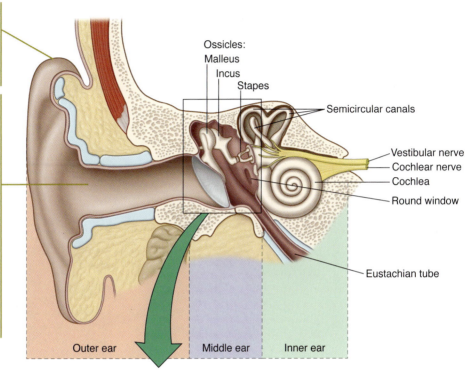

Ossicles:
Malleus
Incus
Stapes
Semicircular canals
Vestibular nerve
Cochlear nerve
Cochlea
Round window
Eustachian tube
Outer ear
Middle ear
Inner ear

Middle Ear

The middle ear consists of these structures:

Auditory ossicles: The three smallest bones in the body connect the eardrum to the inner ear; they are named for their shape:
- **Malleus** (hammer)
- **Incus** (anvil)
- **Stapes** (stirrup)

The stapes fits within the **oval window** of the vestibule, which is where the inner ear begins.

Tympanic membrane (or eardrum): This membranous structure separates the outer ear from the middle ear; it vibrates freely in response to sound waves.

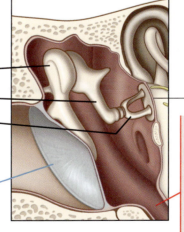

Oval window

The **auditory** or **eustachian tube** is a passageway from the middle ear to the nasopharynx. Its purpose is to equalize pressure on both sides of the tympanic membrane. Unfortunately, it can also allow infection to spread from the throat to the middle ear.

Life lesson: Middle ear infections

Middle ear infections, called *otitis media*, occur commonly in children. The reason is simple: the size and position of the eustachian tube. In children, the eustachian tube is fairly short and horizontal. This short, straight passageway to the nasopharynx allows drainage from the nose to flow easily into the middle ear, spreading infection. As a child grows, the eustachian tube lengthens and slants downward, making the drainage of secretions into the ear, and resultant infection, less likely.

Inner Ear

A complicated system of passageways within the temporal bone contains the inner ear, which explains why this part of the ear is called the **bony labyrinth**. The **membranous labyrinth** lines the inside of the bony labyrinth. Fluid called **perilymph** cushions the space between the two labyrinths, while another fluid, called **endolymph**, occupies the inside of the membranous labyrinth.

Three separate structures form the bony labyrinth:

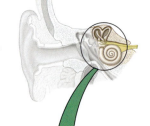

Vestibular nerve

Cochlear nerve

Semicircular canals: These structures are crucial for the maintenance of equilibrium and balance.

Vestibule: This structure, which marks the entrance to the labyrinths, contains organs necessary for the sense of balance.

Cochlea: This snail-like structure contains the structures for hearing.

Oval window

Round window

The spirals of the cochlea are divided into three compartments. The middle compartment is a triangular duct (called the **cochlear duct**) filled with endolymph; the outer two compartments are filled with perilymph.

Perilymph

Cochlear duct (with endolymph)

Resting on the floor (called the **basilar membrane**) of this duct is the **organ of Corti**, the hearing sense organ.

The Body AT WORK

The number of sound waves that occur during a specific time frame, called frequency, determines the pitch of a sound. What we can hear depends on how loud a sound is (the volume) as well as its pitch. Human ears can respond to sounds having a pitch between 20 Hz (vibrations per second) and 16,000 Hz. Many animals, though, can hear sounds the human ear can't detect. For example, cats can hear sounds up to 60,000 Hz, and bats can detect frequencies as high as 120,000 Hz.

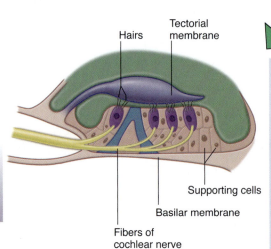

Hairs

Tectorial membrane

Supporting cells

Basilar membrane

Fibers of cochlear nerve

The organ of Corti consists of a layer of epithelium (composed of sensory and supporting cells). Thousands of hair cells project from this epithelial layer and are topped with a gelatin-like membrane called the **tectorial membrane**. Nerve fibers extending from the base of the hairs eventually form the cochlear nerve (cranial nerve VIII).

How Hearing Occurs

Hearing occurs when sound creates vibrations in the air, known as sound waves.

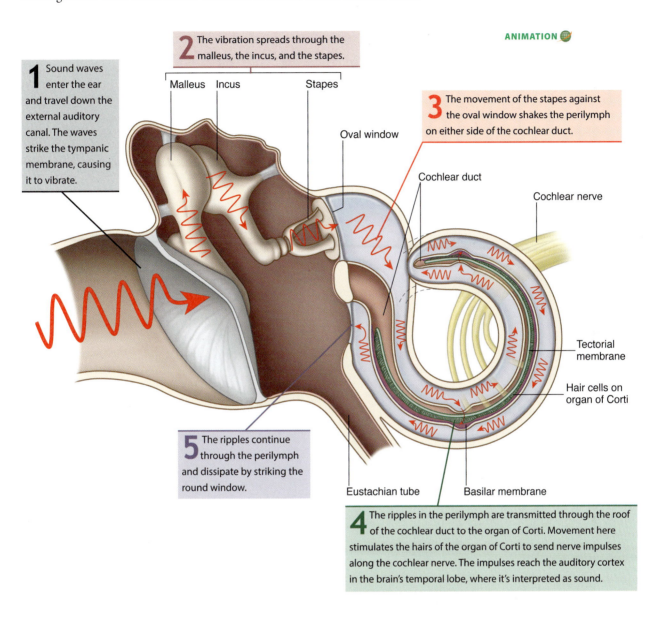

ANIMATION

1 Sound waves enter the ear and travel down the external auditory canal. The waves strike the tympanic membrane, causing it to vibrate.

2 The vibration spreads through the malleus, the incus, and the stapes.

Malleus   Incus   Stapes

Oval window

3 The movement of the stapes against the oval window shakes the perilymph on either side of the cochlear duct.

Cochlear duct

Cochlear nerve

Tectorial membrane

Hair cells on organ of Corti

5 The ripples continue through the perilymph and dissipate by striking the round window.

Eustachian tube   Basilar membrane

4 The ripples in the perilymph are transmitted through the roof of the cochlear duct to the organ of Corti. Movement here stimulates the hairs of the organ of Corti to send nerve impulses along the cochlear nerve. The impulses reach the auditory cortex in the brain's temporal lobe, where it's interpreted as sound.

Life lesson: Hearing loss

Hearing loss can be divided into two main categories:

1. *Conductive hearing loss.* Anything that interferes with the transmission of vibrations to the inner ear will result in a hearing loss. For example, fluid in the middle ear (as a result of an infection, cold, or allergies), impacted cerumen, or a foreign body will all block the transmission of vibrations. When the underlying cause is treated, hearing returns to normal. A more serious type of conductive hearing loss is *otosclerosis*, a condition in which the auditory ossicles fuse together. Because the ossicles can't move, the vibrations stop when they reach the middle ear. Surgical intervention can sometimes restore hearing.
2. *Sensorineural (nerve) hearing loss.* This type of hearing loss most often results from the death of hair cells in the organ of Corti, usually a result of frequent exposure to sustained loud noise (such as that experienced by factory workers and musicians). Once the hairs are damaged, they never grow back, making this type of hearing loss permanent.

Balance

The vestibule and semicircular canals of the inner ear play a key role in the process of balance.

Three fluid-filled semicircular canals lie at right angles to one another. This arrangement allows each canal to be stimulated by a different movement of the head.

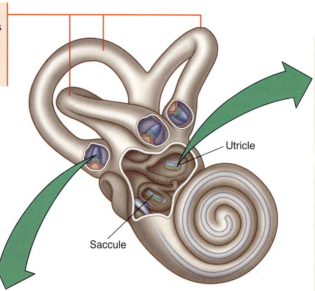

Inside the vestibule are two sense organs: the *utricle* and *saccule*. A patch of hair cells lies inside both these organs. The tips of the hair cells are covered by a gelatin-like material; embedded throughout the gelatin material are heavy mineral crystals called otoliths.

At the end of each canal is a bulb-like area called an **ampulla**. Within each ampulla is a mound of hair cells topped by a gelatinous cone-shaped cap called the cupula. The lightweight cupula floats in the endolymph that fills the semicircular canals.

Utricle

Saccule

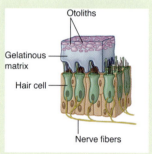

Otoliths

Gelatinous matrix

Hair cell

Nerve fibers

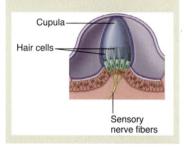

Cupula

Hair cells

Sensory nerve fibers

The Body AT WORK

The semicircular canals and the vestibule monitor different aspects of balance. The semicircular canals are primarily concerned with the speed and direction of head movements (dynamic equilibrium). In contrast, the utricle and saccule share responsibility for detecting the position of the head when the body is stationary and also for the sense of acceleration when moving in a straight line (such as when riding in a car). This is called static equilibrium.

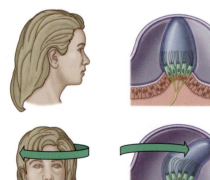

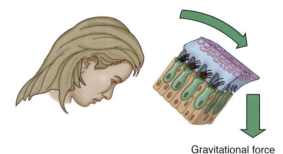

Gravitational force

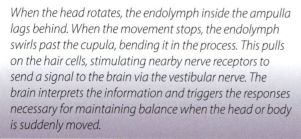

When the head rotates, the endolymph inside the ampulla lags behind. When the movement stops, the endolymph swirls past the cupula, bending it in the process. This pulls on the hair cells, stimulating nearby nerve receptors to send a signal to the brain via the vestibular nerve. The brain interprets the information and triggers the responses necessary for maintaining balance when the head or body is suddenly moved.

Inside the vestibule, the otoliths remain level on the hair cells when the head is level, causing minimal stimulation. When the head tilts (or when the entire body moves forward), the membrane and the otoliths shift, stimulating the hair cells. This, in turn, stimulates nearby receptors of the vestibular nerve to conduct impulses to the brain, which produces a sense of the head's position.

Vision

The most complex of the senses, vision depends on the eye to use light to convert stored energy into nerve impulses; these nerve impulses travel to the brain, where they are interpreted as sight.

Accessory Structures of the Eye

Eyebrow: Perhaps the most significant role of eyebrows is to enhance facial expressions, aiding in nonverbal communication. They also help keep perspiration out of the eye and shield the eye from glare.

Eyelashes: These hairs along the edges of the eyelids help keep debris out of the eye. Touching the eyelashes stimulates the blink reflex.

Eyelids (palpebrae): Formed primarily by the orbicularis oculi muscle covered with skin, the upper and lower eyelids protect the eye from foreign bodies and block light when closed to allow for sleeping. Periodic blinking helps moisten the eyes with tears and wash out debris.

Conjunctiva: The conjunctiva is a transparent mucous membrane that lines the inner surface of the eyelid and covers the anterior surface of the eyeball (except for the cornea). It secretes a thin mucous film to help keep the eyeball moist. It is very vascular, which becomes apparent when eyes are "bloodshot," a result of dilated vessels in the conjunctiva.

Upper eyelid

Lateral canthus

Medial canthus

Palpebral fissure: This is the opening between the lids.

Lower eyelid

Tarsal glands: These glands, which lie along the thickened area at the edge of the eye (called the **tarsal plate**), secrete oil to slow the evaporation of tears and help form a barrier seal when the eyes are closed.

Lacrimal Apparatus

The **lacrimal apparatus** consists of the lacrimal gland and a series of ducts (which are also called tear ducts).

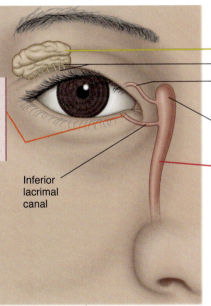

Lacrimal gland: This small gland secretes tears that flow onto the surface of the conjunctiva. Tears clean and moisten the eye's surface and also deliver oxygen and nutrients to the conjunctiva. Furthermore, tears contain a bacterial enzyme called *lysozyme* that helps prevent infection.

Ducts

Superior lacrimal canal

Lacrimal sac

Lacrimal punctum: This tiny pore at the end of each lacrimal canal drains tears into the lacrimal canals and nasolacrimal duct.

Nasolacrimal duct: This passageway carries tears into the nasal cavity (which explains why crying or watery eyes can cause a runny nose).

Inferior lacrimal canal

FAST FACT

The study of the eye and the treatment of its diseases is called **ophthalmology**.

Extrinsic Eye Muscles

Six muscles attach to the bony walls of the orbit and to the surface of the eyeball. This group of muscles—called *extrinsic muscles* because they reside outside the eyeball—moves the eye. Other muscles—called intrinsic muscles—arise from within the eyeball. Intrinsic muscles, which will be discussed later in this chapter, regulate the size of the pupil and change the shape of the lens.

The superior oblique muscle is innervated by the trochlear nerve (cranial nerve IV) and the lateral rectus by the abducens nerve (cranial nerve VI). All the other extrinsic muscles are innervated by the oculomotor nerve (cranial nerve III).

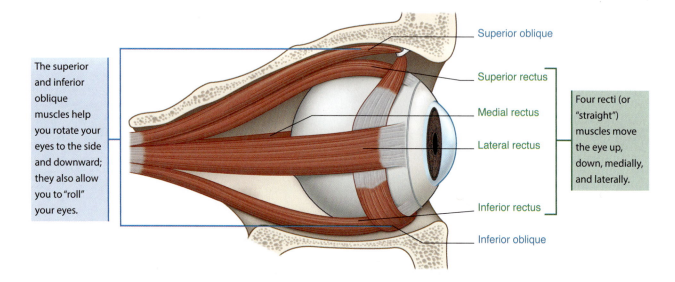

The superior and inferior oblique muscles help you rotate your eyes to the side and downward; they also allow you to "roll" your eyes.

Superior oblique

Superior rectus

Medial rectus

Lateral rectus

Inferior rectus

Inferior oblique

Four recti (or "straight") muscles move the eye up, down, medially, and laterally.

The Body AT WORK

Both eyes work in tandem: when one eye moves, so does the other eye. As a result, when one eye needs to remain still because of an injury or following surgery, it's necessary to patch both eyes.

The Body AT WORK

Human vision is restricted to a band of wavelengths ranging from 400 to 700 nm. Ultraviolet wavelengths lie just above this spectrum, while infrared wavelengths lie just below it. Some animals, though, can detect ultraviolet light, making colors visible that humans are blind to. As an example, a specific species of bird (called the blue tit) distinguish male from female by brilliant ultraviolet feathers, the color of which we can't detect. Also, certain snakes, including rattlesnakes, have a second set of "eyes" that sense infrared radiation, allowing them to spot prey in their vicinity.

FAST FACT

Over half the information in the conscious mind enters through the eyes.

Eye Anatomy

The eye is a sphere about $^3/_4$ to 1 inch (19 to 25 mm) in diameter. It lies within the bony orbit of the skull and is partially surrounded by a layer of fat. Three layers of tissue form the surface of the eye, while the inside is divided into two fluid-filled chambers.

Tissue Layers

The eye is formed by three layers of tissue

- A fibrous outer layer (consisting of the sclera and cornea)
- A vascular middle layer (consisting of the choroid, ciliary body, and iris)
- A neural inner layer (consisting of the retina, optic nerve, and blood vessels)

Fibrous Outer Layer

The **sclera**—formed from dense connective tissue— is the outermost layer of the eye. Most of the sclera is white and opaque; it forms what is called "the white of the eye." Blood vessels and nerves run throughout the sclera.

The **cornea** is a transparent extension of the sclera in the anterior part of the eye. It sits over the iris (the colored portion of the eye) and admits light into the eye. It contains no blood vessels.

Vascular Middle Layer

The **iris** is a ring of colored muscle; it works to adjust the diameter of the pupil (the central opening of the iris) to control the amount of light entering the eye.

The **ciliary body** is a thickened extension of the choroid that forms a collar around the lens. It also secretes a fluid called aqueous humor.

The **choroid** is a highly vascular layer of tissue that supplies oxygen and nutrients to the retina and sclera.

Neural Inner Layer

The **retina** is a thin layer of light-sensitive cells.

Exiting from the posterior portion of the eyeball is the **optic nerve** (cranial nerve II), which transmits signals to the brain.

The Retina

Lining the posterior two-thirds of the eye is the **retina**. Inside the retina are photoreceptors called **rods** and **cones** that are stimulated by light rays to produce an electrical or chemical signal. The retina can be viewed by using a hand-held instrument called an ophthalmoscope to look through the pupil to the back of the eye.

The center point of the retina, as seen through an ophthalmoscope, is a patch of cells called the **macula lutea**.

Inside the macula lutea is a depression called the **fovea centralis**. Most of the cones are concentrated here, making this the area that produces the sharpest vision. (Rods are absent from the fovea centralis; they're mostly clustered along the outside edges of the retina.)

Medial to the macula lutea is the **optic disc**. Nerve fibers leave the retina at this point, converging to become the optic nerve. This is also the spot where blood vessels enter and leave the eye.

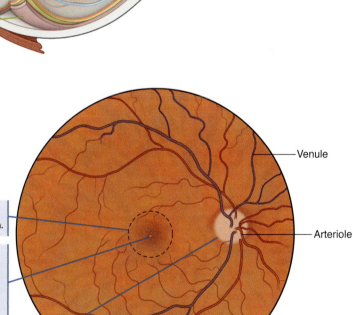

Venule

Arteriole

PART III Regulation and Integration of the Body

That Makes Sense

Remember: The eye consists of three spaces: the anterior chamber, the posterior chamber, and the posterior cavity. The anterior and posterior chambers, together, are known as the anterior cavity.

The Body AT WORK

*The optic disc contains no photoreceptors; consequently, it produces a **blind spot** in the visual field of each eye. To identify your own blind spot, draw a large dot on the left side of a 3" x 5" card and an "X" on the right. Cover your right eye and hold the card about a foot from your face. Focus on the "X" as you move the card slightly forward or to the right and left. At some point, the dot will disappear as it falls on the blind spot of your left eye.*

Chambers and Fluids

The eye is actually a fluid-filled sphere divided into two main cavities.

The space between the lens and the cornea is the **anterior cavity**. This cavity is further divided into an **anterior chamber** (anterior to the iris) and a **posterior chamber** (posterior to the iris but anterior to the lens). A clear, watery fluid called **aqueous humor** fills the anterior cavity.

The **lens** is a transparent disc of tissue just behind the pupil, between the anterior and posterior cavities. The lens changes shape for near and far vision.

The **posterior cavity** is the larger cavity lying posterior to the lens and anterior cavity. It is filled with a jelly-like substance called **vitreous humor**. This semi-solid material helps keep the eyeball from collapsing.

Anterior chamber

Canal of Schlemm

Posterior chamber

The ciliary body secretes aqueous humor that fills the anterior cavity. The fluid flows from the posterior chamber, through the pupil, and into the anterior chamber of the anterior cavity. It then drains into a blood vessel called the **canal of Schlemm**.

Life lesson: Glaucoma

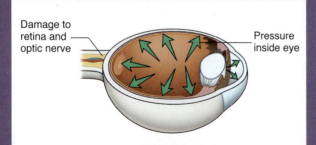

Damage to retina and optic nerve

Pressure inside eye

Normally, the production of aqueous humor by the ciliary body equals the rate of absorption through the canal of Schlemm. If the canal of Schlemm becomes obstructed, aqueous humor accumulates first in the anterior chamber and then in the posterior chamber, causing pressure within the entire anterior cavity to build. Rising pressure in the anterior cavity forces the lens backward, driving the vitreous body against the choroid, which, in turn, obstructs blood flow to the retina and optic nerve. Left untreated, cells in the retina die, the optic nerve atrophies, and blindness may result.

The condition of increased intraocular pressure is called *glaucoma*. Although glaucoma can be easily diagnosed during a routine eye exam, it remains a leading cause of blindness. One reason is that early symptoms are vague (such as flashes of light). Later symptoms include a narrowed field of vision and colored halos around artificial lights. While glaucoma can be treated with drugs or surgery, any resulting vision loss is permanent.

The Process of Vision

For vision to occur, all of the following must happen:

1. Light must enter the eye and focus on the retina to produce a tiny, upside-down image of the object being viewed.
2. The photoreceptors in the retina (rods and cones) must convert that image into nerve impulses.
3. The impulses must be transmitted to the brain for interpretation.

Formation of a Retinal Image

For a retinal image to form, light rays entering the eye must be bent, or *refracted*, so they focus on the retina. Also, if the object being viewed is near rather than far away, other eye adjustments are required. Specifically, the eyes must *converge* on the object being viewed, the pupils must constrict and the lens must change its curvature (*accommodation*).

Refraction

Light rays entering the eye must be bent so they focus precisely on the retina. Bending of light rays is called **refraction**. When light rays strike a substance at an angle other than 90°—such as when light rays strike the curved edge of the cornea—the light rays bend.

Light rays that strike the center of the cornea pass straight through, while light rays that strike off-center, where the cornea is curved, are bent toward the center.

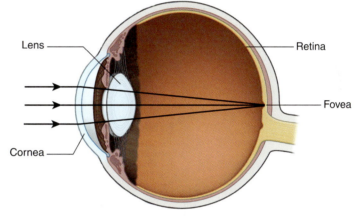

Lens — Retina

Fovea

Cornea

Convergence

Proper vision requires the light rays from an object to fall on the same area of each retina. **Convergence** lines up the visual axis of each eye toward the object so that the light rays fall on the corresponding spots on each retina.

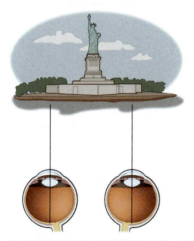

Light rays from distant objects are almost parallel, meaning the eyes require little adjustment.

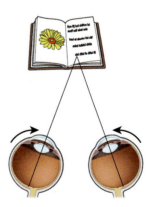

Light waves from close objects diverge more. Therefore, the eyes must move inward, or converge, on the object to align the visual axis with the light rays.

If the eyes fail to converge, light rays from the object will fall on different parts of each retina, resulting in double vision (*diplopia*). To see convergence in action, ask a friend to focus on your finger as you bring it slowly toward his or her nose; soon you'll see the eyes converge on your finger.

220

PART III Regulation and Integration of the Body

Life lesson: Common visual defects

Many people experience less than perfect vision, typically caused by errors in refraction. Special lenses (eyeglasses) can be used to correct these errors. The lenses bend light rays before they reach the cornea so that, by the time the rays reach the back of the eye, they focus on the retina to produce clear vision. The following figures illustrate normal vision as well as common refractive errors.

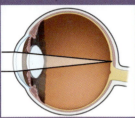

Emmetropia: When light rays focus on the retina without the need of a corrective lens, normal vision results. This is called emmetropia.

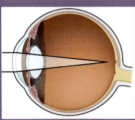

***Myopia* (nearsightedness):** When light rays focus in front of the retina instead of directly on it, distant objects appear blurry while those up close are clear. This condition, called myopia, occurs if the eyeball is too long or the cornea has more curvature than normal. Myopia is the most common refractive vision defect.

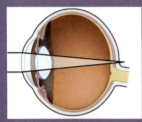

***Hyperopia* (farsightedness):** When light rays focus at a point behind the retina, objects up close appear blurry. Called hyperopia, this condition occurs if the eyeball is too short or the cornea is flatter than normal.

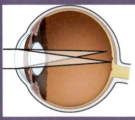

Astigmatism: Astigmatism results from an uneven or asymmetrical curvature of the cornea, causing light to be focused unevenly. People with astigmatism have difficulty viewing fine detail in objects up close as well as at a distance. This refractive defect often accompanies myopia or hyperopia.

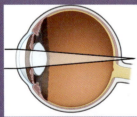

Presbyopia: With age, the lens loses flexibility—interfering with its ability to change shape—and the focusing muscles in the eye weaken. As a result, light focuses behind the retina, creating difficulty focusing on objects up close (such as when reading). Presbyopia usually begins between the ages of 40 and 50 years.

Life lesson: Cataracts

Another common cause of visual disturbances, especially among the elderly, is *cataracts*. A cataract is clouding of the lens, making vision cloudy or blurry. Other common complaints include glare, colors appearing faded, and poor night vision. Cataracts commonly occur as a part of aging, although other risk factors include diabetes mellitus, smoking, and prolonged exposure to sunlight. Treatment includes surgery to remove the lens with the cataract and insertion of an artificial lens.

FAST FACT

The sharpness of visual perception is called **visual acuity**.

Constriction of the Pupil

The center of the cornea—just like the center of any lens—can focus light rays better than the periphery. To reduce blurriness when focusing on a nearby object, the pupil constricts to screen out peripheral light rays. The constriction and dilation of the pupil depends upon muscles inside the iris; these are called the *intrinsic eye muscles*.

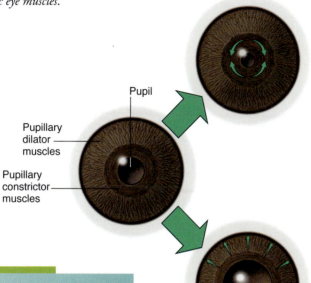

Pupil

Pupillary dilator muscles

Pupillary constrictor muscles

The **pupillary constrictor** muscle encircles the pupil. When stimulated by the parasympathetic nervous system, the muscle constricts, narrowing the pupil to admit less light.

The **pupillary dilator** looks like the spokes of a wheel. When stimulated by the sympathetic nervous system, this muscle contracts, pulling the inside edge of the iris outward. This widens the pupil and admits more light.

FAST FACT

Continually using the eyes for close-up work stresses the ciliary muscles, resulting in eyestrain. Taking periodic breaks to focus on a distant object will help lessen the strain.

The Body AT WORK

Pupils also constrict automatically when exposed to bright light. This is called the **photopupillary reflex***. In fact, both pupils constrict even if only one eye is illuminated, which is why this is sometimes called the* **consensual light reflex***.*

Accommodation of the Lens

While the cornea refracts most of the light rays entering the eye, the lens fine-tunes the rays for sharper focus. Specifically, the curvature of the lens changes to allow the eye to focus on a near object, a process called **accommodation**.

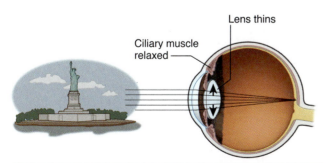

Lens thins

Ciliary muscle relaxed

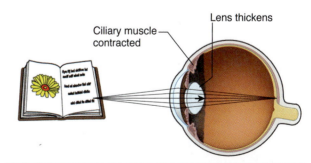

Lens thickens

Ciliary muscle contracted

The nearly parallel light rays from distant objects require little refraction. Consequently, the ciliary muscle encircling the lens relaxes and the lens flattens and thins.

The more divergent light rays from a nearby object require more refraction. To help focus the light rays, the ciliary muscle surrounding the lens contracts. This narrows the lens, causing it to bulge into a convex shape and thicken, giving it more focusing power.

Action of Photoreceptors

Photoreceptor cells (rods and cones) within the retina absorb the incoming light and, in return, trigger an action potential. There are two types of photoreceptors: rods and cones. Rods handle vision in low light but cannot distinguish colors (which explains why it's hard to identify colors in dim light). Cones function in bright light and are responsible for color vision and detail. There are three types of cones—red, green, and blue—each of which responds to the wavelength of light from that particular color. All the colors we perceive result from a mixture of nerve signals from these three types of cones.

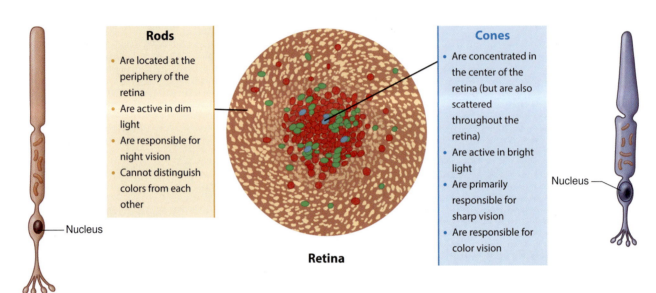

Rods

- Are located at the periphery of the retina
- Are active in dim light
- Are responsible for night vision
- Cannot distinguish colors from each other

Nucleus

Retina

Cones

- Are concentrated in the center of the retina (but are also scattered throughout the retina)
- Are active in bright light
- Are primarily responsible for sharp vision
- Are responsible for color vision

Nucleus

The Body AT WORK

Cones generate the sharpest visual images. Because cones are concentrated in the center of the retina, to see an object clearly in the daytime—or to distinguish between colors—we look at it straight on. At night, or in dim light, we can see more clearly by looking slightly to one side of an object. That's because in those conditions we're using rods, which are concentrated at the periphery of the retina.

That Makes Sense

To distinguish between the actions of rods and cones, remember that "c" (as in cones) stands for "color."

Life lesson: Color blindness

Color blindness results when one or more of the chemicals (photopigments) sensitive to a particular color's wavelength are missing. Contrary to its name, color blindness does not mean that the individual sees everything in shades of gray (except in very rare cases). Rather, the person sees color, but he has difficulty distinguishing certain colors.

The most common form of color blindness is a red-green color deficit. In this case, the person can't distinguish between shades of these two colors. (For example, a person with red-green color blindness would not easily see red flowers in the midst of green leaves.)

Color blindness is an inherited condition, affecting about 8% of males and 0.5% of females.

Transmission of Nervous Impulses

The final step in the visual process involves relaying the nerve impulses to the brain, where the images are interpreted as sight.

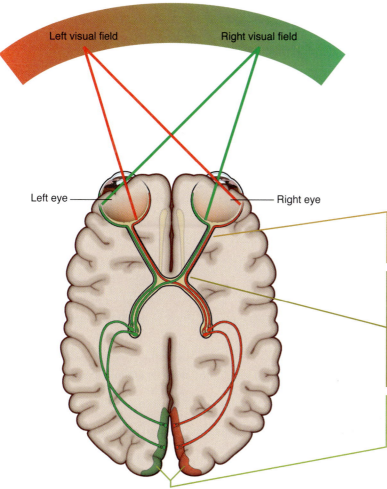

Left visual field

Right visual field

Left eye

Right eye

Nerve impulses generated by the rods and cones leave the eye via the optic nerve.

Half the nerve fibers cross over to the opposite side of the brain at the optic chiasm. Specifically, fibers from the nasal side cross over while the fibers on the temporal side remain on the same side.

The impulses travel to the primary visual cortex in the occipital lobe for interpretation.

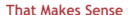

That Makes Sense

It may be confusing to think that images from the right visual field are handled by the left cerebral hemisphere, and that images from the left visual field are handled by the right cerebral hemisphere. It makes more sense, however, when you remember that the right brain controls motor responses on the left side of the body and vice versa. Therefore, each side of the brain needs to "see" what's happening on the side of the body for which it initiates movement.

The Body AT WORK

The optic chiasm is located just anterior to the pituitary gland. That's why an enlargement of the pituitary gland, such as from a tumor, can affect vision.

FAST FACT

A lesion in the brain's occipital lobe can cause blindness, even if the eyes are functioning properly.

Review of Key Terms

Adaptation: The diminishing of a sensation that occurs after continuous exposure to a stimulus

Analgesic: Drug used to relieve pain

Aqueous humor: Clear, watery fluid that fills the anterior cavity of the eye

Bony labyrinth: Complicated system of passageways within the temporal bone that contains the inner ear

Chemoreceptors: Receptors that react to various chemicals, including odors, tastes, and the concentration of various chemicals in the body

Choroid: Highly vascular layer of tissue in the eye that supplies oxygen and nutrients to the sclera and retina

Ciliary body: Thickened extension of the choroid that secretes aqueous humor

Cochlea: Snail-like structure in inner ear that contains the structures for hearing

Cones: Photoreceptors in the retina responsible for color vision

Conjunctiva: Transparent mucous membrane that lines the eyelids and covers the anterior surface of the eyeball (except for the cornea)

Cornea: Transparent extension of sclera that sits over the iris and admits light into the eye

Eustachian tube: Passageway from middle ear to nasopharynx

Fovea centralis: Depressed area in the middle of the macula lutea that contains only cones; it is the area of sharpest vision

Gustation: Sense of taste

Lacrimal gland: Small gland that secretes tears

Macula lutea: Center point of the retina

Mechanoreceptors: Receptors that respond to factors that change the position of a receptor

Membranous labyrinth: Lines the inside of the bony labyrinth

Nociceptors: Pain receptors that respond to tissue damage from trauma as well as from heat, chemicals, pressure, or a lack of oxygen

Olfaction: Sense of smell

Optic chiasm: Point in the brain where half the optic nerve fibers cross to the opposite side of the brain

Optic disc: Spot where nerve fibers leave the retina, converging to become the optic nerve

Organ of Corti: Hearing sense organ

Papillae: Protrusions on the tongue on which taste buds are located

Photoreceptors: Receptors in the eyes that respond to light

Referred pain: Pain originating in a deep organ that is sensed as if it's originating from the body's surface

Refraction: Bending of light rays so they focus on the retina

Retina: Innermost layer of the eye that contains receptors for vision

Rods: Photoreceptors in the retina active in dim light

Sclera: Outermost layer of the eye; formed from dense connective tissue

Thermoreceptors: Receptors activated by a change in temperature

Tympanic membrane: Membrane separating outer ear from middle ear that vibrates in response to sound waves; eardrum

Vestibule: Structure of inner ear that contains organs necessary for sense of balance

Vitreous humor: Jelly-like substance that fills the posterior cavity of the eye

Own the Information

To make the information in this chapter part of your working memory, take some time to reflect on what you've learned. On a separate sheet of paper, write down everything you recall from the chapter. After you're done, log on to the Davis*Plus* website, and check out the Study Group podcast and Study Group Questions for the chapter.

Key Topics for Chapter 11:

- Types and locations of sensory receptors
- Classifications of sensory receptors
- Types and locations of pain receptors
- The main pain pathway
- Characteristics and locations of receptors for temperature and touch
- The location of receptors for taste and the chemical and neural process for experiencing taste
- The location of receptors for smell and the process for experiencing smell
- Structures of the outer, middle, and inner ear
- How hearing occurs
- The role of the vestibule and semicircular canals in the process of balance
- Accessory structures of the eye
- Anatomy of the eye, including the retina and chambers of the eye
- The process of vision
- The action of photoreceptors

Test Your Knowledge

Answers: Chapter 11

1. *Correct answer:* **c.** Chemoreceptors react to chemicals; mechanoreceptors respond to factors (such as pressure, stretch, or vibration) that change the position of a receptor; thermoreceptors respond to changes in temperature.

2. *Correct answer:* **d.** Injured receptors do release several different chemicals, but this has nothing to do with identifying the source of pain. Deep body organs and structures contain slow pain fibers, which produce dull, aching pain. Pain signals that travel to the thalamus proceed to the postcentral gyrus, making the individual aware of pain, while signals that travel to the limbic system trigger emotional responses to pain.

3. *Correct answer:* **a.** Olfaction is the sense of smell. Equilibrium is the sense of balance. Convergence is when the visual axis of each eye lines up properly to the incoming light rays.

4. *Correct answer:* **c.** The vestibule contains organs necessary for the sense of balance. The semicircular canals are crucial for the maintenance of balance and equilibrium. The auricle, or pinna, is the visible part of the external ear.

5. *Correct answer:* **a.** All of the other conditions would interfere with the transmission of vibrations to the inner ear, resulting in a conductive hearing loss.

1. Nociceptors are receptors that respond to:
   a. various chemicals inside and outside the body.
   b. pressure, stretch, or vibration.
   c. pain from tissue damage.
   d. changes in temperature.

2. The true source of pain can be difficult to identify because:
   a. injured tissues release several different chemicals that stimulate the nociceptors and trigger pain.
   b. deep body organs and structures don't contain pain fibers.
   c. some pain signals travel to the thalamus while others travel to the limbic system.
   d. sensory impulses from different areas of the body often travel to the brain over the same pathway.

3. The sense of taste is called:
   a. gustation.
   b. olfaction.
   c. equilibrium.
   d. convergence.

4. Which inner ear structure contains the structures for hearing?
   a. Vestibule
   b. Semicircular canals
   c. Cochlea
   d. Auricle

5. Which condition would cause a sensorineural hearing loss?
   a. Death of hair cells in the organ of Corti
   b. Fluid in the middle ear
   c. Fusion of the auditory ossicles
   d. Impacted cerumen

6. *Correct answer:* **b.** The eustachian tube is a passageway from the middle ear to the nasopharynx; it does not respond to vibrations in the tympanic membrane. The bony labyrinth is the part of the temporal bone containing the structures of the inner ear. Perilymph moves in response to vibrations transmitted by the auditory ossicles through the oval window.

7. *Correct answer:* **b.** Tears do not aid in the refraction or transmission of light rays. Aqueous humor fills the anterior cavity.

8. *Correct answer:* **a.** The ciliary body and choroid are parts of the middle vascular layer. The retina is part of the inner neural layer.

9. *Correct answer:* **d.** Cataracts result from clouding of the lens. Astigmatism results from an uneven or asymmetrical curvature of the cornea. Hyperopia, or farsightedness, results when light rays focus at a point behind the retina.

10. *Correct answer:* **a.** All of the other descriptions pertain to cones.

6. Vibration of the tympanic membrane triggers vibration in the:
  a. eustachian tube.
  b. auditory ossicles.
  c. bony labyrinth.
  d. perilymph.

7. Which is a normal function of tears?
  a. Aid in the refraction of light rays
  b. Deliver oxygen and nutrients to the conjunctiva
  c. Transmit light rays to the cornea
  d. Fill the anterior cavity

8. The outermost layer of the eye is the:
  a. sclera.
  b. ciliary body.
  c. choroid.
  d. retina.

9. What condition results when the rate of absorption of aqueous humor through the canal of Schlemm is less than its production?
  a. Cataracts
  b. Astigmatism
  c. Hyperopia
  d. Glaucoma

10. Rods are:
  a. active in dim light.
  b. concentrated in the center of the retina.
  c. responsible for color vision.
  d. primarily responsible for sharp vision.

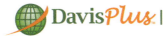 Go to **http://davisplus.fadavis.com** Keyword: Thompson to see all of the resources available with this chapter.

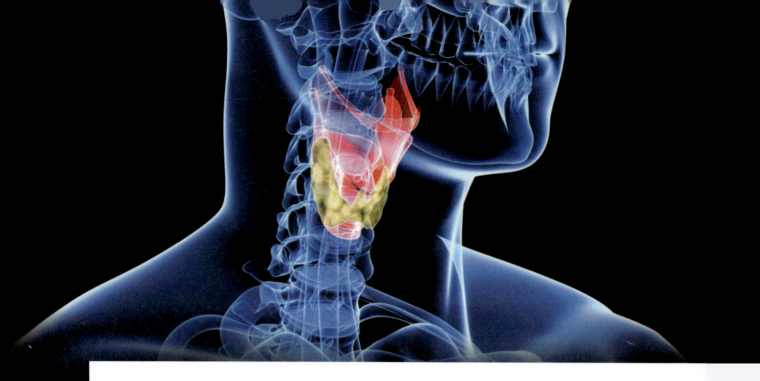

LEARNING OUTCOMES

1. Define *hormone.*

2. List the organs of the endocrine system.

3. Differentiate between the actions of the endocrine system and the nervous system.

4. Compare and contrast the chemical makeup and actions of steroid and nonsteroid hormones.

5. Describe the anatomical relationship between the pituitary gland and hypothalamus.

6. Identify the hormones, as well as the actions of the hormones, secreted by both the pituitary gland and the hypothalamus

7. Explain how pituitary secretions are controlled by the nervous system as well as by negative feedback.

8. Describe the structure and location of the major endocrine glands.

9. Identify the hormones secreted by the major endocrine glands and describe their functions.

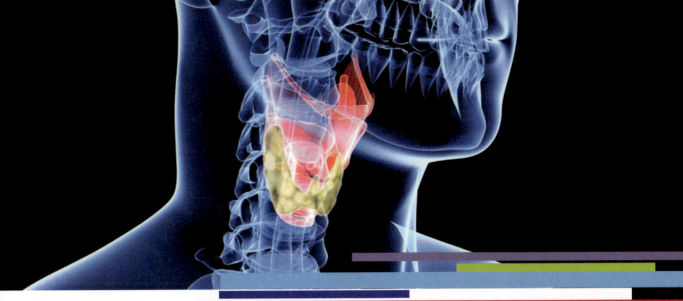

12

ENDOCRINE SYSTEM

The endocrine system produces a multitude of hormones with effects as wide ranging as influencing mood to controlling reproduction.

The endocrine system consists of a variety of glands and specialized cells throughout the body. These glands and cells secrete chemicals (called **hormones**) that influence almost every cell and organ in the body. Hormones determine, among other things, when you feel hungry or full, whether you're fat or thin, how you handle stress, and even how you sleep.

The endocrine and nervous systems often work hand-in-hand to promote communication between cells, allowing them to coordinate and integrate their activities. Although they share a common goal—homeostasis—their methods for accomplishing this vary. For example, the nervous system uses lightning-fast electrical signals to communicate, making it the ideal choice to oversee such time-sensitive processes as breathing and movement. In contrast, the endocrine system communicates through slower-acting hormones, placing it in charge of body processes that happen more slowly, such as cell growth.

FAST FACT

The study of the endocrine system and the diagnosis and treatment of its disorders is called **endocrinology**.

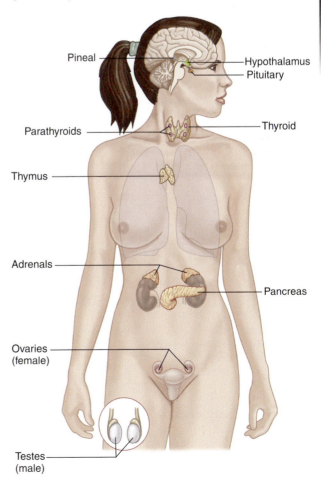

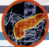

Overview of the Endocrine System

The endocrine system consists of the glands shown in the figure on the previous page as well as clusters of hormone-secreting cells in various organs, including the brain, heart, and small intestine.

The Body AT WORK

*Endocrine glands are ductless glands: they secrete hormones directly into the bloodstream. (In contrast, exocrine glands secrete hormones into ducts, which, in turn, lead to a surface in some other location, such as the body's surface—as in sweat glands—or the digestive tract—as in digestive enzymes.) Once in the bloodstream, each hormone travels throughout the body. In the process, the cells of many different organs are exposed to a particular hormone; however, only cells having receptors for that hormone (called **target cells**) will respond. In other words, a hormone acts only on cells with receptors specific to that hormone; this is called **specificity**.*

FAST FACT

Even after a stimulus ceases, the effects of the endocrine system can persist for days or even weeks.

Comparison of Endocrine and Nervous Systems

The actions of the endocrine and nervous systems complement one another to ensure that the body maintains homeostasis. Their methods of action differ, though, as detailed below.

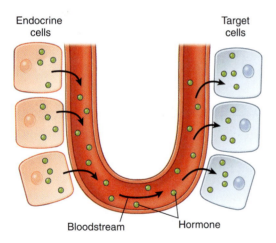

Endocrine cells — Target cells — Bloodstream — Hormone — Target cells — Neuron — Neuro-transmitter

Endocrine system

- Employs hormones to relay messages
- Distributes hormones throughout the body via the bloodstream
- Responds slowly to stimuli (seconds to days)
- Exerts long-lasting effects
- Adapts slowly to continual stimulation

Nervous system

- Employs neurotransmitters to relay messages
- Secretes neurotransmitters into tiny space of a synapse
- Responds to stimuli quickly (milliseconds)
- Exerts short-lived effects
- Adapts quickly to continual stimulation

That Makes Sense

*To differentiate between endocrine and exocrine glands, remember: **EX**ocrine glands have **EX**it routes (ducts) to an environment **EX**ternal to themselves. **END**ocrine glands secrete hormones with**IN** the body that **END** up in the bloodstream.*

Hormones

Hormones can be classified as steroid or nonsteroid. Steroid hormones are synthesized from cholesterol; they include male and female sex hormones as well as aldosterone (secreted by the adrenal cortex). Nonsteroid, or protein-based, hormones are synthesized from amino acids. They can be further divided into protein hormones (such as insulin), peptide hormones (such as antidiuretic hormone), or amino acid derivative hormones (such as epinephrine and norepinephrine). Regardless of classification, hormones travel through the bloodstream to stimulate specific target cells. The target cells may lie anywhere in the body: close to the gland or far from it.

Once a hormone reaches the target cell, it binds with a receptor to trigger changes within the cell. How this occurs, though, depends upon whether the hormone is a steroid or protein-based hormone.

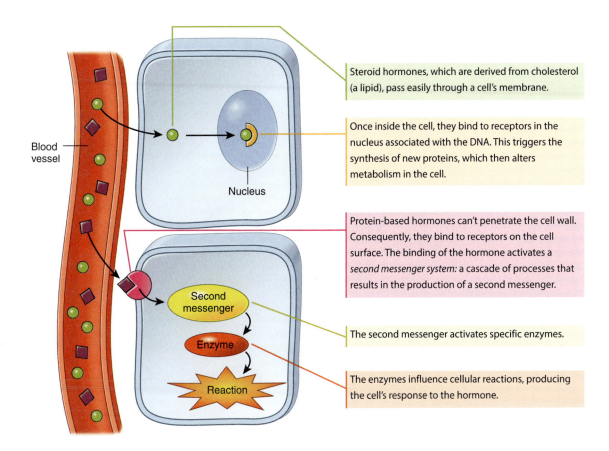

Blood vessel

Nucleus

Second messenger

Enzyme

Reaction

Steroid hormones, which are derived from cholesterol (a lipid), pass easily through a cell's membrane.

Once inside the cell, they bind to receptors in the nucleus associated with the DNA. This triggers the synthesis of new proteins, which then alters metabolism in the cell.

Protein-based hormones can't penetrate the cell wall. Consequently, they bind to receptors on the cell surface. The binding of the hormone activates a *second messenger system:* a cascade of processes that results in the production of a second messenger.

The second messenger activates specific enzymes.

The enzymes influence cellular reactions, producing the cell's response to the hormone.

The Body AT WORK

The more receptors a target cell has, the more sensitive it will be to a hormone. Likewise, the fewer the receptors, the less sensitive it will be. Cells constantly create new receptors to replace older ones. Furthermore, cells can add to their receptors, making them more sensitive to a hormone. As an example, during the final stage of pregnancy, cells in the uterus increase their receptors for oxytocin, the hormone responsible for triggering uterine contractions during childbirth.

FAST FACT

The body employs a number of second messenger molecules; however, the most prominent may be cyclic adenosine monophosphate, or cAMP.

The Pituitary Gland and Hypothalamus

The pituitary gland—especially in conjunction with the nearby hypothalamus—exerts more influence on body processes than any other endocrine gland.

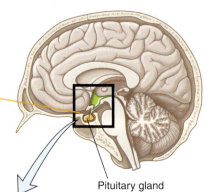

The tiny, pea-sized pituitary gland sits just underneath the hypothalamus. It lies cradled in the sella turcica, a cavity within the sphenoid bone.

Pituitary gland

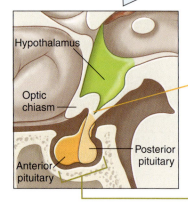

Hypothalamus

Optic chiasm

Posterior pituitary

Anterior pituitary

A stalk called the *infundibulum* connects the hypothalamus and pituitary.

Despite its small size, the pituitary gland is actually two distinct glands: the **anterior pituitary**, or **adenohypophysis**, and the **posterior pituitary**, or **neurohypophysis**. These two glands are made of different tissue, excited by different types of stimuli, and secrete different hormones.

Anterior Pituitary

The anterior pituitary—the larger of the two pituitary glands—consists of glandular tissue. It synthesizes and secretes a number of very important hormones, all under the direction of the hypothalamus.

ANIMATION 🌐

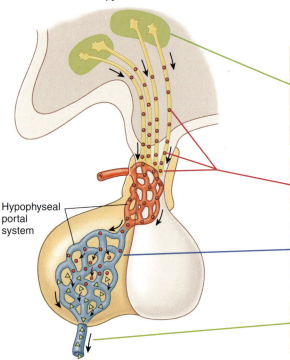

Hypophyseal portal system

Neurons within the hypothalamus synthesize various hormones. Some, called **releasing hormones**, stimulate the anterior pituitary to secrete its hormones. Others, called **inhibiting hormones**, suppress hormone secretion by the anterior pituitary.

The neurons of the hypothalamus release their hormones into a system of blood vessels called the **hypophyseal portal system**.

The blood travels straight to the anterior pituitary, where the hormones from the hypothalamus act on target cells in the anterior pituitary.

This stimulates the anterior pituitary to release, or to suppress the release of, certain hormones into the general circulation.

Hormones of the Anterior Pituitary

Most of the hormones produced and secreted by the anterior pituitary are **tropic** (or **trophic**) hormones (so called because the hormone names end with the suffix *-tropin* or *-tropic*, such as gonado*tropin*, thyro*tropin*, etc.). Tropic hormones stimulate other endocrine cells to release their hormones, as shown in the illustration below.

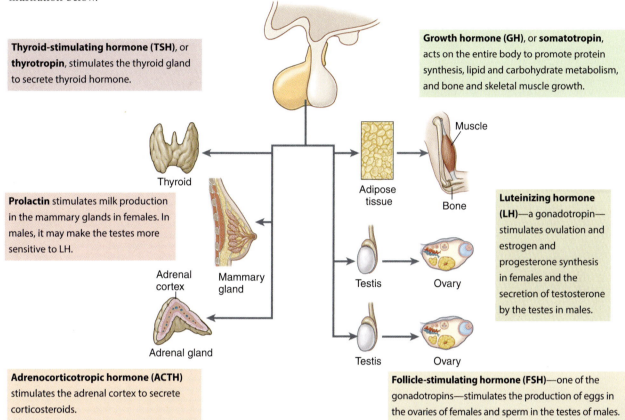

Thyroid-stimulating hormone (TSH), or **thyrotropin**, stimulates the thyroid gland to secrete thyroid hormone.

Growth hormone (GH), or **somatotropin**, acts on the entire body to promote protein synthesis, lipid and carbohydrate metabolism, and bone and skeletal muscle growth.

Muscle

Thyroid

Adipose tissue

Bone

Prolactin stimulates milk production in the mammary glands in females. In males, it may make the testes more sensitive to LH.

Luteinizing hormone (LH)—a gonadotropin—stimulates ovulation and estrogen and progesterone synthesis in females and the secretion of testosterone by the testes in males.

Adrenal cortex

Mammary gland

Testis

Ovary

Adrenal gland

Testis

Ovary

Adrenocorticotropic hormone (ACTH) stimulates the adrenal cortex to secrete corticosteroids.

Follicle-stimulating hormone (FSH)—one of the gonadotropins—stimulates the production of eggs in the ovaries of females and sperm in the testes of males.

Life lesson: Growth hormone abnormalities

The secretion of too much growth hormone (*hypersecretion*) during a child's growth years will trigger rapid, excessive skeletal growth, resulting in a condition called *gigantism*. If the epiphyseal plates have already fused when the hypersecretion occurs, cartilage will form new bone, causing the hands, feet, face, and jaw to enlarge—a disorder called *acromegaly*.

In contrast, a deficiency of growth hormone (*hyposecretion*) while a child is still growing will result in stunted growth. This is sometimes called *pituitary dwarfism*. The condition is usually treated with growth hormone injections.

The Body AT WORK

Following are some of the important hormones released by the hypothalamus. Each acts on the anterior pituitary to release, or suppress, a particular hormone. For example, thyrotropin-releasing hormone stimulates the anterior pituitary to release of thyrotropin, also called thyroid-stimulating hormone; in turn, this hormone stimulates the thyroid to secrete thyroid hormone, or TH.

- Gonadotropin-releasing hormone: *Promotes secretion of FSH and LH*
- Thyrotropin-releasing hormone: *Promotes secretion of TSH*
- Corticotropin-releasing hormone: *Promotes secretion of ACTH*
- Prolactin-releasing hormone: *Promotes secretion of prolactin*
- Prolactin-inhibiting hormone: *Inhibits secretion of prolactin*
- Growth hormone–releasing hormone: *Promotes secretion of GH*
- Somatostatin: *Inhibits secretion of GH and TSH*

Posterior Pituitary

Unlike the anterior pituitary, which is composed of glandular tissue, the posterior pituitary is made of neural tissue. Also, instead of synthesizing hormones as the anterior pituitary does, the posterior pituitary simply stores hormones synthesized by the hypothalamus. The hormones stored by the posterior pituitary are **antidiuretic hormone (ADH)** and **oxytocin (OT)**.

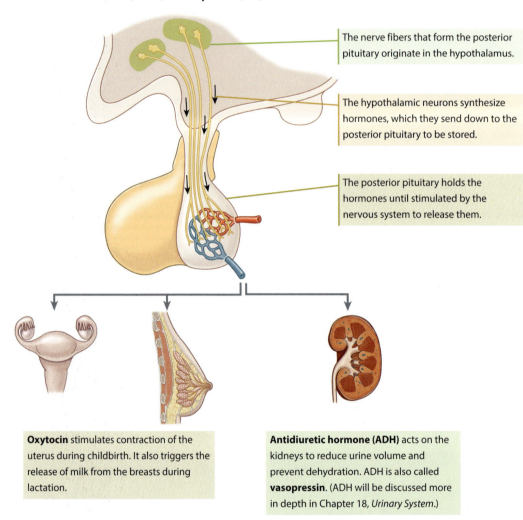

The nerve fibers that form the posterior pituitary originate in the hypothalamus.

The hypothalamic neurons synthesize hormones, which they send down to the posterior pituitary to be stored.

The posterior pituitary holds the hormones until stimulated by the nervous system to release them.

Oxytocin stimulates contraction of the uterus during childbirth. It also triggers the release of milk from the breasts during lactation.

Antidiuretic hormone (ADH) acts on the kidneys to reduce urine volume and prevent dehydration. ADH is also called **vasopressin**. (ADH will be discussed more in depth in Chapter 18, *Urinary System*.)

Hormones of the Pituitary Gland

Hormone	Target	Principal Effects
Anterior pituitary		
GH: Growth hormone (somatotropin)	Throughout body, including liver, bone, muscle, and fat	Growth and the repair of tissue through the breakdown of proteins and fats
PRL: Prolactin	Mammary glands	Milk secretion
TSH: Thyroid-stimulating hormone	Thyroid gland	Growth of the thyroid gland and secretion of thyroid hormone
ACTH: Adrenocorticotropic hormone	Adrenal cortex	Growth of, and secretion of corticosteroids by, the adrenal cortex
FSH: Follicle-stimulating hormone	Ovaries; testes	*Female:* Growth of ovarian follicles and secretion of estrogen *Male:* Sperm production
LH: Luteinizing hormone	Ovaries; testes	*Female:* Ovulation; maintenance of corpus luteum *Male:* Secretion of testosterone
Posterior pituitary		
ADH: Antidiuretic hormone	Kidneys	Water retention
OT: Oxytocin	Uterus; mammary glands	Stimulation of uterine contractions; stimulation of release of milk into ducts of mammary glands

Control of Pituitary Secretions

The pituitary gland does not release a steady flow of hormones. Rather, it releases hormones in phases or pulses. For example, growth hormone is mainly secreted at night, whereas LH surges in the middle of the menstrual cycle. The central nervous system plays a role in controlling hormone secretion. So, too, do the target organs themselves through the process of negative feedback.

Control by the Central Nervous System

The brain constantly monitors conditions both inside and outside the body. In turn, it triggers the release of hormones as needed. For example, when it's cold, it triggers the release of TSH to promote body heat. After a hearty meal, it stimulates the secretion of GH to break down fats for energy and use amino acids to build tissue.

Control by Negative Feedback

When the pituitary stimulates another endocrine gland to secrete its hormone, that hormone is then fed back to the pituitary, telling it to stop further release of the tropic hormone. This process is called **negative feedback**. Negative feedback loops are used extensively to regulate hormones in the hypothalamic-pituitary axis. The following figure illustrates the negative feedback process as it relates to the regulation of body temperature.

ANIMATION 🌐

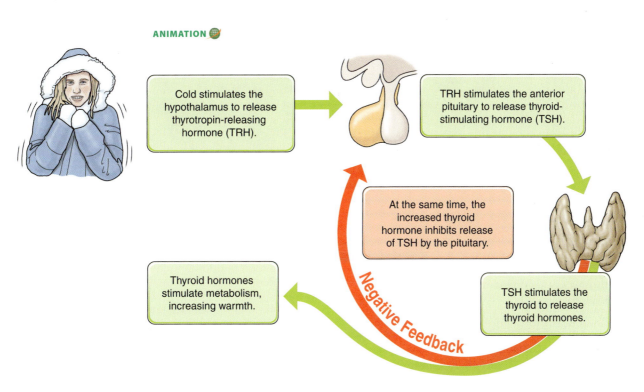

Cold stimulates the hypothalamus to release thyrotropin-releasing hormone (TRH).

TRH stimulates the anterior pituitary to release thyroid-stimulating hormone (TSH).

At the same time, the increased thyroid hormone inhibits release of TSH by the pituitary.

Thyroid hormones stimulate metabolism, increasing warmth.

TSH stimulates the thyroid to release thyroid hormones.

Negative Feedback

FAST FACT

The use of negative feedback to control hormone secretion, combined with the fact that hormones have a limited lifespan, causes most hormones to be secreted in "pulses."

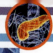
Pineal Gland

The pineal gland produces **melatonin,** a hormone that rises at night, when sunlight is absent, and falls during the day. High melatonin levels trigger sleepiness, making it a key factor in the sleep-wake cycle. Although yet to be proven, scientists speculate that the pineal gland may also regulate the timing of puberty.

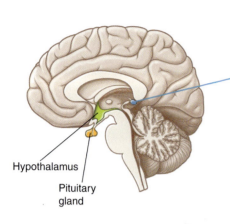

Tucked in the center of the brain, on the roof of the brain's third ventricle, is the tiny, cone-shaped pineal gland.

Hypothalamus

Pituitary gland

FAST FACT

A number of people take supplemental melatonin orally to combat jet lag or other sleep disorders. While the supplements are generally regarded as safe for short-term use, taking too much can increase one's risk for blood clots and seizures.

Life lesson: Seasonal affective disorder

Low levels of melatonin have been linked to mood disorders, particularly *seasonal affective disorder (SAD)*. Occurring during winter months, when exposure to sunlight is limited, people with SAD complain of sleepiness, depression, irritability, and carbohydrate cravings. Exposure to special high-intensity lights for several hours each day often relieves symptoms.

Thymus

The thymus secretes **thymosin** and **thymopoietin,** two hormones having a role in the development of the immune system. Although it secretes hormones, making it a member of the endocrine system, the actions of the hormones make the thymus part of the immune system. (For more information on the thymus gland, see Chapter 16, *Lymphatic & Immune Systems.*)

The thymus lies in the mediastinum just beneath the sternum.

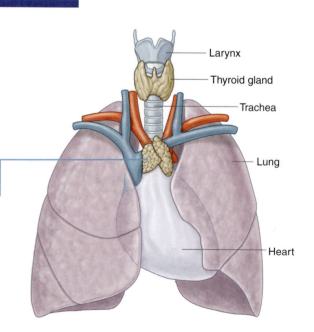

Larynx

Thyroid gland

Trachea

Lung

Heart

In children, the thymus gland is large. Beginning in puberty, though, the gland starts to shrink. By the time one reaches old age, the gland consists of mostly fat and fibrous tissue.

Thyroid Gland

The largest endocrine gland, the thyroid, consists of two large lobes connected by a narrow band of tissue called the isthmus.

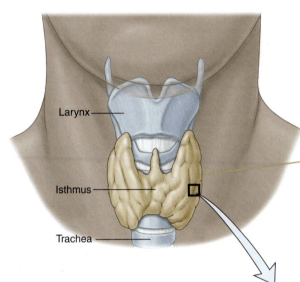

Larynx

Isthmus

Trachea

The thyroid gland resides in the neck, just below the trachea, where it is wrapped around the anterior and lateral portions of the trachea.

Thyroid tissue is made of tiny sacs called **thyroid follicles**. Each follicle is filled with a thick fluid called **thyroid colloid**. The cells lining the sacs secrete the two main thyroid hormones: **T_3 (triiodothyronine)** and **T_4 (thyroxine)**. Unlike other glands, the thyroid gland can store the hormones for later use.

Cells between the thyroid follicles, called **parafollicular cells**, secrete another hormone called **calcitonin**. Secreted in response to rising blood calcium levels, calcitonin triggers the deposition of calcium in bone, thus promoting bone formation. The effects of calcitonin are particularly important in children.

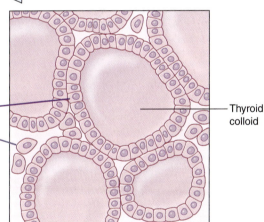

Thyroid colloid

The Body AT WORK

As previously described, TSH (released from the anterior pituitary) stimulates the release of thyroid hormone (TH) from the thyroid gland. The overall effect of TH is to increase the body's metabolic rate, which, in turn, increases heat production. (This explains why TH is released when the body is exposed to cold.) Just a few of the other effects of TH are increased rate and strength of heart contractions, increased respiratory rate, and increased appetite. TH is also crucial for growth and development: it promotes the development of bone; the nervous system; and skin, hair, nails, and teeth.

FAST FACT

The abbreviations T_3 and T_4 refer to the number of iodine atoms in each hormone: T_3 has three iodine atoms while T_4 has four.

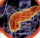

Life lesson: Thyroid disorders

A number of significant disorders develop from hyper- or hyposecretion of thyroid hormone. If a child is born without a thyroid gland, the lack of thyroid hormone (TH) leads to *cretinism*: a condition characterized by retarded growth and sexual development, a low metabolic rate, and mental retardation. If the hyposecretion develops later in life, a lowered metabolic rate causes weight gain, hair loss, and fatigue. If hypothyroidism is severe or prolonged, a condition called *myxedema* may result, which involves swelling and firmness of the skin.

Hypersecretion of TH stimulates the body's metabolism, resulting in a condition called *Graves' disease*. Thought to be due to an autoimmune disorder, Graves' disease causes unexplained weight loss, increased heart rate, nervousness, and *exophthalmos*—a protrusion of the eyeballs due to swelling of tissue behind the eye.

An enlarged thyroid gland due to a dietary deficiency of iodine is called *simple goiter*. Iodine is the basis for TH. Without enough iodine, the production of TH falls. Consequently, the anterior pituitary never receives a negative feedback message to stop producing TSH. Not only that, because TH levels are low, the anterior pituitary tries to stimulate the thyroid even more by secreting greater levels of TSH. Instead of triggering the production of TH (which the thyroid gland can't do without enough iodine), the TSH stimulates growth of thyroid tissue, leading to thyroid enlargement and goiter.

Parathyroid Glands

Located on the posterior surface of the thyroid are four **parathyroid glands**. These glands secrete **parathyroid hormone (PTH)** in response to low blood levels of calcium.

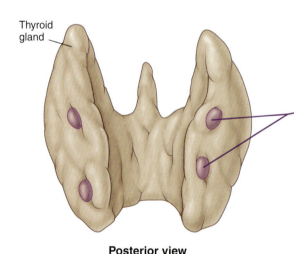

Thyroid gland

The parathyroid glands are embedded in the posterior lobes of the thyroid. Most people have four parathyroid glands, but the number of glands, as well as their locations, can vary.

Posterior view

FAST FACT

The margin of safety for blood calcium levels is so narrow that a drop in blood calcium levels as small as 1% causes the secretion of PTH to double.

PTH is the main hormone the body uses to maintain normal levels of calcium in the blood. Normal nerve and muscle function, blood clotting, cell membrane permeability, and the function of certain enzymes all depend on adequate levels of calcium.

In an effort to achieve calcium homeostasis, PTH exerts its influence on the bones, kidneys, and intestines:

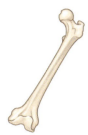

PTH inhibits new bone formation while stimulating the breakdown of old bone, causing calcium (and phosphate) to move out of bone and into the blood.

PTH encourages the kidneys to reabsorb calcium—blocking its excretion into the urine—while promoting the secretion of phosphate. PTH also prompts the kidneys to activate vitamin D, necessary for intestinal absorption of calcium.

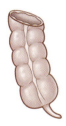

After its activation by the kidneys, vitamin D allows the intestines to absorb calcium from food; the calcium is transported through intestinal cells and into the blood.

FAST FACT
Ninety-nine percent of the body's calcium is found in the bones.

Calcium Homeostasis

Calcitonin (secreted by the thyroid) has antagonistic effects on PTH. The interaction of these two hormones helps the body achieve calcium homeostasis.

ANIMATION

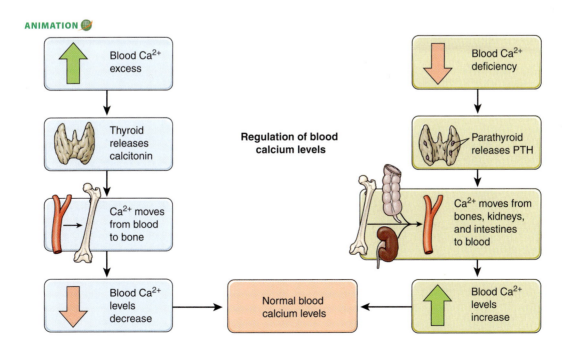

Life lesson: Calcium abnormalities

Calcium ions normally contribute to the difference in polarity across the cell membrane (with the outer surface of the membrane having a positive charge and the interior having a negative). When calcium is in short supply, the charge difference lessens, and sodium ions can more easily enter the cell. As was discussed in the last chapter, it's the inflow of sodium that excites nerve and muscle cells.

So, in a calcium deficiency (*hypocalcemia*), nerve and muscle cells become more

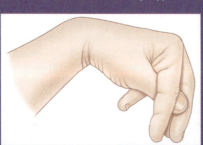

excitable. The excessive excitation leads to muscle tremors, spasms, or *tetany*—the sustained contraction of a muscle. In fact, a cardinal sign of hypocalcemia is a tetany of the hands and feet called *carpopedal spasm*. As shown here, the muscles of the hands contract tightly, unable to relax. (Similar contractions occur in the feet.) If calcium levels drop further, the muscles of the larynx can spasm enough to stop airflow.

When the blood contains too many calcium ions (*hypercalcemia*), the excess calcium ions bind to the cell's surface. Fewer sodium ions flow in and the cell becomes less responsive, resulting in such symptoms as muscle weakness, sluggish reflexes, and, in severe cases, cardiac arrest.

FAST FACT

Tetany from hypocalcemia typically occurs following the accidental removal of the parathyroid glands during thyroid surgery.

Hormones of the Thyroid and Parathyroid Glands

Hormone	Target	Principal Effects
Thyroid		
Triiodothyronine (T_3) and thyroxine (T_4)	Most tissues	Increases rate of metabolism
Calcitonin	Bone	Increases deposition of Ca^{2+} in bones, lowering blood Ca^{2+} levels
Parathyroid		
Parathyroid hormone (PTH)	Bone, kidneys	Increases blood Ca^{2+} levels by increasing removal of Ca^{2+} from bone, reducing urinary excretion of Ca^{2+}, and increasing absorption of Ca^{2+} by the intestines

Adrenal Glands

The adrenal glands perch on the top of each kidney. Instead of being one gland, though, each adrenal gland is actually two distinct glands. The inner portion—called the **adrenal medulla**—consists of modified neurons and functions as part of the sympathetic nervous system. The outer portion—called the **adrenal cortex**—is glandular tissue and secretes steroid hormones called **corticosteroids**.

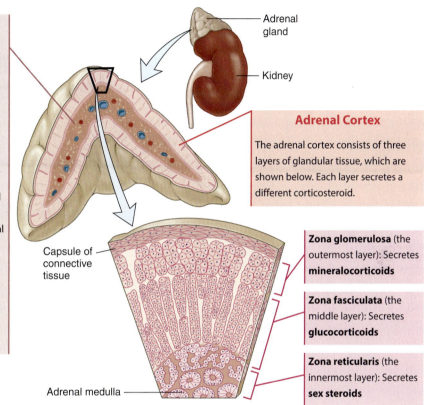

Adrenal Medulla

The adrenal medulla contains modified neurons (called *chromaffin cells*) that act as part of the sympathetic nervous system. These cells secrete **catecholamines** (specifically, epinephrine and norepinephrine) in response to stimulation. Catecholamines:

- Prepare the body for physical activity by increasing heart rate and blood pressure, stimulating circulation to the muscles, and dilating the bronchioles; to maximize blood flow to the areas needed for physical activity, they also inhibit digestion and urinary production.
- Boost glucose levels (a source of fuel) by breaking down glycogen into glucose (**glycogenolysis**) and converting fatty acids and amino acids into glucose (**gluconeogenesis**).

Adrenal gland

Kidney

Adrenal Cortex

The adrenal cortex consists of three layers of glandular tissue, which are shown below. Each layer secretes a different corticosteroid.

Capsule of connective tissue

Adrenal medulla

Zona glomerulosa (the outermost layer): Secretes **mineralocorticoids**

Zona fasciculata (the middle layer): Secretes **glucocorticoids**

Zona reticularis (the innermost layer): Secretes **sex steroids**

Classes of Hormones Secreted by Adrenal Cortex

The hormones secreted by the adrenal cortex fall into one of the following three classes.

Mineralocorticoids

- The principal mineralocorticoid is **aldosterone**.
- Aldosterone acts on the kidneys to promote Na^+ retention and K^+ excretion.
- In turn, it also causes water retention.

(For more information on aldosterone, see Chapter 19, *Fluid, Electrolyte, & Acid-Base Balance*.)

Glucocorticoids

- The principal glucocorticoid is **cortisol**.
- Glucocorticoids help the body adapt to stress and repair damaged tissue by stimulating the breakdown of fat and protein, converting fat and protein to glucose, and releasing fatty acids and glucose into the blood.
- They have an anti-inflammatory effect.
- They also suppress the immune system if secreted over a long term.
- Glucocorticoids are essential for maintaining a normal blood pressure.

Sex Steroids

- Sex steroids include a weak form of **androgen** that is converted to the more potent androgen **testosterone**.
- The testes produce much more testosterone, making this an unimportant source of testosterone in men.
- Androgens stimulate development of pubic and axillary hair and sustain sex drive (libido) in both sexes.

- The sex steroids also include small amounts of **estrogen**.
- Because the amount is small, it has little importance during reproductive years.
- However, it is the only source of estrogen after menopause.

FAST FACT

Glucocorticoids affect nearly every cell in the body.

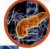

Life lesson: Adrenal disorders

Hypersecretion of cortisol from the adrenal gland results in a collection of symptoms called *Cushing syndrome*. Classic symptoms include a "moon face" (a rounded face) and a "buffalo hump" (a hump between the shoulders resulting from a redistribution of body fat). Because excess cortisol also disrupts carbohydrate and protein metabolism, other symptoms include hyperglycemia, muscle weakness, and edema. The breakdown of protein causes muscle wasting and loss of bone mass, while the retention of sodium and water leads to hypertension.

The hypersecretion of adrenal androgens often accompanies Cushing syndrome. This results in premature puberty in children and the development of masculine characteristics (deepening voice, increased body hair, and the development of facial hair) in women.

Hyposecretion of mineralocorticoids and glucocorticoids occurs in a disorder called *Addison's disease*, also called adrenal cortical insufficiency. Symptoms include a loss of fluid and electrolytes, weakness, muscle wasting, dehydration, and weight loss. Without treatment, adrenal insufficiency is life threatening.

Hormones of the Adrenal Glands

Hormone	Target	Principal Effects
Adrenal medulla		
Epinephrine	Most tissues	Enhances the effects of the sympathetic nervous system
Norepinephrine	Most tissues	Enhances the effects of the sympathetic nervous system
Adrenal cortex		
Aldosterone	Kidney	Promotes Na^+ retention and K^+ excretion, which leads to water retention
Cortisol	Most tissues	Stimulates the breakdown of fat and protein and the conversion of fat and protein to glucose; enhances tissue repair; anti-inflammatory; in large amounts, inhibits the immune system
Adrenal androgens	Sex organs	Promotes growth of pubic and axillary hair; sex drive
Adrenal estrogens	Sex organs	Physiologically insignificant

FAST FACT

Prolonged stress results in increased blood levels of cortisol, which, in turn, leads to immune system dysfunction. One reason this occurs is that high concentrations of cortisol cause lymphatic tissues to atrophy and the numbers of white blood cells to decline.

Life lesson: Changes with Aging

With age, some target tissues become less sensitive to their controlling hormone. The amount of hormone secreted may change, and the hormone may be metabolized more slowly. Following are some common effects of age on the endocrine system:

- The thyroid gland becomes more nodular, leading to a decrease in secretion of thyroid hormones and a decrease in metabolism.
- Changes in levels of parathyroid hormone may contribute to osteoporosis.
- Cells become less sensitive to insulin after age 50, which leads to a gradual rise in fasting blood glucose levels.
- Secretion of growth hormone decreases, resulting in decreased muscle mass and an increase in fat storage.

Pancreas

The pancreas is somewhat unique in that it contains both endocrine and exocrine tissues. The vast majority of the pancreas acts as an exocrine gland, but a small percentage serves an important endocrine function. (For more information on the role of the pancreas as an exocrine gland, see Chapter 20, *Digestive System*.)

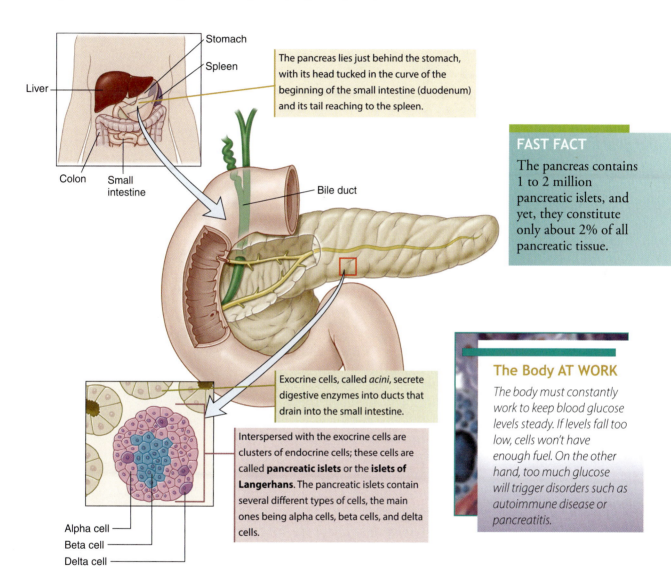

Liver

Stomach

Spleen

Colon

Small intestine

The pancreas lies just behind the stomach, with its head tucked in the curve of the beginning of the small intestine (duodenum) and its tail reaching to the spleen.

Bile duct

Exocrine cells, called *acini*, secrete digestive enzymes into ducts that drain into the small intestine.

Interspersed with the exocrine cells are clusters of endocrine cells; these cells are called **pancreatic islets** or the **islets of Langerhans**. The pancreatic islets contain several different types of cells, the main ones being alpha cells, beta cells, and delta cells.

Alpha cell

Beta cell

Delta cell

FAST FACT

The pancreas contains 1 to 2 million pancreatic islets, and yet, they constitute only about 2% of all pancreatic tissue.

The Body AT WORK

The body must constantly work to keep blood glucose levels steady. If levels fall too low, cells won't have enough fuel. On the other hand, too much glucose will trigger disorders such as autoimmune disease or pancreatitis.

Alpha Cells

Alpha cells secrete the hormone **glucagon**. Between meals, when blood glucose levels fall, glucagon stimulates liver cells to convert glycogen into glucose and also to convert fatty acids and amino acids into glucose (gluconeogenesis). The resulting glucose is released into the bloodstream, causing blood glucose levels to rise.

Beta Cells

Beta cells secrete the hormone **insulin**. After eating, the levels of glucose and amino acids in the blood rise. Insulin stimulates cells to absorb both of these nutrients, causing blood glucose levels to fall.

Delta Cells

Delta cells secrete **somatostatin**, a hormone that works within the pancreas to regulate the other endocrine cells. Specifically, it inhibits the release of both glucagon and insulin. It also inhibits the release of growth hormone.

Regulation of Blood Glucose

Two of the major pancreatic hormones—insulin and glucagon—have opposite effects on levels of blood glucose, which helps maintain blood glucose levels within a normal range.

ANIMATION

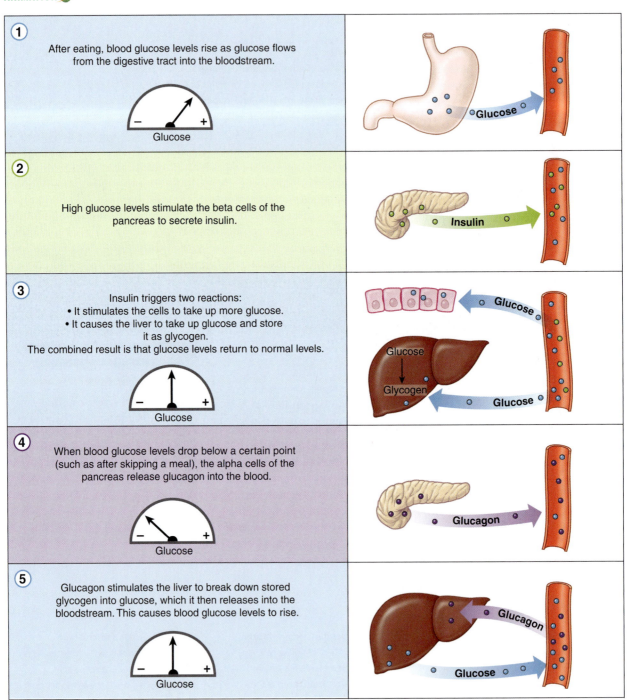

1. After eating, blood glucose levels rise as glucose flows from the digestive tract into the bloodstream.

Glucose

Glucose

2. High glucose levels stimulate the beta cells of the pancreas to secrete insulin.

Insulin

3. Insulin triggers two reactions:
• It stimulates the cells to take up more glucose.
• It causes the liver to take up glucose and store it as glycogen.
The combined result is that glucose levels return to normal levels.

Glucose

Glucose

Glucose
↓
Glycogen

Glucose

Glucose

4. When blood glucose levels drop below a certain point (such as after skipping a meal), the alpha cells of the pancreas release glucagon into the blood.

Glucose

Glucagon

5. Glucagon stimulates the liver to break down stored glycogen into glucose, which it then releases into the bloodstream. This causes blood glucose levels to rise.

Glucose

Glucagon

Glucose

Life lesson: Diabetes mellitus

One of the most common endocrine disorders, the incidence of diabetes in the United States continues to rise. According to the American Diabetes Association, over 29 million Americans, or 9.3% of the population, have diabetes. Of those, thousands experience serious complications: 810 people die, 230 undergo an amputation of a lower limb, 120 begin kidney dialysis or receive a kidney transplant, and 55 go blind *each day*. What's more, it's estimated that about 6 million of the people with diabetes don't even know they have the disease.

Diabetes results from an inadequate amount of insulin or from a diminished number of normal insulin receptors. Either way, without enough insulin, or without enough insulin receptors, glucose can't enter cells. As a result, cells are deprived of their main energy source, and glucose builds up in the blood. This produces high levels of blood glucose (*hyperglycemia*)—one of the cardinal signs of diabetes.

High levels of blood glucose trigger a number of physiological changes that produce the classic signs of this disease. For example, the kidneys normally filter blood plasma and convert it to urine; as it does, it removes glucose and returns it to the bloodstream. In hyperglycemia, the high levels of glucose overwhelm the kidneys, and excess glucose "spills over" into the urine (*glycosuria*).

To flush out this extra load of glucose, the kidneys produce more urine (*polyuria*). In turn, this dehydrates the body, triggering excessive thirst (*polydipsia*). In addition to drinking excessive quantities of fluids, people with untreated diabetes also experience continuous hunger (*polyphagia*). That's because, even though the blood is carrying an overabundant supply of glucose, the cells are starving because the glucose can't enter.

If left untreated, the body begins to burn protein and fat for energy. Besides causing fatigue and weight loss, this abnormal metabolism produces an acidic byproduct called *ketone bodies*. As ketones accumulate, blood pH drops, causing acidosis. Unchecked, this will progress to *diabetic ketoacidosis*, causing symptoms such as nausea, vomiting, fruity odor of the breath, and possibly coma and death.

Diabetes also damages blood vessels (resulting in heart attacks, strokes, decreased circulation in the extremities, and even blindness from damaged blood vessels in the retina) as well as nerves (resulting in numbness and tingling). Kidney disease is another common complication.

FAST FACT

Adults with diabetes have heart disease death rates two to four times higher than adults without diabetes.

There are two main types of diabetes: **type 1** and **type 2**. The characteristics of each type are outlined in the table below.

Characteristics of Type 1 and Type 2 Diabetes Mellitus

	Type 1 Diabetes Characteristics	Type 2 Diabetes Characteristics
Average age at onset	Before age 30	Usually after age 40
Rate of onset	Rapid	Gradual
Percent of all diabetics	10%	90%
Cause	Deficiency of insulin resulting from the destruction of beta cells of the pancreatic islets	Loss of insulin receptors on target cells, leading to insulin resistance
Contributing factors	Uncertain; may be caused by autoimmune disease	Heredity combined with excess body weight and sedentary lifestyle; also more prevalent in Native Americans, Hispanics, and African Americans
Treatment	Daily insulin injections	Lifestyle changes may control disease; if not, oral diabetic medications or insulin injections may be used
	Type 1 diabetes was formerly called juvenile-onset diabetes or insulin-dependent diabetes mellitus (IDDM)	*Type 2 diabetes was formerly called maturity-onset diabetes or non–insulin-dependent diabetes mellitus (NIDDM)*

That Makes Sense

Routine screening for diabetes includes checking the urine for glucose and asking about the "three polys": polyuria, polydipsia, and polyphagia. To make sense of the names of the "three polys," remember this:

- *Poly- is a prefix meaning "much."*
- *The suffix -uria sounds like urine, so polyuria means "much urine."*
- *The suffix -phagia comes from a Greek word meaning "eating." For example, dysphagia means "difficulty eating," while polyphagia means "much, or excessive eating."*
- *The suffix -dipsia comes from a Greek suffix meaning "thirst." Think of taking a "dip" in a body of water; then make the connection to polydipsia, or "drinking much water."*

FAST FACT

About 1 in 50 women develops diabetes during pregnancy. Called *gestational diabetes*, this form of diabetes usually disappears after the woman gives birth.

FAST FACT

Every year, 1.6 million new cases of diabetes are diagnosed in people aged 20 years and older.

The Body AT WORK

Diabetes damages both the cardiovascular and nervous systems. While experts remain unclear as to why this occurs, it appears that chronic hyperglycemia triggers a metabolic reaction that damages cells in small to medium-sized blood vessels. Vascular walls become thicker, restricting blood flow. Nerves, which require an adequate supply of blood to function, suffer ischemia and damage results.

Sixty to seventy percent of people with diabetes have some form of nerve damage. Nerve damage can occur anywhere in the body, although nerves in the legs and feet are most frequently affected. The resulting loss of sensation in these areas makes patients unaware of minor injuries. Left untreated, these wounds can become infected and even gangrenous, often requiring amputation.

Hormones of the Pancreatic Islets

Hormone	Target	Principal Effects
Glucagon	Primarily liver	Stimulates the breakdown of the stored form of glucose for release into the bloodstream
Insulin	Most tissues	Stimulates the movement of glucose from the bloodstream into cells
Somatostatin	Pancreatic cells	Mainly helps regulate the secretion of other hormones of the pancreas

Gonads

Gonads—the testes in males and the ovaries in females—are the primary sex organs. They produce sex hormones, which stimulate the production of sperm (in males) and eggs (in females). They also influence the development of secondary sex characteristics during puberty. (For further information, see Chapter 23, *Reproductive Systems*.)

The cells of the ovarian follicle secrete **estrogen**. Estrogen promotes the development of female characteristics (such as breast development) and also contributes to the development of the reproductive system.

After ovulation, the corpus luteum (the tissue left behind after a rupture of a follicle during ovulation) secretes **progesterone**. Progesterone, in combination with estrogen, helps maintain the uterine lining during pregnancy.

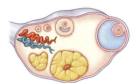

Ovary

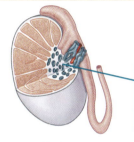

Specialized cells within the testes secrete **testosterone**. Testosterone triggers the development of male sexual characteristics; it also sustains sperm production.

Testis

Other Endocrine Cells and Chemicals

Not all hormones are secreted from specific, well-defined glands. In fact, organs such as the heart, liver, kidneys, stomach, small intestines, and placenta contain clusters of cells that secret hormones. Just a few examples:

- When stretched by rising blood pressure, heart muscle cells secrete *atrial natriuretic peptide (ANP),* a hormone that triggers changes to lower blood pressure.
- The placenta secretes estrogen, progesterone, and other hormones that help maintain a woman's pregnancy.
- The stomach secretes several hormones that help regulate the digestive process.

Also realize that hormones and neurotransmitters are not the only chemical messengers in the body. Certain cells in the body secrete other chemicals that help regulate function. Perhaps the most significant of these is prostaglandins.

Prostaglandins

Made by cells throughout the body, prostaglandins are lipid molecules that, like hormones, integrate the activities of other cells. Unlike hormones—which are released into the bloodstream so they can influence the activities of widely separated organs—prostaglandins are released within the tissue where they are produced. As a result, instead of influencing activities in distant organs, prostaglandins influence the activities of neighboring cells.

The body manufactures a multitude of different prostaglandins. The various prostaglandins play many roles. For example, some prostaglandins promote pain and fever, while others act as vasodilators and vasoconstrictors. They also are involved in inflammation, blood clotting, uterine contraction, reproduction, and digestion.

FAST FACT

Nonsteroidal anti-inflammatory drugs (NSAIDS), such as ibuprofen, relieve pain and fever by blocking the synthesis of certain prostaglandins.

Review of Key Terms

Adenohypophysis: Anterior pituitary gland

Adrenal cortex: Outer portion of the adrenal gland that secretes corticosteroids

Adrenal gland: Gland perched on top of the kidney; consists of two distinct glands (the adrenal medulla and the adrenal cortex)

Adrenal medulla: Inner portion of adrenal gland that functions as part of the sympathetic nervous system

Catecholamines: Epinephrine and norepinephrine; secreted by the adrenal medulla

Corticosteroids: Steroid hormones secreted by the adrenal cortex

Endocrine gland: Ductless glands that secrete hormones directly into the bloodstream

Gonads: Primary sex organs, which are the testes in males and ovaries in females

Graves' disease: Disorder resulting from hypersecretion of thyroid hormone

Hormones: Chemicals secreted by glands and specialized cells of the endocrine system

Neurohypophysis: Posterior pituitary gland

Pancreas: Secretes digestive enzymes (exocrine function) as well as hormones used to regulate blood glucose levels (endocrine function)

Parathyroid glands: Glands embedded on the posterior surface of the thyroid gland that secrete a hormone used to regulate blood calcium levels

Pineal gland: Produces the hormone melatonin, which increases at night and decreases during the day

Pituitary gland: Small gland attached to the lower surface of the hypothalamus that secretes a number of hormones that regulate many bodily processes; consists of an anterior and posterior lobe

Target cells: Cells having receptors for a particular hormone

Tetany: Sustained muscle contraction; may result from hypocalcemia

Thymus: Secretes hormones having a role in the development of the immune system

Thyroid gland: Gland in the neck that secretes hormones that affect the body's metabolic rate

Own the Information

To make the information in this chapter part of your working memory, take some time to reflect on what you've learned. On a separate sheet of paper, write down everything you recall from the chapter. After you're done, log on to the Davis*Plus* website, and check out the Study Group podcast and Study Group Questions for the chapter.

Key Topics for Chapter 12:
- Function of the endocrine system
- Comparison of the endocrine and nervous systems
- The classification and actions of hormones
- The relationship of the pituitary gland and hypothalamus
- Hormones of the hypothalamus and pituitary gland
- Control of pituitary secretions by the central nervous system and negative feedback
- The location, structure, and function of the pineal gland, thymus, thyroid gland, parathyroid glands, adrenal glands, pancreas, and gonads
- Other endocrine tissues and chemicals

Test Your Knowledge

1. Which is a characteristic of exocrine glands?
   a. They secrete hormones into the bloodstream.
   b. Ducts carry their secretions to the body's surface.
   c. They exert a long-lasting effect.
   d. They respond slowly to stimuli.

2. Which endocrine gland influences more body processes than any other endocrine gland?
   a. Thyroid
   b. Pituitary
   c. Adrenal cortex
   d. Limbic system

3. A key difference between the anterior and posterior pituitary is that the posterior pituitary:
   a. consists of glandular tissue.
   b. secretes hormones under the direction of the hypothalamus.
   c. receives hormones from the hypothalamus via the hypophyseal portal system.
   d. stores hormones released from the hypothalamus.

4. Negative feedback is a process by which:
   a. a hormone is fed back to the pituitary, telling it to stop further release of that hormone.
   b. the deficiency of a certain hormone stimulates a gland to release more of that hormone.
   c. the central nervous system monitors the conditions inside and outside of the body and, in turn, triggers the release of hormones as needed.
   d. hormone levels fall precipitously, triggering shock.

5. Cold temperatures are most likely to stimulate the release of which hormone by the anterior pituitary?
   a. Growth hormone
   b. ACTH
   c. Thyroid-stimulating hormone
   d. Prolactin

6. Following thyroid surgery, a patient is most at risk for which disorder?
   a. Graves' disease
   b. Goiter
   c. Hypercalcemia
   d. Hypocalcemia

7. To help the body cope with stress, the adrenal cortex secretes which class of hormones?
   a. Mineralocorticoids
   b. Catecholamines
   c. Glucocorticoids
   d. Sex steroids

8. Which gland has more exocrine than endocrine tissue?
   a. Thyroid gland
   b. Adrenal gland
   c. Pancreas
   d. Thymus

9. The chief role of insulin is to:
   a. stimulate cells to take up more glucose.
   b. stimulate the liver to break down stored glycogen into glucose.
   c. stimulate the pancreas to release glucagon into the blood.
   d. trigger the conversion of fatty acids and amino acids into glucose.

10. A hypersecretion of growth hormone during adulthood causes:
    a. gigantism.
    b. pituitary dwarfism.
    c. acromegaly.
    d. myxedema.

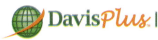

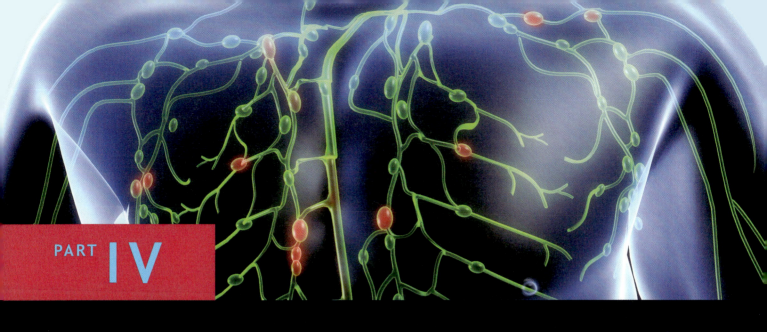

PART **IV**

MAINTENANCE
OF THE BODY

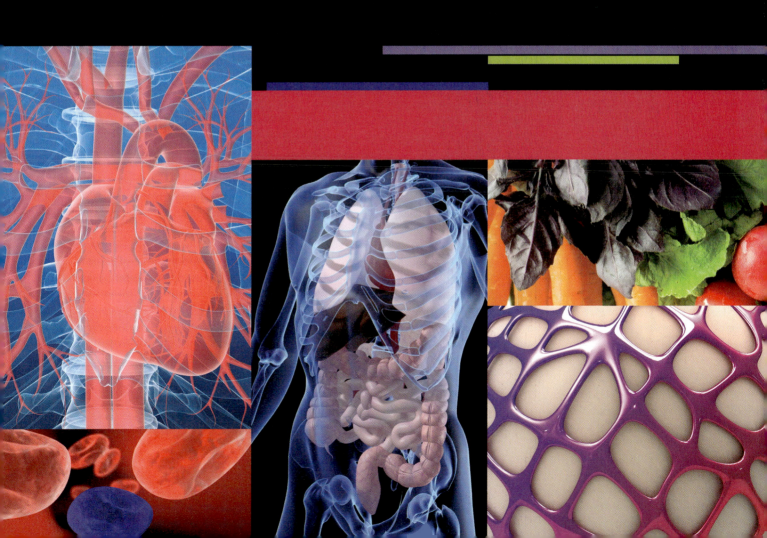

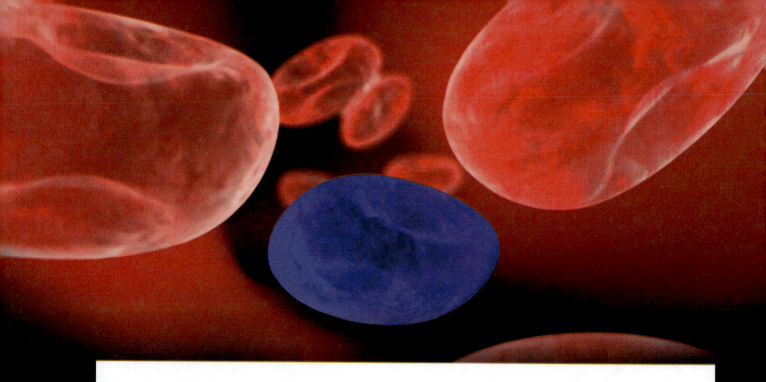

CHAPTER OUTLINE

Components of Blood

Blood Cell Formation

Red Blood Cells

White Blood Cells

Platelets and the Control of Bleeding

Blood Types

LEARNING OUTCOMES

1. List the major components of blood.

2. Explain how blood cells are produced.

3. Describe the structure and function of red blood cells.

4. Describe the structure and function of hemoglobin.

5. Summarize the life cycle of red blood cells.

6. Explain the function of white blood cells in general as well as the specific role of each type of white blood cell.

7. Describe the formation and function of platelets.

8. Discuss the mechanisms for controlling bleeding.

9. Describe the two pathways that result in the formation of a blood clot.

10. Explain how a blood clot is dissolved.

11. List the ABO and Rh blood types and explain how blood type relates to transfusion compatibility.

12. Describe the effects of Rh incompatibility between a mother and a fetus.

13

BLOOD

The blood of an average adult measures about 5 liters and accounts for 7% of body weight.

For centuries, scientists and philosophers alike have regarded blood as the fluid of life. It has only been since the invention of the microscope, however, that the complexity of this vital fluid has become apparent. Blood is actually a connective tissue consisting of several types of cells in combination with fluid: a tissue with a fluid matrix. Its fluid composition allows blood to function as no other connective tissue can. Instead of staying fixed in one location, blood can *move*. In fact, its main function is to serve as a transport medium as it makes endless, frequent laps around the body. Blood delivers oxygen and removes waste products from the body's cells; it delivers nutrients, hormones, enzymes, and many other critical substances to points throughout the body; it plays multiple roles in protecting the body against infection; it helps stabilize the body's acid-base balance; it also helps regulate body temperature.

By analyzing the components of blood, one can gain clues about diseases and disorders throughout the body, which is why blood tests are performed more often than any other medical test. Interpreting those results, though, depends upon a solid understanding of the components and functions of blood.

Components of Blood

When a sample of blood is spun down in a centrifuge, its two main components become apparent.

The main component of plasma is water; however, plasma also contains proteins (the main one being **albumin**), nutrients, electrolytes, hormones, and gases. Plasma proteins play roles in blood clotting, the immune system, and the regulation of fluid volume. Plasma without the clotting proteins (which occurs when blood is allowed to clot and the solid portion is removed) is called **serum**.

Plasma is the clear, extracellular matrix of this liquid connective tissue. It accounts for 55% of blood.

WBCs and platelets form a narrow buff-colored band just underneath the plasma. Called the *buffy coat*, these cells constitute 1% or less of the blood volume.

Formed elements—which include cells and cell fragments—make up 45% of blood. Specific blood cells include **erythrocytes** (red blood cells, or RBCs), **leukocytes** (white blood cells, or WBCs), and **platelets**.

RBCs are the heaviest of the formed elements and sink to the bottom of the sample. They account for most of the formed elements. This value—the percentage of cells in a sample of blood—is called the **hematocrit**.

The Body AT WORK

*An important property of blood—determined by the combination of plasma and blood cells—is **viscosity**. Basically, viscosity refers to how thick or sticky a fluid is. The more viscous a fluid, the thicker it is. (For example, honey is more viscous than water.) Whole blood is normally five times as thick as water, mainly due to the presence of RBCs. If the number of RBCs drops, blood becomes "thinner," or less viscous, causing it to flow too rapidly. Too many RBCs increase viscosity, making blood flow sluggish. Left untreated, either condition can cause cardiovascular problems.*

Blood Cell Formation

The body works continually to replace blood cells that are old or damaged or that have been used up in body processes. The production of blood is called **hemopoiesis**; tissues that produce blood cells are called hemopoietic tissues. The body has two types of **hemopoietic** tissue: red bone marrow and lymphatic tissue.

- Red bone marrow—found in the ends of long bones and in flat irregular bones such as the sternum, cranial bones, vertebrae, and pelvis—produces all types of blood cells.
- Lymphatic tissue—found in the spleen, lymph nodes, and thymus gland—supplement blood cell production by producing lymphocytes, a specific type of WBC.

FAST FACT

An adult normally produces 400 billion platelets, 200 billion RBCs, and 20 billion WBCs *every day*.

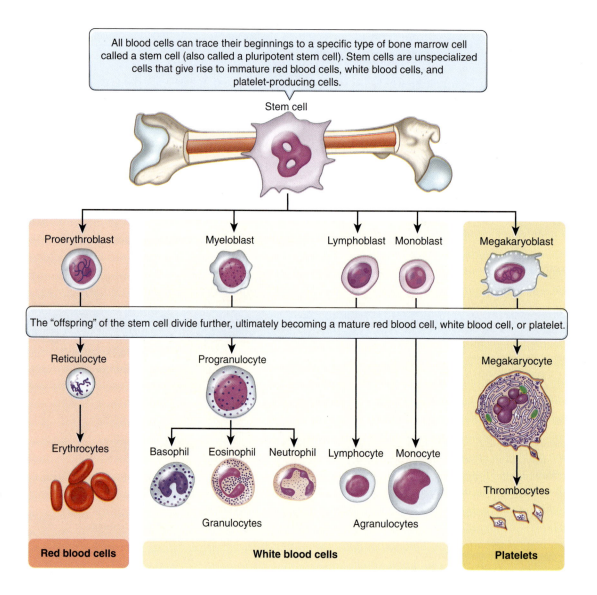

All blood cells can trace their beginnings to a specific type of bone marrow cell called a stem cell (also called a pluripotent stem cell). Stem cells are unspecialized cells that give rise to immature red blood cells, white blood cells, and platelet-producing cells.

Stem cell

Proerythroblast   Myeloblast   Lymphoblast   Monoblast   Megakaryoblast

The "offspring" of the stem cell divide further, ultimately becoming a mature red blood cell, white blood cell, or platelet.

Reticulocyte   Progranulocyte   Megakaryocyte

Erythrocytes   Basophil   Eosinophil   Neutrophil   Lymphocyte   Monocyte   Thrombocytes

Granulocytes   Agranulocytes

Red blood cells   **White blood cells**   **Platelets**

Red Blood Cells

Charged with delivering oxygen to cells and removing carbon dioxide, red blood cells, or **erythrocytes**, are critical to survival. Blood contains more RBCs than any other formed element.

A normal RBC is shaped like a disc with a sunken center. This shape gives the cell a large surface area through which oxygen and carbon dioxide can readily diffuse.

RBCs lose almost all of their organelles during development. Because they lack a nucleus and DNA, they cannot replicate themselves.

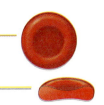

The cytoskeleton of the RBC contains stretchable fibers that make it flexible, allowing it to fold and stretch as it squeezes through tiny capillaries. When the cell emerges from the tight confines of a narrow vessel, it springs back to its original shape.

Hemoglobin

Over a third of the interior of a RBC is filled with **hemoglobin**—a red pigment that gives blood its color.

Hemoglobin consists of four ribbon-like protein chains called **globins**.

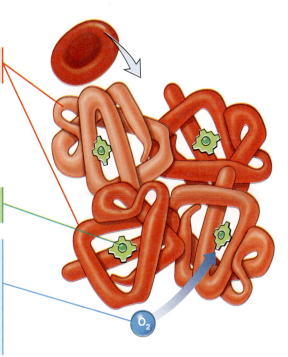

Bound to each globin is an iron-containing molecule called **heme**.

Each heme molecule can combine with one molecule of oxygen; therefore, one hemoglobin molecule can unite with four molecules of oxygen to form **oxyhemoglobin**. (Hemoglobin also carries CO_2, but, instead of binding with heme, CO_2 binds with globin.) (For more information about gas transport by hemoglobin, see Chapter 17, *Respiratory System*.)

O_2

The Body AT WORK

How much oxygen the blood can carry depends on the quantity of red blood cells and hemoglobin it contains. That's why some of the most commonly performed blood tests measure hematocrit, hemoglobin concentration, and RBC count. Normal values vary between men and women, as shown below:

- ***Hematocrit:*** *Female: 37%–48%;* **Male:** *45%–52%*
- ***Hemoglobin:*** *Female: 12–16 g/dl;* **Male:** *13–18 g/dl*
- ***RBC count:*** *Female: 4.2–5.4 million/mcL;* **Male:** *4.6–6.2 million/mcL*

Differences in blood values between men and women result because of several factors. Men have higher levels of androgens, and androgens stimulate RBC production. Also, women of reproductive age lose blood through menstruation, which lowers blood cell counts. Finally, women typically have more body fat than men, and the higher the body fat content, the lower the hematocrit level.

FAST FACT

The study of blood is called **hematology.**

FAST FACT

The color of blood always remains within the red spectrum: bright red when oxygenated and a deep maroon when deoxygenated. Blood is never blue.

The Body AT WORK

The oxygen-carrying component of hemoglobin contains iron. Consequently, an adequate supply of dietary iron is crucial for hemoglobin synthesis. Because of the loss of blood through menstruation, women of reproductive age have the highest nutritional requirement for iron. Other nutritional requirements for red blood cell formation include vitamin B_{12}, folic acid, and vitamin C.

Life lesson: Sickle cell disease

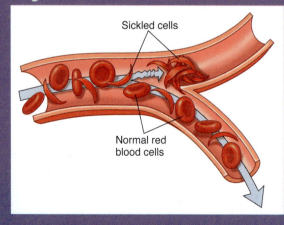

Sickled cells

Normal red blood cells

Sickle cell disease is an inherited blood disorder involving hemoglobin. Affected RBCs are stiff rather than flexible; as they try to squeeze into narrow blood vessels, they can't fold over like a normal RBC. Instead, their shape becomes distorted: the cells elongate and the ends point, making them look somewhat like a sickle (which is where the disease gets its name). These distorted cells are also sticky, causing them to clump together and block small blood vessels. This deprives tissues of necessary oxygen, resulting in intense pain. Other complications of sickle cell disease include kidney or heart failure or stroke.

If a person inherits the gene for the disease from only one parent, he will have *sickle cell trait*. People with sickle cell trait are generally healthy. If a person inherits the defective gene from both parents, sickle cell disease will result. The disease occurs mostly among people of African descent.

Life Cycle of Red Blood Cells

Red blood cells circulate for about 120 days before they die, break up, and are consumed by phagocytic cells in the spleen and the liver. In fact, 2.5 million RBCs are destroyed every second. While this is only a fraction of the trillions of RBCs in the body, the body must constantly produce new RBCs to maintain homeostasis. The process of producing new erythrocytes—called **erythropoiesis**—is maintained through a negative feedback loop.

ANIMATION

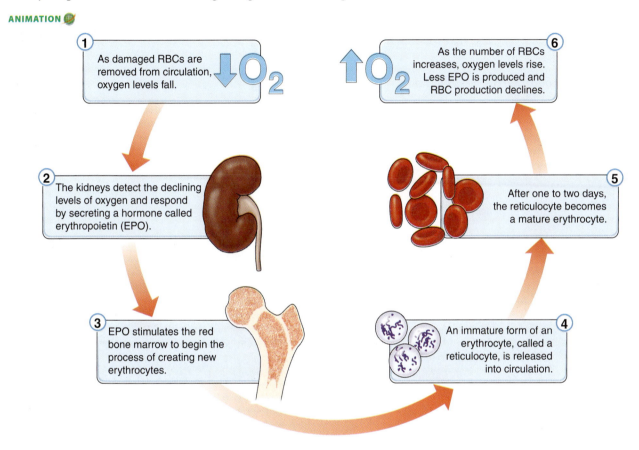

1 As damaged RBCs are removed from circulation, oxygen levels fall. ↓O_2

2 The kidneys detect the declining levels of oxygen and respond by secreting a hormone called erythropoietin (EPO).

3 EPO stimulates the red bone marrow to begin the process of creating new erythrocytes.

4 An immature form of an erythrocyte, called a reticulocyte, is released into circulation.

5 After one to two days, the reticulocyte becomes a mature erythrocyte.

6 As the number of RBCs increases, oxygen levels rise. Less EPO is produced and RBC production declines. ↑O_2

FAST FACT

The process of erythropoiesis takes three to five days.

The Body AT WORK

At any given time, reticulocytes comprise about 0.5% to 1.5% of the circulating RBCs. This number rises, though, in certain situations. For example, following blood loss, the body tries to produce more RBCs to make up for those that were lost. In its effort to catch up, the bone marrow releases an increased number of reticulocytes into the circulation. Another common cause of increased RBC production is a move to higher altitude, where the atmosphere contains less oxygen. The body compensates for the lower atmospheric oxygen by producing more red blood cells.

In contrast, a low reticulocyte count may mean that fewer RBCs are being made by the bone marrow, which may result from certain types of anemia or bone marrow disorders.

Breakdown of Red Blood Cells

As an RBC ages, its membrane weakens, becoming fragile. As it passes through the narrow capillaries in the spleen, it begins to break down.

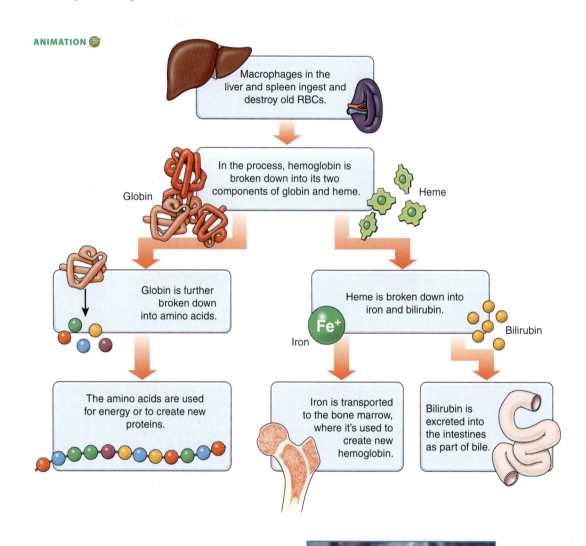

ANIMATION

Macrophages in the liver and spleen ingest and destroy old RBCs.

In the process, hemoglobin is broken down into its two components of globin and heme.

Globin

Heme

Globin is further broken down into amino acids.

Heme is broken down into iron and bilirubin.

Fe⁺

Iron

Bilirubin

The amino acids are used for energy or to create new proteins.

Iron is transported to the bone marrow, where it's used to create new hemoglobin.

Bilirubin is excreted into the intestines as part of bile.

FAST FACT

Bile in the intestines gives feces its brown color. Another pigment resulting from the breakdown of hemoglobin (called urochrome) gives urine its yellow color.

The Body AT WORK

When the destruction of RBCs becomes excessive (hemolysis), the body can't readily assimilate the increased amounts of bilirubin being produced. Instead of being excreted into the intestines, the excess bilirubin enters the tissues, causing the skin and sclera to take on a yellowish hue. This condition is called jaundice.

Jaundice may also result from conditions such as liver disease or bile duct obstruction that interfere with the flow of bile into the intestines. Newborns, too, often develop jaundice shortly after birth (a condition called physiological jaundice). This occurs as their immature livers begin the task of clearing bilirubin from the blood.

Life lesson: Polycythemia

When the rate at which new RBCs are being created exceeds the rate at which old ones are being destroyed, an imbalance results. The state in which the body has an excess of RBCs is called *polycythemia*.

An abnormality in the red bone marrow, such as cancer, is one possible cause of polycythemia. In this instance, the diseased marrow triggers overproduction of RBCs; this condition is called *polycythemia vera*. Another type of polycythemia—*secondary polycythemia*—results when the body attempts to compensate for conditions that have caused the amount of oxygen in the blood to drop. For example, smoking, lung or heart diseases, and air pollution all lower oxygen levels in the blood. In an attempt to maintain its delivery of oxygen to the tissues, the body increases production of RBCs. (Living at a high altitude also causes polycythemia as the body compensates for lower levels of atmospheric oxygen.)

An increased number of RBCs increases blood volume as well as viscosity. Symptoms include headache, ruddiness, and itchiness. Unchecked, complications such as high blood pressure, blood clots, and even heart failure may occur.

FAST FACT

To ensure adequate erythropoiesis, we must consume 5 to 20 mg of iron in our food each day to cover the amount lost through the urine, feces, and bleeding.

FAST FACT

"Packaging" hemoglobin inside red blood cells ensures that the hemoglobin remains within the confines of the blood vessels instead of leaking out into the surrounding tissues.

Life lesson: Anemia

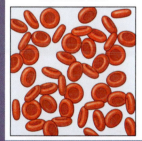
Normal number of red blood cells

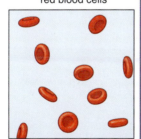
Anemic number of red blood cells

Anemia is a deficiency of RBCs or hemoglobin. Sometimes anemia occurs because of a loss of RBCs, such as from a hemorrhage, or when too many RBCs are being destroyed (*hemolytic anemia*). More commonly, anemia results from an insufficient supply of iron in the diet. Because iron is a key component of hemoglobin, an insufficient supply of this nutrient leads to **iron-deficiency anemia**. (Another nutritional anemia—*pernicious anemia*—results from a lack of vitamin B_{12}. In this instance, the anemia typically occurs because the body can't assimilate the vitamin due to a lack of a chemical produced in the stomach called *intrinsic factor*.) Another cause of anemia is an insufficient supply of the hormone erythropoietin (EPO). Without EPO, red bone marrow isn't stimulated to create new erythrocytes, which explains why anemia usually accompanies kidney disease.

Without enough RBCs or hemoglobin, the oxygen-carrying capacity of blood is diminished, causing fatigue, pallor, and, possibly, shortness of breath. Blood viscosity is also reduced, resulting in a faster heart rate and lower blood pressure.

White Blood Cells

White blood cells (WBCs) or **leukocytes** are the fewest of the formed elements. (A microliter of blood contains between 5000 and 10,000 WBCs and 5 million RBCs.) Regardless, WBCs are crucial to life: they are the body's line of defense against invasion by infectious pathogens. The body contains five types of WBCs, all different in size, appearance, abundance, and function.

All leukocytes—unlike RBCs—contain a nucleus. They also contain a number of other internal structures, some of which look like granules when stained and examined under a microscope. The presence or absence of granules identifies the two classifications of WBCs: **granulocytes** (those having obvious granules) and **agranulocytes** (those having few or no granules).

Granulocytes

Besides containing granules in the cytoplasm, granulocytes also contain a single multilobular nucleus. The three types of granulocytes are **neutrophils**, **eosinophils**, and **basophils**.

Types of Granulocytes

	Neutrophils	**Eosinophils**	**Basophils**
Quantity	Most abundant of the WBCs, neutrophils make up 60% to 70% of all the WBCs in circulation.	Eosinophils account for 2% to 5% of circulating WBCs.	The fewest of the WBCs, basophils comprise only 0.5% to 1% of the WBC count.
Characteristics	The nucleus of young neutrophils looks like a band or a stab wound; therefore, they are sometimes called *band cells* or *stab cells*. They are also called polymorphonuclear leukocytes (PMNs) because the shape of the nucleus varies between neutrophils.	While few exist in the bloodstream, eosinophils are numerous in the lining of the respiratory and digestive tracts.	Basophils possess little or no phagocytic ability.
Function	Highly mobile, neutrophils quickly migrate out of blood vessels and into tissue spaces, where they engulf and digest foreign materials. Worn-out neutrophils left at the site of infection form the main component of pus.	Eosinophils are involved in allergic reactions; they also kill parasites.	Basophils secrete heparin (an anticoagulant), which prevents clotting in the infected area so WBCs can enter; they also secrete histamine, a substance that causes blood vessels to leak, which attracts WBCs.
Life cycle	All granulocytes circulate for 5 to 8 hours and then migrate into the tissues, where they live another 4 or 5 days.		

Agranulocytes

Unlike granulocytes, agranulocytes lack cytoplasmic granules; the nuclei of these WBCs also lack lobes. There are two types of agranulocytes: **lymphocytes** and **monocytes**.

Types of Agranulocytes

	Lymphocytes	Monocytes
Quantity	The second most numerous of the WBCs, lymphocytes constitute 25% to 33% of the WBC count.	Monocytes comprise 3% to 8% of the WBC count.
Characteristics	Lymphocytes are the smallest of the WBCs.	Monocytes are the largest of the WBCs.
Function	Lymphocytes are responsible for long-term immunity. There are two types: • *T lymphocytes,* which directly attack an infected or cancerous cell • *B lymphocytes,* which produce antibodies against specific antigens	Monocytes are highly phagocytic and can engulf large bacteria and viral-infected cells.
Life cycle	All lymphocytes begin in the bone marrow; while some mature there, others migrate to the thymus to finish developing. After maturing, all lymphocytes colonize the organs and tissues of the lymph system (such as the spleen and lymph nodes). Afterward, they continually cycle between the bloodstream and lymph system. Lymphocytes may survive from a few weeks to decades. (For more information on lymphocytes, see Chapter 16, *Lymphatic & Immune Systems*.)	After circulating in the bloodstream for 10 to 20 hours, monocytes migrate into tissues, where they transform into macrophages: aggressive phagocytic cells that ingest bacteria, cellular debris, and cancerous cells. Macrophages can live as long as a few years.

FAST FACT

When cells become inflamed from a bacterial infection, they release chemicals that attract neutrophils and other phagocytic WBCs to the infection site.

Life lesson: Changes with aging

The volume and composition of blood remain relatively constant with age. Abnormal blood values that do occur usually result from disorders in other systems. For example, elderly individuals are more likely to form unwanted blood clots or develop chronic types of leukemia. However, these disorders usually occur because of changes in blood vessels (in the case of blood clots) or the immune system (in the case of leukemia). Elderly individuals also have a greater risk for developing pernicious anemia due to the fact that the stomach mucosa, which produces intrinsic factor, atrophies with age.

262

PART IV Maintenance of the Body

The Body AT WORK

*An abnormally low WBC count (called **leukopenia**) may result from certain viral illnesses, including AIDS, as well as lead poisoning. An elevated WBC count (called **leukocytosis**) usually indicates infection or an allergy. Because each WBC has a slightly different function, knowing the count of each WBC (called a differential WBC count) can be useful. For example, an increased number of neutrophils indicate a bacterial infection. A high eosinophil count signals an allergy or a parasitic infection.*

FAST FACT

The most commonly performed blood test is the complete blood count (CBC). It provides information about all the formed elements of the blood: RBCs (including hemoglobin, hematocrit, and reticulocytes), WBCs (including a differential), and platelets.

Life lesson: Leukemia

A cancer of the blood or bone marrow, *leukemia* is characterized by an extremely high WBC count. The term *leukemia* encompasses a number of varieties of the disease. To differentiate between types, leukemia is subdivided into several large groups.

The first differentiation is between acute and chronic forms of the disease. *Acute leukemia*—the form occurring most commonly in children—appears suddenly and involves the rapid increase of immature WBCs. In contrast, *chronic leukemia*, which involves the proliferation of relatively mature but still abnormal WBCs, develops more slowly. It occurs most often in older people, although it may occur at any age.

The next major classification of leukemia is based on the type of blood cell affected. *Lymphocytic leukemia* involves the rapid proliferation of lymphocytes; *myeloid leukemia* involves uncontrolled granulocyte production.

In all types, the proliferation of abnormal WBCs crowds out normal bone marrow cells, resulting in deficiencies of normal WBCs, RBCs, and platelets. The deficiency of normal WBCs leads to a weakened immune system, placing the individual at risk for infection. The deficiency of RBCs leads to anemia, which may cause fatigue and pallor. Finally, the deficiency of platelets results in an increased risk for bleeding and bruising.

Acute lymphocytic leukemia—the most common form of leukemia in children—has the highest cure rate. Treatment includes chemotherapy, radiation, and bone marrow transplants.

FAST FACT

An increased number of band cells (typically a sign of an infection) is often called a shift to the left. That's because, historically, paper laboratory slips used for differential WBC counts listed the count for band cells to the left of the counts for mature neutrophils.

Platelets and the Control of Bleeding

Platelets (also called *thrombocytes*) are the second most abundant of the formed elements, with each microliter of blood containing between 150,000 and 400,000 platelets. Platelets play a key role in stopping bleeding (**hemostasis**).

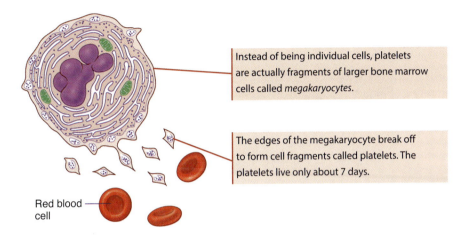

Instead of being individual cells, platelets are actually fragments of larger bone marrow cells called *megakaryocytes*.

The edges of the megakaryocyte break off to form cell fragments called platelets. The platelets live only about 7 days.

Red blood cell

Hemostasis

When a blood vessel is cut, the body must react quickly to stop the flow of blood. It does so through the following sequence of events: vascular spasm, the formation of a platelet plug, and the formation of a blood clot.

Vascular Spasm

As soon as a blood vessel is injured, smooth muscle fibers in the wall of the vessel spasm. This constricts the blood vessel and slows the flow of blood. (This response is only temporary but gives the other hemostatic mechanisms time to activate.)

Formation of a Platelet Plug

The break in the blood vessel exposes collagen fibers, creating a rough spot on the vessel's normally slick interior. This rough spot triggers changes in the passing platelets, transforming them into *sticky platelets*.

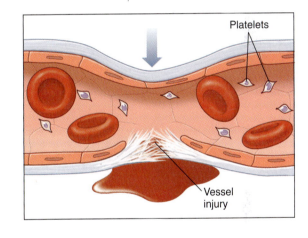

Platelets

Vessel injury

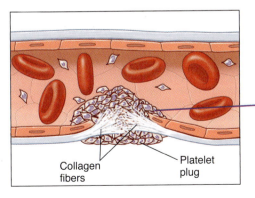

Collagen fibers

Platelet plug

The sticky platelets do as their name implies: stick to the vessel wall and to each other, forming a mass of platelets called a **platelet plug**. The platelets facilitate their clumping by secreting several chemicals—some cause the vessel to constrict further while others attract even more platelets. The platelet plug forms a temporary seal in the vessel wall. A more stable solution requires the formation of a clot.

Formation of a Blood Clot

Blood clotting, or **coagulation**, involves a complex series of chemical reactions using proteins called clotting factors. (See "The Body at Work" on this page.)

The first several reactions in the clotting process vary, depending upon whether the process has been stimulated by factors inside or outside the blood. Specifically, when the damaged blood vessel and surrounding tissues—areas outside or *extrinsic* to the blood—release clotting factors, this kicks off a cascade of events called the **extrinsic pathway**. When the clotting factors are activated within the blood—such as by the platelets as they adhere to the collagen in the damaged vessel wall—this sets off a different cascade of events called the **intrinsic pathway**.

ANIMATION

Both the extrinsic and intrinsic pathways result in the formation of factor X. (This occurs in a single reaction in the extrinsic pathway, whereas, in the intrinsic pathway, four different reactions are required to activate factor X.) Either way, once factor X is activated, the formation of a blood clot follows a common pathway, as shown here.

Sticky platelets

Injured cells

Intrinsic pathway

Extrinsic pathway

The end result of both the extrinsic and intrinsic pathways is the production of an enzyme called **prothrombin activator**.

Prothrombin activator acts on a globulin called **prothrombin** (factor II)…

…converting it to the enzyme **thrombin**. Thrombin transforms the soluble plasma protein fibrinogen into fine threads of insoluble **fibrin**.

Prothrombin activator

Prothrombin

Thrombin

Fibrin

Fibrin

The sticky fibrin threads form a web at the site of the injury. Red blood cells and platelets flowing through the web become ensnared, creating a clot of fibrin, blood cells, and platelets. A blood clot can effectively seal breaks in a smaller vessel; however, blood clotting alone may not stop a hemorrhage from a large blood vessel.

FAST FACT

Normal clotting requires adequate blood levels of calcium. That's because many of the reactions in the clotting process use calcium.

The Body AT WORK

The blood contains numerous proteins called clotting factors. Under normal conditions, these factors are inactive. However, the activation of one factor sets off a chain of reactions, with the product of the first reaction triggering another reaction in the next factor on a set pathway. A series of reactions in which each depends on the product of the preceding reaction is called a **reaction cascade**.

The process of coagulation involves more than 30 chemical reactions, with one following the other in a precise order. Many of the clotting factors involved in this process are identified by Roman numerals, such as factor VIII, factor X, etc. The numerals indicate the order in which they were discovered, not their order in the reaction cascade.

The Body AT WORK

Because the liver synthesizes most of the clotting factors, abnormal liver function interferes with normal blood clotting. Even more interesting is that seemingly mild disorders, such as gallstones, can also interfere with blood clotting. That's because the synthesis of clotting factors requires vitamin K. Vitamin K is absorbed into the blood from the intestine but, because vitamin K is fat soluble, it can be absorbed only if bile is present. Bile is secreted by the liver. If the bile ducts become blocked, such as by liver disease or gallstones, vitamin K can't be absorbed and bleeding tendencies develop.

FAST FACT

The extrinsic pathway leads to clot formation in about 15 seconds, whereas the intrinsic pathway takes 3 to 6 minutes. To stop bleeding more quickly, massage the tissues surrounding the wound. Stimulating the cells in the area will trigger the extrinsic pathway and speed up clot formation.

Dissolution of Blood Clots

The blood clotting process doesn't stop with the formation of the clot.

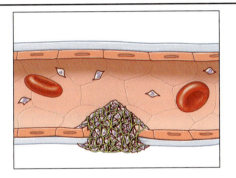

Soon after the blood clot forms, the platelets trapped within the fibrin web contract, pulling the edges of the damaged vessel closer together.

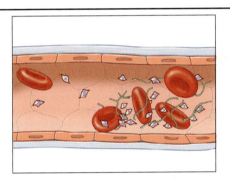

Later, after the vessel has healed, a small chain of reactions converts an inactive plasma protein (**plasminogen**) into plasmin. **Plasmin** works to dissolve the fibrin meshwork, and the clot breaks up. This process is called **fibrinolysis**.

Prevention of Blood Clots

When a blood vessel has broken, speedy clot formation is essential to stop the bleeding. However, it's just as crucial to prevent clots from forming when they aren't needed. The following factors discourage blood clot formation.

- **Smooth endothelium:** The inner lining of undamaged blood vessels is very smooth, which helps prevent platelets from sticking.
- **Blood flow:** The blood normally produces small amounts of thrombin. When blood is circulating normally, the rapidly moving bloodstream dilutes the thrombin before a clot can form. If blood flow decreases—such as when blood pools in the legs during prolonged sitting or lying down—thrombin can accumulate to the point that a clot develops.
- **Anticoagulants:** Basophils and mast cells normally secrete the anticoagulant **heparin**, which prevents blood clots by blocking the action of thrombin. Heparin is also given by injection to inhibit clot formation in patients who are susceptible to developing unwanted blood clots.

Life lesson: Blood clotting disorders

The formation of unwanted blood clots is the most common, and perhaps the most serious, of clotting disorders. In fact, about 650,000 Americans die every year from blood clots that have lodged in arteries in the brain, heart, or lungs. Once lodged, the clot shuts off blood flow, often resulting in sudden death.

An unwanted blood clot inside of a vessel is called a *thrombus*. If a piece of the clot breaks off and circulates through the bloodstream, it's called an *embolus*. Such clots may be treated with injections of heparin or the oral anticoagulant warfarin (Coumadin). While heparin blocks the action of thrombin, Coumadin blocks the effects of vitamin K on the liver. This causes the liver to produce less prothrombin, which, in turn, leads to less thrombin. Either way, blood clotting diminishes.

A more rare disorder—*hemophilia*—results from a deficiency of one of the clotting factors. Because hemophilia is a sex-linked recessive disorder, it affects primarily males. (Specifically, it afflicts about 1 out of 30,000 males.) People with hemophilia may be deficient in any one of several different clotting factors, but the most common missing factor is factor VIII. Because people with hemophilia lack the ability to form blood clots, even minor injuries can become life threatening. The disorder is treated with infusions of the missing clotting factor.

FAST FACT

Tissue plasminogen activator (t-PA)—one of the substances that stimulates the conversion of plasminogen into plasmin—can be administered as a drug. It's often given as an early treatment to dissolve clots causing strokes and heart attacks.

Blood Types

For centuries, people have realized that excessive blood loss often proved fatal. However, when they tried to fight the effects of hemorrhage by transfusing blood from one person into another, they were mystified as to why some recovered while others died. It wasn't until 1900, when a scientist discovered the blood types A, B, and O, that the matter became clear.

This scientist discovered that the surface of each red blood cell carries a protein called an **antigen** (also called **agglutinogen**). There are two antigens: A and B.

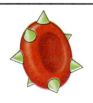

Blood type A

People with type A blood have the A antigen on their RBCs.

△ A antigen
♀ B antigen

Blood type B

People with type B blood have the B antigen.

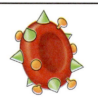

Blood type AB

People with type AB blood have both A and B antigens.

Blood type O

People with type O blood have neither antigen.

FAST FACT

In the United States, about 45% of the population has O blood, 40% has A blood, 11% has type B blood, and 4% has type AB blood.

While the blood cell carries antigens, the blood plasma carries **antibodies** (called **agglutinins**) against the antigens of the other blood types. (See "The Body at Work" on this page for further explanation of antigens and antibodies.)

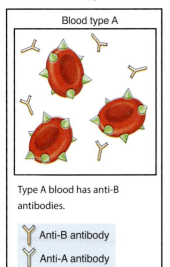

Blood type A

Type A blood has anti-B antibodies.

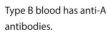
Anti-B antibody

Anti-A antibody

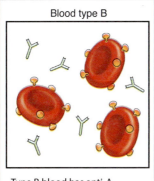

Blood type B

Type B blood has anti-A antibodies.

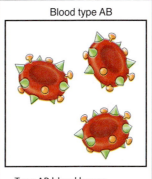

Blood type AB

Type AB blood has no antibodies.

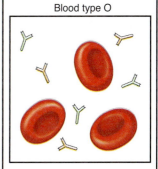

Blood type O

Type O blood has both anti-A and anti-B antibodies.

Transfusions are successful as long as the recipient's plasma doesn't contain antibodies against the ABO type being transfused. If such antibodies are present, they will attack the donor's RBCs, causing a **transfusion reaction.**

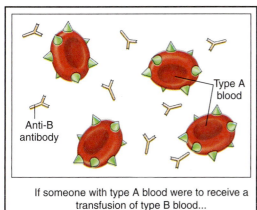

Anti-B antibody

Type A blood

If someone with type A blood were to receive a transfusion of type B blood...

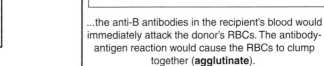

Type B blood

...the anti-B antibodies in the recipient's blood would immediately attack the donor's RBCs. The antibody-antigen reaction would cause the RBCs to clump together (**agglutinate**).

The clumping of RBCs blocks blood vessels, cutting off the flow of oxygen. The RBCs also burst (called **hemolysis**) and release their hemoglobin into the bloodstream. The free hemoglobin could block tubules in the kidneys, leading to renal failure and possibly death.

The Body AT WORK

Every cell in the body carries antigens on its surface. The antigens, which are unique to each individual, allow the body to distinguish its own cells from foreign invaders. When the body detects a substance with an unfamiliar antigen, it launches an immune response to destroy it.

*The first step in the attack occurs when antibodies in the blood plasma bind to the foreign cells (or the cells containing the foreign material). Next, antibodies bind to more than one antigen molecule in an effort to "corral" the foreign invaders until the immune system can break them down. This process, which produces large clumps of antigen-antibody molecules, is called **agglutination**. (Antigens and antibodies will be discussed more fully in Chapter 16, Lymphatic & Immune Systems.)*

FAST FACT

ABO antibodies are not present at birth. Rather, they first appear during infancy and build, reaching maximum concentration between the ages of 8 and 10 years.

The Body AT WORK

Because type O blood contains neither antigens A or B, it has been referred to as **universal donor blood**, *implying that it can be given to any recipient. This isn't true, however, because the donor's plasma contains both anti-A and anti-B antibodies; this means that the type O blood would agglutinate the RBCs of a type A, B, or AB recipient. Usually this doesn't occur because only the RBCs are transfused. Traces of plasma still remain, however, so a reaction is possible, although unlikely. The only way to be certain is to perform a test in which a sample of the donor's blood is mixed (or cross-matched) with a sample of the recipient's blood to ensure that agglutination won't occur.*

Likewise, type AB blood is sometimes called the **universal recipient**— *implying that a person with this blood type can receive a transfusion of any type of blood—because it contains neither anti-A nor anti-B antibodies. However, the donor's plasma may contain either of those antibodies; if transfused, they would agglutinate the recipient's RBCs. Again, the only way to ensure that won't happen is to cross-match the samples.*

FAST FACT

In the United States, type O blood is the most common, while type AB is the most rare.

FAST FACT

The ABO type and Rh type are both used when classifying blood. For example, O⁺ blood refers to type O, Rh positive; B⁻ blood refers to type B, Rh negative.

The Rh Group

Besides being classified according to ABO type, blood is also classified as being *Rh positive* or *Rh negative.* Rh-positive blood contains the Rh antigen; Rh-negative blood lacks this specific antigen. About 85% of white Americans and 95% of African Americans have Rh-positive blood.

Blood does not normally contain anti-Rh antibodies; however, it's possible for someone with Rh-negative blood to develop anti-Rh antibodies. There are two ways this can occur. The first way is when someone with Rh-negative blood receives a transfusion of Rh-positive blood. The second way is when an Rh-negative mother becomes pregnant with an Rh-positive fetus.

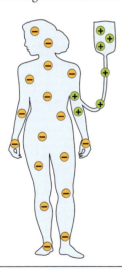

In the case of a transfusion, if a person with Rh-negative blood receives a transfusion of Rh-positive blood, the recipient's body interprets the Rh antigen as something foreign.

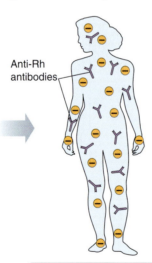

Anti-Rh antibodies

To protect itself, the body develops antibodies against the Rh antigen (anti-Rh antibodies).

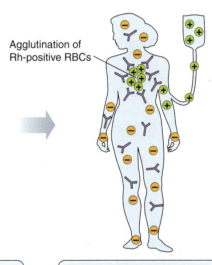

Agglutination of Rh-positive RBCs

Difficulty arises if the recipient encounters the Rh antigen again, such as through a subsequent infusion of Rh-positive blood. If that occurs, the anti-Rh antibodies that formed during the first transfusion will attack the Rh antigen in the donor blood, causing agglutination.

A similar condition may result when a woman with Rh-negative blood and a man with Rh-positive blood conceive a baby who is Rh positive.

ANIMATION

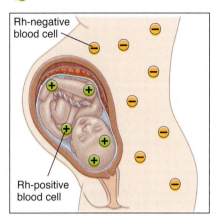

Because maternal and fetal blood doesn't mix, the first pregnancy with an Rh-positive fetus will proceed normally.

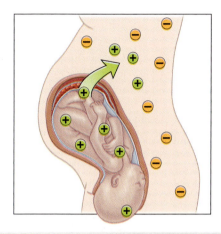

However, during delivery (or miscarriage), the fetus' blood often mixes with that of the mother, thus introducing Rh antigens into the mother's bloodstream.

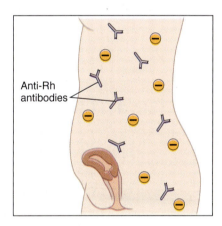

The mother's body responds by forming anti-Rh antibodies against this foreign substance.

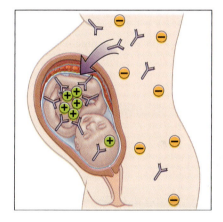

If the mother later becomes pregnant with another Rh-positive baby, the anti-Rh antibodies can pass through the placenta even if the RBCs can't. When they do, they attack the fetal RBCs, causing agglutination and hemolysis. The infant develops a severe hemolytic anemia called **erythroblastosis fetalis**.

FAST FACT

All Rh-negative women who become pregnant with an Rh-positive baby should be treated with an Rh immune globulin called RhoGAM. The immune globulin prevents the formation of anti-Rh antibodies by the mother, thus preventing an attack on the fetus's RBCs.

Review of Key Terms

Anemia: A deficiency of red blood cells or hemoglobin

Basophil: The fewest of the WBCs; secretes heparin

Coagulation: Blood clotting

Eosinophils: White blood cells that protect against parasites; also involved in allergic reactions

Erythrocytes: Red blood cells

Erythropoietin: Hormone secreted by the kidneys that stimulates the production of erythrocytes

Fibrin: Insoluble protein fibers involved in forming a blood clot

Fibrinolysis: Process of dissolution of a blood clot

Hematocrit: The percentage of red blood cells in a sample of blood

Hemoglobin: Iron-containing pigment of red blood cells that carries oxygen

Hemolysis: The destruction of red blood cells

Hemopoiesis: The production of blood

Hemostasis: An arrest of bleeding

Leukocytes: White blood cells

Leukocytosis: Elevated white blood cell count

Leukopenia: Abnormally low white blood cell count

Lymphocytes: Second most numerous of the WBCs; responsible for long-term immunity

Monocytes: Largest and most long-lived of the WBCs; highly phagocytic

Neutrophils: Most abundant of the white blood cells; highly mobile

Plasma: The clear extracellular matrix of blood

Platelets: Blood cell fragments that play a key role in stopping bleeding

Reticulocyte: An immature form of an erythrocyte

Serum: Plasma without the clotting proteins

Viscosity: The thickness or stickiness of blood

Own the Information

To make the information in this chapter part of your working memory, take some time to reflect on what you've learned. On a separate sheet of paper, write down everything you recall from the chapter. After you're done, log on to the Davis*Plus* website, and check out the Study Group podcast and Study Group Questions for the chapter.

Key Topics for Chapter 13:
- The components of blood
- The formation of blood cells
- The structure and function of red blood cells and hemoglobin
- The life cycle of red blood cells
- The structure and function of white blood cells
- The structure and function of platelets
- Mechanisms for the formation of a blood clot
- The dissolution of a clot
- ABO and Rh blood types
- The results of blood incompatibility from a transfusion or in utero

Test Your Knowledge

Answers: Chapter 13

1. *Correct answer:* **c.** WBCs help the body fight infection, so an analysis of these cells would reflect that ability. Platelets allow the blood to clot, so a measurement of platelets would reflect that ability. Iron is a key component of hemoglobin; therefore, a low hemoglobin level could possibly reflect a deficiency of iron.

2. *Correct answer:* **d.** Erythropoietin is a hormone secreted by the kidneys to stimulate the production of RBCs. Thrombin (an enzyme) stimulates the formation of fibrin, an insoluble protein used to form a blood clot.

3. *Correct answer:* **a.** Reticulocytes are immature RBCs; as the body compensates for lower levels of atmospheric oxygen, it would increase production of RBCs. As a result, the number of immature RBCs (reticulocytes) would increase rather than decrease. Neutrophils are WBCs, and a change in altitude alone would not affect their rate of production.

4. *Correct answer:* **a.** A lack of red blood cells and hemoglobin may cause pallor and cyanosis; however, the initial response from hemolysis would be to produce jaundice. Ruddiness would result from an excessive number of red blood cells, not hemolysis.

5. *Correct answer:* **d.** Basophils have little or no phagocytic ability. Eosinophils are mostly involved in allergic reactions, but they also kill parasites. Lymphocytes colonize the organs and tissues of the lymph system, where they are involved in long-term immunity.

6. *Correct answer:* **d.** All granulocytes (which includes neutrophils, eosinophils, and basophils) circulate for 5 to 8 hours and then migrate into the tissues, where they live another 4 or 5 days. In contrast, macrophages (into which monocytes transform) can live as long as a few years.

7. *Correct answer:* **c.** A thrombus is an unwanted blood clot inside a blood vessel. The other answers are all a part of hemostasis.

8. *Correct answer:* **d.** None of the other answers are correct.

9. *Correct answer:* **b.** Blood plasma carries antibodies against the other blood types. Hemoglobin is the red pigment with blood cells. Globin is the ribbon-like protein chain that helps form hemoglobin.

10. *Correct answer:* **c.** Leukocytosis is an elevated number of white blood cells. Polycythemia is an increased number of red blood cells. Fibrinolysis is the dissolution of a blood clot. None of these occur in a transfusion reaction.

1. What does a hematocrit reveal?
   a. The ability of the body to fight infection
   b. The ability of the blood to clot
   c. How much oxygen the blood can carry
   d. The amount of iron in the blood

2. Which substance allows RBCs to transport oxygen?
   a. Erythropoietin (EPO)
   b. Thrombin
   c. Fibrin
   d. Hemoglobin

3. A move to high altitude would trigger which change in the blood?
   a. An increased number of reticulocytes
   b. A decreased number of reticulocytes
   c. An increased number of neutrophils
   d. A decreased number of neutrophils

4. Hemolysis may produce which physical sign?
   a. Jaundice
   b. Pallor
   c. Cyanosis
   d. Ruddiness

5. When an infecting organism pierces the skin, which of the following WBCs would quickly migrate out of the blood vessels and into the tissues to ingest the foreign invader?
   a. Basophils
   b. Eosinophils
   c. Lymphocytes
   d. Neutrophils

6. Which of the following WBCs have the longest life span?
   a. Neutrophils
   b. Eosinophils
   c. Basophils
   d. Monocytes

7. Which of the following is an unwanted part of hemostasis?
   a. Vascular spasm
   b. Formation of fibrin
   c. Formation of a thrombus
   d. Formation of thrombin

8. How would someone experiencing a heart attack caused by a blood clot benefit from a drug that stimulates the conversion of plasminogen into plasmin?
   a. Plasmin encourages the growth of new blood vessels that can bypass the clot.
   b. Plasmin increases the oxygen-carrying capacity of RBCs.
   c. Plasmin inhibits the formation of new blood clots.
   d. Plasmin dissolves the fibrin meshwork around blood clots.

9. What substance, carried by each red blood cell, determines blood type?
   a. Antibody
   b. Antigen
   c. Hemoglobin
   d. Globin

10. Which of the following will occur if someone with type A blood receives a transfusion with type B blood?
    a. Leukocytosis
    b. Polycythemia
    c. Agglutination
    d. Fibrinolysis

Go to http://davisplus.fadavis.com Keyword: Thompson to see all of the resources available with this chapter.

DavisPlus

CHAPTER OUTLINE

Structures of the Heart

Heart Sounds

Blood Flow through the Heart

Coronary Circulation

Cardiac Conduction

Cardiac Cycle

Cardiac Output

LEARNING OUTCOMES

1. Describe the size and location of the heart.

2. Describe the layers of the pericardial sac surrounding the heart.

3. Identify the three layers of the heart wall and describe the characteristics of each.

4. Name the four chambers of the heart.

5. Describe the basic role and characteristics of each of the heart's chambers.

6. Identify the name, location, and function of each of the heart's four valves.

7. Identify the purpose of the skeleton of the heart.

8. Identify the locations on the chest where the various heart sounds can be heard and explain how the sounds are created.

9. Trace the flow of blood through the heart.

10. Identify the two main coronary arteries and describe the parts of the myocardium nourished by each.

11. Explain the process of coronary circulation.

12. Describe the unique electrical characteristics of the cardiac muscle.

13. Discuss the heart's conduction system.

14. Identify the basic components of an electrocardiogram and describe what each part of the waveform represents.

15. Describe in detail all the events of the cardiac cycle.

16. Define *cardiac output* and identify the variables that affect it.

17. Discuss how the nervous system can affect heart rate.

18. Describe how changes in activity, blood pressure, the levels of certain chemicals, and emotion affect heart rate.

19 Define what is meant by the terms *stroke volume* and *ejection fraction*.

20. Define *preload, contractility,* and *afterload,* and describe how each affects stroke volume.

21. Define Starling's law of the heart and describe how it affects stroke volume.

22. Describe the physiological consequences, and resulting symptoms, of both right and left ventricular failure.

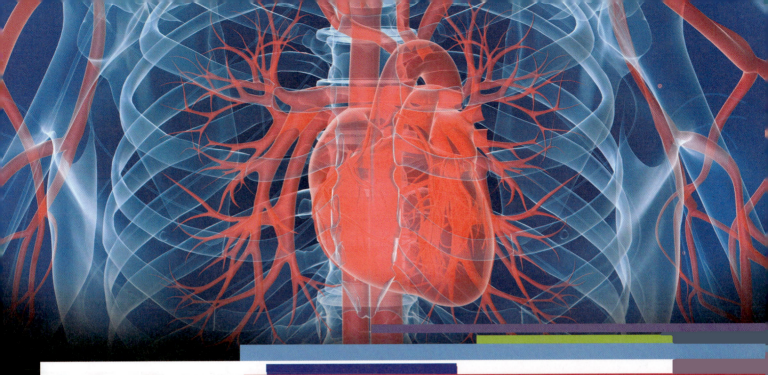

14

HEART

The human heart beats about 100,000 times in one day and about 35 million times in a year. During an average lifetime, the human heart will beat more than 2.5 billion times.

The heart could be called the engine of life. This incredibly powerful organ works constantly, never pausing. Composed of a type of muscle found nowhere else in the body, the heart works to pump blood throughout the body, delivering oxygen-rich blood to organs and tissues and returning oxygen-poor blood to the lungs.

About the size of a fist, the heart lies in the thoracic cavity in the **mediastinum**, a space between the lungs and beneath the sternum. The heart tilts toward the left, so that two-thirds of it extends to the left of the body's midline. The broadest part of the heart, called the **base**, is at the upper right, while the pointed end, called the **apex**, is at the lower left.

Base: Where the great vessels enter and leave the heart

Fifth intercostal space

Apex: The point of maximum impulse, where the strongest beat can be felt or heard

Right midclavicular line   Midline   Left midclavicular line

FAST FACT

The study of the heart and the treatment of related disorders is called **cardiology**.

Structures of the Heart

Key structures of the heart include the pericardium, the heart wall, the chambers, and the valves.

The Pericardium

Surrounding the heart is a double-walled sac called the **pericardium**. Anchored by ligaments and tissue to surrounding structures, the pericardium has two layers: the fibrous pericardium and serous pericardium.

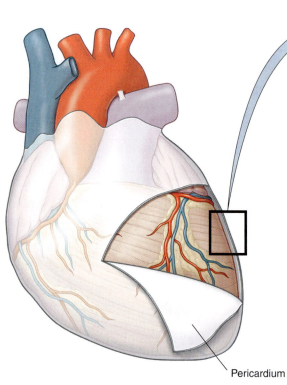

Pericardium

The **fibrous pericardium**—a loose-fitting sac of strong connective tissue—is the outermost layer.

The **serous pericardium**, which consists of two layers, covers the heart's surface.

At the heart's base, the serous pericardium folds back on itself to form the:

- **parietal layer**, which lines the inside of the fibrous pericardium, and the
- **visceral layer**, which covers the heart's surface.

Between these two layers is the **pericardial cavity**. This cavity contains a small amount of serous fluid, which helps prevent friction as the heart beats.

The Heart Wall

The heart wall consists of three layers:

The **endocardium** lines the heart's chambers, covers the valves, and continues into the vessels. It consists of a thin layer of squamous epithelial cells.

The **myocardium**, composed of cardiac muscle, forms the middle layer. It's the thickest of the three layers and performs the work of the heart.

The **epicardium**, which consists of a thin layer of squamous epithelial cells, covers the heart's surface. Also known as the visceral layer of the serous pericardium, the epicardium is closely integrated with the myocardium.

FAST FACT

The endocardium is very smooth, an important characteristic that helps keep blood from clotting as it fills the heart's chambers.

The Heart Chambers and Great Vessels

The heart contains four hollow chambers. The two upper chambers are called **atria** (singular: **atrium**); the two lower chambers are called **ventricles**.

Attached to the heart are several large vessels that transport blood to and from the heart. Called **great vessels**, they include the superior and inferior vena, pulmonary artery (which branches into a right and left pulmonary artery), four pulmonary veins (two for each lung), and the aorta.

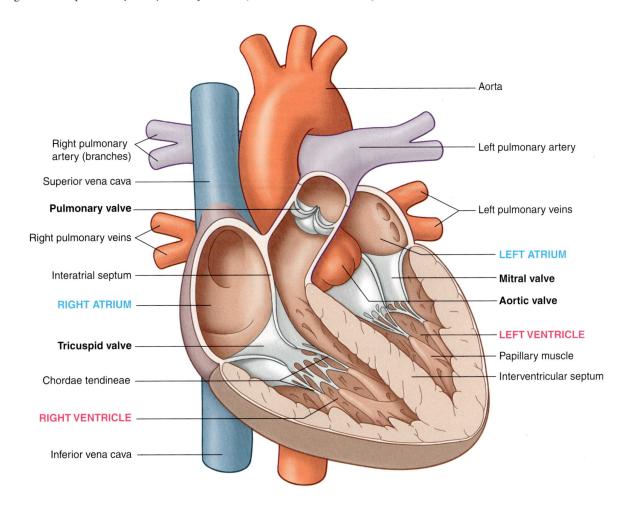

- Aorta
- Left pulmonary artery
- Left pulmonary veins
- **LEFT ATRIUM**
- **Mitral valve**
- **Aortic valve**
- **LEFT VENTRICLE**
- Papillary muscle
- Interventricular septum

- Right pulmonary artery (branches)
- Superior vena cava
- **Pulmonary valve**
- Right pulmonary veins
- Interatrial septum
- **RIGHT ATRIUM**
- **Tricuspid valve**
- Chordae tendineae
- **RIGHT VENTRICLE**
- Inferior vena cava

Atria

The atria serve primarily as reservoirs, receiving blood from the body or lungs. The right and left atria are separated by a common wall of myocardium called the **interatrial septum**. Because the atria move blood only a short distance—from the atria to the ventricles—they don't have to generate much force. Consequently, the walls of the atria are not very thick.

Ventricles

The ventricles serve as pumps, receiving blood from the atria and then pumping it either to the lungs (right ventricle) or the body (left ventricle). The right and left ventricles are separated by the **interventricular septum**. Because the ventricles pump rather than receive blood, they must generate more force than the atria. Therefore, the walls of the ventricles are thicker than those of the atria. Furthermore, because the left ventricle must generate enough force to push blood throughout the body, rather than just to the lungs, its walls are thicker than those of the right ventricle.

The Heart Valves

To ensure that blood moves in a forward direction through the heart, the heart contains four valves: one between each atrium and its ventricle and another at the exit of each ventricle. Each valve is formed by two or three flaps of tissue called **cusps** or **leaflets**.

The **atrioventricular (AV) valves** regulate flow between the atria and the ventricles.

- The right AV valve—also called the **tricuspid valve** (because it has three leaflets)—prevents backflow from the right ventricle to the right atrium.
- The left AV valve—also called the **bicuspid valve** (because it has two leaflets), or, more commonly, the **mitral valve**—prevents backflow from the left ventricle to the left atrium.

The **semilunar valves** regulate flow between the ventricles and the great arteries. There are two semilunar valves:

- The **pulmonary valve** prevents backflow from the pulmonary artery to the right ventricle.
- The **aortic valve** prevents backflow from the aorta to the left ventricle.

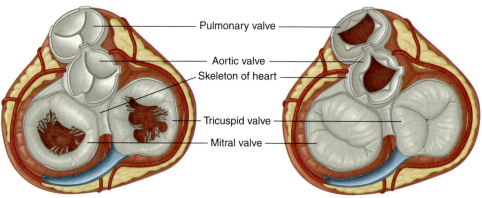

Ventricles relaxed   **Ventricles contracted**

The Heart Skeleton

A semi-rigid, fibrous, connective tissue called the **skeleton of the heart** encircles each valve. Besides offering support for the heart, the skeleton keeps the valves from stretching; it also acts as an insulating barrier between the atria and the ventricles, preventing electrical impulses from reaching the ventricles other than through a normal conduction pathway.

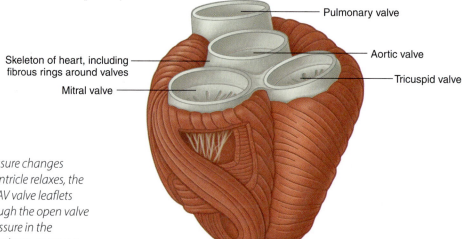

Posterior view

The Body AT WORK

Valves open and close in response to pressure changes within the heart. For example, when a ventricle relaxes, the pressure within that ventricle drops. The AV valve leaflets hang limply, allowing blood to flow through the open valve into the ventricle. As the ventricle fills, pressure in the ventricle rises. After filling, the ventricle begins to contract and the pressure rises even more. This increased pressure pushes against the cusps of the AV valve, causing it to snap closed. When pressure in the ventricle exceeds the pressure "downstream," the semilunar valve pops open, allowing blood to flow out into the area of lower pressure.

Heart Sounds

When the heart valves close, they produce vibrations that can be heard with a stethoscope on the body's surface. (Think of a door, which is silent as it opens but produces a sound as it closes.) By listening in key areas, the sounds made by individual valves can be identified. The illustration here shows the relationship between each valve and the surface area where its sound is heard the loudest. (Heart sounds will be discussed in more detail in the section, "Cardiac Cycle," which appears later in this chapter.)

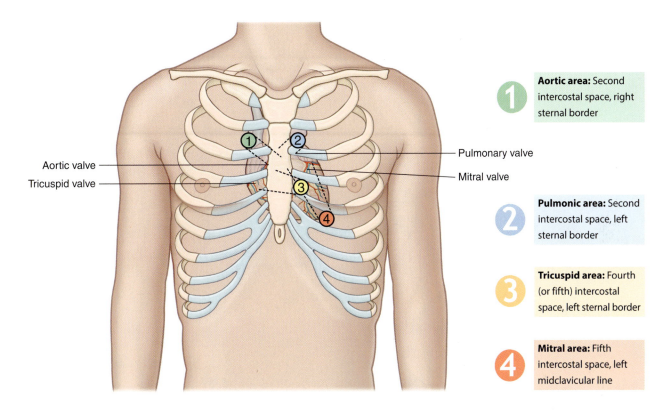

Aortic valve

Tricuspid valve

Pulmonary valve

Mitral valve

1 **Aortic area:** Second intercostal space, right sternal border

2 **Pulmonic area:** Second intercostal space, left sternal border

3 **Tricuspid area:** Fourth (or fifth) intercostal space, left sternal border

4 **Mitral area:** Fifth intercostal space, left midclavicular line

Life lesson: Valvular disease

A heart valve that fails to prevent the backflow of blood during contraction is called *incompetent*, and the condition is known as *valvular insufficiency*. Valvular insufficiency allows blood to leak backward, or *regurgitate*, into the chamber from which it was just pumped. For example, aortic insufficiency allows blood to leak back into the left ventricle after being pumped into the aorta. As a result, the left ventricle has to work harder: pumping out the blood flowing into it from the left atrium as well as the blood flowing back into it from the aorta.

A *stenotic* valve is one that's become narrowed, such as from scar tissue; this condition is called *valvular stenosis*. Stenotic valves also force the heart to work harder, causing it to strain to pump blood through the narrowed opening.

The backflow of blood through an incompetent valve, or the force of the blood moving through a stenotic valve, creates turbulence. This turbulence produces an abnormal sound called a *heart murmur*, which can be heard through a stethoscope.

Depending upon the severity of the defect, incompetent and stenotic valves can eventually lead to heart failure. In these instances, the defective valves can be replaced with either artificial valves or valves transplanted from a pig's heart.

Blood Flow through the Heart

No connection exists between the right and left sides of the heart, and the flow of blood through each side is kept separate from each other. Even so, the two sides, or pumps, work together to ensure that the organs and tissues of the body receive an adequate supply of oxygenated blood.

ANIMATION

1 The right atrium receives deoxygenated blood returning from the body through the superior and inferior vena cavae.

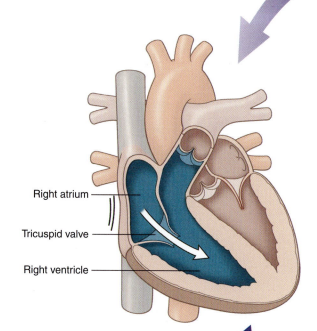

Right atrium

Tricuspid valve

Right ventricle

Superior
vena cava

Right atrium

Unoxygenated
blood

Tricuspid valve

Right ventricle

Inferior vena cava

2 Once the right atrium is full, it contracts. This forces the tricuspid valve open and blood flows into the right ventricle. When the right ventricle is full, the tricuspid valve snaps closed to prevent blood from flowing backward into the atria.

The Body AT WORK

*To prevent the tricuspid valve from inverting like a windblown umbrella during ventricular contraction, strands of fibrous connective tissue (called **chordae tendineae**) extend from conical **papillary muscles** on the floor of the ventricle to the valve cusps. The papillary muscles contract along with the ventricles, pulling on the chordae tendineae and anchoring the valve cusps in the proper position to prevent the regurgitation of blood into the atrium.*

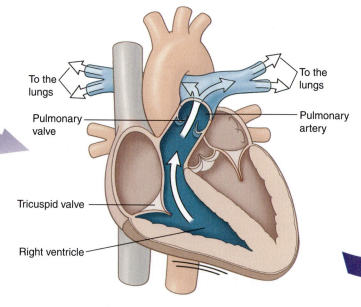

To the
lungs

Pulmonary
valve

Tricuspid valve

Right ventricle

To the
lungs

Pulmonary
artery

3 After filling, the right ventricle contracts, forcing the pulmonary valve open. Blood is pumped into the right and left pulmonary arteries and onto the lungs. After the right ventricle empties, the pulmonary valve closes to prevent the blood from flowing backward into the ventricle.

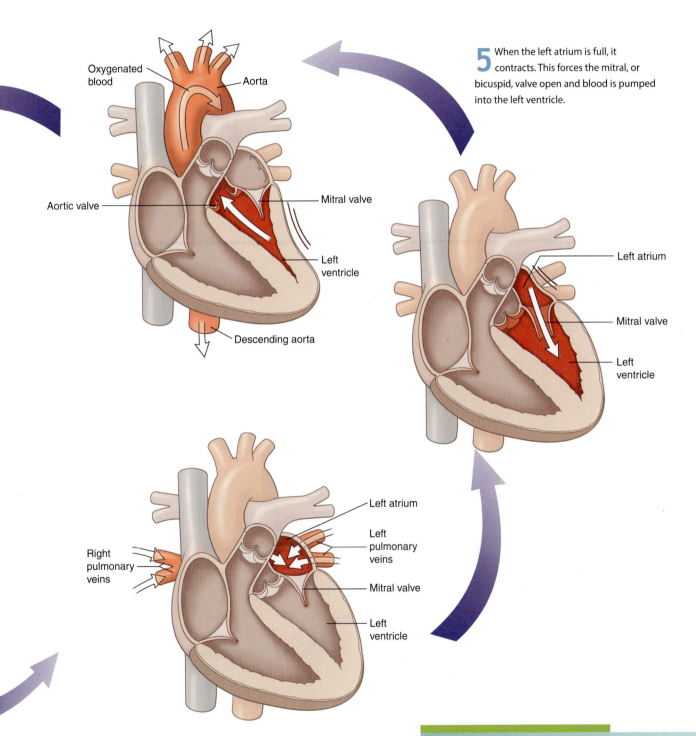

6 When the left ventricle is full, the mitral valve closes to prevent backflow. The ventricle then contracts, forcing the aortic valve to open, allowing blood to flow into the aorta. From there, oxygenated blood is distributed to every organ in the body.

Oxygenated blood

Aorta

Aortic valve

Mitral valve

Left ventricle

Descending aorta

5 When the left atrium is full, it contracts. This forces the mitral, or bicuspid, valve open and blood is pumped into the left ventricle.

Left atrium

Mitral valve

Left ventricle

Left atrium

Left pulmonary veins

Mitral valve

Left ventricle

Right pulmonary veins

4 After replenishing its supply of oxygen (and cleansing itself of carbon dioxide) in the lungs, the blood enters the pulmonary veins and returns to the heart through the left atrium.

FAST FACT

Although the right and left sides of the heart act as separate pumps, they perform their work simultaneously. Both the right and left atria contract at the same time, as do both ventricles.

Coronary Circulation

Just like any other organ or tissue in the body, the heart muscle requires an abundant supply of oxygen and nutrients. Because of its high demands, the heart has its own vascular system, known as the coronary circulation, to keep it well supplied with oxygenated blood. **Coronary arteries** deliver oxygenated blood to the myocardium, while cardiac veins collect the deoxygenated blood.

Two main coronary arteries—the right and the left—arise from the ascending aorta and serve as the principle routes for supplying blood to the myocardium.

The **right coronary artery** supplies blood to the right atrium, part of the left atrium, most of the right ventricle, and the inferior part of the left ventricle.

The **left coronary artery**, which branches into the **anterior descending** and **circumflex arteries**, supplies blood to the left atrium, most of the left ventricle, and most of the interventricular septum

Anterior

FAST FACT

The most abundant blood supply goes to the myocardium of the left ventricle. That's because the left ventricle does most of the work and therefore needs more oxygen and nutrients than the rest of the myocardium.

The Body AT WORK

Unlike the rest of the body, coronary arteries receive their supply of blood when the ventricles relax. That's because myocardial contraction compresses the coronary arteries, restricting blood flow. Also, as the aortic valve opens during contraction, the cusps of the valve cover the openings to the coronary arteries, blocking the flow of blood. When the ventricles relax, the coronary arteries fill with the blood needed to nourish the heart muscle. Knowing this, can you see why a sustained elevated heart rate can be harmful?

Life lesson: Angina and myocardial infarction

Coronary artery disease is the leading cause of death in America today, causing almost one-half million deaths each year. The disease results when the coronary arteries become blocked or narrowed by a buildup of cholesterol and fatty deposits (*atherosclerosis*). Any interruption in blood supply to the myocardium deprives the heart tissue of oxygen (*ischemia*), causing pain. Within minutes, cell death (*necrosis*) occurs.

Sometimes the interruption is temporary, such as in angina pectoris. What happens in this condition is that a partially blocked vessel spasms—or the heart demands more oxygen than the narrowed vessel can supply (such as during a period of exertion). When the demand for oxygen exceeds the supply, ischemia and chest pain result. With rest, the heart rate slows and adequate circulation resumes. Chest pain stops and permanent myocardial damage is avoided.

A more serious condition is a *myocardial infarction (MI)*. In this situation, blood flow is completely blocked by a blood clot or fatty deposit, resulting in the death of myocardial cells in the area fed by the artery. Once the cells die, they produce an area of necrosis.

Symptoms of a MI, or "heart attack," vary widely, particularly between women and men. Men commonly experience chest pain or pressure, discomfort in the upper body (including either arm, the back, neck, jaw, or stomach), shortness of breath, nausea, profuse sweating, or anxiety. Women are more likely to complain of sudden extreme fatigue (not explained by a lack of sleep), abdominal pain or "heartburn," dizziness, or weakness.

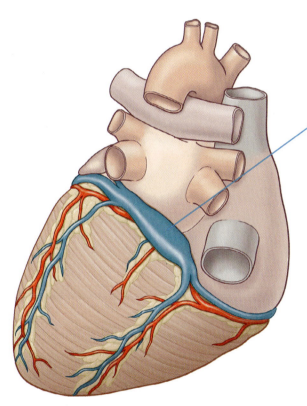

Posterior

Most cardiac veins empty into the **coronary sinus**, a large transverse vein on the heart's posterior, which returns the blood to the right atrium. (The exception is the anterior cardiac veins, which empty directly into the right atrium.)

The Body AT WORK

When a blockage occurs gradually, a narrowed coronary artery may develop "collateral circulation." Collateral circulation is when new blood vessels develop to reroute blood flow around a blockage. Even so, the new arteries may not supply enough blood to the myocardium during times of increased oxygen demand, such as during exertion or stress. The good news, however, is that studies have shown that regular exercise promotes the development of even greater collateral circulation.

FAST FACT

Heart disease kills twice as many women as all cancers combined. In addition, women are more likely to die from their first heart attack than men are.

Cardiac Conduction

Cardiac muscle is unique in that it doesn't depend upon stimulation by extrinsic nerves to contract. Rather, it contains special pacemaker cells that allow it to contract spontaneously, an ability called **automaticity**. Also, because the heart beats regularly, it is said to have **rhythmicity**. (Although extrinsic nerves don't *cause* the heart to beat, the nervous system and certain hormones can affect the heart's rate and rhythm.)

The electrical impulses generated by the heart follow a very specific route through the myocardium, as shown below.

ANIMATION

1 Normal cardiac impulses arise in the **sinoatrial (SA) node** from its spot in the wall of the right atrium just below the opening of the superior vena cava.

2 An interatrial bundle of conducting fibers rapidly conducts the impulses to the left atrium, and both atria begin to contract.

3 The impulse travels along three internodal bundles to the **atrioventricular (AV) node** (located near the right AV valve at the lower end of the interatrial septum). There, the impulse slows considerably to allow the atria time to contract completely and the ventricles to fill with blood. The heart's skeleton insulates the ventricles, ensuring that only impulses passing through the AV node can enter.

4 After passing through the AV node, the impulse picks up speed. It then travels down the **bundle of His**, also called the **atrioventricular (AV) bundle**.

5 The AV bundle soon branches into **right** and **left bundle branches**.

6 **Purkinje fibers** conduct the impulses throughout the muscle of both ventricles, causing them to contract almost simultaneously.

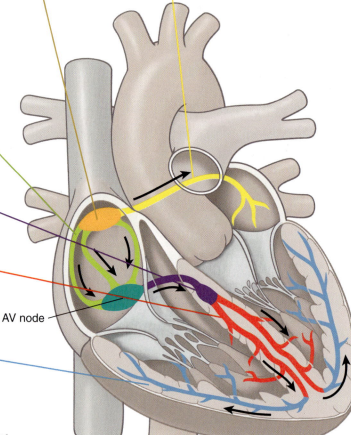

AV node

The Body AT WORK

The SA node is the heart's primary pacemaker. If the SA node fails to fire, pacemaker cells in the AV node or Purkinje fibers can initiate impulses, although at a slower rate. Pacemakers other than the SA node are called **ectopic** *pacemakers. The heart's pacemakers, and their firing rates when the heart is at rest, are as follows:*

- *SA node: Fires at 60 to 80 beats per minute*
- *AV node: Has a firing rate of 40 to 60 beats per minute*
- *Purkinje fibers: Have a firing rate of 20 to 40 beats per minute*

FAST FACT

Because the signals triggering the heart's contractions originate within itself, even if the heart is removed from the body, it will continue to beat for hours as long as it's kept in a protected environment.

Electrocardiogram

Cardiac impulses generate electrical currents in the heart. These currents spread through surrounding tissue and can be detected by electrodes placed on the body's surface. The record of these signals is called an **electrocardiogram (ECG)**. An ECG records the electrical activity or impulses; it does *not* record the heart's contractions. An ECG that appears normal is called **normal sinus rhythm**, meaning that the impulse originates in the SA node. An irregular heartbeat is called an **arrhythmia**.

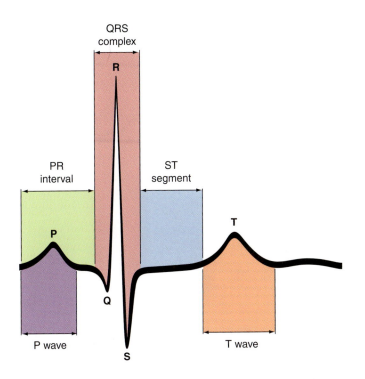

The **P wave** represents atrial depolarization: the transmission of electrical impulses from the SA node through the atria. This occurs right before the atria contract.

The **PR interval** represents the time it takes for the cardiac impulse to travel from the atria to the ventricles.

The **QRS complex** represents ventricular depolarization: the spread of electrical impulses throughout the ventricles.

The **ST segment** represents the end of ventricular depolarization and the beginning of ventricular repolarization.

The **T wave** represents ventricular repolarization.

Life Lesson: Arrhythmias

Arrhythmias result when part of the conduction pathway is injured or when a part of the myocardium other than the SA node (called an *ectopic focus*) generates a beat. Common cardiac arrhythmias include atrial flutter, premature ventricular contractions, and ventricular fibrillation.

Atrial flutter occurs when an ectopic focus in the atria fires rapidly, causing the atria to contract between 200 and 400 times per minute. The AV node blocks impulses in excess of 180 beats/minute, which helps protect the heart from a life-threatening ventricular response. Because proper atrial function isn't as crucial as proper ventricular function, atrial flutter isn't usually life-threatening.

Premature ventricular contractions (PVCs)—which may occur as a single beat or in bursts of several beats—result from the firing of an ectopic focus in the ventricles. While PVCs may indicate a serious underlying condition, more benign causes of PVCs include a lack of sleep, caffeine, or emotional stress.

Ventricular fibrillation, on the other hand, is a life-threatening emergency. Resulting from electrical signals arising from different regions of the myocardium, fibrillation causes the heart to quiver rather than contract. Since a fibrillating heart can't pump blood, cardiac output plummets and cardiac arrest may quickly follow.

Ventricular fibrillation requires immediate defibrillation. In this procedure, a strong electrical jolt is delivered to the heart through a pair of large electrodes, causing the entire myocardium to depolarize. If the first part of the heart to recover from depolarization is the SA node, sinus rhythm can resume. Keep in mind that defibrillation treats only the symptom of fibrillation; it doesn't treat its cause. However, once sinus rhythm is restored, other treatments can be implemented to correct the cause of the arrhythmia.

Cardiac Cycle

The series of events that occur from the beginning of one heartbeat to the beginning of the next is called the cardiac cycle. The cardiac cycle consists of two phases: **systole** (contraction) and **diastole** (relaxation). Both atria contract simultaneously; then, as the atria relax, both ventricles contract.

The vibrations produced by the contraction of the heart and the closure of the valves produce the "lub-dub" heart sounds that can be heard with a stethoscope. The first heart sound (S_1) is louder and longer; the second sound (S_2) is a little softer and sharper.

Here's what happens during one heartbeat:

ANIMATION

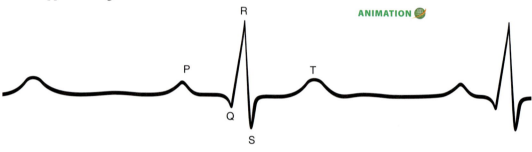

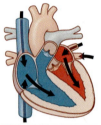 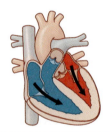 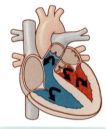 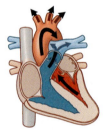 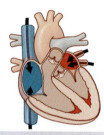

1 Passive ventricular filling

- Returning venous blood has filled the atria, causing their pressure to rise above that in the ventricles.
- The AV valves open and blood flows into the ventricles.
- The P wave appears on the ECG, marking the end of atrial depolarization.

2 Atrial systole

- The AV valves are open and the semilunar valves are closed.
- The atria contract to eject their remaining volume of blood.
- The ventricles are relaxed, filling with blood.

3 Isovolumetric contraction

- This is the brief period during which the ventricles are beginning to contract but the semilunar valves haven't yet opened. (*Note:* The prefix *iso-* means "equal"; *volumetric* refers to volume. Therefore, *isovolumetric* refers to something having the same or equal volume.)
- The volume of blood in the ventricles remains constant, but the pressure rises rapidly as the ventricles begin to contract.
- The R wave appears on the ECG.
- **The first heart sound (S_1) can be heard.**

4 Ventricular ejection

- When the pressure in the ventricles exceeds the pressure in the pulmonary artery and aorta, the semilunar valves open.
- Blood spurts out of each ventricle: rapidly at first and then more slowly as the pressure drops.
- The ventricles don't eject all of their blood. The blood remaining in the ventricles at the end of the ejection period is the **residual volume**.
- The T wave occurs late in this phase, beginning at the moment of peak ventricular pressure.

5 Isovolumetric ventricular relaxation

- This is the period at the end of ventricular ejection—before the AV valves have opened but after the semilunar valves have closed to prevent blood from reentering the ventricles.
- The volume of blood in the ventricles remains unchanged, but the pressure falls dramatically as the ventricles relax.
- The T wave ends on the ECG.
- **The second heart sound (S_2) can be heard as blood rebounds against the closed semilunar valves.**

The Body AT WORK

*The right and left ventricles receive about 70% of their blood passively: it simply flows from the right and left atria after the mitral and tricuspid valves open. Late in the filling process, both atria contract. Known as **atrial kick**, this contraction supplies the ventricles with the remaining 30% of the blood.*

In contrast, the ventricles must actively pump all their blood to the arteries. Knowing this, it becomes clear why properly functioning ventricles are more crucial to survival than properly functioning atria.

Cardiac Output

Cardiac output (CO) refers to the amount of blood the heart pumps in 1 minute. To determine cardiac output multiply the **heart rate** (HR)—the number of times the heart beats in 1 minute— by the **stroke volume** (SV)—the amount of blood ejected with each heartbeat.

CO The amount of blood pumped by the heart in 1 minute	=	**HR** The number of times the heart beats in 1 minute	X	**SV** The amount of blood ejected by the heart with each beat

A typical resting heart rate is 75 beats per minute. The heart ejects about 70 ml each time it beats: that's its stroke volume. To determine cardiac output, multiply 75 × 70; that equals 5250 ml, or over 5 liters, each minute. That is a typical cardiac output.

Cardiac output increases with activity, but the average resting cardiac output is between 5 and 6 liters per minute. If an individual's heart has a greater stroke volume (such as the well-conditioned heart of an athlete), the heart would have to beat fewer times to maintain a cardiac output of 5 liters per minute. This explains why athletes tend to have slower pulse rates.

Because cardiac output equals heart rate times stroke volume, the only two ways to affect cardiac output are:

1. Change the heart rate
2. Change the stroke volume

Keep in mind, though, that these two factors are interdependent. When heart rate increases, stroke volume decreases. That's because the faster the heart rate, the less time the ventricles have to fill.

That Makes Sense

To help clarify the variables affecting cardiac output, envision yourself pumping water out of an old-fashioned hand pump. The more times you pump (HR), the more water you'll produce (CO). Of course, the number of buckets you'll fill for every 100 pumps on the handle will vary, depending upon the volume of flow (SV). For example, if the water pressure is low and each pump produces a trickle, 100 pumps may barely fill a bucket. However, if the water flow is strong, 100 pumps may fill several buckets.

Heart Rate

A person's heart rate, or pulse, is the number of times the heart beats each minute. Newborn infants have heart rates of about 120 beats per minute. Young adult females tend to have heart rates of 72 to 80 beats per minute; young adult males have heart rates of 64 to 72 beats per minute.

A persistent pulse rate slower than 60 beats per minute is called **bradycardia**, although this commonly occurs during sleep or in athletes. A persistent, resting heart rate greater than 100 beats per minute is called **tachycardia**.

FAST FACT

The body's total volume of blood is 4 to 6 liters. Since a normal cardiac output is 5 liters per minute, that means the body's total volume of blood passes through the heart every minute.

Factors Affecting Heart Rate

The heart generates and maintains its own beat. However, the nervous system—even though it doesn't initiate the heartbeat—can alter the heart's rhythm and force of contractions. Specifically, the medulla in the brain detects changes in the body and sends messages to the sympathetic or parasympathetic nervous system (divisions of the autonomic nervous system) to raise or lower heart rate. Here's how it works:

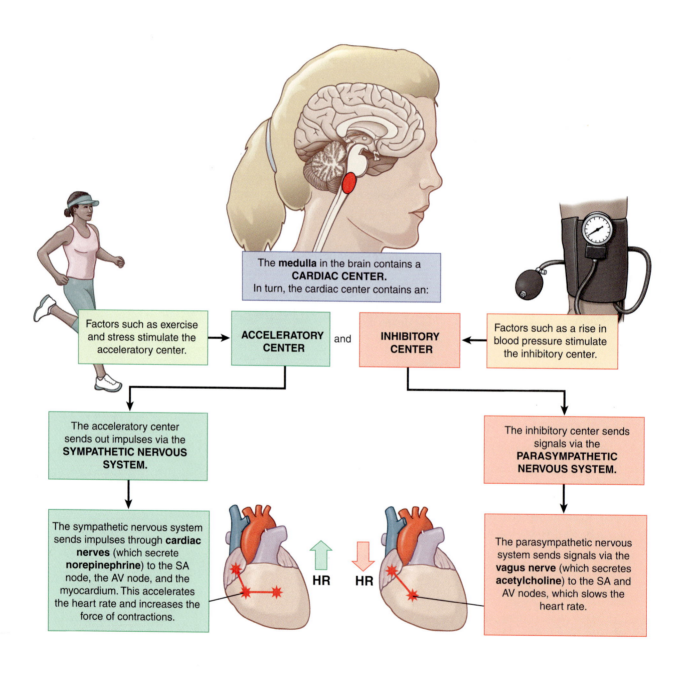

The **medulla** in the brain contains a **CARDIAC CENTER.** In turn, the cardiac center contains an:

Factors such as exercise and stress stimulate the acceleratory center.

ACCELERATORY CENTER

and

INHIBITORY CENTER

Factors such as a rise in blood pressure stimulate the inhibitory center.

The acceleratory center sends out impulses via the **SYMPATHETIC NERVOUS SYSTEM.**

The inhibitory center sends signals via the **PARASYMPATHETIC NERVOUS SYSTEM.**

The sympathetic nervous system sends impulses through **cardiac nerves** (which secrete **norepinephrine**) to the SA node, the AV node, and the myocardium. This accelerates the heart rate and increases the force of contractions.

↑ HR   ↓ HR

The parasympathetic nervous system sends signals via the **vagus nerve** (which secretes **acetylcholine**) to the SA and AV nodes, which slows the heart rate.

For more information, see Chapter 10, *Nervous System.*

Input to the Cardiac Center

The cardiac center in the medulla receives input from multiple sources to initiate changes in heart rate. These include receptors in the muscles, joints, arteries, and brainstem. For example:

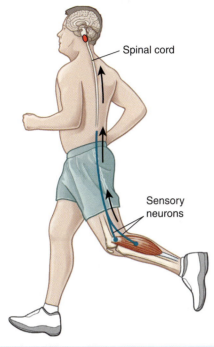

Spinal cord

Sensory neurons

1 Proprioceptors

Proprioceptors in the muscles and joints signal the cardiac center of changes in physical activity. This allows the heart to increase output even before the muscles demand more blood flow.

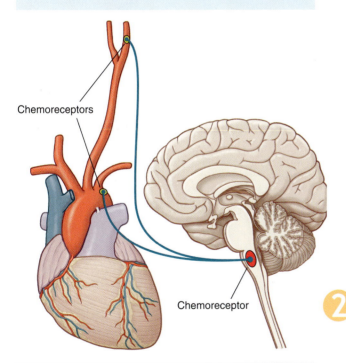

Chemoreceptors

Chemoreceptor

3 Chemoreceptors

Chemoreceptors—found in the aortic arch, carotid arteries, and medulla—detect increases in carbon dioxide, decreases in oxygen, and decreases in pH. In response, the sympathetic nervous system increases heart rate and stroke volume so as to circulate more oxygen. (Note: A cluster of chemoreceptors near the fork of the carotid artery is called a **carotid body**. A similar cluster in the aorta is called an **aortic body**.)

Life lesson: Emotions and heart rate

Emotions such as fear, pain, grief, and anger all affect heart rate. This occurs because two almond-shaped areas of the brain, called amygdalae, are key players in the formation and storage of memories associated with emotion. It's thought that stimulation of the amygdalae (such as by emotion) causes it to send impulses to the autonomic nervous system.

Anxiety, fear, and anger all cause the heart to beat faster. In contrast, grief slows the heart rate. It's also interesting that just the *thought* of doing something frightening—such as sky diving or taking a plunge off the high dive—can make your heart beat faster.

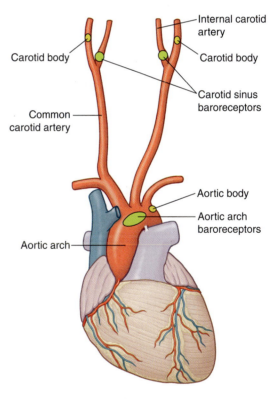

Internal carotid artery

Carotid body

Carotid body

Carotid sinus baroreceptors

Common carotid artery

Aortic body

Aortic arch baroreceptors

Aortic arch

2 Baroreceptors

Baroreceptors (pressoreceptors)—pressure sensors in the aorta and internal carotid arteries—detect changes in blood pressure. If blood pressure falls, cardiac output drops; therefore, the cardioacceleratory center will stimulate the heart to beat faster and maintain cardiac output. Vice versa, if blood pressure suddenly rises, impulses will be sent to slow the heart rate, decreasing cardiac output, and lowering blood pressure.

Stroke Volume

Stroke volume—the second factor affecting cardiac output—is never 100% of the volume in the ventricles. Typically, the ventricles eject 60% to 80% of their blood volume. This percentage is called the **ejection fraction**. An ejection fraction significantly lower than this indicates that the ventricle is weak and may be failing.

Factors Affecting Stroke Volume

Stroke volume is affected by three factors—**preload**, **contractility**, and **afterload**:

ANIMATION 🌐

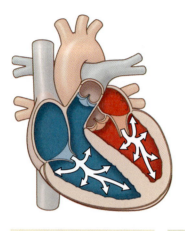 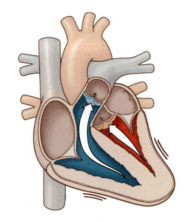 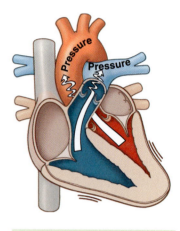

Preload

- Preload is the amount of tension, or stretch, in the ventricular muscle just before it contracts.
- The more blood entering the heart, the more the ventricle stretches.
- *Example:* Think of shooting a rubber band. The tension, or stretch, placed on the rubber band before you shoot it is its preload.

Contractility

- Contractility is the force with which ventricular ejection occurs.
- The more the ventricle is stretched (within limits), the more forcefully it will contract. This is known as **Starling's law of the heart**.
- Because the amount of blood in the ventricle at the end of diastole determines how much the ventricle is stretched, the more blood returned to the heart each minute, the more forcefully it will contract. Too much blood, however, can overstretch the heart's muscle, causing it to lose elasticity.
- *Example:* The more you stretch the rubber band, the more it will contract when it's released, and the farther it will fly. Likewise, an old rubber band that has been overstretched isn't as elastic as a new one and won't fly as far when released.

Afterload

- The forces the heart must work against (such as the pressure of the blood in the arteries) to eject its volume of blood is called the afterload.
- An increase in afterload (such as high blood pressure) opposes the ejection of blood from the ventricles, which decreases stroke volume.
- *Example:* If you try to shoot a rubber band under water, the pressure of the water (the afterload) will resist the forward movement of the rubber band.

That Makes Sense

*Factors that affect contractility are called **inotropic** agents. (Tip: To help remember this term, think "in." An IN-otropic agent affects the myocardium's ability to contract IN-ward.) Agents that increase contractility (positive inotropic agents) include excess calcium and epinephrine. Agents that decrease contractility (negative inotropic agents) include a calcium deficiency as well as a potassium excess.*

*Factors that influence heart rate are called **chronotropic** agents. (Tip: The prefix chron- refers to time, as in a chronology. Therefore, chronotropic refers to how many times the heart beats within a certain time period.) Agents that increase heart rate (positive chronotropic agents) include epinephrine and low levels of calcium. Agents that decrease heart rate (negative chronotropic agents) include acetylcholine and excess levels of potassium.*

Life lesson: Congestive heart failure

Congestive heart failure (CHF) results when either ventricle fails to pump blood effectively. This can occur because the ventricle is weakened from a myocardial infarction. Also, prolonged high blood pressure or incompetent heart valves, both of which force the heart to work harder, can weaken the ventricles. Chronic lung disease places a strain on the right ventricle, because diseased lungs make it more difficult for the right ventricle to pump blood into pulmonary circulation. Over time, this can lead to failure of the right ventricle, called right-sided heart failure. Failure of the left ventricle is called left-sided heart failure.

Symptoms of congestive heart failure vary according to the side of the heart affected. Keep in mind, however, that the failure of one ventricle places an added strain on the other ventricle. Eventually, both ventricles fail.

Left Ventricular Failure

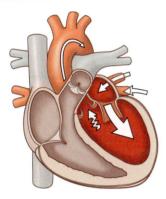

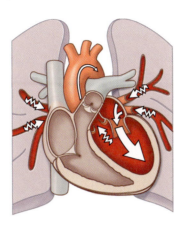

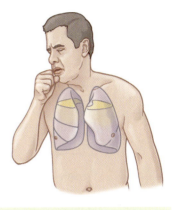

If the left ventricle fails, it falls behind in ejecting all of the blood it receives from the lungs.

Consequently, blood backs up in the lungs.

This causes:
- Shortness of breath
- A buildup of fluid in the lungs (pulmonary edema)
- Coughing

Right Ventricular Failure

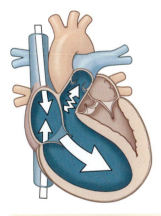

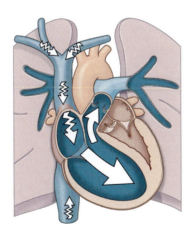

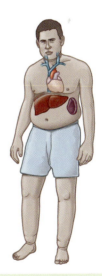

If the right ventricle fails, it falls behind in ejecting all of the blood it receives from the systemic circulation.

Blood backs up into the vena cava and throughout the peripheral vascular system.

This results in:
- Generalized swelling throughout the body (systemic edema)
- Enlargement of the liver and spleen
- Pooling of fluid in the abdomen (**ascites**)
- Distension of the jugular veins
- Swelling of the ankles, feet, and fingers

FAST FACT

Adults with diabetes have a two to eight times greater risk of developing heart failure. That's partly because the disease process of diabetes damages the heart muscle.

Review of Key Terms

Afterload: The forces that impede the flow of blood out of the heart

Aortic valve: Heart valve that prevents backflow from the aorta to the left ventricle

Apex: Pointed end of the heart, the location of the point of maximum impulse

Atrioventricular (AV) node: Group of pacemaker cells in the interatrial septum that relays impulses from the atria to the ventricles

Atrium: The upper chamber of each half of the heart

Automaticity: The unique ability of the cardiac muscle to contract without nervous stimulation

Baroreceptors: Pressure sensors in the aorta and carotid arteries that detect changes in blood pressure; also called pressoreceptors

Base: Broadest part of the heart; where great vessels enter and leave

Cardiac cycle: The series of events that occur from the beginning of one heartbeat to the beginning of the next

Cardiac output: The amount of blood pumped by the heart in 1 minute

Chemoreceptors: Sensors in the aortic arch, carotid arteries, and medulla that detect increased levels of carbon dioxide, decreased levels of oxygen, and decreases in pH

Chordae tendineae: Tendinous cords that connect the edges of the AV valves to the papillary muscles to prevent inversion of the valve during ventricular systole

Coronary arteries: Vessels that deliver oxygenated blood to the myocardium

Coronary sinus: Large transverse vein on the heart's posterior that returns blood to the right atrium

Diastole: The period of cardiac muscle relaxation

Electrocardiogram (ECG): Record of the electrical currents in the heart

Endocardium: The endothelial membrane that lines the chambers of the heart

Epicardium: The serous membrane on the surface of the myocardium

Mediastinum: Space between the lungs and beneath the sternum

Mitral valve: The valve that regulates blood flow between the left atrium and left ventricle

Myocardium: The middle layer of the heart wall; composed of cardiac muscle

Pericardial cavity: Space between the visceral and parietal layers of the serous pericardium that contains a small amount of serous fluid

Pericardium: The membranous fibroserous sac enclosing the heart and the bases of the great vessels

Preload: The amount of tension, or stretch, in the ventricular muscle just before it contracts

Proprioceptors: Sensors in muscles and joints that signal the cardiac center of changes in physical activity

Pulmonary valve: Heart valve that prevents backflow from the pulmonary artery to the right ventricle

Purkinje fiber: Nerve-like processes that extend from the bundle branches to the ventricular myocardium; form the last part of the cardiac conduction system

Rhythmicity: Term applied to the heart's ability to beat regularly

Semilunar valves: The two valves that regulate flow between the ventricles and the great arteries

Sinoatrial node: The heart's primary pacemaker, where normal cardiac impulses arise

Stroke volume: The amount of blood ejected by the heart with each beat

Systole: Contraction of the chambers of the heart

Tricuspid valve: The right atrioventricular valve, which regulates flow between the right atrium and right ventricle

Ventricles: The two lower chambers of the heart

Own the Information

To make the information in this chapter part of your working memory, take some time to reflect on what you've learned. On a separate sheet of paper, write down everything you recall from the chapter. After you're done, log on to the DavisPlus website, and check out the Study Group podcast and Study Group Questions for the chapter.

Key Topics for Chapter 14:
- The size, location, and key structures of the heart
- Sounds made by the heart
- Heart chambers, valves, and great vessels
- Blood flow through the heart
- Coronary circulation
- Cardiac conduction and ECGs
- Cardiac cycle
- Cardiac output and the factors affecting cardiac output

Test Your Knowledge

1. The point of maximum impulse of the heart is at the:
   a. mediastinum.
   b. base.
   c. apex.
   d. aorta.

2. The portion of the heart wall that lines the heart's chambers is the:
   a. myocardium.
   b. pericardium.
   c. endocardium.
   d. epicardium.

3. Which heart valve controls the flow of blood between the left atrium and the left ventricle?
   a. Pulmonary valve
   b. Aortic valve
   c. Tricuspid valve
   d. Mitral valve

4. What is the name of the great vessel that supplies blood to the right atrium?
   a. Superior and inferior vena cavae
   b. Aorta
   c. Pulmonary artery
   d. Pulmonary veins

5. How does the myocardium receive its blood supply?
   a. It receives its supply of blood from the left ventricle.
   b. It receives its blood through the coronary sinus.
   c. It doesn't require any additional blood other than what flows through the chambers.
   d. It receives its blood through the right and left coronary arteries.

6. What is the heart's primary pacemaker?
   a. The atrioventricular (AV) node
   b. The Purkinje fibers
   c. The sympathetic nervous system
   d. The sinoatrial (SA) node

7. On an electrocardiogram, the QRS complex represents:
   a. atrial depolarization.
   b. ventricular depolarization.
   c. ventricular repolarization.
   d. impulse transmission from the atria to the ventricles.

8. The cardiac cycle is:
   a. the amount of blood pumped by the heart in 1 minute.
   b. the heart's ability to beat spontaneously.
   c. the period of time when the left ventricle ejects its volume of blood.
   d. the series of events that occur from the beginning of one heartbeat to the beginning of the next.

9. Cardiac output equals:
   a. heart rate times stroke volume.
   b. stroke volume times ejection fraction.
   c. age times heart rate.
   d. the percentage of blood ejected by the ventricles with each contraction.

10. The parasympathetic nervous system sends impulses to the heart via the vagus nerve, which:
    a. slows the heart rate.
    b. increases the heart rate.
    c. doesn't affect the heart rate.
    d. raises the blood pressure, which, in turn, slows the heart rate.

11. What is the term used to describe the amount of tension, or stretch, in the ventricular muscle just before it contacts?
    a. Contractility
    b. Afterload
    c. Ascites
    d. Preload

CHAPTER OUTLINE

Vessel Structure

Arteries

Veins

Capillaries

Circulatory Routes

Principles of Circulation

LEARNING OUTCOMES

1. Trace the route taken by blood as it leaves, and then returns to, the heart.

2. Describe the structure of the walls of arteries and veins.

3. Discuss the structure and function of the three classes of arteries.

4. Describe the characteristics that make veins distinct from arteries.

5. Discuss the structure and function of the three classes of veins.

6. Describe the structure, function, and organization of capillaries.

7. Explain the methods of capillary exchange: diffusion, filtration, and colloid osmotic pressure.

8. Identify and explain three main causes of edema.

9. Trace the path of pulmonary circulation.

10. Name the regions of the aorta and the major arteries arising from each region.

11. Describe the blood supply to the head and neck.

12. Identify the principal veins of systemic circulation.

13. Discuss hepatic portal circulation.

14. Discuss the principles of a pressure gradient and how it relates to blood pressure and circulation.

15. Summarize how cardiac output, blood volume, and resistance affect blood pressure.

16. Explain the relationship between blood pressure, peripheral resistance, and blood flow.

17. Discuss why blood flow through capillaries is slower than in any other part of the vascular system.

18. Describe the neural and hormonal regulation of blood pressure and flow.

19. Describe how the skeletal muscle pump and the respiratory pump aid venous return.

chapter 15

VASCULAR SYSTEM

The vascular system of the average adult is more than 60,000 miles long: enough to circle the earth twice.

FAST FACT

When the body is at rest, only 4% of the blood is in the heart; the rest is in the blood vessels. Of that, about 13% is in circulation in the brain.

Every organ, every tissue, and every cell in the body depends upon a continual supply of blood to provide it with oxygen and nutrients and to remove waste products. The body has an elaborate system of vessels—the vascular system—to meet this need.

The demands on this system are great: it must penetrate every square inch of the body, from the skin's surface to the deepest recesses of the internal structures. It must adapt to changes in body position (from lying down to standing up…or even being upside down), changes in activity, and changes in fluid volume. It must also work with the heart to keep the blood constantly moving.

The framework of this system consists of three types of blood vessels:

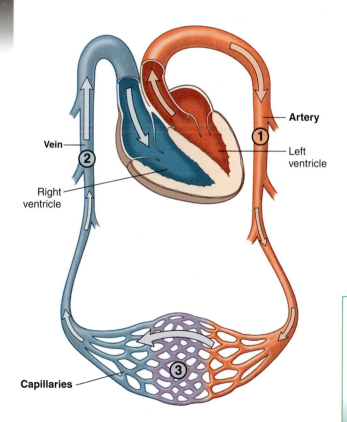

Vein

②

Right ventricle

Artery

①

Left ventricle

Capillaries

③

① **Arteries** carry blood *away* from the heart.

② **Veins** *return* blood to the heart.

③ **Capillaries** *connect* the smallest arteries to the smallest veins.

That Makes Sense

To remember the difference between the various blood vessels, remember:
- ***A**rteries **A**way: arteries carry blood away from the heart.*
- ***C**apillaries **C**onnect: capillaries serve to connect arteries and veins.*

Vessel Structure

The walls of both arteries and veins consist of three layers, called **tunics.** The basic layers include the **tunica intima, tunica media,** and **tunica externa.**

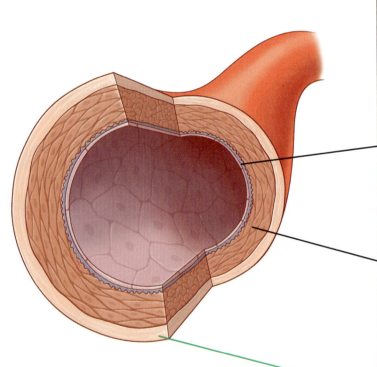

Tunica intima, the innermost layer, is exposed to the blood. It consists of a simple squamous epithelium—called **endothelium**—that is continuous with the endothelium that lines the heart. Its smooth surface keeps blood flowing freely, without sticking to the vessel wall. This layer also produces chemicals that cause blood vessels to dilate or constrict.

Tunica media, the middle layer, is the thickest layer. Composed of smooth muscle and elastic tissue, it allows the blood vessel to change diameter. The smooth muscle in this layer is innervated by the autonomic nervous system.

Tunica externa, the outer layer, is made of strong, flexible, fibrous connective tissue. This layer supports and protects the blood vessel. In veins, this is the thickest of the three layers. In arteries, it's usually a little thinner than the middle layer.

Life lesson: Aneurysm

The blood flowing through arteries is under high pressure. If a portion of the arterial wall weakens, the blood inside the artery will push against the weakened area, causing it to bulge. This is called an *aneurysm*. The most common cause of aneurysm development is atherosclerosis combined with high blood pressure, although they may also result from a congenital weakness of the vessel wall, trauma, or a bacterial infection.

The most common sites for aneurysms include the aorta, the renal arteries, and a circle of arteries at the base of the brain. If the aneurysm ruptures, massive hemorrhage will result. Even without rupturing, the aneurysm can cause pain and even death by putting pressure on surrounding nerves, tissues, and organs.

Arteries

Arteries carry blood away from the heart. Every time the heart contracts, it forcefully ejects blood into the arteries. Therefore, arteries must be strong as well as resilient to withstand these high pressures.

The arteries closest to the heart are the largest. As they travel farther away from the heart, the arteries branch and divide, becoming ever smaller. Finally, they become **arterioles,** which are the smallest arteries. Arteries can be divided into conducting arteries, distributing arteries, and arterioles.

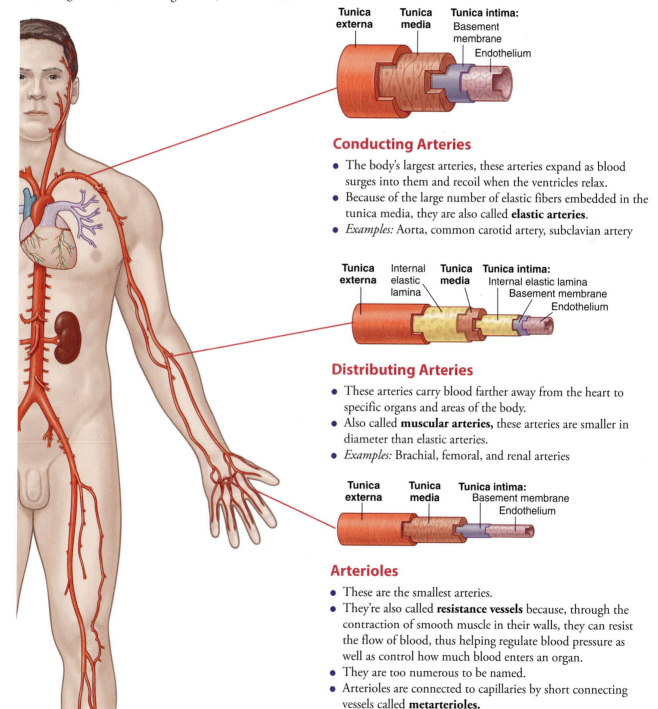

Conducting Arteries

- The body's largest arteries, these arteries expand as blood surges into them and recoil when the ventricles relax.
- Because of the large number of elastic fibers embedded in the tunica media, they are also called **elastic arteries**.
- *Examples:* Aorta, common carotid artery, subclavian artery

Distributing Arteries

- These arteries carry blood farther away from the heart to specific organs and areas of the body.
- Also called **muscular arteries,** these arteries are smaller in diameter than elastic arteries.
- *Examples:* Brachial, femoral, and renal arteries

Arterioles

- These are the smallest arteries.
- They're also called **resistance vessels** because, through the contraction of smooth muscle in their walls, they can resist the flow of blood, thus helping regulate blood pressure as well as control how much blood enters an organ.
- They are too numerous to be named.
- Arterioles are connected to capillaries by short connecting vessels called **metarterioles.**

Veins

Blood returns to the heart through veins. In contrast to arteries that branch and divide, forming progressively smaller vessels as they lead away from the heart—veins converge, forming progressively larger and fewer vessels as they lead back to the heart. Either way, the vessels closest to the heart are the largest. Veins are distinct from arteries in other ways:

- Because they aren't subjected to the same high pressures as arteries, the walls of veins are thinner.
- Veins have a great ability to stretch, which allows them to carry varying amounts of blood with almost no change in pressure. Because of this great capacity for storing blood, they're sometimes called **capacitance vessels.**
- Veins can constrict extensively. This helps the body maintain blood pressure when blood volume drops, such as from a hemorrhage.

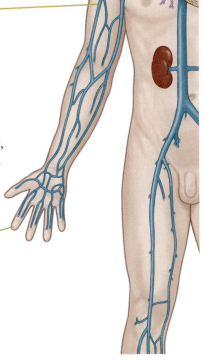

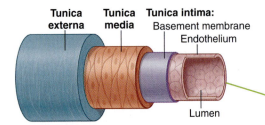

Large Veins

- Formed as medium-sized veins converge, these veins have a thick tunica externa.
- *Examples:* Vena cavae, pulmonary veins, internal jugular veins

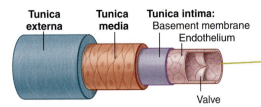

Medium-Sized Veins

- Formed by the convergence of venules on their route toward the heart, medium-sized veins have thicker, more elastic walls.
- These veins contain one-way valves. Formed from the thin endothelium lining, valves keep blood moving toward the heart and prevent backflow. Veins in the legs, which must fight the forces of gravity as they transport blood to the heart, contain the most valves.
- *Examples:* Radial and ulnar veins of the forearm, saphenous veins in the legs

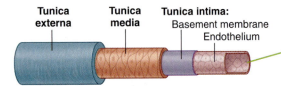

Venules

- These are the smallest veins and collect blood from capillaries.
- The endothelium consists of squamous epithelial cells and acts as a membrane; the tunica media is poorly developed, giving venules thinner walls.
- They are porous and can exchange fluid with surrounding tissues.

Capillaries

Capillaries are microscopic vessels that link arterioles to venules. More importantly, it's within capillaries that nutrients, wastes, and hormones are transferred between blood and tissues. These are the **exchange vessels** of the circulatory system. Properly functioning capillaries are as vital to survival as a properly beating heart. For this reason, no cell in the body is more than four or six cell-widths from a capillary.

Capillaries aren't evenly distributed, however. Tissues with high metabolic rates—such as the liver, kidneys, and myocardium—contain large numbers of capillaries. Fibrous connective tissues, such as tendons, have lower metabolic rates and contain fewer capillaries. Still other tissues—such as the epidermis, cartilage, and the lens and cornea of the eye—don't have any capillaries.

> **FAST FACT**
> Veins contain over 50% of the blood in circulation; in comparison, arteries contain 11%. (The rest is contained in the lungs, heart, and capillaries.)

Composed of only an endothelium and basement membrane, capillaries have extremely thin walls through which substances can filter.

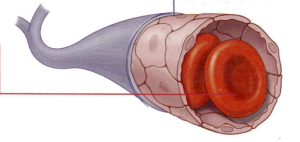

Capillaries have very small diameters, barely wide enough for blood cells to pass.

Capillary Organization

Capillaries are organized into networks called **capillary beds**. Connecting arterioles to venules, capillaries form what is called the **microcirculation**.

> **The Body AT WORK**
> *The body doesn't contain enough blood to fill the entire vascular system at once. During periods of rest, about 90% of the capillaries in skeletal muscles shut down. During exercise, when muscles demand an abundance of blood, the vascular system diverts blood from other areas, such as the intestines.*

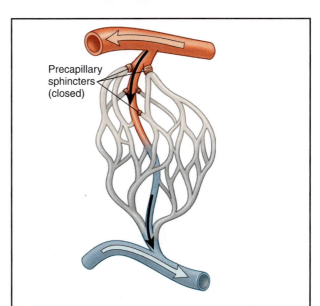

Arteriole

Precapillary sphincters (open)

Arterial capillaries

Venous capillaries

Venule

Precapillary sphincters (closed)

At the beginning of each capillary bed is a **precapillary sphincter** that regulates the flow of blood into the network. During exercise, when skeletal muscles require more oxygen, the precapillary sphincters open, blood fills the capillary network, and the exchange of oxygen, nutrients, and wastes occurs with the tissue fluid.

During a time of rest, the precapillary sphincters close. Blood bypasses the capillary bed and flows directly into a venule to begin its journey back to the heart and lungs.

Sinusoid

Some organs—such as the liver, bone marrow, and spleen—contain a unique capillary called a **sinusoid**. These irregular, blood-filled spaces are more permeable, allowing for the passage of large substances such as proteins and blood cells. This is how blood cells formed in bone marrow as well as clotting factors and other proteins synthesized in the liver enter the bloodstream.

Capillary Exchange

Capillary walls allow for a two-way exchange of substances and fluid.

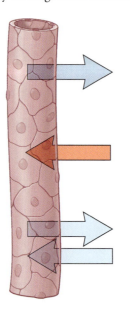

Capillaries release chemicals, including oxygen, glucose, hormones, and nutrients that will be used by surrounding tissues.

Capillaries take up waste, such as carbon dioxide and ammonia. They also take up substances that need to be transported to other parts of the body. These include glucose (released by the liver), calcium (released from bone), antibodies (released from immune cells), and hormones (released from endocrine glands).

Water moves into and out of capillaries.

Mechanisms of Capillary Exchange

The mechanisms used to move substances into and out of capillaries are diffusion, filtration, and osmosis. (See Chapter 3, *Cells*, for a review of these mechanisms.)

Diffusion

In diffusion—the most important mechanism of capillary exchange—substances move from areas of greater to lesser concentration. What occurs is this: Blood flows into the capillaries from the arterial system, carrying a supply of oxygen. Therefore, the concentration of oxygen inside capillaries is greater than that in surrounding tissue fluid. As a result, oxygen diffuses out of capillaries and into the surrounding fluid.

At the same time, carbon dioxide, which is more concentrated in the fluid of the surrounding tissue, diffuses into the capillary.

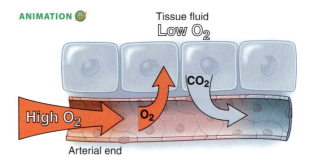

ANIMATION

Tissue fluid
Low O_2

CO_2

High O_2

O_2

Arterial end

FAST FACT

Capillaries make up in number what they lack in size. It's estimated that the body has over 1 billion capillaries.

Filtration and Colloid Osmotic Pressure

Filtration—another method of capillary exchange—occurs close to the arterial side of the capillary bed, while colloid osmotic pressure operates toward the venous side. Of all the fluid filtered at the arterial end of the capillary bed, about 85% is reabsorbed at the venous end. The remaining 15% of fluid is absorbed and returned to the blood by the lymphatic system. (This will be discussed further in Chapter 16, *Lymphatic & Immune Systems.*)

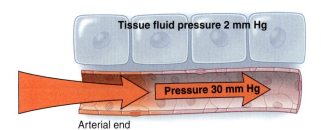

Blood enters the capillary through the metarteriole. The pressure here is about 30 to 35 mm Hg, while the pressure of the fluid in surrounding tissues is about 2 mm Hg.

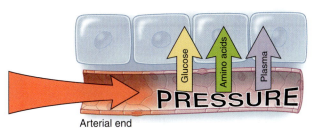

The higher pressure in the capillary pushes plasma and dissolved nutrients (such as glucose and amino acids) through the capillary wall and into the fluid in the surrounding tissues. This is **filtration**.

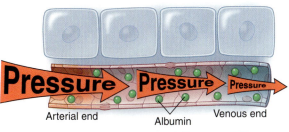

Meanwhile, as the blood continues to move toward the venous end of the capillary, blood pressure inside the capillary drops to about 10 mm Hg.

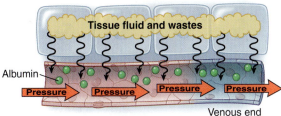

The lower pressure allows proteins in the blood, such as albumin, to exert what's known as **colloid osmotic pressure**. In this mechanism, the albumin in the blood pulls tissue fluid, along with the cells' waste products, into the capillaries.

Life lesson: Edema

When fluid filters out of the capillaries faster than it's reabsorbed, it accumulates in the tissues. Called *edema*, this accumulation of fluid appears as swelling in the ankles, fingers, abdomen, or face. It may also occur in internal organs. Edema has three main causes:

1. *Increased capillary filtration:* Because capillary pressure drives filtration, a rise in capillary pressure would increase filtration. Causes of increased capillary pressure include kidney failure, poor venous return from inactivity, or failure of the right ventricle—all of which allow blood to accumulate in the veins and capillaries, driving up pressure.
2. *Reduced capillary reabsorption:* Capillary reabsorption depends on albumin; therefore, a deficiency of albumin would slow reabsorption, causing edema. Albumin deficiency may result from liver disease (because albumin is produced by the liver), severe burns (which allow protein to be lost from the skin surface), and kidney disease (which allows albumin to be lost in the urine).
3. *Obstructed lymphatic drainage:* Because the body depends on the lymphatic system to absorb 15% of the fluid filtered by the capillaries, an obstruction here would cause fluid to accumulate. Besides an obstruction, the surgical removal of lymph nodes can also interfere with fluid drainage, leading to edema.

Circulatory Routes

In general, blood flows from the heart through arteries, then capillaries, then veins, and back to the heart. Typically, blood passes through only one network of capillaries before returning to the heart. An exception is a **portal system,** in which blood flows through two networks of capillaries. (The body's main portal system occurs in the liver.) Another exception is when two vessels join together; this is called an **anastomosis**. An anastomosis may cause blood to flow directly from an artery to a vein (**arteriovenous anastomosis**) or from one vein to another vein (**venous anastomosis**). Anastomoses provide alternative routes of blood flow in case a vessel becomes obstructed.

   The body contains two major pathways of circulation, pulmonary circulation and systemic circulation. **Pulmonary circulation** begins at the right ventricle and involves the circulation of blood through the lungs. **Systemic circulation** begins at the left ventricle and involves the circulation of blood through the body.

   Specialized circulatory systems include hepatic portal circulation (which routes blood from the digestive organs to the liver), circulation to the brain, and fetal circulation. (Because fetal circulation involves pathways that are only present before birth, this system will be discussed in Chapter 24, *Pregnancy & Human Development.*)

Pulmonary Circulation

Pulmonary circulation routes blood to and from the lungs to exchange carbon dioxide for oxygen. It doesn't supply the lung tissue itself with oxygen. Those needs are met through systemic circulation.

ANIMATION

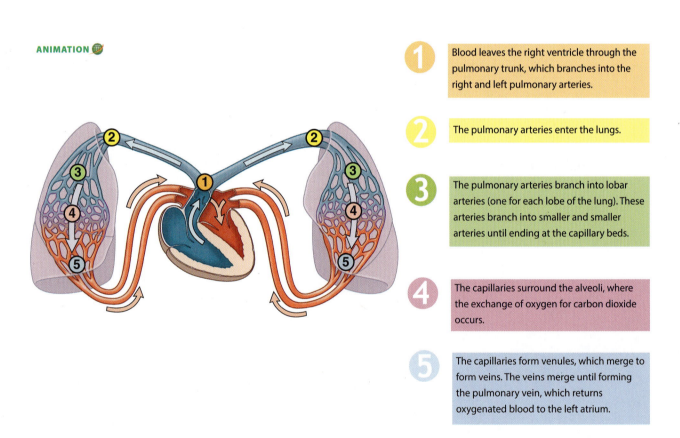

1 Blood leaves the right ventricle through the pulmonary trunk, which branches into the right and left pulmonary arteries.

2 The pulmonary arteries enter the lungs.

3 The pulmonary arteries branch into lobar arteries (one for each lobe of the lung). These arteries branch into smaller and smaller arteries until ending at the capillary beds.

4 The capillaries surround the alveoli, where the exchange of oxygen for carbon dioxide occurs.

5 The capillaries form venules, which merge to form veins. The veins merge until forming the pulmonary vein, which returns oxygenated blood to the left atrium.

Systemic Circulation

Systemic circulation supplies oxygen and nutrients to organs and removes wastes. This, of course, involves both arteries and veins. All systemic arteries arise, either directly or indirectly, from the **aorta**. The aorta, which originates in the left ventricle, is divided into three regions: (1) the **ascending aorta**, (2) the **aortic arch**, and (3) the **descending aorta**. It branches into several major arteries.

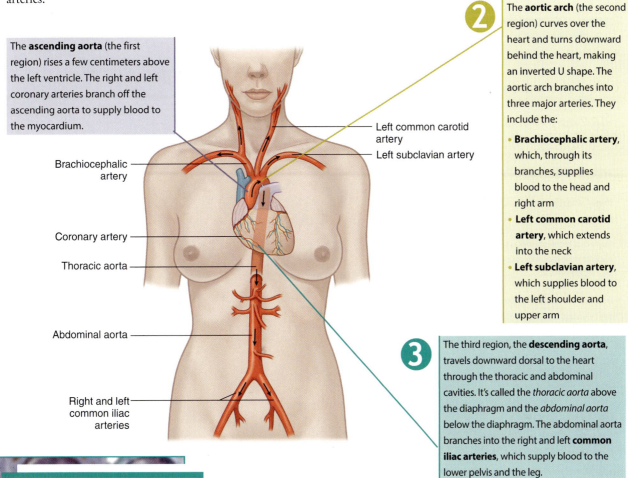

1 The **ascending aorta** (the first region) rises a few centimeters above the left ventricle. The right and left coronary arteries branch off the ascending aorta to supply blood to the myocardium.

Brachiocephalic artery

Coronary artery

Thoracic aorta

Abdominal aorta

Right and left common iliac arteries

Left common carotid artery

Left subclavian artery

2 The **aortic arch** (the second region) curves over the heart and turns downward behind the heart, making an inverted U shape. The aortic arch branches into three major arteries. They include the:

- **Brachiocephalic artery**, which, through its branches, supplies blood to the head and right arm
- **Left common carotid artery**, which extends into the neck
- **Left subclavian artery**, which supplies blood to the left shoulder and upper arm

3 The third region, the **descending aorta**, travels downward dorsal to the heart through the thoracic and abdominal cavities. It's called the *thoracic aorta* above the diaphragm and the *abdominal aorta* below the diaphragm. The abdominal aorta branches into the right and left **common iliac arteries**, which supply blood to the lower pelvis and the leg.

The Body AT WORK

Each beat of the heart produces a surge of pressure that can be felt at points where an artery comes close to the body's surface. Perhaps the most common site used to measure a person's pulse is the radial artery in the wrist. However, pulses can be palpated in a number of other locations, including those shown here.

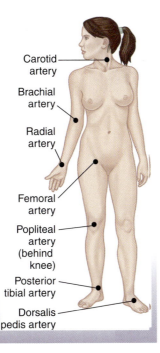

Carotid artery

Brachial artery

Radial artery

Femoral artery

Popliteal artery (behind knee)

Posterior tibial artery

Dorsalis pedis artery

FAST FACT

Arteries and veins are typically named for their location in the body (such as the femoral or axillary artery), the organ they supply (such as the renal artery), or a nearby bone (such as the radial or ulnar artery). Arteries change names as they leave one body region and enter another. For example, the axillary artery becomes the brachial artery as it travels distally from the body.

Principal Arteries

As previously mentioned, all of the systemic arteries arise, either directly or indirectly, from the aorta.

The **thoracic aorta** and its branches supply the chest wall and the organs within the thoracic cavity.

The **abdominal aorta** gives rise to the:

- **Celiac trunk**, which divides into the **gastric artery** (which supplies the stomach), the **splenic artery** (which supplies the spleen), and the **hepatic artery** (which supplies the liver)

- **Renal arteries**, which supply the kidneys

- **Superior mesenteric artery**, which supplies most of the small intestine and part of the large intestine

- **Inferior mesenteric artery**, which supplies the other part of the large intestine

The distal end of the abdominal aorta splits into the right and left **common iliac arteries**, which supply the pelvic organs, thigh, and lower extremities.

Major arteries branching off the iliac arteries include the:

- **Internal iliac artery**

- **External iliac artery**

- **Femoral artery**

- **Popliteal artery**

- **Anterior tibial artery**

- **Posterior tibial artery**

- **Dorsalis pedis artery**

Branching off the aortic arch is the:

- **Subclavian artery**, which supplies blood to the arm

- **Axillary artery**, which is the continuation of the subclavian artery in the axillary region

- **Brachial artery**, which is the continuation of the axillary artery and the artery most often used for routine blood pressure measurement

- **Radial artery**, which is often palpated to measure a pulse

Arteries of the Head and Neck

The brain requires a constant supply of blood. An interruption of blood flow for just a few seconds causes loss of consciousness. If the brain is deprived of oxygen for 4 or 5 minutes, irreversible brain damage occurs. Because of this critical need for oxygen, two arteries supply blood to the brain. Remember: Arterial blood flows from the heart. So, to trace the path of blood to the brain, begin at the bottom of the illustration and work upward.

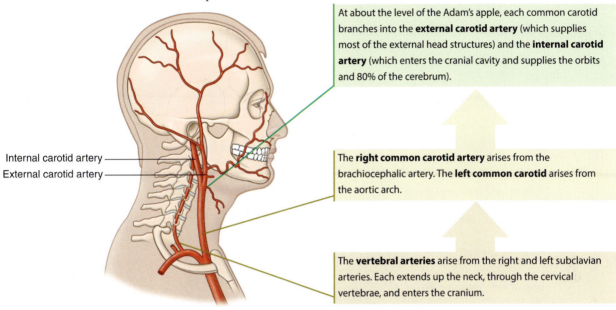

Internal carotid artery

External carotid artery

At about the level of the Adam's apple, each common carotid branches into the **external carotid artery** (which supplies most of the external head structures) and the **internal carotid artery** (which enters the cranial cavity and supplies the orbits and 80% of the cerebrum).

The **right common carotid artery** arises from the brachiocephalic artery. The **left common carotid** arises from the aortic arch.

The **vertebral arteries** arise from the right and left subclavian arteries. Each extends up the neck, through the cervical vertebrae, and enters the cranium.

Circle of Willis

On the undersurface of the brainstem, the two vertebral arteries unite to form a single **basilar artery**. Branches from the internal carotids and basilar artery form several anastomoses to create a circle of arteries at the base of the brain. This circle of arteries, called the **circle of Willis**, helps ensure that the brain receives an adequate supply of blood.

The complete circle of Willis consists of:

- A single anterior communicating artery
- Two anterior cerebral arteries
- Two posterior communicating arteries
- Two posterior cerebral arteries

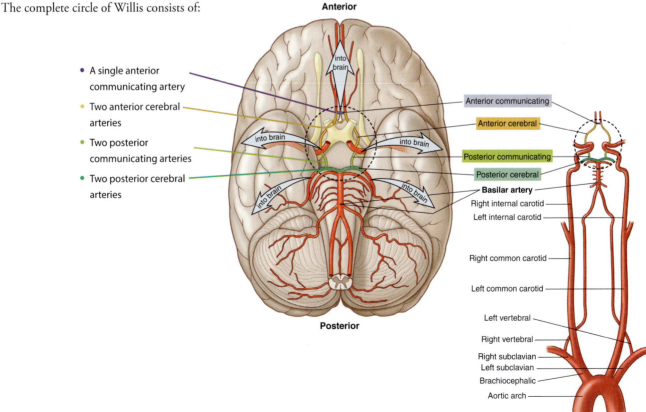

Principal Veins

The veins drain blood from the organs and other parts of the body and carry it to the vena cava, which, in turn, delivers it to the heart's right atrium. The vena cava is the body's main vein. It's divided into the:

- **Superior vena cava (SVC)**, which receives blood from the head, shoulders, and arms
- **Inferior vena cava (IVC)**, which receives blood from the lower part of the body

Some veins, like the brachiocephalic, drain directly into the SVC. Others drain into a second vein, which may merge with still another vein, before draining into the vena cava. For example, the axillary vein drains into the subclavian vein, which drains into the brachiocephalic vein, which then drains into the SVC.

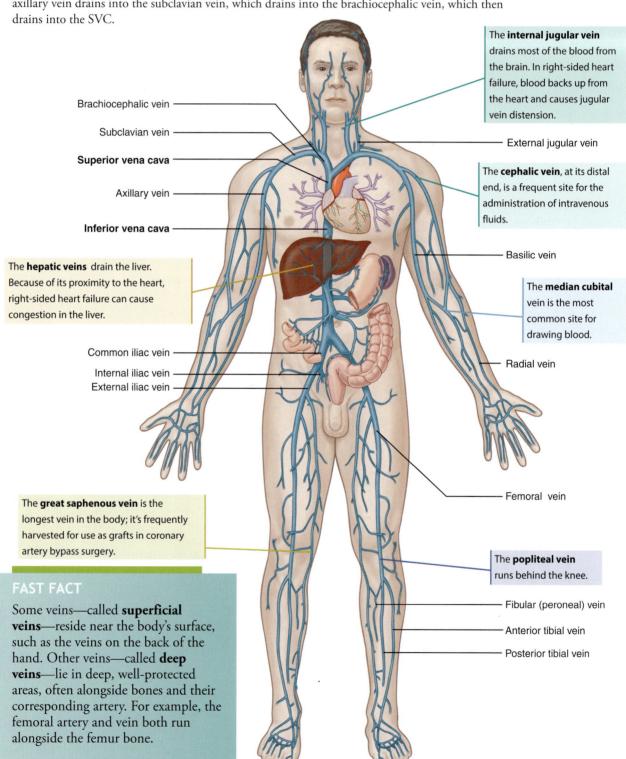

The **internal jugular vein** drains most of the blood from the brain. In right-sided heart failure, blood backs up from the heart and causes jugular vein distension.

Brachiocephalic vein

Subclavian vein

Superior vena cava

Axillary vein

Inferior vena cava

External jugular vein

The **cephalic vein**, at its distal end, is a frequent site for the administration of intravenous fluids.

Basilic vein

The **hepatic veins** drain the liver. Because of its proximity to the heart, right-sided heart failure can cause congestion in the liver.

The **median cubital** vein is the most common site for drawing blood.

Common iliac vein

Internal iliac vein

External iliac vein

Radial vein

The **great saphenous vein** is the longest vein in the body; it's frequently harvested for use as grafts in coronary artery bypass surgery.

Femoral vein

The **popliteal vein** runs behind the knee.

Fibular (peroneal) vein

Anterior tibial vein

Posterior tibial vein

FAST FACT

Some veins—called **superficial veins**—reside near the body's surface, such as the veins on the back of the hand. Other veins—called **deep veins**—lie in deep, well-protected areas, often alongside bones and their corresponding artery. For example, the femoral artery and vein both run alongside the femur bone.

Veins of the Head and Neck

Most of the blood of the head and neck is drained by the internal jugular, external jugular, and vertebral veins.

The **internal jugular vein** receives most of the blood from the brain as well as from the face. The internal jugular vein merges into the subclavian vein, which, in turn, becomes the brachiocephalic vein. The brachiocephalic vein drains into the superior vena cava.

The **external jugular vein**—the more superficial of the jugular veins—drains blood from the scalp, facial muscles, and other superficial structures. It, too, drains into the subclavian vein.

The **vertebral vein** drains the cervical vertebrae, spinal cord, and some of the muscles of the neck.

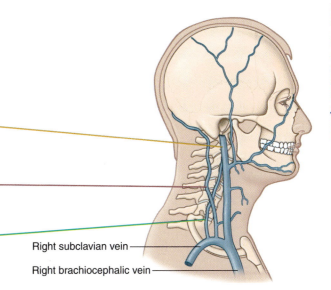

Right subclavian vein ——

Right brachiocephalic vein ——

Hepatic Portal Circulation

Unlike the veins of other abdominal organs, veins from the digestive organs and spleen don't empty into the inferior vena cava. Rather, they send their blood through the hepatic portal vein to the liver. This circulatory pathway allows the liver to modify the blood returning to the heart. For example, after a meal, blood glucose levels rise dramatically. This circulatory pathway allows the liver to remove excess glucose, which it then stores as glycogen. Toxins, such as bacteria or alcohol, can also be partially removed before the blood is distributed to the rest of the body. Here's the specific route:

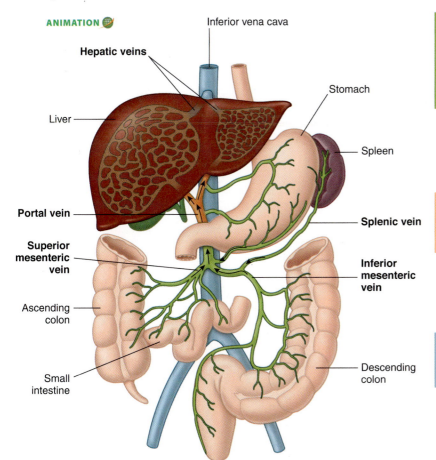

ANIMATION

Inferior vena cava

Hepatic veins

Liver —

Portal vein —

Superior mesenteric vein —

Ascending colon

Small intestine

Stomach

Spleen

Splenic vein

Inferior mesenteric vein

Descending colon

Blood from the capillaries of the spleen, stomach, pancreas, gallbladder, and intestines flows into the superior mesenteric vein and the splenic vein, which converge to form the portal vein. (Blood from the left and right gastric veins empty into the hepatic portal vein.)

The portal vein channels blood into the liver; the blood is then distributed to innumerable microscopic sinusoids (the capillaries of the liver).

Blood flows out of the sinusoids into the hepatic veins and, from there, into the inferior vena cava, where it is returned to the heart.

Principles of Circulation

The purpose of the circulatory system is to deliver oxygen and nutrients to tissues and to remove wastes. A deficiency of oxygen or nutrients, or an accumulation of waste products—even for a few minutes—can cause tissue necrosis and, possibly, even death of the individual. Therefore, it's imperative that blood constantly circulate, or flow.

Blood flows for the same reason that any fluid (including the water in a river or the fluid in an intravenous tubing) flows: because of differences in pressure between two structures. This is called a **pressure gradient**. Fluid always flows from an area with higher pressure toward an area with lower pressure.

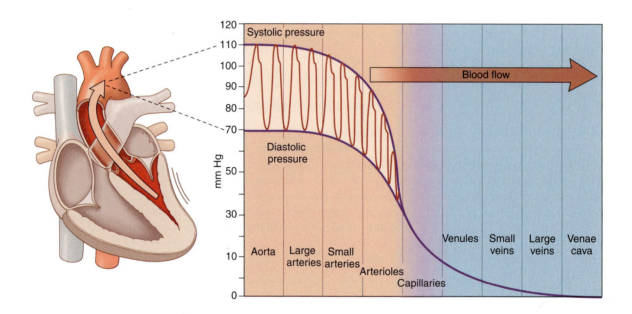

As the left ventricle contracts (systole), it ejects blood into the aorta, producing a typical, normal pressure of 110 mm Hg. This is the **systolic pressure**. When the ventricle relaxes (diastole), the pressure drops to an average of 70 mm Hg. This is the **diastolic pressure**.

As blood moves away from the heart, blood pressure declines until, in the vena cava, it is about 1 mm Hg. The greater the pressure difference between two points, the greater the flow. However, as blood flows, it also meets resistance, and the greater the resistance, the less the flow. Therefore, to understand the flow of blood, we must consider these two factors: **blood pressure** and **resistance**.

The Body AT WORK

The pressure gradient principle applies to blood flow throughout the entire body, including the flow in organs and tissues. For example, pressure in the arteries and arterioles of the kidney must be higher than the pressure in the capillaries and veins of the kidney for blood to flow through the kidney's tissues. The pressure gradient requires a certain balance, however. If the pressure gradient between the arterial and venous ends of the capillary network is too low, filtration won't occur. If it's too high, the thin-walled capillaries will rupture.

FAST FACT

The ability of arteries to expand and recoil with the force of ejected blood helps maintain a certain pressure: blood vessels expand to absorb the force of ejected blood and then recoil to prevent the pressure from dropping to zero.

Blood Pressure

The maintenance of a proper **blood pressure**—the force exerted by the blood against a vessel wall—is crucial for proper body functioning. Blood pressure is determined by three factors: cardiac output, blood volume, and resistance.

Three Factors That Affect Blood Pressure		How Factors Affect Blood Pressure
Cardiac output	When the heart beats harder, such as during exercise, cardiac output increases. When cardiac output increases, blood pressure increases. When cardiac output falls, such as when exercise ends or the heart is weak, blood pressure falls.	↑CO = ↑BP ↓CO = ↓BP
Blood volume	When blood volume declines, such as from dehydration or a hemorrhage, blood pressure falls. To try and preserve blood pressure, the kidneys reduce urine output, which helps boost blood volume and raise blood pressure.	↓Volume = ↓BP ↑Volume = ↑BP
Resistance	Also called peripheral resistance, this is the opposition to flow resulting from the friction of moving blood against the vessel walls. The greater the resistance, the slower the flow and the higher the pressure. The lower the resistance, the faster the flow and the lower the pressure.	↑Resistance = ↓Flow and ↑Pressure ↓Resistance = ↑Flow and ↓Pressure

Life lesson: Blood pressure

Routinely, blood pressure (BP) is measured with a sphygmomanometer connected to an inflatable cuff wrapped around the upper arm, the location of the brachial artery. The brachial artery is close enough to the heart that it reflects the blood pressure found elsewhere in the body. Arterial blood pressure is written as a ratio of systolic pressure (the peak arterial pressure during ventricular contraction, or systole) over diastolic pressure (the minimum arterial pressure during ventricular relaxation, or diastole).

A normal systolic pressure ranges from 90 to 120 millimeters of mercury (mm Hg), while a normal diastolic pressure ranges from 60 to 80 mm Hg. A lower than normal blood pressure is called *hypotension*. If blood pressure drops too low, blood flow to the organs is diminished and, if severe, can lead to shock and even death.

Higher than normal blood pressure, called *hypertension*, is a major risk factor for heart disease, the chief risk factor for stroke and heart failure, and a cause of kidney damage.

In fact, studies show that the risk of death from heart disease and stroke begins to rise at blood pressures as low as 115 over 75 and that it doubles for each 20 over 10 mm Hg increase. Hypertension affects 67 million Americans—one in 3 adults.

The difference between systolic and diastolic pressure is called *pulse pressure*. For a BP of 110/70 mm Hg, the pulse pressure would be 40 mm Hg. Pulse pressure reflects the stress on the small arteries by the pressure surges during systole.

Ranges for Blood Pressure	
Normal	Less than 120/80 mm Hg
Prehypertension	120-139/80-89 mm Hg
Stage I hypertension	140-159/90-99 mm Hg
Stage II hypertension	160/100 mm or Hg or greater

Peripheral Resistance

Peripheral resistance is the resistance to blood flow resulting from the friction of blood against the walls of vessels. The amount of friction depends upon the viscosity of the blood and the diameter of the blood vessel.

Blood Viscosity

Viscosity refers to the thickness, or "stickiness," of blood. The greater the viscosity, the slower the flow; likewise, the lower the viscosity, the faster the flow. (Think of the difference between the speed of a milkshake flowing through a straw versus the speed of water.) The chief cause of increased blood viscosity is an increased number of red blood cells, but it may also result from an increased amount of protein (albumin) or dehydration.

Vessel Diameter

The muscular layer of arterioles allows them to constrict or dilate, changing the amount of resistance to blood flow. Because blood viscosity remains stable in healthy individuals, adjusting the diameter of vessels is the body's chief way of controlling peripheral resistance, and therefore blood pressure. Adjusting the diameter of blood vessels is called **vasomotion**.

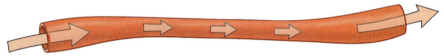

Vasoconstriction = ↑ pressure and ↓ flow

A reduction of the diameter of a vessel—called **vasoconstriction**—increases the resistance to blood flow. Because blood is being squeezed into a smaller space, pressure rises. Also, because the amount of blood allowed to enter the vessel is reduced, blood flow into tissues decreases.

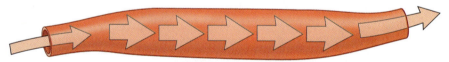

Vasodilation = ↓ pressure and ↑ flow

An increase in vessel diameter caused by the relaxation of vascular muscles—called **vasodilation**—decreases resistance to blood flow. Blood pressure declines and blood flow into tissues increases.

The Body AT WORK

The elastic property of healthy arteries allows them to expand with each beat of the heart to absorb some of the force of the ejected blood. Then, when the heart's in diastole, the arteries recoil, shrinking their diameter. This expansion and recoil propels blood steadily downstream toward the capillaries; it also helps smooth out the surges of pressure that occur with systole, protecting smaller arteries.

Because of their distance from the beating heart, capillaries and veins don't need to be protected from pressure surges. Consequently, blood in these vessels flows at a steady speed without pulsation. That's why an injured vein produces a steady flow of blood while an injured artery squirts blood intermittently.

FAST FACT

Arteries become less elastic with age and absorb less systolic force. As a result, blood pressure rises. Atherosclerosis also stiffens arteries and raises blood pressure.

The diameter of a vessel affects how fast blood flows: its velocity. The greater the diameter of the vessel, the faster blood flows. The velocity of blood in the aorta is about 1200 mm/sec; in capillaries, it's about 0.4 mm/sec.

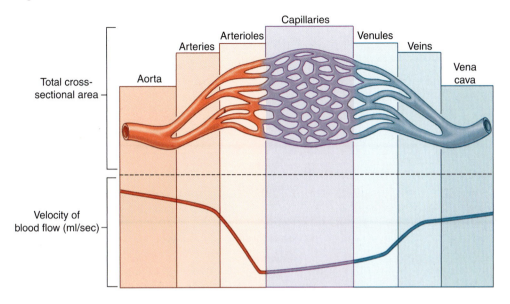

Flow is fastest in the aorta. Besides being a large vessel, it's also close to the left ventricle.

By the time the blood reaches the capillaries, it has slowed considerably. That's because:

- Capillaries are far removed from the left ventricle.
- Friction along the way has slowed the flow.
- The smaller diameter of arterioles and capillaries has put up more resistance.
- The number of vessels has become greater, giving capillaries a greater total cross-sectional area. (See "That Makes Sense!" on this page.)

Blood flow through capillaries is slower than in any other part of the vascular system. This slow flow rate allows capillaries time to exchange nutrients, wastes, and gases with surrounding tissues.

From the capillaries to the vena cava, velocity rises again. That's because:

- Veins have larger diameters than capillaries, so they create less resistance.
- Many capillaries converge on one venule, and many venules converge on one vein, creating a smaller cross-sectional area.

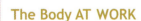

That Makes Sense

To understand how cross-sectional area affects flow rate, think of a raging river. As the river travels farther from its headwaters, it begins to slow, both because it's farther from its source and because the friction of the water against the shore creates resistance. After a while, the river begins to branch repeatedly into a number of smaller streams, spreading water over a larger area. The flow rate in these smallest streams (like the capillary network) is much slower than the flow rate in the larger streams or the river. That's because the water now covers a greater cross-sectional area. Then, if these streams converge (like capillaries into venules and venules into veins), the water picks ups speed as a greater volume of water is forced into a smaller space (a smaller cross-sectional area).

The Body AT WORK

Changing the diameter of blood vessels also allows the body to redistribute blood flow according to its needs. For example, after eating, blood vessels to the skeletal muscles and kidneys constrict while those to the gastrointestinal system dilate. This directs a larger amount of blood to the gastrointestinal system, giving it the blood it needs for digestion and nutrient absorption. When the digestion process ends, the body reverses the process to redirect blood back to the kidneys and other organs. The body can greatly alter flow in specific regions while general circulation patterns remain unchanged.

Regulation of Blood Pressure and Flow

The vascular system can quickly adjust blood pressure and alter blood flow to respond to the body's changing needs. This occurs because of input from the nervous system as well as the influence of certain hormones.

Neural Regulation of Blood Pressure

- The **vasomotor center** (an area of the medulla in the brain) sends impulses via the autonomic nervous system to alter blood vessel diameter and, therefore, blood pressure.

- **Baroreceptors** in the carotid sinus and aortic arch detect changes in blood pressure and transmit signals along the glossopharyngeal and vagus nerves to the cardiac control center and the vasomotor center in the medulla.

ANIMATION 🌐

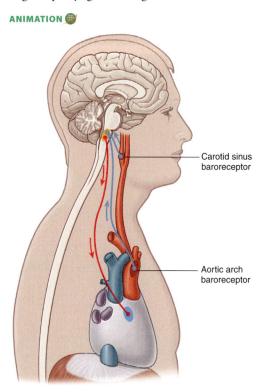

Carotid sinus
baroreceptor

Aortic arch
baroreceptor

If pressure is too **HIGH**:

- The medulla increases its output of **parasympathetic impulses**.
- **Vasodilation** occurs; heart rate and stroke volume decrease.
- **Blood pressure drops**.

If pressure is too **LOW**:

- The medulla increases its output of **sympathetic impulses**.
- **Vasoconstriction** occurs; heart rate and stroke volume increase.
- **Blood pressure rises**.

The Body AT WORK

Baroreceptors mostly regulate BP on a short-term basis, such as adjusting for changes in posture. For example, if you jump up after lying down, gravity will draw blood into your legs and away from your brain and heart and you'll feel dizzy. When this happens, baroreceptors respond quickly to restore blood flow to the brain. However, baroreceptors aren't effective at controlling chronic hypertension.

Hormonal Regulation of Blood Pressure

A number of hormones also influence blood pressure.

	⬆ Cause blood pressure to RISE ⬆
Hormone	**Actions**
Renin, angiotensin I, and angiotensin II	• Cause vasoconstriction and water retention through an interactive mechanism
	• Because renin is released by the kidneys, this mechanism is discussed in Chapter 18, *Urinary System*.
Aldosterone	• Secreted by the adrenal medulla when blood pressure falls
	• Stimulates the kidneys to retain sodium
	• Water follows sodium, increasing blood volume
Antidiuretic hormone (ADH)	• Secreted by the posterior pituitary gland when the water content of the body falls
	• Promotes vasoconstriction and water retention
Epinephrine and norepinephrine	• Secreted by the adrenal medulla when the body is under stress
	• Cause vasoconstriction
	• Increases heart rate and force of contraction (epinephrine only)
	⬇ Causes blood pressure to FALL ⬇
Hormone	**Actions**
Atrial natriuretic peptide (ANP)	• Released by the heart's atria when elevated blood pressure stretches the walls of the heart
	• Causes vasodilation
	• Stimulates the kidneys to excrete sodium (and, therefore, water), reducing blood volume

Venous Return

After making its way through the arterial system, blood must return to the heart by way of the venous system. However, because gravity pulls blood into the legs and away from the heart whenever someone stands, veins must fight the forces of gravity to deliver blood back to the heart. (The only exceptions are the veins in the head and neck.) Two key mechanisms aid in venous return: the **skeletal muscle pump** and the **respiratory pump**.

Skeletal Muscle Pump

Muscles surrounding leg veins aid in venous return.

- When leg muscles contract, they massage the veins in the legs, propelling blood toward the heart.
- The valves in veins ensure the blood flows upward, toward the heart.
- When the muscles relax, the blood flows backward, pulled by the force of gravity.
- Blood puddles in valve flaps, keeping the valve closed and preventing further backward flow.

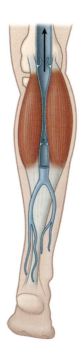
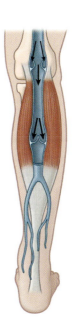

Respiratory Pump

The process of breathing also promotes the flow of venous blood in the thoracic and abdominal cavities.

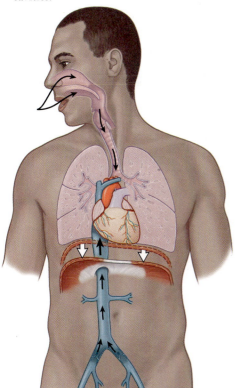

- During inhalation, the chest expands and the diaphragm moves downward. This causes the pressure in the chest cavity to drop and the pressure in the abdominal cavity to rise.
- The rising abdominal pressure squeezes the inferior vena cava, forcing blood upward toward the thorax.
- Lower pressure in the thorax helps draw blood toward the heart.
- Valves in the veins in the legs ensure that blood doesn't flow backward.

Life lesson:
Aging and the vascular system

With age, blood vessels become less elastic, causing blood pressure to rise. In fact, blood pressure rises steadily throughout the adult years. Veins also weaken and stretch. This pulls the cusps of the valves apart, allowing blood to flow backward. The veins become distended, which leads to an increased incidence of varicose veins in elderly adults.

Review of Key Terms

Anastomosis: A natural connection between two vessels

Arteries: Blood vessels that carry blood away from the heart

Arteriole: The smallest arteries; also called resistance vessels

Baroreceptors: Sensory nerve endings in the aortic arch and carotid arteries that sense changes in pressure

Capillary: Microscopic vessels that link arterioles to venules; site where nutrients, wastes, and hormones are exchanged between blood and tissue

Circle of Willis: Circle of arteries at the base of the brain

Colloid osmotic pressure: Process whereby albumin in the blood pulls tissue fluid into capillaries

Conducting arteries: The body's largest arteries; also called elastic arteries

Diastolic pressure: Pressure within arteries when the ventricle relaxes

Diffusion: Process by which molecules of a substance move from an area of higher to lower concentration

Distributing arteries: Carry blood to specific organs and tissues; also called muscular arteries

Filtration: Process of removing particles from a solution by allowing the liquid portion to pass through a membrane

Hypertension: Blood pressure consistently higher than 140 mm Hg systolic over 90 mm Hg diastolic

Peripheral resistance: Resistance to blood flow resulting from the friction of the blood against the walls of the vessels

Portal system: System of vessels in which blood passes through a capillary network, a large vessel, and then another capillary network before returning to the systemic circulation

Pressure gradient: Difference in pressure between two structures

Sinusoid: Large, permeable capillary found in organs such as the liver, spleen, and bone marrow that allows for the passage of large cells and proteins

Systolic pressure: Pressure in arteries when the ventricle ejects blood

Tunica externa: Outer layer of blood vessels; composed of strong, flexible, fibrous connective tissue

Tunica intima: Innermost layer of blood vessels; consists of simple squamous epithelium

Tunica media: Middle layer of blood vessels; composed of smooth muscle and elastic tissue

Vasoconstriction: Reduction in the diameter of a vessel

Vasodilation: Increase in the diameter of a vessel

Vasomotor center: Area in the medulla of the brain that sends impulses to alter blood vessel diameter and therefore blood pressure

Veins: Blood vessels that return blood to the heart; called capacitance vessels because of their capacity for storing blood

Vena cava: The body's chief vein, which serves to return blood to the heart

Venule: The smallest veins; serve to collect blood from the capillaries

Own the Information

To make the information in this chapter part of your working memory, take some time to reflect on what you've learned. On a separate sheet of paper, write down everything you recall from the chapter. After you're done, log on to the Davis*Plus* website, and check out the Study Group podcast and Study Group Questions for the chapter.

Key Topics for Chapter 15:
- The structure of the walls of arteries and veins
- The structure and function of three classes of arteries
- The structure and function of three classes of veins
- The structure, function, and organization of capillaries
- Mechanisms of capillary exchange
- The route of pulmonary circulation
- Principal arteries of systemic circulation
- Arteries of the head and neck
- Principal veins of systemic circulation
- Veins of the head and neck
- Hepatic portal circulation
- The relationship between blood pressure and peripheral resistance in producing blood flow
- The influence of the nervous system and hormones on the regulation of blood pressure and flow
- Mechanisms that aid venous return

Test Your Knowledge

1. The vessels that carry blood away from the heart are:
   a. capillaries.
   b. sinusoids.
   c. veins.
   d. arteries.

2. The innermost layer of blood vessels is composed of what type of material?
   a. Simple squamous epithelium
   b. Smooth muscle
   c. Connective tissue
   d. Elastic tissue

3. Which arteries are called elastic arteries because of their ability to expand when blood surges into them?
   a. Distributing arteries
   b. Conducting arteries
   c. Arterioles
   d. Metarterioles

4. Veins are called capacitance vessels because they have the:
   a. capacity to pulsate with the heart's contractions.
   b. capacity to dilate and constrict to regulate blood pressure.
   c. ability to stretch, giving them a great capacity for storing blood.
   d. capacity to direct blood flow to organs and tissues in need.

5. What is the purpose of the valves in veins?
   a. Keep oxygenated blood from mixing with unoxygenated blood
   b. Prevent the backflow of blood
   c. Aid in the redirection of blood flow
   d. Aid in the pumping of blood

6. What are the exchange vessels of the circulatory system, where nutrients, wastes, and hormones are transferred between blood and tissues?
   a. Arterioles
   b. Capillaries
   c. Veins
   d. Venules

7. The most important mechanism for capillary exchange is:
   a. filtration.
   b. colloid osmotic pressure.
   c. gravity.
   d. diffusion.

8. All systemic arteries arise, directly or indirectly, from the:
   a. aorta.
   b. inferior vena cava.
   c. subclavian artery.
   d. carotid artery.

9. The reason blood constantly circulates is because of:
   a. the beating of the heart.
   b. low blood viscosity.
   c. pressure gradients.
   d. vasoconstriction and dilation.

10. What is the main reason blood flow is slowest in the capillaries?
    a. Capillaries have a greater cross-sectional area.
    b. Capillaries have a higher osmotic pressure.
    c. Capillary blood has a higher viscosity than venous blood.
    d. Capillaries have to fight the pull of gravity.

Answers: Chapter 15

1. *Correct answer:* **d.** Capillaries act as the exchange vessels. Sinusoids are specialized capillaries found in the liver, spleen, and bone marrow. Veins return blood to the heart.
2. *Correct answer:* **a.** The middle layer of blood vessels is composed of smooth muscle and elastic tissue. The outer layer consists of strong, flexible connective tissue.
3. *Correct answer:* **b.** Distributing arteries are also called muscular arteries. Arterioles are called resistance vessels. Metarterioles are short vessels that connect arterioles to capillaries.
4. *Correct answer:* **c.** Arteries pulsate, not veins. Arteries dilate and constrict to redirect blood flow to organs and tissues and to regulate blood pressure.
5. *Correct answer:* **b.** The valves do not function to keep oxygenated blood from mixing with unoxygenated blood or to redirect blood flow. They also do not aid in the pumping of blood.
6. *Correct answer:* **b.** Arterioles (the smallest arteries) aid in regulating blood pressure and in controlling blood flow into organs. Veins and venules (the smallest veins) return blood to the heart.
7. *Correct answer:* **d.** Filtration and colloid osmotic pressure are both mechanisms used in capillary exchange, but neither are the most important mechanism. Gravity does not influence capillary exchange.
8. *Correct answer:* **a.** The inferior vena cava is the body's largest vein and doesn't directly connect to arteries. The subclavian and carotid arteries both branch off the aortic arch.
9. *Correct answer:* **c.** The beating of the heart helps propel arterial blood, but it is not a key factor in venous flow. Blood viscosity affects the velocity of blood flow, but it is not the reason blood constantly circulates. Vasoconstriction and dilation help direct flow and influence blood pressure, not general circulation.
10. *Correct answer:* **a.** Colloid osmotic pressure influences capillary exchange, not blood velocity. Blood viscosity is constant throughout the circulatory system. Gravity does not have a direct affect on the velocity of capillary flow.

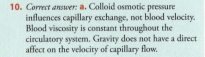 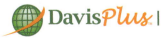 Go to **http://davisplus.fadavis.com** Keyword: Thompson to see all of the resources available with this chapter.

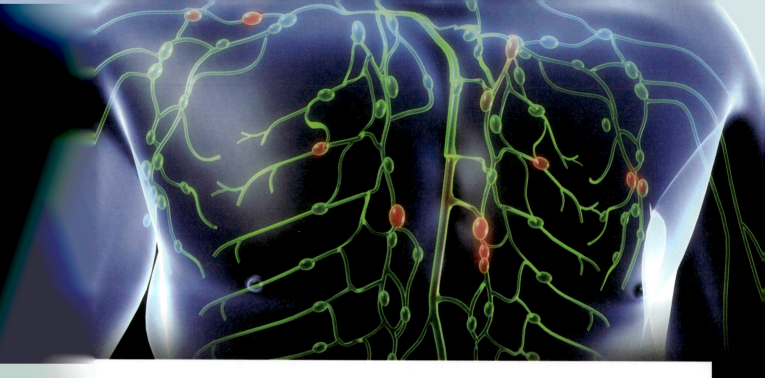

CHAPTER OUTLINE

Lymphatic System

Overview of the Immune System

Nonspecific Immunity

Specific Immunity

Immune System Disorders

LEARNING OUTCOMES

1. List three functions of the lymphatic system.

2. Describe the formation and flow of lymph.

3. Describe the structure of lymphatic vessels.

4. Differentiate between lymphatic tissues and organs.

5. Identify the location and function of the thymus, lymph nodes, tonsils, and spleen.

6. Describe the body's three lines of defense against infection.

7. Explain the difference between specific and nonspecific immunity.

8. Describe the process of phagocytosis and identify the body's two main phagocytes.

9. Discuss the role of antimicrobial proteins in immunity.

10. Summarize the process of inflammation.

11. Describe the process of fever and explain its role in fighting infection.

12. Compare and contrast active and passive immunity.

13. Explain how T and B lymphocytes develop.

14. Describe the role of antibodies in the immune system.

15. Compare and contrast cellular and humoral immunity.

16. Explain how hypersensitivity develops.

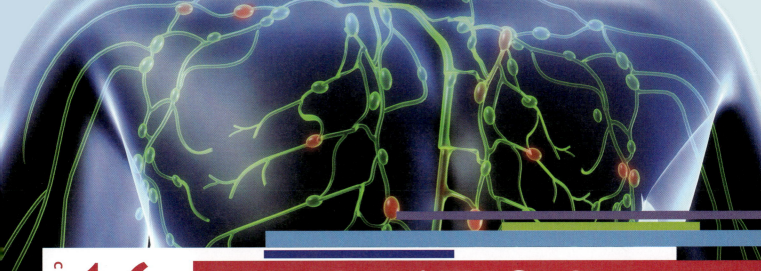

16 LYMPHATIC & IMMUNE SYSTEMS

One hundred trillion microorganisms live on or inside the human body.

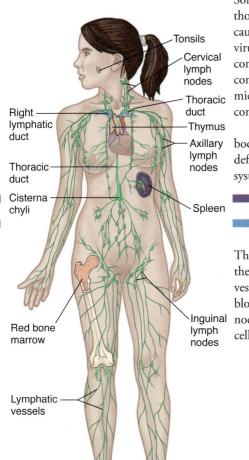

Tonsils

Cervical lymph nodes

Thoracic duct

Thymus

Axillary lymph nodes

Right lymphatic duct

Thoracic duct

Cisterna chyli

Spleen

Red bone marrow

Inguinal lymph nodes

Lymphatic vessels

Some of the millions of microorganisms living inside the body—such as those in the intestines—are necessary for health. Many others, however, can cause disease. If not for the immune system, the body would be overrun by viruses and bacteria. To illustrate the importance of the immune system, consider that when someone dies, the immune system stops working completely. Within hours, bacteria and parasites invade; within a few weeks, microorganisms can completely consume the body. Although morbid to consider, this illustrates the incredible effectiveness of the immune system.

The lymphatic and immune systems work hand-in-hand to protect the body. The immune system basically consists of a population of cells that defend the body against disease. Most of these cells exist within the lymphatic system—a network of organs and vessels that extend throughout the body.

Lymphatic System

The lymphatic system consists of lymphatic vessels, lymph (the fluid within the vessels), lymphatic tissue, and lymphatic organs. As shown here, the vessels of the lymphatic system cover the body in much the same way as blood vessels. The tissues and organs of the lymphatic system—the lymph nodes, thymus, tonsils, spleen, and red bone marrow—produce immune cells.

FAST FACT

Lymphatic vessels are found in almost every tissue, except for bone marrow, cartilage, and the central nervous system.

The Body AT WORK

The lymphatic system has three functions: the maintenance of fluid balance, the absorption of fat, and immunity.

- *Maintenance of fluid balance: Fluid continually seeps out of capillaries into surrounding tissues. The capillaries reabsorb about 85% of the fluid, leaving about 15% behind. This amount may seem minimal, but, over the course of a day, the remaining fluid would total as much as 4 liters, enough to cause massive swelling and even death. One of the roles of the lymphatic system is to absorb this fluid and return it to the bloodstream.*
- *Absorption of fats: Specialized lymphatic vessels in the small intestines absorb fats and fat-soluble vitamins.*
- *Immunity: The lymphatic system is a key component of the immune system. Lymph nodes and other lymphatic organs filter lymph (the fluid inside the lymphatic vessels) to remove microorganisms and foreign particles.*

FAST FACT
Unlike blood vessels, lymphatic vessels carry fluid in one direction only: away from the tissues.

Lymph

Lymphatic vessels are filled with lymph: a clear, colorless fluid similar to plasma but with a lower protein content. Lymph originates in the tissues as the fluid left behind following capillary exchange. Depending upon its location in the body, lymph may contain lipids (after draining the small intestines), lymphocytes (after leaving the lymph nodes), hormones, bacteria, viruses, and cellular debris.

Lymphatic Vessels

Similar to veins, lymphatic vessels—also called lymphatic capillaries—have thin walls and valves to prevent backflow. Lymphatic vessel walls are formed by a thin layer of epithelial cells. However, unlike the cells in veins (which are tightly joined), the cells forming lymphatic vessel walls overlap loosely, allowing gaps to exist between the cells.

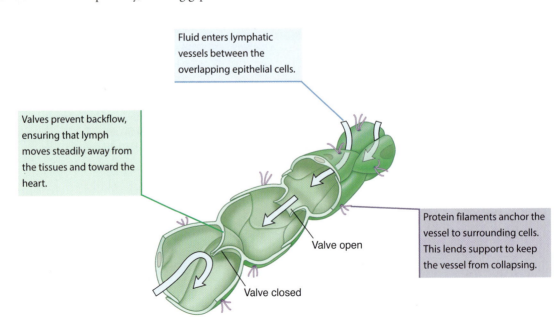

Fluid enters lymphatic vessels between the overlapping epithelial cells.

Valves prevent backflow, ensuring that lymph moves steadily away from the tissues and toward the heart.

Protein filaments anchor the vessel to surrounding cells. This lends support to keep the vessel from collapsing.

Valve open

Valve closed

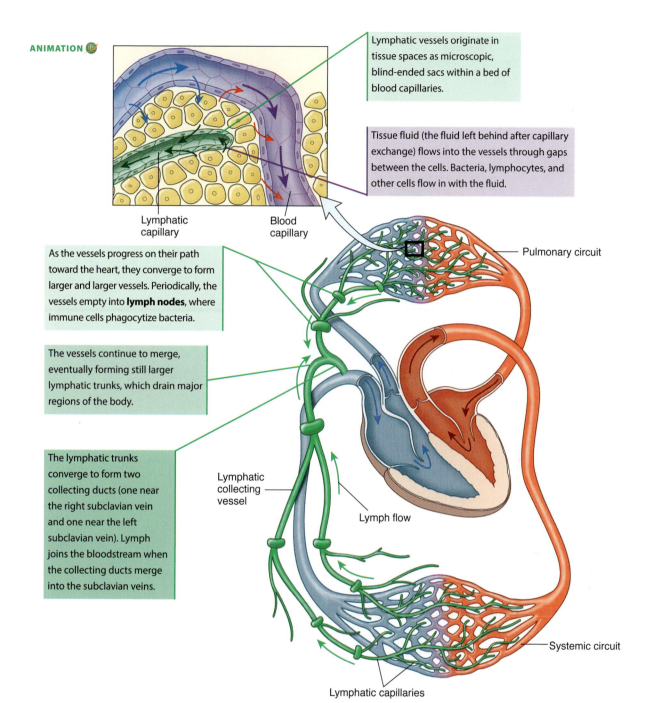

ANIMATION

Lymphatic vessels originate in tissue spaces as microscopic, blind-ended sacs within a bed of blood capillaries.

Tissue fluid (the fluid left behind after capillary exchange) flows into the vessels through gaps between the cells. Bacteria, lymphocytes, and other cells flow in with the fluid.

Lymphatic capillary

Blood capillary

As the vessels progress on their path toward the heart, they converge to form larger and larger vessels. Periodically, the vessels empty into **lymph nodes**, where immune cells phagocytize bacteria.

The vessels continue to merge, eventually forming still larger lymphatic trunks, which drain major regions of the body.

The lymphatic trunks converge to form two collecting ducts (one near the right subclavian vein and one near the left subclavian vein). Lymph joins the bloodstream when the collecting ducts merge into the subclavian veins.

Pulmonary circuit

Lymphatic collecting vessel

Lymph flow

Systemic circuit

Lymphatic capillaries

The Body AT WORK

In the cardiovascular system, the heart acts as a pump to help propel blood through the blood vessels. The lymphatic system, however, has no pump. Instead, the fluid moves passively, aided primarily by the rhythmic contractions of the lymphatic vessels themselves. The valves within the vessels prevent backflow. Flow is aided further by the contraction of skeletal muscles, which squeeze the lymphatic vessels. Finally, respiration causes pressure changes that help propel lymph from the abdominal to the thoracic cavity.

The Body AT WORK

The lymphatic system has two collecting ducts: the right lymphatic duct and the thoracic duct.

- *The **right lymphatic duct** drains lymph for the upper right quadrant of the body into the right subclavian vein.*
- *The **thoracic duct** (which originates at a dilated portion of a lymphatic vessel in the abdomen called the cisterna chyli) drains lymph from the rest of the body into the left subclavian vein.*

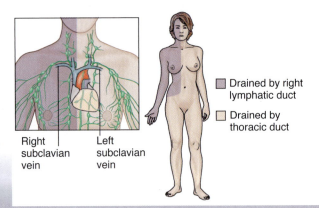

Right subclavian vein

Left subclavian vein

☐ Drained by right lymphatic duct

☐ Drained by thoracic duct

Lymphatic Tissues and Organs

Patches of specialized tissue containing lymphocytes exist throughout the body. Passages that open to the outside of the body (such as the respiratory, digestive, urinary, and reproductive tracts) contain a scattering of lymphocytes throughout their mucosa linings. In other parts of the body, lymphatic tissue exists in masses called **lymphatic nodules**. An example of this is *Peyer's patches*, lymphatic nodules residing in the small intestines.

Lymphatic organs, on the other hand, are well defined. These organs include red bone marrow, the thymus, lymph nodes, the tonsils, and the spleen. Red bone marrow and the thymus—called *primary lymphatic organs*—provide a location for B and T lymphocytes to mature. The lymph nodes, tonsils, and spleen—called *secondary lymphatic organs*—contain lymphocytes that have matured in either the red bone marrow or the thymus.

Thymus

Located in the mediastinum, the size of the thymus varies with age. Quite large in children, it begins to shrink about age 14. By adulthood, it is a fraction of its former size. The thymus also produces a hormone called *thymosin* that promote the development of lymphocytes.

The thymus is divided into lobules that extend inward from a fibrous outer capsule. Each lobule consists of a dense outer cortex and a less dense medulla filled with T lymphocytes.

ANIMATION 🌐

1. Immature T lymphocytes travel from the red bone marrow to the outer cortex of the thymus. Inside the thymus, the cells are protected from antigens in the blood, giving them a chance to divide and mature.

2. The developing T lymphocytes migrate toward the inner medulla. As they do, they encounter other lymphoid cells (such as macrophages and dendritic cells). This process "trains" the new lymphocytes to distinguish between the cells of its host body and foreign cells.

3. Once the training is complete, the lymphocytes are released into the bloodstream.

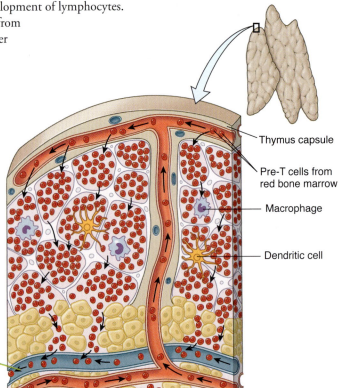

Thymus capsule

Pre-T cells from red bone marrow

Macrophage

Dendritic cell

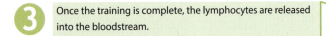

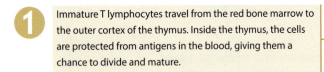

Lymph Nodes

As lymph flows along its course, it passes through multiple lymph nodes. When it reaches a node, the fluid slows to a trickle as the lymph node removes pathogens and other foreign material. Besides cleansing lymph, lymph nodes also serve as sites for final maturation of some types of lymphocytes and monocytes.

The body contains hundreds of lymph nodes. Shaped like a bean, some lymph nodes are tiny: only $^1/_{25}''$ (1 mm) long; others are over an inch (25 mm).

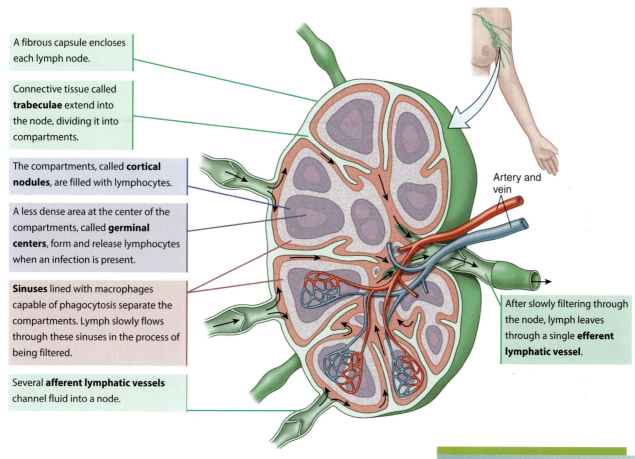

A fibrous capsule encloses each lymph node.

Connective tissue called **trabeculae** extend into the node, dividing it into compartments.

The compartments, called **cortical nodules**, are filled with lymphocytes.

A less dense area at the center of the compartments, called **germinal centers**, form and release lymphocytes when an infection is present.

Sinuses lined with macrophages capable of phagocytosis separate the compartments. Lymph slowly flows through these sinuses in the process of being filtered.

Several **afferent lymphatic vessels** channel fluid into a node.

Artery and vein

After slowly filtering through the node, lymph leaves through a single **efferent lymphatic vessel**.

FAST FACT
Lymph nodes remove 99% of the impurities in lymph before it returns the fluid to the bloodstream.

The Body AT WORK

Lymph nodes tend to occur in clusters in certain areas. The major lymph node groups are listed below.

- *Cervical lymph nodes, found in the neck, monitor lymph coming from the head and neck.*
- *Axillary lymph nodes, clustered in the armpit, receive lymph from the arm and breast.*
- *Inguinal lymph nodes occur in the groin; they receive lymph from the legs.*

Life lesson: Lymph nodes and cancer

Cancer often spreads (*metastasizes*) through the lymphatic system. When cancerous cells break free of the original tumor, they often enter the lymphatic vessels and travel to the nearest lymph node. (The first lymph node reached by metastasizing cancer cells is called the *sentinel lymph node*.) There, the cells multiply, eventually destroying the node. From that point, more cancerous cells may break off and travel to next node.

As an example, more than 85% of the lymph of the breast enters the axillary lymph nodes, making these nodes the most common route for breast cancer metastasis. That's why, during surgery to remove a cancerous breast tumor, the nearby axillary lymph nodes are typically also removed. Closely examining the nodes for cancerous cells following removal signals whether the cancer has spread and helps determine future treatment. Sometimes surgery disrupts normal lymph flow, causing lymph to accumulate in surrounding tissues. This produces swelling called *lymphedema*. Typically, new lymphatic vessels develop to reestablish normal flow.

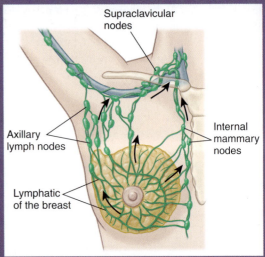

Supraclavicular nodes

Axillary lymph nodes

Internal mammary nodes

Lymphatic of the breast

Tonsils

Masses of lymphoid tissue, the tonsils form a protective circle at the back of the throat. They guard against pathogens entering the body through the nose or throat. There are three sets of tonsils:

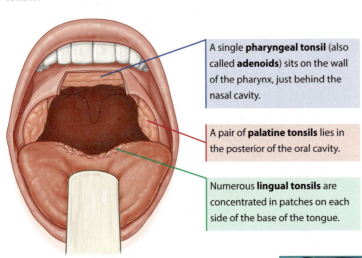

A single **pharyngeal tonsil** (also called **adenoids**) sits on the wall of the pharynx, just behind the nasal cavity.

A pair of **palatine tonsils** lies in the posterior of the oral cavity.

Numerous **lingual tonsils** are concentrated in patches on each side of the base of the tongue.

The Body AT WORK

The ring of tonsils at the back of the throat filters air flowing in through the nose and mouth. The white blood cells within the lymphoid tissue of the tonsils can then destroy any viruses or bacteria before they enter the body. Occasionally, the tonsils themselves—particularly the palatine tonsils—become infected by a virus or bacteria. When this happens, the tonsils swell and become inflamed, a condition known as tonsillitis. Symptoms of tonsillitis include a sore throat, painful swallowing, and fever. When caused by a virus, the condition usually resolves on its own after a few days. When it's caused by a bacteria (usually the streptococcal bacteria that causes strep throat), antibiotics are required. Surgical removal of the tonsils is recommended only when tonsillitis resists treatment or repeatedly recurs.

Spleen

About the size of a fist, the **spleen** is the body's largest lymphatic organ. It resides in the upper left quadrant of the abdomen, just inferior to the diaphragm, where it's protected by the lower ribs. Just like lymph nodes, the spleen is surrounded by a fibrous capsule; inward extensions of the capsule divide the spleen into compartments. The spleen contains two types of tissue: red pulp and white pulp.

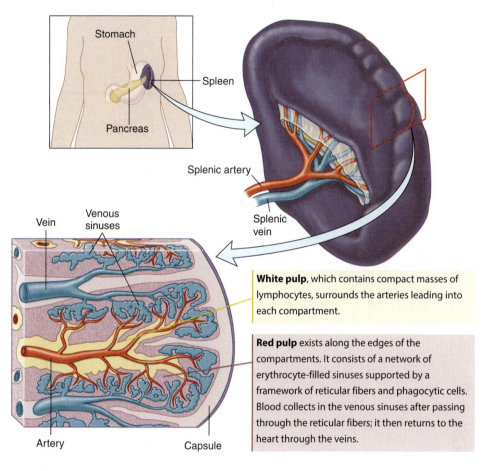

White pulp, which contains compact masses of lymphocytes, surrounds the arteries leading into each compartment.

Red pulp exists along the edges of the compartments. It consists of a network of erythrocyte-filled sinuses supported by a framework of reticular fibers and phagocytic cells. Blood collects in the venous sinuses after passing through the reticular fibers; it then returns to the heart through the veins.

The Body AT WORK

The spleen fulfills many functions in the body, including those described below.

- *Immunity: Lymphocytes and macrophages in the white pulp screen passing blood for foreign antigens while phagocytic cells in the sinuses ingest and destroy any microorganisms.*
- *Destruction of old red blood cells: Macrophages in the sinuses digest worn-out RBCs and imperfect platelets. Macrophages also recycle hemoglobin from the destroyed RBCs, salvaging the iron and globin and returning it to the bone marrow and liver for later use.*
- *Blood storage: The spleen stores 20% to 30% of the body's platelets. Consequently, it can help stabilize blood volume by rapidly adding blood back into general circulation.*
- *Hematopoiesis: The spleen produces red blood cells in the fetus. After birth, it does so only in cases of severe anemia. Throughout life, the spleen provides a location for monocytes and lymphocytes to mature.*

Life lesson: Splenic rupture

The spleen's location makes it vulnerable to injury from trauma. Because it is highly vascular, a severe injury or rupture can produce a fatal hemorrhage. The spleen is also difficult to repair, which is why it is usually removed surgically (called a *splenectomy*) when injured. A person can live without a spleen but may be more vulnerable to infection.

Overview of the Immune System

A person's survival depends on the body's ability to protect itself against the hordes of microorganisms—including viruses, bacteria, fungi, and protozoa—that constantly surround us. Other threats from which the body needs protection include toxic chemicals, radiation, and even allergens, like pollen. All the threats aren't external, however. Some arise from inside the body. For example, abnormal cells often develop as a part of daily life. Left unchecked, these cells will continue to grow and divide, resulting in a tumor or even cancer.

The body has three lines of defense for taking care of the threats it encounters on a daily basis.

First line of defense

External barriers, such as the skin and mucous membranes, keep most of the pathogens we encounter at bay.

Second line of defense

If a pathogen penetrates the first line of defense, the body launches several mechanisms geared at repelling a wide variety of threats, including the production of phagocytic white blood cells and triggering inflammation and fever. Because these responses are aimed at a broad range of attackers, rather than one specific pathogen, the response is called **nonspecific immunity**. Another term is *innate immunity* because the mechanisms are present from birth, allowing the body to repel pathogens to which it has never been exposed.

Third line of defense

The last line of defense is **specific immunity**. This occurs when the body retains a memory of a pathogen after defeating it. If exposed to the same pathogen in the future, the body can quickly recognize it, targeting a response at this one specific invader.

That Makes Sense

Remember that specific immunity is aimed at a specific *pathogen. For the immune system to recognize that pathogen, it must have been previously "introduced" (or exposed) to that pathogen. (The same thing goes for us: to recognize someone, you need to have been previously introduced.)*

Nonspecific Immunity

Nonspecific immunity protects against a broad range of pathogens, using a variety of mechanisms, such as external barriers, phagocytosis, antimicrobial proteins, natural killer cells, inflammation, and fever.

External Barriers

The skin and mucous membranes provide the first line of defense against microorganisms. The skin, composed of tough protein, repels most pathogens, while its surface, which is dry and lacking in nutrients, makes a hostile environment for bacteria. Further inhibiting bacterial growth is the *acid mantle*, a thin layer of acid produced by sweat.

The mucous membranes lining the digestive, respiratory, urinary, and reproductive tracts (which are open to the exterior) produce mucus that physically traps pathogens. In the respiratory tract, the mucus is then swallowed, and the pathogens are destroyed by stomach acid. Mucus, tears, and saliva also contain an enzyme called **lysozyme**, which destroys bacteria.

Phagocytosis

If a pathogen makes its way past the skin or mucous membranes and enters the body, it will immediately confront a key player in the second line of defense: phagocytes.

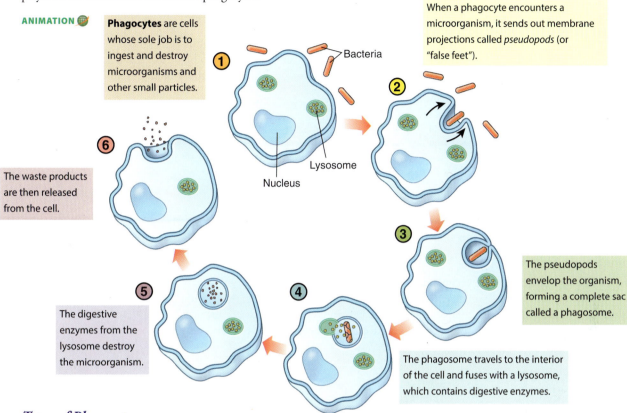

ANIMATION

Phagocytes are cells whose sole job is to ingest and destroy microorganisms and other small particles.

When a phagocyte encounters a microorganism, it sends out membrane projections called *pseudopods* (or "false feet").

Bacteria

Lysosome

Nucleus

The pseudopods envelop the organism, forming a complete sac called a phagosome.

The phagosome travels to the interior of the cell and fuses with a lysosome, which contains digestive enzymes.

The digestive enzymes from the lysosome destroy the microorganism.

The waste products are then released from the cell.

Types of Phagocytes

The most important phagocytes are **neutrophils** and **macrophages**. While neutrophils roam the body, seeking out bacteria, most macrophages remain fixed within strategic areas.

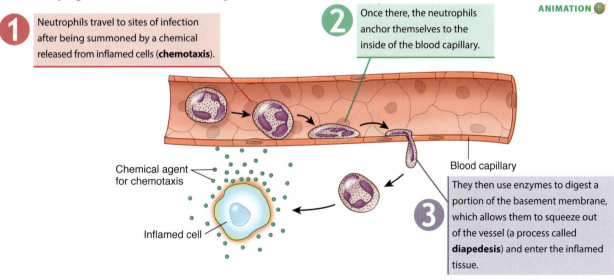

1 Neutrophils travel to sites of infection after being summoned by a chemical released from inflamed cells (**chemotaxis**).

2 Once there, the neutrophils anchor themselves to the inside of the blood capillary.

ANIMATION

Chemical agent for chemotaxis

Inflamed cell

Blood capillary

3 They then use enzymes to digest a portion of the basement membrane, which allows them to squeeze out of the vessel (a process called **diapedesis**) and enter the inflamed tissue.

Macrophages evolve from monocytes (another type of phagocytic WBC). Monocytes migrate into connective tissues, where they grow several times larger than their original size and transform into macrophages. (The name *macrophage* actually means "large eater.") Macrophages congregate in areas where microbial invasion is likely to occur: the alveolus of the lungs, the liver, nerve tissue, bone, and the spleen.

Antimicrobial Proteins

Two types of proteins help provide nonspecific resistance against bacterial and viral invasion: interferons and the complement system.

Interferons

Some cells respond to viral invasion by producing a protein called **interferon**. When a virus infects a cell, the cell produces interferon, which it releases to nearby cells. The interferon binds to surface receptors on neighboring cells. This triggers the production of enzymes within the cells that would prevent the virus from replicating if it managed to invade.

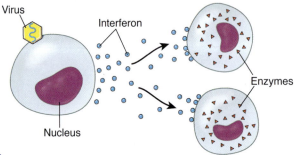

Complement System

Over 20 different proteins (called **complement**) circulate in the bloodstream in an inactive form, waiting to assist in the immune response. A bacteria, or antibodies against the bacteria, activate the complement. Once a complement reaction begins, it continues as a cascade of chemical reactions, with one complement protein activating the next (similar to what occurs in blood clotting).

ANIMATION

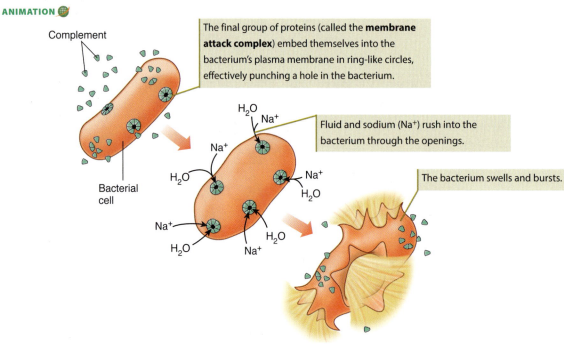

The final group of proteins (called the **membrane attack complex**) embed themselves into the bacterium's plasma membrane in ring-like circles, effectively punching a hole in the bacterium.

Fluid and sodium (Na^+) rush into the bacterium through the openings.

The bacterium swells and bursts.

Complement also aids the immune system by coating pathogens, making them attractive to phagocytes, and stimulating inflammation (which summons neutrophils through chemotaxis).

Natural Killer Cells

A unique group of lymphocytes called **natural killer (NK) cells** continually roam the body, seeking out pathogens or diseased cells. They recognize and destroy any foreign cells, including cancer cells, virus-infected cells, and bacteria—as well as the cells of transplanted organs and tissues. The NK cells use several methods to destroy the cells. Most of them involve the secretion of chemicals that causes the cell to die and break apart (*lysis*).

Inflammation

Tissue injury, whether from trauma, ischemia, or infection, produces inflammation. Inflammation stimulates the body's defense system to begin fighting the infection while instigating measures to contain the pathogen. Furthermore, the inflammatory response includes processes that clean up and repair the damaged tissue.

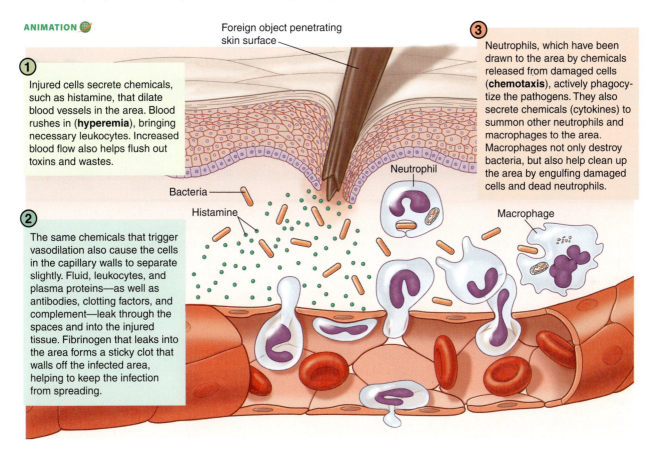

ANIMATION 🌐

Foreign object penetrating skin surface

① Injured cells secrete chemicals, such as histamine, that dilate blood vessels in the area. Blood rushes in (**hyperemia**), bringing necessary leukocytes. Increased blood flow also helps flush out toxins and wastes.

② The same chemicals that trigger vasodilation also cause the cells in the capillary walls to separate slightly. Fluid, leukocytes, and plasma proteins—as well as antibodies, clotting factors, and complement—leak through the spaces and into the injured tissue. Fibrinogen that leaks into the area forms a sticky clot that walls off the infected area, helping to keep the infection from spreading.

③ Neutrophils, which have been drawn to the area by chemicals released from damaged cells (**chemotaxis**), actively phagocytize the pathogens. They also secrete chemicals (cytokines) to summon other neutrophils and macrophages to the area. Macrophages not only destroy bacteria, but also help clean up the area by engulfing damaged cells and dead neutrophils.

Bacteria

Histamine

Neutrophil

Macrophage

Most of the phagocytes (especially the neutrophils) die during the process of fighting the infection. The dead cells pile up, along with tissue debris and fluid, to create a thick yellowish fluid called **pus**. When pus accumulates in a tissue cavity, it's called an **abscess**.

The Body AT WORK

Redness, swelling, heat, and pain are the four classic signs of inflammation.

- *Swelling results from fluid leaking out of the capillaries.*
- *Redness results from hyperemia.*
- *Heat also results from hyperemia.*
- *Pain may result from injured nerves, pressure on the nerves from swelling, or stimulation of nerves by bacterial toxins.*

The signs of inflammation also facilitate healing.

- *Swelling compresses veins—reducing venous drainage—while forcing the capillary valves open to promote capillary drainage. This helps healing because lymphatic capillaries are more adept at removing bacteria, dead cells, and tissue debris than are blood capillaries.*
- *Hyperemia brings materials necessary for healing, including oxygen and amino acids.*
- *Heat in the area increases the metabolic rate, and thus, the rate of tissue repair.*
- *Pain signals that an injury has occurred and serves as a reminder to rest the area to allow healing.*

Fever

Also known as **pyrexia**, fever is an abnormal elevation of body temperature. (A person with a fever is said to be **febrile**.) Experts now believe that fever is beneficial during an illness. Besides promoting the activity of interferon, an elevated body temperature inhibits the reproduction of bacteria and viruses. Following is the normal sequence of events during a fever:

1. As neutrophils and macrophages phagocytize bacteria, they secrete a fever-producing substance called a **pyrogen**. The pyrogen stimulates the anterior hypothalamus to secrete prostaglandin E (PGE).
2. PGE resets the body's set point for temperature. For example, it may raise it from a normal of 98.6° F (37° C) to 102° F (39° C).
3. When the set point rises, the body needs to generate heat, which it does through shivering and constricting blood vessels in the skin. The result: chills and cold, clammy skin.
4. The temperature rises until it reaches its new set point, where it remains as long as the pathogen is present.
5. When the pathogen is no longer a threat, the phagocytes stop producing the pyrogen and the body's set point for temperature returns to normal. When this happens, the body needs to lose the excess heat, which it does through sweating and dilating blood vessels in the skin. The result: warm and flushed skin.

Even though most fevers are beneficial, excessively high temperatures are dangerous. Temperatures above 105° F (40.5° C) can cause convulsions; those above 111° F to 115° F (44° C to 46° C) typically result in irreversible brain damage or death.

The Body AT WORK

A body temperature of 98.6° F (37° C) is commonly considered to be normal. However, body temperature varies during the course of a day, with different activity levels, and even from person to person. A temperature deemed normal in one person may represent a fever in another.

Temperature also varies according to the part of the body being tested: measurements taken inside a body cavity, such as orally or rectally, are higher than those measured on the skin. Specifically, a temperature taken rectally is usually 1° F (0.6° C) higher than an oral reading, whereas a reading taken under the arm (axillary) is 1° F (0.6° C) lower than an oral reading.

Specific Immunity

In contrast to nonspecific immunity, specific immunity is directed against a specific pathogen. After being exposed to a pathogen, the immune system retains a memory of the encounter. If that particular pathogen enters the body in the future, the immune system will recognize it immediately, allowing it to destroy the pathogen before symptoms even develop.

For this third line of defense, the body employs two mechanisms. One aims to destroy foreign cells or host cells that have become infected with a pathogen. This is called **cellular (cell-mediated) immunity**. The other mechanism, which focuses on pathogens outside the host cells, sends out antibodies to "mark" a pathogen for later destruction. This is called **humoral (antibody-mediated) immunity**.

Understanding these two forms of immunity requires an understanding of their weapons: lymphocytes and antibodies.

FAST FACT

Humoral immunity is so named because antibodies exist in body fluids, and body fluids were once called humors.

The Body AT WORK

The body routinely makes its own antibodies or T cells against a pathogen; this is called **active immunity**. It's also possible to achieve immunity after receiving an injection of antibodies from another person or an animal; this is called **passive immunity**. Active immunity is permanent, or at least long lasting. In passive immunity, the body doesn't develop a memory for the pathogen, so the immunity lasts only a few months.

Following are the four classes of immunity:

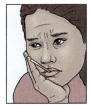

Natural active immunity: This type of immunity occurs when the body produces antibodies or T cells after being exposed to a particular antigen. (For example, if you become ill with the measles, your body will produce antibodies to this particular virus, making you immune to infection in the future.)

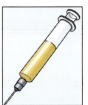

Artificial active immunity: This results when the body makes T cells and antibodies against a disease as a result of a vaccination (such as for tetanus or influenza). By injecting a vaccine containing dead or weakened (attenuated) pathogens, the recipient's body produces an immune response without actually developing the illness.

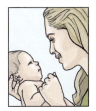

Natural passive immunity: This form of immunity results when a fetus acquires antibodies from the mother through the placenta, or when a baby acquires them through breastfeeding.

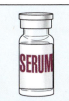

Artificial passive immunity: This form of immunity involves obtaining serum from a person or animal that has produced antibodies against a certain pathogen and then injecting it into someone else. This is typically used in emergencies for the treatment of rabies and botulism.

Lymphocytes

The immune system relies on lymphocytes to wage war against invading pathogens. Lymphocytes fall into one of three classes: natural killer cells (which have already been discussed), T lymphocytes, and B lymphocytes.

T Lymphocytes

Commonly called **T cells**, T lymphocytes develop from stem cells in red bone marrow.

Before the T cells have fully matured, they leave the bone marrow and travel to the thymus gland, where they remain until fully functional.

Once the T cells are *immunocompetent*—that is, capable of recognizing antigens—they leave the thymus and migrate to lymphatic organs and tissues throughout the body (such as the lymph nodes, spleen, and tonsils).

B Lymphocytes

Commonly called **B cells**, B lymphocytes also begin life as stem cells in red bone marrow. Unlike T cells, B cells remain in bone marrow until they are fully mature.

Once mature, *B* cells leave the bone marrow for lymphatic organs and tissues, particularly the lymph nodes, spleen, bone marrow, and mucous membranes.

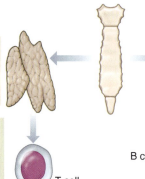

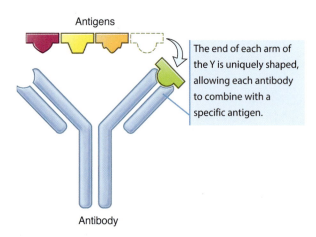

T cell

B cell

Lymph node

Tonsils

Spleen

That Makes Sense

To differentiate between T cells and B cells, remember that T cells mature in the Thymus while B cells mature in the Bone marrow.

Antibodies

Key players in the body's immune system, antibodies are gamma globulin proteins formed by B cells and found in plasma and body secretions. Also known as **immunoglobulins (Ig)**, antibodies consist of chains of protein joined in a way that resembles a capital letter Y or T.

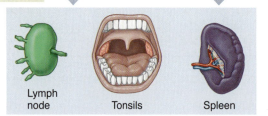

Antigens

The end of each arm of the Y is uniquely shaped, allowing each antibody to combine with a specific antigen.

Antibody

An **antigen** is any molecule that triggers an immune response. Any foreign substance is said to be antigenic. The immune system learns to distinguish between "self" and "non-self" cells before birth so that it attacks only those substances that aren't part of the body.

The Body AT WORK

The body manufactures five classes of antibodies: IgA, IgD, IgE, IgG, and IgM.

- *IgA: Populates mucous membranes in the intestines, respiratory tract, and urinary tract; also found in saliva, tears, and breast milk*
- *IgD: Exists in the blood in very small amounts; may activate basophils and mast cells*
- *IgE: Involved in allergic reactions*
- *IgG: Is the primary antibody of the secondary immune response; also the most abundant of all the immunoglobulins, making up 80% of all circulating antibodies*
- *IgM: Active in the primary immune response; also involved in agglutination of incompatible blood types*

Cellular Immunity

Cellular immunity destroys pathogens that exist within a cell. To accomplish this, it employs three classes of T cells:

- **Cytotoxic T cells** (also called killer T cells—not to be confused with natural killer cells), which carry out the attack
- **Helper T cells**, which play a supportive role
- **Memory T cells**, which remember the pathogen in case of future invasion

ANIMATION 🌐

1 The immune process begins when a phagocyte (such as a macrophage, reticular cell, or B cell) ingests an antigen.

2 The phagocyte, called an **antigen-presenting cell (APC)**, displays fragments of the antigen on its surface—a process called **antigen presentation**—which alerts the immune system to the presence of a foreign antigen. When a T cell spots the foreign antigen, it binds to it.

3 This activates (or sensitizes) the T cell, which begins dividing repeatedly to form clones: identical T cells already sensitized to the antigen. Some of these T cells become effector cells (such as cytotoxic T cells and helper T cells), which will carry out the attack, while others become memory T cells.

4 The cytotoxic T cell binds to the surface of the antigen and delivers a toxic dose of chemicals that will kill it.

5 Helper T cells support the attack by secreting the chemical **interleukin**, which attracts neutrophils, natural killer cells, and macrophages. It also stimulates the production of T and B cells.

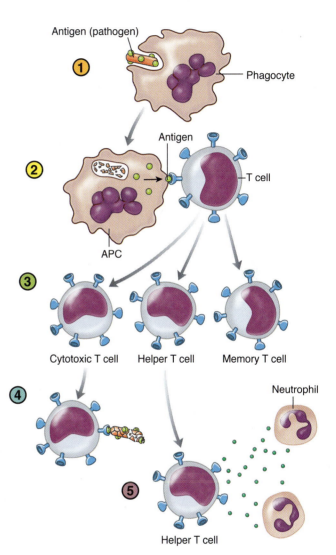

Following the attack, some of the cytotoxic T cells and helper T cells become memory T cells. These numerous, long-lived cells retain a memory of this particular pathogen. If re-exposure to the same antigen occurs, these cells can launch a quick attack.

FAST FACT

IgG is the only antibody that can cross the placenta to impart temporary immunity to the fetus.

FAST FACT

Because the cellular immune system is programmed to attack any cell not identified with the "self," it also attacks and tries to destroy transplanted organs and tissues.

Humoral Immunity

Humoral immunity differs from cellular immunity in that it focuses on pathogens outside the cell. Also, instead of destroying the antigen directly, it uses antibodies to mark them for later destruction.

ANIMATION 🌐

 1 The surface of a B cell contains thousands of receptors for a specific antigen. When the antigen specific to that receptor comes along, it binds to the B cell.

 2 The B cell then engulfs the antigen, digests it, and displays some of the antigen's fragments on its surface. A helper T cell binds to the presented antigen and secretes interleukins, which activate the B cell.

 3 The B cell begins to rapidly reproduce, creating a clone, or family, of identical B cells that are programmed against the same antigen.

 4 Some of these cloned B cells become effector B cells or memory B cells; most, though, become plasma cells.

5 The plasma cells secrete large numbers of antibodies. Antibodies stop the antigens through a number of different means. (See "The Body at Work" on this page.)

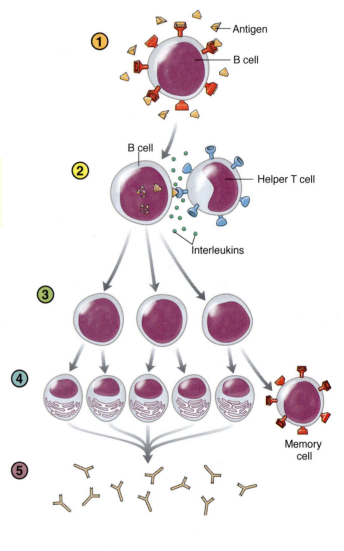

The Body AT WORK

Antibodies use a range of tactics to defeat antigens, including:

- *Binding to the antigen's attachment points, preventing it from attaching to a human cell*
- *Triggering agglutination (as in the antigen-antibody reaction), thus helping to contain the antigen and also make it easier for phagocytes to do their work*
- *Promoting the binding of complement proteins to the invading cell, thus setting off the complement cascade, which ends with the destruction of the invading microorganism*

FAST FACT

A single plasma cell secretes 2000 antibody molecules a second during the few days that it lives.

The Body AT WORK

*When the body is exposed to a particular antigen for the first time, the immune system must complete a number of different tasks before it can attack the invading antigens. For example, it must create B cells that, in turn, must differentiate into plasma cells. Once that is completed, the plasma cells can begin producing antibodies. This initial reaction is called the **primary response**. The amount of time between exposure to a new antigen and a rising level of blood antibodies against that antigen (called the **antibody titer**) ranges from three to six days.*

*Once the attack is over and the antigen has been removed from the body, memory B cells remain. Even though the number of antibodies decline, if the same antigen should invade again, the memory B cells can immediately begin to divide. This allows for rapid production of memory and plasma cells, which can then create large numbers of antibodies against the antigen. This response, called the **secondary response**, takes only hours as opposed to days. Consequently, the body can attack the antigen before it has time to produce symptoms.*

FAST FACT

The human immune system can produce billions of different antibodies, each of which responds to a different antigen.

Immune System Disorders

Maintaining immunity requires a series of complex interactions between cells. Disorders occur when the immune system overreacts to an antigen (hypersensitivity) or, the opposite, fails to react (as occurs in immunodeficiency disorders). At times, the immune system directs its actions at its own tissues, producing an autoimmune disease.

Hypersensitivity

Hypersensitivity involves an inappropriate or excessive response of the immune system. The most common type of hypersensitivity is called an **allergy**, a condition in which the immune system reacts to environmental substances (called **allergens**) that most people can tolerate. Common allergens include mold, dust, pollen, animal dander, and foods such as chocolate, shellfish, nuts, or milk. Certain drugs, particularly penicillin, tetracycline, or sulfa, can also trigger an allergic response in some individuals. Allergic responses may occur within seconds, or they may be delayed for several days.

Immediate Allergic Reactions

Immediate allergic reactions include common allergies, such as those to pollen or bee stings.

ANIMATION

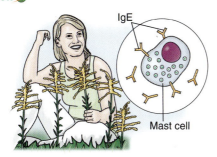
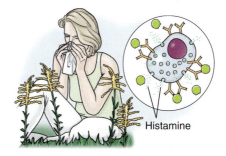

When someone with a genetic predisposition to an allergy (such as ragweed) is first exposed to the allergen, the body responds by producing large amounts of the antibody IgE specific to ragweed. These antibodies bind to mast cells. (Mast cells reside in the skin, lungs and upper airways, and the lining of the stomach.) While this response doesn't produce an allergic reaction, the person is now *sensitized* to ragweed. (More than one exposure may be necessary before someone is sensitized to an allergen.)

When the person encounters ragweed at a later date, the allergen binds to the antibodies already in the body. If the allergen links two or more antibodies, the mast cells release histamine and other inflammatory chemicals. Histamine causes inflammatory responses that produce the symptoms of an allergy, such as runny nose, watery eyes, congestion, and hives.

The Body AT WORK

A severe, immediate allergic reaction that affects the whole body is called **anaphylaxis**. *The release of huge amounts of histamine causes constriction of the airways—making breathing difficult—and vasodilation—causing blood pressure to drop. Other possible symptoms include a red, itchy, raised rash and swelling of the face, lips, and tongue.*

*   **Anaphylactic shock** occurs when symptoms worsen to the point that circulatory shock and even sudden death may occur. Mild anaphylaxis can often be relieved with antihistamines. Anaphylactic shock, however, is a medical emergency, requiring emergency treatment with epinephrine. Allergens often linked to anaphylaxis include foods such as peanuts or shellfish, medicines such a penicillin, and bee venom.*

FAST FACT

One in six Americans is genetically predisposed to some type of an allergy.

Delayed Allergic Reaction

Unlike immediate allergic reactions, which involve an antigen-antibody reaction, delayed allergic reactions involve cell-mediated immunity. A common example of a delayed allergic response is contact dermatitis following exposure to poison ivy or soaps. In this situation, T cells trigger a mixture of nonspecific and immune responses that result in local skin inflammation 12 to 72 hours after exposure.

Autoimmune Diseases

Sometimes the body's immune system fails to differentiate between self-antigens—the molecules native to a person's body—and foreign antigens. When this occurs, the body produces antibodies that attack its own tissues. The process may begin when antibodies produced in response to an infection react not only to the bacteria but also to self-antigens. For example, in rheumatic fever, the antibodies against a streptococcal infection react to the bacteria as well as to the heart's myocardium, causing scarring of the mitral and aortic valves. In other instances, a virus may change the structure of a self-antigen (such as those of the insulin-producing pancreatic islets), causing the immune system to attack those cells as foreign invaders. Some experts believe that this is the underlying cause of type 1 diabetes mellitus. In most cases, though, an exact cause cannot be identified. Inheritance seems to play a role, however, because autoimmune diseases tend to run in families.

There are more than 80 types of autoimmune diseases. These include systemic lupus erythematosus (which affects multiple organs, including the kidneys, skin, heart, and joints), scleroderma (which affects the skin, intestines, and lungs), Graves' disease (which affects the thyroid gland), and ulcerative colitis (which affects the gastrointestinal tract).

Immunodeficiency Diseases

In immunodeficiency diseases, the immune system fails to adequately protect the body against pathogens. Rarely, the deficiency may be present at birth, such as in **severe combined immunodeficiency disease (SCID)**, in which children have few or no T and B cells. As a result, their bodies can't fight off pathogens, forcing them to live in a protective environment.

More common is **acquired immunodeficiency syndrome (AIDS)**, which results from infection with the **human immunodeficiency virus (HIV)**. The virus invades helper T cells (also called CD4 cells), eventually destroying them. Because helper T cells are a key player in both humoral and cellular immunity, their loss places the host at risk for infections and cancers that a healthy immune system easily rebuffs. For example, a protozoal infection called *Pneumocystis carinii pneumonia* and a type of skin cancer called *Kaposi sarcoma* rarely occur in healthy people but occur frequently in persons with AIDS.

Review of Key Terms

Active immunity: Immunity that results when the body manufactures its own antibodies or T cells against a pathogen

Allergen: Environmental substance that triggers an allergic response

Anaphylaxis: Severe, immediate hypersensitivity reaction affecting the entire body

Antibody: Substance produced by B lymphocytes in response to a specific antigen

Antigen: Any molecule that triggers an immune response

Cellular immunity: Immune response that targets foreign cells or host cells that have become infected with a pathogen

Chemotaxis: The movement of white blood cells to an area of inflammation in response to the release of chemicals from the injured cells

Complement: A group of proteins in the blood that, through a cascade of chemical reactions, participate in nonspecific immunity

Diapedesis: Process in which neutrophils enzymatically digest a portion of the capillary basement membrane, allowing them to leave the vessel and enter inflamed tissue

Histamine: Substance secreted by injured or irritated cells that produces local vasodilation, among other effects

Humoral immunity: Immune response that uses antibodies to target pathogens outside the host cells

Hyperemia: Increased blood flow to an area

Immunoglobulins: Antibodies

Inflammation: An immunological response to injury, infection, or allergy, marked by increases in regional blood flow, immigration of white blood cells, and release of chemical toxins

Interferon: Protein released from virus-infected cells that helps protect nearby cells from invasion

Lymph: Clear, colorless fluid filling lymphatic capillaries

Lymph nodes: Kidney-shaped masses of lymphatic tissue that lie along lymphatic vessels

Macrophage: Important phagocyte that remains fixed in strategic areas

Natural killer cells: Unique group of lymphocytes that continually roam the body seeking out pathogens or diseased cells

Neutrophils: Phagocytes that accumulate rapidly at sites of acute injury

Nonspecific immunity: First and second lines of defense; immune response aimed at a broad range of pathogens

Passive immunity: Immunity that results when someone receives antibodies from another person or animal

Phagocytosis: Process by which phagocytes engulf and destroy microorganisms

Pyrexia: Fever

Specific immunity: The third line of defense; immune response targeted at a specific pathogen

Spleen: The body's largest lymphatic organ; contains masses of lymphocytes

T lymphocytes: Lymphocytes that participate in both cellular and humoral immunity; also called T cells

Thymus gland: Lymphoid organ where T cells mature; located in the mediastinal cavity

Tonsils: Masses of lymphoid tissue that form a protective circle at the back of the throat

Own the Information

To make the information in this chapter part of your working memory, take some time to reflect on what you've learned. On a separate sheet of paper, write down everything you recall from the chapter. After you're done, log on to the Davis*Plus* website, and check out the Study Group podcast and Study Group Questions for the chapter.

Key Topics for Chapter 16:
- Functions of the lymphatic system
- The formation and flow of lymph
- Structure of lymphatic vessels
- Location, structure, and function of the thymus, lymph nodes, tonsils, and spleen
- The body's three lines of defense against infection

- Types of nonspecific immunity
- The process of phagocytosis
- The role of interferons and the complement system in fighting infection
- The process and role of inflammation
- The process and role of fever
- Classes of specific immunity
- The formation of T and B lymphocytes
- The role of antibodies and antigens
- The process of cellular immunity
- The process of humoral immunity
- The development of hypersensitivity
- Autoimmune and immunodeficiency diseases

Test Your Knowledge

Answers: Chapter 16

1. *Correct answer:* **b.** The lymphatic system has three functions: immunity, the absorption of fats, and maintenance of fluid balance. It does not contribute to electrolyte balance.

2. *Correct answer:* **a.** None of the other answers is correct.

3. *Correct answer:* **d.** T cells evolve from stem cells in red bone marrow, but they leave the bone marrow before maturity. Both tonsils and the spleen are lymphatic organs; however, they play no role in T-cell maturity.

4. *Correct answer:* **c.** Lymph nodes filter lymphatic fluid, not plasma. Lymph nodes have no role in the production of lymphatic fluid. Antibodies are produced by B lymphocytes.

5. *Correct answer:* **c.** Macrophages are important white blood cells that remain fixed in strategic areas. Phagocytes are a group of white blood cells that ingest and destroy microorganisms; both macrophages and neutrophils are phagocytes. A phagosome is the sac formed around a microorganism when it's ingested by a phagocyte.

6. *Correct answer:* **b.** Natural active immunity results following an illness, in which the body produces antibodies or T cells against that particular pathogen. Natural passive immunity results when a fetus acquires antibodies from the mother across the placenta or through breastfeeding. Artificial passive immunity results following an injection of antibodies to a specific pathogen.

1. What are the key functions of the lymphatic system?
   a. Immunity and electrolyte balance
   b. Immunity, absorption of fats, and the maintenance of fluid balance
   c. Immunity only
   d. Maintenance of fluid balance only

2. What forms the basis of lymphatic fluid?
   a. Tissue fluid left behind following capillary exchange
   b. Secretions of lymph nodes
   c. Secretions from the cells lining lymphatic capillaries
   d. Plasma

3. In which lymphatic organ do T cells mature?
   a. Red bone marrow
   b. Tonsils
   c. Spleen
   d. Thymus

4. Which statement most correctly describes the main function of lymph nodes?
   a. The filtration of blood plasma to remove excess white blood cells
   b. The production of lymphatic fluid
   c. The removal of pathogens and foreign material from lymphatic fluid
   d. The production of antibodies

5. Which important white blood cells travel throughout the bloodstream seeking out bacteria?
   a. Macrophages
   b. Phagocytes
   c. Neutrophils
   d. Phagosomes.

6. A tetanus shot creates what type of immunity?
   a. Natural active immunity
   b. Artificial active immunity
   c. Natural passive immunity
   d. Artificial passive immunity

7. *Correct answer:* **d.** Lymphocytes and monocytes in the white pulp screen passing blood for foreign antigens while phagocytic cells in the sinuses ingest and destroy microorganisms. It does not produce immunoglobulins, B and T cells, or interferon.

8. *Correct answer:* **b.** An allergen is an environmental substance capable of triggering an allergic reaction in susceptible individuals. An antibody is an immunoglobulin that protects the body against certain antigens. A macrophage is a phagocytic white blood cell.

9. *Correct answer:* **a.** Humoral immunity focuses on pathogens outside of the cell. Passive immunity occurs when someone receives antibodies against a specific antigen from another person or an animal. Nonspecific immunity uses mechanisms such as external barriers, phagocytosis, antimicrobial proteins, natural killer cells, inflammation, and fever to protect against a broad range of pathogens.

10. *Correct answer:* **a.** Complement is an antimicrobial protein that attacks bacteria. Interferon is also an antimicrobial protein that is secreted by an infected cell to help protect neighboring cells. Lysozyme is a bacteria-destroying enzyme found in mucus, tears, and saliva.

7. How does the spleen contribute to immunity?
   a. It produces immunoglobulins
   b. It produces B and T lymphocytes
   c. It produces interferon
   d. It screens passing blood for foreign antigens

8. A substance capable of causing disease is called:
   a. an allergen.
   b. an antigen.
   c. an antibody.
   d. a macrophage.

9. Which type of immunity uses T cells to destroy pathogens within a cell?
   a. Cellular immunity
   b. Humoral immunity
   c. Passive immunity
   d. Nonspecific immunity

10. Humoral immunity triggers the production of _____ to fight pathogens.
    a. antibodies
    b. complement
    c. interferon
    d. lysozyme

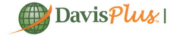

Go to **http://davisplus.fadavis.com** Keyword: Thompson to see all of the resources available with this chapter.

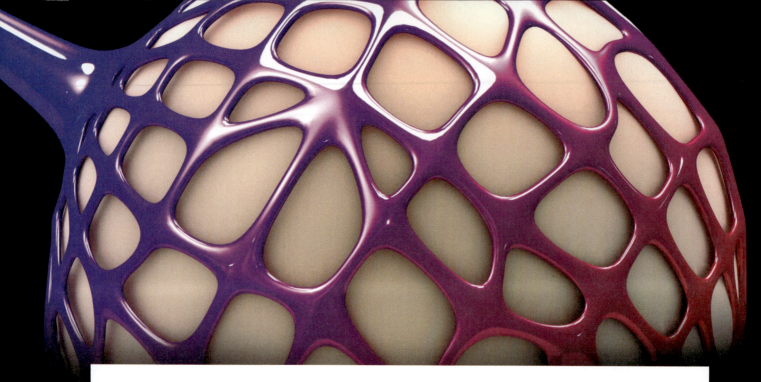

CHAPTER OUTLINE

Upper Respiratory Tract

Lower Respiratory Tract

Pulmonary Ventilation

LEARNING OUTCOMES

1. List the roles of the respiratory system.

2. Name and describe the functions of the organs of the respiratory system.

3. Trace the flow of air from the nostrils to the alveoli.

4. Name the muscles used for breathing and state their role in inspiration and expiration.

5. Identify the respiratory centers in the medulla and explain how they control breathing.

6. Identify the various factors that alter the rate and depth of breathing.

7. Describe how pressure gradients affect the flow of air into and out of the lungs.

8. Discuss how pulmonary compliance and alveolar surface tension affect airflow.

9. List and describe the measurements of ventilation.

10. Explain the process of gas exchange along the circulatory route.

11. Describe the transport of oxygen and carbon dioxide.

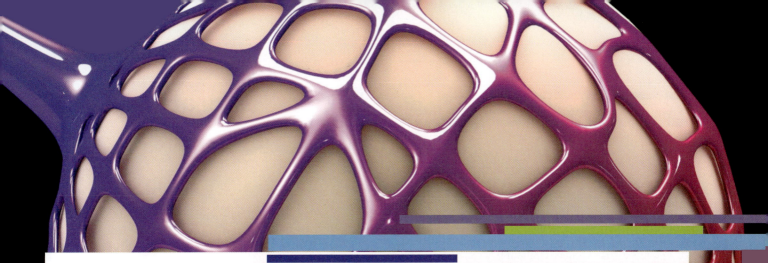

17

RESPIRATORY SYSTEM

During a 24-hour period, the average person will breathe 23,040 times.

Oxygen plays a powerful role in overall health and well-being. Most metabolic processes of the body—including the digestion of food, the fighting of infection and disease, and the production of energy—depend on oxygen. Your ability to think, feel, and act depend upon the availability of oxygen.

The respiratory and cardiovascular systems work closely together to provide the body with oxygen and to remove carbon dioxide. The respiratory system assumes other roles as well: it influences sound production and speech; it makes the sense of smell (and therefore taste) possible; and, as will be discussed in Chapter 19, it helps the body maintain homeostasis through the regulation of acid-base balance. The respiratory system is divided into two tracts:

FAST FACT
You can live about 40 days without food, about 7 days without water, but only minutes without oxygen.

The **upper respiratory tract** consists of structures located outside the thoracic cavity.

The **lower respiratory tract** consists of structures located inside the thoracic cavity.

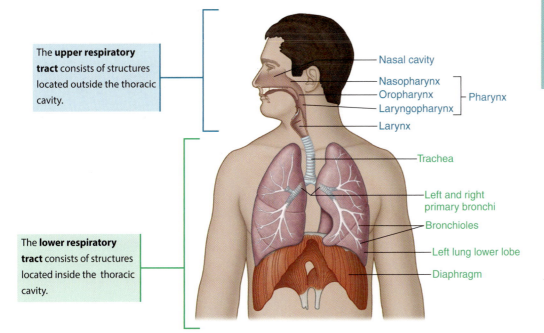

- Nasal cavity
- Nasopharynx
- Oropharynx — Pharynx
- Laryngopharynx
- Larynx
- Trachea
- Left and right primary bronchi
- Bronchioles
- Left lung lower lobe
- Diaphragm

Upper Respiratory Tract

Functionally, the respiratory system also includes the:

- Oral cavity
- Rib cage
- Respiratory muscles (including the diaphragm)

The structures of the **upper respiratory tract**—consisting of the nose, nasopharynx, oropharynx, laryngopharynx, and larynx—warm and humidify inspired air. They're also responsible for the senses of smell and taste as well as chewing and swallowing food.

Nose and Nasal Cavities

Air enters and leaves the respiratory system through the nose. Just inside the nostrils are small hairs called **cilia** that filter out dust and large foreign particles.

The nasal cavity lies just over the mouth, separated from that orifice by a bony structure called the **palate**. A vertical plate of bone and cartilage—called the **septum**—separates the cavity into two halves. The cavity is lined with epithelium rich in goblet cells that produce mucus.

> **FAST FACT**
> Spontaneous nosebleeds (that result without trauma or irritation) can be an early sign of hypertension.

Projecting from the lateral wall of each cavity are three bones called **conchae**. These bones create narrow passages, ensuring that most air contacts the mucous membrane on the way through. As it does, the air picks up moisture and heat from the mucosa. At the same time, dust sticks to the mucus, which is then swallowed.

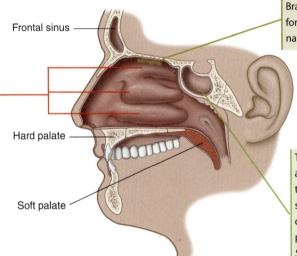

Frontal sinus

Hard palate

Soft palate

Branches of the olfactory nerve (responsible for the sense of smell) penetrate the upper nasal cavity and lead to the brain.

The sphenoid sinus (shown here), as well as the other paranasal sinuses (including the frontal, maxillary, and ethmoidal sinuses), drain mucus into the nasal cavity. (For further discussion of the paranasal sinuses, see Chapter 7, *Skeletal System*).

Pharynx

Just behind the nasal and oral cavities is a muscular tube called the **pharynx**. Commonly called the throat, the pharynx can be divided into three regions:

> **The Body AT WORK**
> *Only air passes through the nasopharynx, while both food and air pass through the oropharynx and laryngopharynx.*

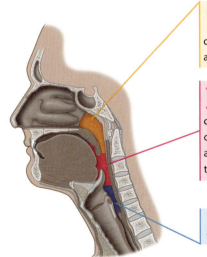

1 The **nasopharynx** extends from the posterior nares to the soft palate. It contains openings for the right and left auditory (eustachian) tubes.

2 The **oropharynx** is a space between the soft palate and the base of the tongue. It contains the palatine tonsils (the ones most commonly removed by tonsillectomy) as well as the lingual tonsils, found at the base of the tongue.

3 The **laryngopharynx** passes dorsal to the larynx and connects to the esophagus.

Larynx

Lying between the root of the tongue and the upper end of the trachea, the **larynx** is a chamber formed by walls of cartilage and muscle. Because it contains the vocal cords, it's often called the voice box; however, it actually has three functions:

1. It prevents food and liquids from entering the trachea.
2. It acts as an air passageway between the pharynx and trachea.
3. It produces sound.

The larynx is formed by nine pieces of cartilage that keep it from collapsing; a group of ligaments bind the pieces of cartilage together and to adjacent structures in the neck.

- The **epiglottis**—which closes over the top of the larynx during swallowing to direct food and liquids into the esophagus—is the uppermost cartilage.
- The largest piece of cartilage is the **thyroid cartilage**, which is also known as the Adam's apple.

- The mucous membrane lining the larynx forms two pairs of folds. The superior pair—called **vestibular folds**, or, occasionally, false vocal cords—play no role in speech. They close the glottis (the opening between the vocal cords) during swallowing to keep food and liquids out of the airway.
- The inferior pair, the **vocal cords**, produces sound when air passes over them during exhalation.
- The opening between the cords is called the **glottis**.

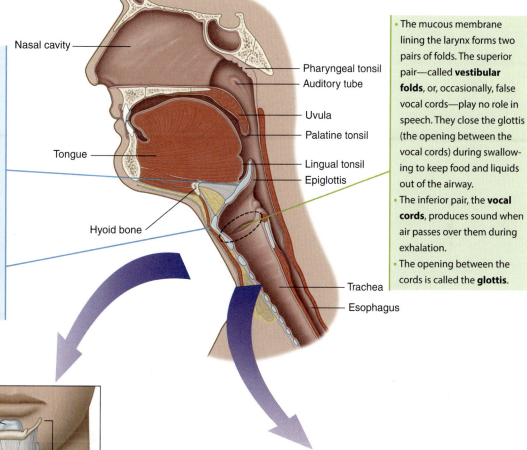

Nasal cavity

Pharyngeal tonsil
Auditory tube

Uvula

Palatine tonsil

Tongue

Lingual tonsil
Epiglottis

Hyoid bone

Trachea

Esophagus

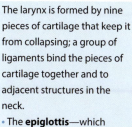

Epiglottis

Hyoid bone

Thyroid cartilage

Larynx

Trachea

Base of tongue

Epiglottis

Vestibular fold

Vocal cord

Glottis

Vocal cords in the closed position

Vocal cords in the open position

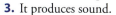

The Body AT WORK

Air passing between the vocal cords during exhalation produces sound. Loudness depends upon the force of the air: the more forceful the air, the louder the sound. Only the vocal cords produce sound; however, the pharynx, oral cavity, tongue, and lips shape the sounds to form words.

High-pitched sounds result when the cords are relatively taut; more relaxed cords produce lower-pitched sounds. The vocal cords in adult males are usually longer and thicker and vibrate more slowly, producing lower-pitched sounds than in females.

Lower Respiratory Tract

The lower respiratory tract consists of the trachea, bronchi, and lungs. The trachea and the bronchi distribute air to the interior of the lungs; deep within the lungs is where gas exchange occurs.

FAST FACT

The trachea and the two bronchi with their many branches resemble an inverted tree: that's why it's often called the bronchial tree.

Trachea

Lying just in front of the esophagus, the trachea is a rigid tube about 4.5 inches (11 cm) long and 1 inch (2.5 cm) wide. C-shaped rings of cartilage encircle the trachea to reinforce it and keep it from collapsing during inhalation. The open part of the "C" faces posteriorly, giving the esophagus room to expand during swallowing.

The trachea extends from the larynx to a cartilaginous ridge called the **carina**.

Bronchial Tree

At the carina, the trachea branches into two **primary bronchi**. Like the trachea, the primary bronchi are supported by C-shaped rings of cartilage. (All of the divisions of the bronchial tree also consist of elastic connective tissue.)

The right bronchus is slightly wider and more vertical than the left, making this the most likely location for aspirated (inhaled) food particles and small objects to lodge.

Immediately after entering the lungs, the primary bronchi branch into **secondary bronchi**: one for each of the lung's lobes. Since the left lung consists of two lobes, it has two secondary bronchi; the right lung has three lobes, so it has three bronchi.

Secondary bronchi branch into smaller **tertiary bronchi**. The cartilaginous rings around the bronchi become irregular and disappear entirely in the smaller bronchioles.

Tertiary bronchi continue to branch, resulting in very small airways called **bronchioles**. Less than 1 mm wide and lacking any supportive cartilage, bronchioles divide further to form thin-walled passages called **alveolar ducts**.

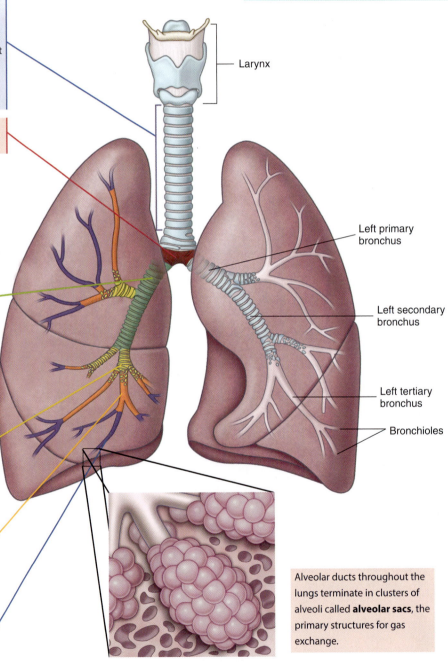

Larynx

Left primary bronchus

Left secondary bronchus

Left tertiary bronchus

Bronchioles

Alveolar ducts throughout the lungs terminate in clusters of alveoli called **alveolar sacs**, the primary structures for gas exchange.

Alveoli

The lung passages all exist to serve the alveoli because it's within the alveoli that gas exchange occurs.

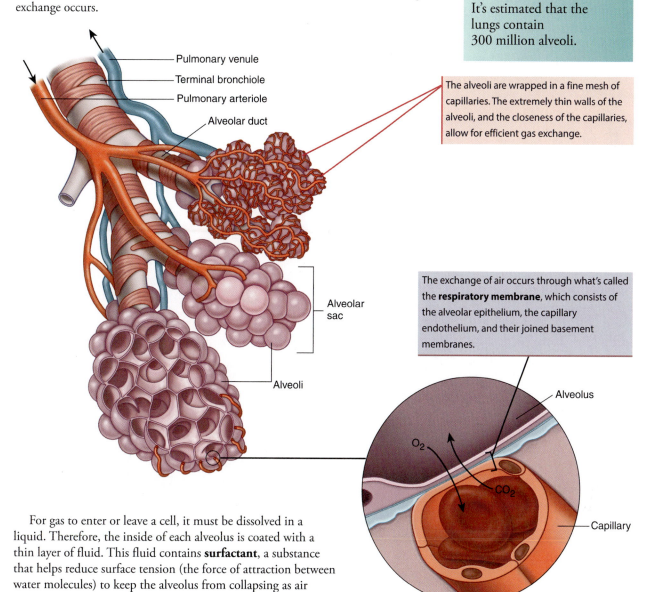

- Pulmonary venule
- Terminal bronchiole
- Pulmonary arteriole
- Alveolar duct

Alveolar sac

Alveoli

The alveoli are wrapped in a fine mesh of capillaries. The extremely thin walls of the alveoli, and the closeness of the capillaries, allow for efficient gas exchange.

The exchange of air occurs through what's called the **respiratory membrane**, which consists of the alveolar epithelium, the capillary endothelium, and their joined basement membranes.

Alveolus

O_2

CO_2

Capillary

For gas to enter or leave a cell, it must be dissolved in a liquid. Therefore, the inside of each alveolus is coated with a thin layer of fluid. This fluid contains **surfactant**, a substance that helps reduce surface tension (the force of attraction between water molecules) to keep the alveolus from collapsing as air moves in and out during respiration. (For more information, see "Alveolar Surface Tension" in this chapter.)

The Body AT WORK

A large portion of the membrane lining the bronchial tree is covered with a layer of protective mucus, which serves to purify the air entering the respiratory tract. This cleansing mucus moves up from the lower portions of the bronchial tree toward the pharynx, propelled along by millions of hair-like cilia that line the respiratory mucosa. The cilia beat in one direction— upward—so that the mucus will move toward the pharynx. Cigarette smoke paralyzes these cilia. As a result, mucus accumulates in the lower portions of the bronchial tree, causing the typical "smoker's cough" as the lungs attempt to rid themselves of the excess mucus.

Lungs

The lungs fill the pleural cavity: they extend from just above the clavicles to the diaphragm and lie against the anterior and posterior ribs. The medial portion of each lung is concave to allow room for the heart and great vessels. The primary bronchi and pulmonary blood vessels enter each lung through an opening on the lung's medial surface called the **hilum**.

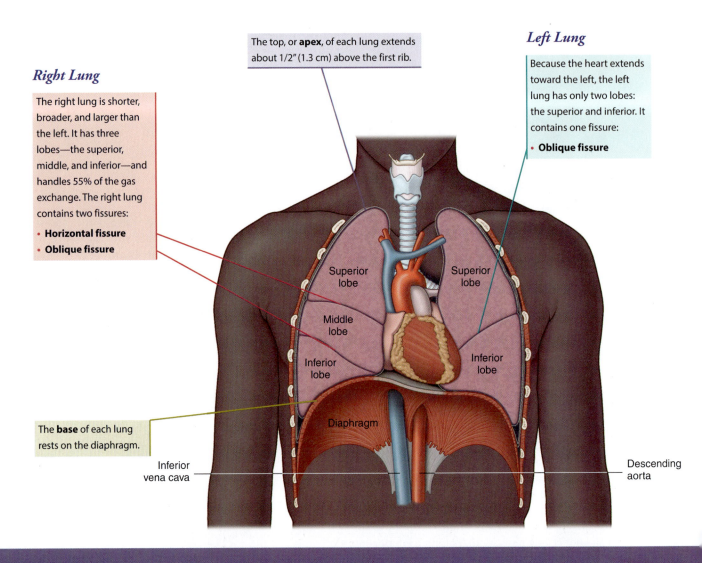

The top, or **apex**, of each lung extends about 1/2" (1.3 cm) above the first rib.

Left Lung

Because the heart extends toward the left, the left lung has only two lobes: the superior and inferior. It contains one fissure:

- **Oblique fissure**

Right Lung

The right lung is shorter, broader, and larger than the left. It has three lobes—the superior, middle, and inferior—and handles 55% of the gas exchange. The right lung contains two fissures:

- **Horizontal fissure**
- **Oblique fissure**

Superior lobe

Superior lobe

Middle lobe

Inferior lobe

Inferior lobe

The **base** of each lung rests on the diaphragm.

Diaphragm

Inferior vena cava

Descending aorta

Life lesson: Asthma

Asthma is the most common chronic illness in children; what's more, the number of people afflicted with asthma is on the rise. In the United States, about 5% of all adults and 10% of all children have asthma.

Typically, when someone with asthma is exposed to an allergen or other respiratory irritant (such as dust or fumes), the bronchioles constrict and spasm. These narrowed airways trigger coughing and wheezing—sometimes severe— as the person struggles to breathe. Inflammation in the airways also causes excessive production of thick, sticky mucus that further clogs the airways. Airway obstruction can become severe enough to cause suffocation and death.

Treatment involves dilating the airways through the administration of epinephrine and beta-adrenergic stimulants. Also, anti-inflammatory medications and inhaled corticosteroids are often prescribed to treat inflammation and minimize scarring.

Pleurae

A serous membrane—the **visceral pleura**—covers the surface of the lungs, extending into the fissures.

The **parietal pleura** lines the entire thoracic cavity.

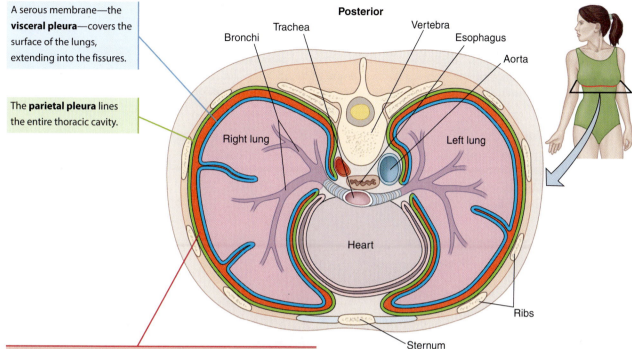

Posterior

Bronchi Trachea Vertebra Esophagus Aorta

Right lung Left lung

Heart

Ribs

Sternum

Anterior

The space between the visceral and parietal pleurae is called the **pleural cavity**. The pleural cavity is only a **potential** space; the two membranes are normally separated only by a film of slippery pleural fluid.

The fluid in the pleural cavity serves two purposes:

• It lubricates the pleural surfaces, allowing the two surfaces to glide painlessly against each other as the lungs expand and contract.

• Because the pressure in the pleural cavity is lower than atmospheric pressure, it creates a pressure gradient that assists in lung inflation.

Life lesson: Changes with aging

As the body ages, numerous changes occur in the respiratory system—all leading to a general reduction in respiratory efficiency. Here are a few of those changes:

• Decreased mobility of the chest wall
• Increased lung rigidity
• Decreased number and dilation of alveoli
• Weakened respiratory muscles
• Reduced volume of protective respiratory fluids

These changes reduce an older person's ability to perform vigorous exercise. They also lead to increased risk for developing pneumonia following a bacterial or viral illness. In addition, these changes can compound the effects of heart and lung diseases.

Pulmonary Ventilation

Pulmonary ventilation is simply breathing: the repetitive process of inhaling (called **inspiration**) and exhaling (called **expiration**). Both actions depend on the function of respiratory muscles and a difference between the air pressure within the lungs and the air pressure outside the body. One inspiration and one expiration comprise one **respiratory cycle**.

Respiratory Muscles

The lungs depend on the skeletal muscles of the trunk (especially the diaphragm and the intercostal muscles) to expand and contract to create airflow. The main muscle responsible for pulmonary ventilation is the diaphragm: the dome-shaped muscle separating the thoracic and pelvic cavities.

> ### FAST FACT
> In adults, normal respiratory rates range from 12 to 20 breaths per minute.

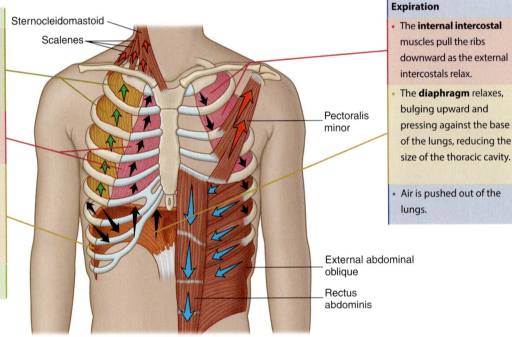

Inspiration

- The **external intercostal** muscles pull the ribs upward and outward, widening the thoracic cavity.
- The **internal intercostals** help elevate the ribs.
- The **diaphragm** contracts, flattens, and drops, pressing the abdominal organs downward and enlarging the thoracic cavity.
- Air rushes in to equalize pressure.

Sternocleidomastoid

Scalenes

Pectoralis minor

External abdominal oblique

Rectus abdominis

Expiration

- The **internal intercostal** muscles pull the ribs downward as the external intercostals relax.
- The **diaphragm** relaxes, bulging upward and pressing against the base of the lungs, reducing the size of the thoracic cavity.
- Air is pushed out of the lungs.

Accessory Muscles of Respiration

During times of forced or labored breathing, additional muscles, called **accessory muscles of respiration**, join in to assist with breathing. For example:

- During **deep inspiration**, muscles of the neck (the sternocleidomastoids and scalenes) and the chest (the pectoralis minor) contract to help elevate the chest (see red arrows in figure).
- During **forced expiration**—such as when singing or shouting—the rectus abdominis and external abdominal obliques contract to pull down the ribs and sternum, further reducing chest size and expelling air more rapidly (see blue arrows in figure).

> ### The Body AT WORK
> *People having difficulty breathing may depend heavily on accessory muscles to breathe. For example, in emphysema, lungs lose their elasticity and exhaling is no longer a passive process. Patients must use their accessory muscles to exhale, making exhaling an active, exhausting process. In other patients, the use of accessory muscles can indicate acute respiratory distress, signaling a medical emergency.*

Neural Control of Breathing

Unlike cardiac muscle, which contains intrinsic pacemakers, the muscles used for breathing are skeletal muscles—and skeletal muscles require nervous stimulation to contract. Although a variety of factors affect the rate and rhythm of breathing, the respiratory centers responsible for automatic, unconscious breathing reside in the medulla and pons—parts of the brainstem.

The medulla contains two interconnected centers that control breathing: the **inspiratory center** and the **expiratory center.**

The **inspiratory center** is the primary respiratory center. It controls inspiration and, indirectly, expiration as well. Here's how it works:

1. The inspiratory center sends impulses to the intercostal muscles (via the intercostal nerves) and to the diaphragm (via the phrenic nerves).
2. The inspiratory muscles contract, causing inhalation.
3. Nerve output then ceases abruptly, causing the inspiratory muscles to relax. The elastic recoil of the thoracic cage produces exhalation.

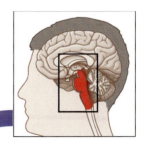

Although the medulla is the main breathing center, the pons contains two centers that can influence basic breathing rhythm:

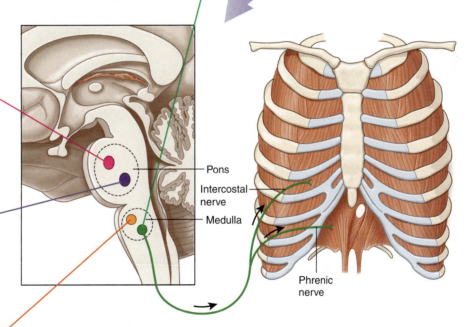

- The **apneustic center** stimulates the inspiratory center to increase the length and depth of inspiration.

- The **pneumotaxic center** inhibits both the apneustic center and the inspiratory center; this contributes to a normal breathing rhythm and prevents overinflation of the lungs.

Pons

Intercostal nerve

Medulla

Phrenic nerve

When more forceful exhalations are needed, such as during exercise, the **expiratory center** sends impulses to the abdominal and other accessory muscles.

The Body AT WORK

The cerebral cortex allows you to voluntarily change your breathing rate or rhythm, such as to sing or blow out a candle, or even to hold your breath. However, when you hold your breath, CO_2 isn't expelled through breathing and the CO_2 level in the blood rises. CO_2 is a powerful respiratory stimulant. When CO_2 rises to a certain level, the respiratory centers override your voluntary action and breathing resumes.

Variations in Breathing

Despite neural input, breathing patterns don't remain constant. Respiratory rate and rhythm vary: with pain, emotion (such as fear, anger, or anxiety), exercise, and changes in the body's physical state. These variations occur because the respiratory centers receive input from a number of sensory receptors throughout the body, alerting it to the body's changing needs.

FAST FACT

Carbon dioxide—NOT oxygen—is the primary regulator of respiration. That's because carbon dioxide easily crosses the blood-brain barrier.

Factors Influencing Breathing

Factor		Sensory Receptor	Action
Oxygen	$\downarrow O_2$	Peripheral chemoreceptors (located in the carotid and aortic bodies)	Low blood levels of oxygen cause peripheral chemoreceptors to send impulses to the medulla to increase the rate and depth of respirations. This brings more air, and therefore oxygen, into the lungs.
Hydrogen ions (pH)	pH	Central chemoreceptors (located in the brainstem)	Central chemoreceptors monitor the pH of cerebrospinal fluid (CSF), which mirrors the level of carbon dioxide in the blood. Falling pH levels indicate an excess of carbon dioxide. When this occurs, central chemoreceptors signal the respiratory centers to increase the rate and depth of breathing. This helps the body "blow off" excess carbon dioxide, raising the pH.
Stretch		Receptors in the lungs and chest wall	As the lungs inflate during inspiration, receptors detect the stretching and signal the respiratory centers to exhale and inhibit inspiration. Called the **Hering-Breuer reflex**, this mechanism prevents lung damage from overinflation.
Pain and emotion		Hypothalamus and limbic system	These areas of the brain send signals that affect breathing in response to pain and emotions (such as fear, anger, and anxiety).
Irritants (such as smoke, dust, pollen, noxious chemicals, and mucus)		Nerve cells in the airway	Nerve cells respond to irritants by signaling the respiratory muscles to contract, resulting in a cough or a sneeze. Coughing or sneezing propels air rapidly from the lungs, helping to remove the offending substance.

Pressure and Airflow

Air moves into and out of the lungs for the same reason that blood flows: because of a pressure gradient. The pressure that drives respiration is **atmospheric pressure**: the weight of the air around us.

When the pressure within the lungs drops lower than atmospheric pressure, air flows from the area of higher pressure—the air outside the body—to an area of lower pressure—the lungs; this is **inspiration**. When the pressure within the lungs rises above atmospheric pressure, air flows out of the lungs **(expiration)** until the two pressures equalize. Whereas inspiration is an active process, requiring the use of muscles, normal expiration is a passive process, resulting from the recoil of healthy lungs.

ANIMATION

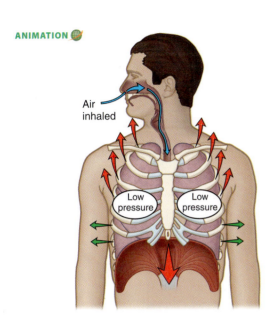

Inspiration

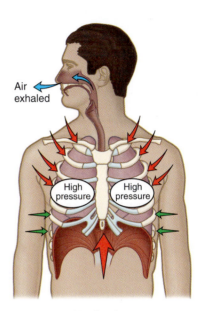

Expiration

- The intercostal muscles contract, pulling the ribs up and out; the diaphragm contracts and moves downward. This enlarges the chest cavity in all directions.
- The lungs expand along with the chest because of the two layers of the pleurae.
  - The parietal pleura is firmly attached to the ribs; the visceral pleura covers the lungs.
  - Although not attached to each other, the thin film of fluid between the two pleurae causes them to cling together like two pieces of wet paper.
  - Furthermore, the potential space between the two pleurae maintains a pressure slightly less than atmospheric pressure (negative pressure). This is the **intrapleural pressure**. When the ribs expand and the parietal pleura pulls away, intrapleural pressure becomes even more negative. This has a suction-like effect, causing the visceral pleura to cling even tighter to the parietal pleura.
  - The visceral pleura follows the parietal pleura, pulling the lung along with it.
- When the lungs expand, the volume of air in the lungs spreads throughout the enlarging space. This causes the pressure within the bronchi and alveoli (the **intrapulmonic pressure**) to drop. (See "That Makes Sense!")
- When the intrapulmonic pressure drops lower than the atmospheric pressure, air flows down the pressure gradient into the lungs.

- The diaphragm and external intercostal muscles relax, and the thoracic cage springs back to its original size.
- The lungs are compressed by the thoracic cage.
- Intrapulmonary pressure rises.
- Air flows down the pressure gradient and out of the lungs.

> **!**
>
> ## That Makes Sense
>
> *A law of physics called Boyle's Law explains why intrapulmonic pressure drops as the lungs expand. **Boyle's Law** states, "At a constant temperature, the pressure of a given quantity of gas is inversely proportional to its volume." In other words, a given volume of gas will exert more pressure in a smaller space than it will in a larger space.*
>
> *To illustrate, imagine tying off the end of a large plastic bag. The air in the bag would cause the bag to balloon slightly but the bag would still be soft to touch. The air inside the bag would have a low pressure. Now imagine twisting the end of the bag, making the volume of the bag smaller. This would force the air in the bag into a smaller space and the bag would become firm to touch—exhibiting a higher pressure. If you continued to twist, making the bag even smaller, the pressure could become great enough to pop the bag.*

Life lesson: Pneumothorax

If the thoracic wall is punctured, air from the atmosphere will rush in to the pleural cavity, transforming what is normally a potential space into a space filled with air. As a result, the negative pressure that characterizes the pleural cavity is lost, and the lung recoils and collapses. This is called a *pneumothorax*. Air can also enter the pleural space when a weakened or diseased alveoli ruptures. This causes a disruption in the visceral pleura, and air from the lung enters the pleural cavity, again resulting in a pneumothorax.

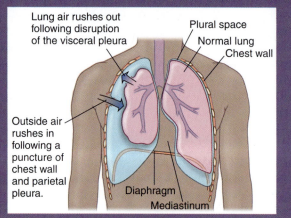

Lung air rushes out following disruption of the visceral pleura

Plural space

Normal lung
Chest wall

Outside air rushes in following a puncture of chest wall and parietal pleura.

Diaphragm
Mediastinum

Factors Affecting Airflow

Effective pulmonary ventilation depends on several factors. Two particularly important factors are pulmonary compliance and alveolar surface tension.

Pulmonary Compliance

Pulmonary compliance refers to the elasticity of lung tissue. Ventilation can't occur unless the lungs and thorax can stretch and, just as important, recoil. Some diseases (such as tuberculosis or black lung disease) cause scarring, which makes the lungs stiffer, or less compliant. The lungs have difficulty expanding, and ventilation is impaired.

Alveolar Surface Tension

The inner surface of each alveoli is covered with a thin film of water. The water is necessary for gas exchange. However, water molecules are also electrically attracted to each other, just like weak magnets. Left alone, the water molecules inside the alveolus will move toward each other, creating a force that will collapse the alveoli. If the alveoli collapse, gas exchange can't occur. To avoid this problem, alveolar cells secrete surfactant, a lipoprotein that disrupts the electrical attraction between the water molecules. This lowers surface tension and prevents alveolar collapse.

Life lesson: Emphysema

Emphysema is a progressive lung disease in which lung tissue surrounding alveoli is destroyed. This leaves alveoli unsupported, allowing them to enlarge and eventually rupture. Alveolar walls fuse into large irregular spaces that offer less area available for gas exchange. The alveoli also lose elasticity and the ability to recoil. Consequently, air becomes trapped in the lungs. Over time, the trapped air causes the diameter of the chest to enlarge, and the chest assumes the shape of a barrel. (A person with emphysema is often said to be "barrel-chested.") Persons with emphysema must work to exhale; they can expend three to four times the normal amount of energy just to breathe.

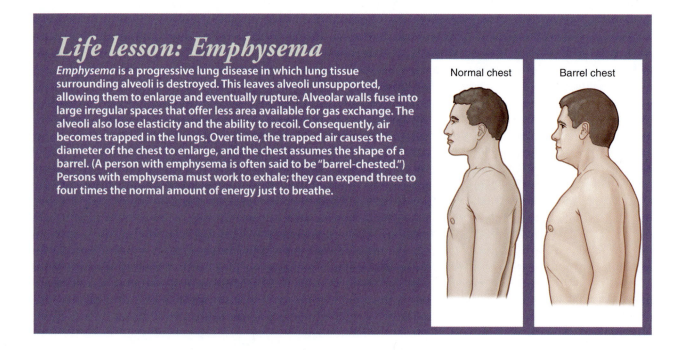

Normal chest

Barrel chest

Measurements of Ventilation

Measuring lung capacity can provide information about the health of a person's lungs. This information is usually obtained by having the person breathe through a device called a **spirometer**. (The values shown in the following spirographic record are typical for a healthy young adult.)

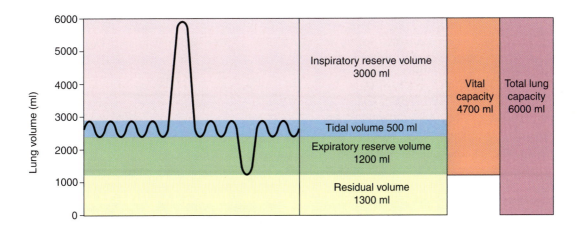

The amount of air inhaled and exhaled during quiet breathing is known as **tidal volume**.

After taking a normal breath, it's still possible to inhale even more air. This amount of air—inhaled using maximum effort *after* a normal inspiration—is called the **inspiratory reserve volume**.

Likewise, after a normal expiration, it's possible to exhale even more air. The amount of air that can be exhaled after a normal expiration by using maximum effort is the **expiratory reserve volume**.

Even after a forced expiration, about 1300 ml of air remains in the lungs. Called the **residual volume**, this air ensures that gas exchange continues even between breaths.

The amount of air that can be inhaled and exhaled with the deepest possible breath is the **vital capacity**. (Vital capacity is the tidal volume combined with the inspiratory and expiratory reserve volumes.)

Total lung capacity is the maximum amount of air that the lungs can contain: the vital capacity plus the residual volume.

With every breath, about 150 ml of air remains in the conducting airways. Since this air doesn't reach the alveoli, it can't participate in gas exchange. The air is said to be in the **anatomical dead space:** in the passageways instead of the alveoli. Anatomical dead space occurs normally as air makes its way to the alveoli.

Physiological dead space includes all the air in conducting airways (the anatomical dead space) plus the air in any alveoli that are poorly perfused and, therefore, less efficient in gas exchange. Certain diseases cause portions of the lung to be poorly perfused, leading to increased physiological dead space.

The Body AT WORK

Vital capacity depends on several factors, including an individual's size, posture, and overall health. In general, a tall person has larger lungs, and therefore a larger vital capacity, than does a short person. Also, standing erect increases vital capacity, while slouching or lying down decreases it.

Certain diseases also affect vital capacity. For example, excess fluid in the abdomen or pleura encroaches upon the space occupied by the lungs, diminishing vital capacity. Congestive heart failure causes blood to back up in the lungs, filling alveolar air space and decreasing vital capacity. On the other hand, exercise programs and yoga have been shown to help increase vital capacity.

Variations in Respiratory Rhythm

A variety of conditions, including exercise, anxiety, and various disease states, influence respiratory rate and rhythm. The following table lists the names for common variations in breathing.

Common Respiratory Terms

Term	Type of Breathing
Apnea	Temporary cessation of breathing
Cheyne-Stokes respirations	Breathing pattern marked by a period of apnea followed by gradually increasing rate and depth of respirations; often seen in terminally ill or brain-damaged adults
Dyspnea	Labored or difficult breathing
Eupnea	Relaxed, quiet breathing
Hyperventilation	Increased rate and depth of respirations resulting in lowered blood levels of carbon dioxide; often results from anxiety
Hypoventilation	Reduced rate and depth of respirations, resulting in increased blood levels of carbon dioxide
Kussmaul respiration	Very deep, gasping respirations associated with diabetic ketoacidosis
Orthopnea	Labored breathing that occurs when a person is lying flat but improves when standing or sitting up; a classic symptom of left ventricular heart failure
Tachypnea	Rapid breathing

FAST FACT

Regular exercise promotes development of respiratory muscles, which leads to an increase in vital capacity.

Gas Exchange

The goal of respiration is the delivery of oxygen to the organs and tissues of the body and the removal of carbon dioxide. This exchange of gases—both in the lungs and the tissues of the body—depends on differences in pressure.

The air we breathe has a pressure of 760 mm Hg; this is known as total atmospheric pressure. The atmosphere consists of about 78% nitrogen, 21% oxygen, and about 1% other gases, of which 0.03% is carbon dioxide. Each one of these gases contributes to the total atmospheric pressure. The contribution of a single gas in any mixture of gases is called **partial pressure**. A gas's partial pressure is symbolized by the letter "P" followed by the formula for the gas, such as PCO_2.

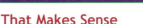

That Makes Sense

The partial pressure of a gas directly relates to its concentration in a mixture. For example, oxygen constitutes approximately 21% of atmospheric air. To determine its partial pressure, multiply 0.21 (the percentage of oxygen) by 760 (the total pressure of the atmosphere). The resulting number of 159.6 is the partial pressure of oxygen in the air we breathe.

Life lesson: Heimlich maneuver

The *Heimlich maneuver* is an effective maneuver for dislodging a foreign object in someone who is choking. The maneuver uses the residual volume of air already in the lungs to expel an object in the trachea. If someone appears to be choking, always ask, "Can you speak?" Someone with an obstructed airway won't be able to talk, even though he's conscious. (Remember: Air has to pass between the vocal cords for someone to talk.) If the airway is indeed obstructed, follow these steps:

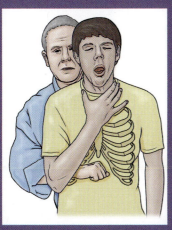

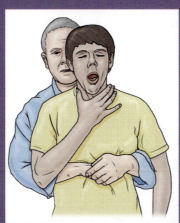

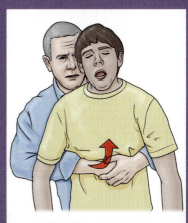

1. Stand or kneel behind the person who is choking. Make a fist with one hand and wrap your arm around the person's waist. Place your fist (thumb inward) in the person's abdomen, above the navel and below the ribcage.

2. Wrap your other arm around the person from the other side, placing your other hand over your fist.

3. Use your outer hand to force your fist into the abdomen. Make quick, hard movements inward and upward to force air out of the person's lungs. Repeat the maneuver several times if necessary to dislodge the object.

Process of Gas Exchange

The partial pressures of oxygen and carbon dioxide vary between the air we breathe, the alveoli, arterial blood, and venous blood. It's these variations in pressure that allow the body to absorb oxygen and expel carbon dioxide. *The key point to remember is that gas diffuses from an area of higher pressure to an area of lower pressure until the pressures are equalized.*

Follow the path of blood along the circulatory route, noting the differences in the partial pressures of oxygen and carbon dioxide.

ANIMATION

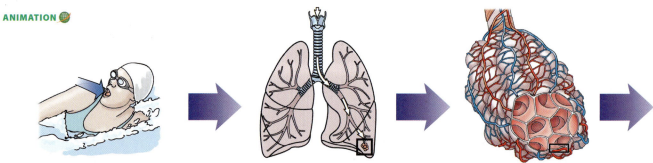

Inspired air has a PO_2 of 159 and a PCO_2 of 0.3.

When it arrives at the alveoli, air has a PO_2 of 104 and a PCO_2 of 40.

On the other side of the alveoli's thin membrane are pulmonary capillaries that contain venous blood. This blood has a PO_2 of 40 and a PCO_2 of 46.

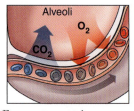

The differences in partial pressures of O_2 and CO_2 on either side of the respiratory membrane cause O_2 to move out of the alveoli and into the capillaries and CO_2 to move out of the capillaries into the alveoli. (In other words, the red blood cells in the capillaries *unload* CO_2 and *load* oxygen.) The CO_2 is later exhaled through the lungs.

Blood in the capillaries now has a PO_2 of 100 and a PCO_2 of 40.

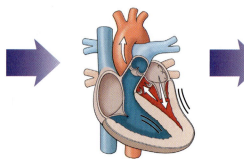

This oxygen-enriched blood travels to the heart's left ventricle, where it's pumped to the body's tissues.

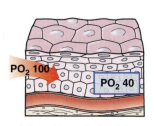

Meanwhile, cells in the body's tissues have been using oxygen for energy production and producing CO_2 as a by-product. The fluid surrounding the cells has a PO_2 of 40 and a PCO_2 of 46.

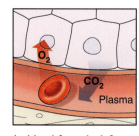

When the blood from the left ventricle (with a PO_2 of 100) arrives at the tissues (with a PO_2 of 40), oxygen diffuses out of the blood and into the tissues. Simultaneously, carbon dioxide diffuses from the tissues (PCO_2 of 46) and into the blood (PCO_2 of 40).

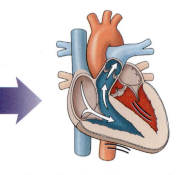

Once it has released oxygen to the tissues and absorbed CO_2, the capillary blood has a PO_2 of 40 and a PCO_2 of 46. Systemic capillaries carry this oxygen-depleted blood away from the tissues and toward the heart's right ventricle, where it will be pumped back to the lungs.

The Body AT WORK

Optimal gas exchange obviously depends upon a number of factors, including those listed in the table below. A disruption in any one of these factors can profoundly affect oxygenation.

Factor Necessary for Oxygenation	Potential Disruption
Pressure gradient between the oxygen in alveolar air and the oxygen in incoming pulmonary blood	At high altitudes, the partial pressure of oxygen in inspired air is less than at sea level. As a result, alveolar PO_2 is decreased and less oxygen enters the blood.
Adequate alveolar surface area	Certain disorders—such as emphysema, pneumothorax, and surfactant disorders—decrease the functional surface area of the lung. Less area is available for gas diffusion, and blood oxygen levels decline.
Adequate respiratory rate	For gas diffusion to occur, alveoli must receive a steady supply of oxygen through inspired air. Anything that decreases the respiratory rate (such as the narcotic morphine) lessens the amount of oxygen entering the blood.

How the Blood Transports Gases

The process of carrying gases from the alveoli to the tissues and back is known as gas transport.

Transport of Oxygen

Of the oxygen entering the body, only 1.5% is dissolved in blood plasma. Here's what happens to the remaining 98.5% of oxygen:

- In the lungs, the oxygen forms a weak bond with the iron portion of hemoglobin, creating **oxyhemoglobin.**
- Oxyhemoglobin travels through the circulatory system to the tissue cells.
- Once there, the difference in pH between the arterial and venous blood is enough to break the bond between the oxygen and the hemoglobin.
- The oxygen is then released to the tissues.

Transport of Carbon Dioxide

Carbon dioxide is transported from the tissues to the lungs in three ways:

1. About 10% is dissolved in the plasma.
2. Another 20% is bound to hemoglobin, forming **carbaminohemoglobin.** (Hemoglobin can transport both O_2 and CO_2 at the same time because they bind to different sites on the hemoglobin molecule.)
3. The vast majority—about 70%—is carried in the form of bicarbonate ions (HCO_3^-). This occurs because when CO_2 dissolves in plasma, it reacts with the water in the plasma to form carbonic acid. Carbonic acid then dissociates into bicarbonate and hydrogen ions.

FAST FACT

Hemoglobin has a stronger affinity for carbon monoxide than it does for oxygen. That's why exposure to carbon monoxide can be deadly: once bound to carbon monoxide, hemoglobin can't transport oxygen.

Review of Key Terms

Alveolus: Air sac in the lungs

Bronchi: The two main branches leading from the trachea to the lungs that serve as passageways for air

Bronchioles: One of the smaller subdivisions of the bronchial tubes

Epiglottis: The uppermost cartilage of the larynx; closes during swallowing to direct food and liquids into the esophagus

Glottis: The opening between the vocal cords

Hilum: Opening on the lung's medial surface through which primary bronchi and pulmonary blood vessels pass

Intrapleural pressure: The pressure between the visceral and parietal pleurae, which assists with lung expansion

Larynx: Structure made of cartilage and muscle at the upper end of the trachea; part of the airway and the vocal apparatus

Palate: Bony structure separating the mouth from the nasal cavity

Partial pressure: The contribution of a single gas in a mixture of gases toward the total pressure of the gas mixture

Pharynx: Muscular tube behind the oral and nasal cavities; commonly called the throat

Pleura: Serous membrane covering the lungs and the thoracic cavity

Surfactant: Lipoprotein secreted by alveolar cells that decreases surface tension of the fluid lining the alveoli, permitting expansion of alveoli

Tidal volume: The amount of air inhaled and exhaled during quiet breathing

Trachea: Portion of the respiratory tract that carries air through the neck and upper chest

Ventilation: The movement of air into and out of the lungs

Vital capacity: The amount of air that can be inhaled and exhaled with the deepest possible breath

Own the Information

To make the information in this chapter part of your working memory, take some time to reflect on what you've learned. On a separate sheet of paper, write down everything you recall from the chapter. After you're done, log on to the Davis*Plus* website, and check out the Study Group podcast and Study Group Questions for the chapter.

Key Topics for Chapter 17:
- Structures of the upper respiratory tract
- Structures of the lower respiratory tract
- Structure and function of the muscles used in pulmonary ventilation
- Neural control of breathing
- Factors influencing breathing
- How a pressure gradient influences the flow of air into and out of the lungs
- How pulmonary compliance and alveolar surface tension affect airflow
- Measurements of ventilation
- Variations in respiratory rhythm
- The process of gas exchange along the circulatory route
- How the blood transports oxygen and carbon dioxide

Test Your Knowledge

1. Which of the following is a function of the nasopharynx?
   a. Filter dust
   b. Warm and moisten inspired air
   c. Provide openings for the right and left eustachian tubes
   d. Contain olfactory receptors responsible for the sense of smell

2. Which structure is responsible for directing food and liquids into the esophagus during swallowing?
   a. Glottis
   b. Epiglottis
   c. Adam's apple
   d. Conchae

3. What purpose do the cartilaginous rings around the trachea serve?
   a. Keep the trachea from collapsing during inhalation
   b. Attach the trachea firmly to the esophagus
   c. Protect the trachea from trauma
   d. They serve no purpose

4. Inhaled food or foreign objects are most likely to lodge in which part of the respiratory system?
   a. Pharynx
   b. Right bronchus
   c. Left bronchus
   d. Bronchioles

5. What is the purpose of surfactant?
   a. Facilitate in the diffusion of oxygen across the respiratory membrane
   b. Transport oxygen to the alveoli
   c. Purify the air entering the respiratory tract
   d. Keep alveoli from collapsing

6. What is one of the purposes of the fluid in the pleural cavity?
   a. Lubricate the pleural surfaces to allow them to glide painlessly during lung expansion and contraction
   b. Warm and moisten lung tissue
   c. Prevent bacteria from entering lung tissue
   d. Assist in the diffusion of oxygen across the respiratory membrane

7. The main muscle responsible for pulmonary ventilation is:
   a. the abdominals.
   b. the external intercostals.
   c. the diaphragm.
   d. the internal intercostals.

8. Which gas is the primary regulator of respiration?
   a. Oxygen
   b. Carbon dioxide
   c. Nitrogen
   d. Bicarbonate

9. When pressure in the lungs drops lower than atmospheric pressure, what occurs?
   a. Air flows out of the lungs.
   b. Air flows into the lungs.
   c. A pneumothorax forms, collapsing the lungs.
   d. The bronchioles constrict, causing respiratory distress.

10. The primary way oxygen is transported in the blood is:
    a. in the form of bicarbonate.
    b. in the form of carbaminohemoglobin.
    c. in the form of oxyhemoglobin.
    d. dissolved in plasma.

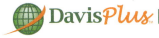

Go to **http://davisplus.fadavis.com** Keyword: Thompson to see all of the resources available with this chapter.

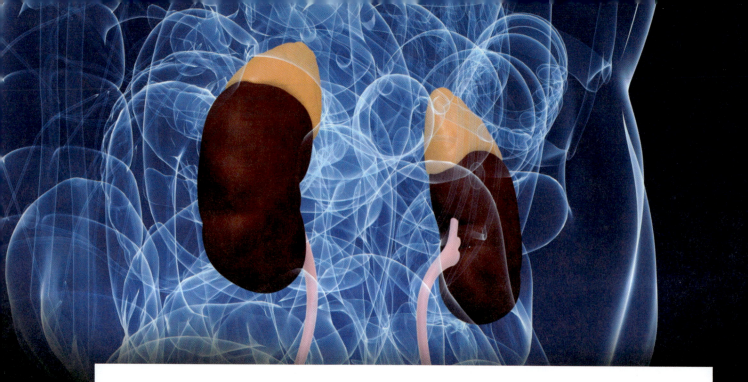

CHAPTER OUTLINE

Overview of the Urinary System

The Kidneys

Urine Formation

Composition of Urine

Storage and Elimination of Urine

LEARNING OUTCOMES

1. Identify the location of the kidneys.

2. Name the internal and external structures of the kidneys.

3. Trace the flow of blood through the kidney.

4. Describe the nerve supply to the kidney.

5. Trace the flow of fluid through the renal tubule.

6. Describe the processes that occur in each section of the renal tubule.

7. Discuss the mechanisms that drive glomerular filtration.

8. Identify the mechanisms used by the kidneys to ensure a steady glomerular filtration rate.

9. Describe the steps in the renin-angiotensin-aldosterone system.

10. Discuss the tubular reabsorption and secretion that occurs in the different parts of the renal tubule.

11. Name the hormones that affect the urinary system and identify their actions.

12. Describe the characteristics and components of urine.

13. Identify the structure and function of the ureters, urinary bladder, and urethra.

14. Describe how the structure of the urethra varies between males and females.

15. Explain the process of urination.

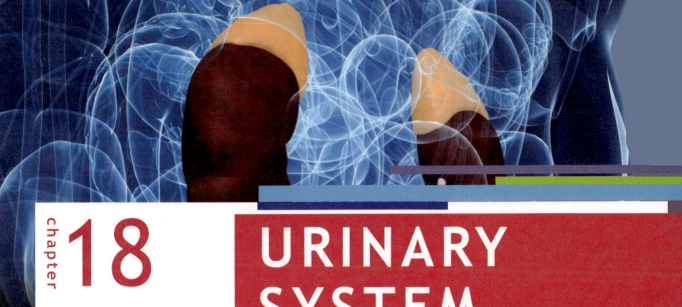

18

URINARY SYSTEM

Every hour, the kidneys filter up to 12 pints (5.7 liters) of fluid from the blood.

Throughout the body, cells continually perform a variety of metabolic processes. Each of these processes produces waste as a by-product. Cleansing the blood of these toxic substances is the job of the kidneys—the principal organs of the urinary system. As blood filters through the kidneys, these mighty organs remove potential poisons, adjust the water content of blood, tweak the levels of sodium and potassium, and adjust the pH level. What's more, the kidneys also play a role in the regulation of blood pressure and the production of red blood cells.

Overview of the Urinary System

The urinary system consists of the kidneys, ureters, urinary bladder, and urethra.

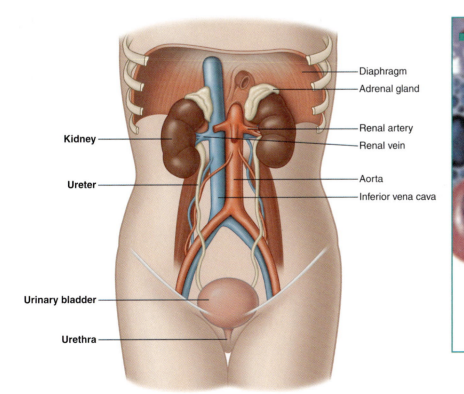

- Diaphragm
- Adrenal gland
- Renal artery
- Renal vein
- Aorta
- Inferior vena cava

Kidney

Ureter

Urinary bladder

Urethra

The Body AT WORK

*The process of eliminating wastes from the body is called **excretion**. Four organ systems perform excretory processes:*

- *The respiratory system excretes carbon dioxide and water.*
- *The integumentary system excretes water, electrolytes, lactic acid, and urea through sweat.*
- *The digestive system excretes water, carbon dioxide, lipids, bile pigments, and other metabolic wastes.*
- *The urinary system excretes metabolic wastes, drugs, hormones, salts, and water.*

The Kidneys

The kidneys lie against the posterior abdominal wall and underneath the 12th rib. They are also retroperitoneal, meaning that they are posterior to the parietal peritoneum. The ribs offer some protection to the kidneys, as does a heavy cushion of fat encasing each organ.

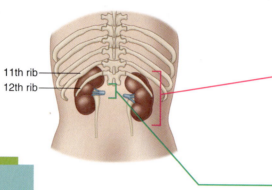

11th rib
12th rib

Each kidney measures about 4 inches (10 cm) long, 2 inches (5 cm) wide, and 1 inch (2.5 cm) thick; they extend from the level of the T12 vertebra to the L3 vertebra.

Structures (such as blood vessels, the ureters, and nerves) enter and leave the kidney through a slit called the **hilum**—located in a concave notch on the medial side.

FAST FACT

The right kidney sits lower than the left because of the space occupied by the liver just above it.

A tough, fibrous capsule surrounds each kidney. The interior of the kidney consists of two regions: the renal cortex (the site of urine production) and the renal medulla (the site of urine collection).

The **renal cortex** forms the outer region of the kidney.

The **renal medulla** forms the inner region.

Extensions from the renal cortex, called **renal columns**, divide the interior region into cone-shaped sections.

The cone-shaped sections are called **renal pyramids**. Consisting of tubules for transporting urine away from the cortex, the base of each pyramid faces outward toward the cortex. The point of the pyramid, called the **renal papilla**, faces the hilum.

The renal papilla extends into a cup called a **minor calyx**. The calyx collects urine leaving the papilla.

Two or three minor calyces join together to form a **major calyx**.

The major calyces converge to form the **renal pelvis**, which receives urine from the major calyces. The renal pelvis continues as the **ureter**, a tube-like structure that channels urine to the urinary bladder.

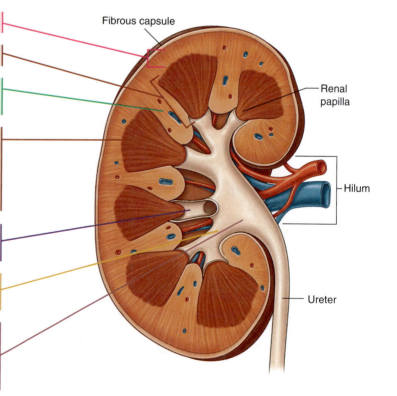

Fibrous capsule

Renal papilla

Hilum

Ureter

Renal Circulation

The **renal artery**—which branches off the abdominal aorta—brings blood to the kidney.

As it enters the kidney, the renal artery divides, branching into smaller and smaller arteries. The arteries pass through the renal columns and extend into the renal cortex.

Blood eventually leaves the kidney through the **renal vein**, which empties into the inferior vena cava.

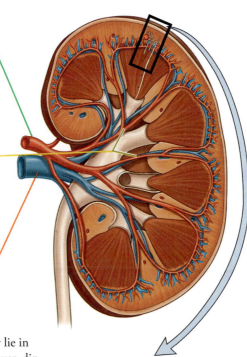

Nephrons—the filtration units of the kidney—primarily lie in the kidney's outer region; loops from the nephrons, however, dip into the inner region of the medulla. Each nephron is well supplied with blood.

FAST FACT
Over 20% of all the blood pumped by the heart each minute goes to the kidneys.

1 In the cortex, a series of **afferent arterioles** arise from the smaller arteries. Each afferent arteriole supplies blood to one nephron.

2 Each afferent arteriole branches into a cluster of capillaries called a **glomerulus**. The glomerulus is enclosed by Bowman's capsule, which will be discussed later in this chapter.

3 Blood leaves the glomerulus through an **efferent arteriole**.

4 The efferent arteriole leads to a network of capillaries around the renal tubules called **peritubular capillaries**. These capillaries pick up water and solutes reabsorbed by the renal tubules.

5 Blood flows from the peritubular capillaries into larger and larger veins that eventually feed into the renal vein.

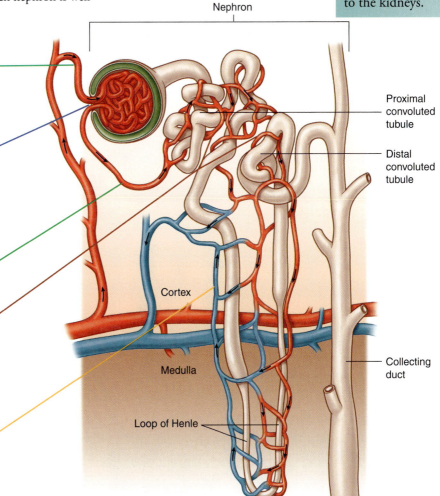

Nephron

Proximal convoluted tubule

Distal convoluted tubule

Cortex

Medulla

Collecting duct

Loop of Henle

Renal Innervation

Along with blood vessels, nerves also enter the kidney at the hilum. These mainly sympathetic fibers stimulate the afferent and efferent arterioles, controlling the diameter of the vessels, which, in turn, regulate the rate of urine formation. Also, if blood pressure drops, the nerves stimulate the release of renin, an enzyme that triggers processes for restoring blood pressure.

Nephron

The outer regions of the kidney are packed with over 1 million nephrons: the microscopic functional units of the kidney. These tiny structures consist of two main components: a *renal corpuscle*—which filters blood plasma—and a *renal tubule*—where urine is formed.

Renal Corpuscle

Known as the beginning of the nephron, a **renal corpuscle** consists of a **glomerulus** and **Bowman's capsule**.

Bowman's capsule—also called a glomerular capsule—consists of two layers of epithelial cells that envelop the glomerulus in an open-ended covering. (To understand the structure of a renal corpuscle, imagine pushing your fist into an inflated balloon. Your fist represents the glomerulus. The balloon, which folds around your fist in two layers, represents Bowman's capsule.)

Fluid filters out of the glomerulus and collects in the space between the two layers of Bowman's capsule. From there, it flows into the proximal renal tubule on the other side of the capsule.

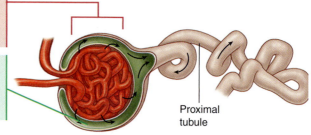

Proximal tubule

Renal Tubule

Leading away from the glomerulus are a series of tube-like structures that, collectively, are called the **renal tubule**. The renal tubule can be divided into four regions: the proximal convoluted tubule, nephron loop, distal convoluted tubule, and collecting duct. The renal tubule has been stretched out in the following figure to more clearly show the different regions.

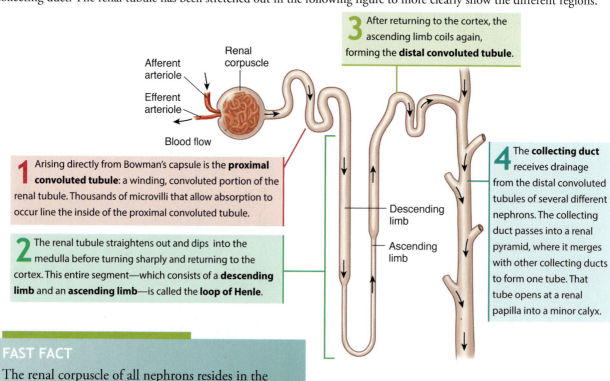

3 After returning to the cortex, the ascending limb coils again, forming the **distal convoluted tubule**.

Renal corpuscle

Afferent arteriole

Efferent arteriole

Blood flow

1 Arising directly from Bowman's capsule is the **proximal convoluted tubule**: a winding, convoluted portion of the renal tubule. Thousands of microvilli that allow absorption to occur line the inside of the proximal convoluted tubule.

2 The renal tubule straightens out and dips into the medulla before turning sharply and returning to the cortex. This entire segment—which consists of a **descending limb** and an **ascending limb**—is called the **loop of Henle**.

Descending limb

Ascending limb

4 The **collecting duct** receives drainage from the distal convoluted tubules of several different nephrons. The collecting duct passes into a renal pyramid, where it merges with other collecting ducts to form one tube. That tube opens at a renal papilla into a minor calyx.

FAST FACT

The renal corpuscle of all nephrons resides in the renal cortex. The loop of Henle dips into the renal medulla; some dip in only slightly whereas others extend deep into the medulla.

Urine Formation

The creation of urine by the nephrons involves three processes: glomerular filtration, tubular reabsorption, and tubular secretion.

Glomerular Filtration

The first step in the creation of urine from blood plasma occurs in the glomerulus as water and small solutes filter out of the blood and into the surrounding space of Bowman's capsule. Filtration in the glomerulus occurs for the same reason filtration occurs in other blood capillaries: the existence of a pressure gradient.

ANIMATION

1 Blood flows into the glomerulus through the afferent arteriole, which is much larger than the efferent arteriole. Consequently, blood flows in faster than it can leave, which contributes to higher pressure within the glomerular capillaries.

2 The walls of glomerular capillaries are dotted with pores, allowing water and small solutes (such as electrolytes, glucose, amino acids, vitamins, and nitrogenous wastes) to filter out of the blood and into Bowman's capsule. Blood cells and most plasma proteins, however, are too large to pass through the pores.

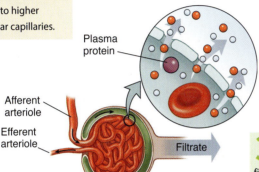

Plasma protein

Afferent arteriole

Efferent arteriole

Filtrate

3 The fluid that has filtered into Bowman's capsule flows into the renal tubules. The amount of fluid filtered by both kidneys—called the **glomerular filtration rate (GFR)**—equals about 180 liters each day, which is 60 times more than the body's total blood volume. The body reabsorbs about 99% of this filtrate, leaving 1 to 2 liters to be excreted as urine.

FAST FACT

Most of the calcium, iron, and thyroid hormone in the blood is bound to plasma proteins, which prevents these solutes from being filtered out of the blood in the glomerulus.

The Body AT WORK

*Some kidney diseases damage the endothelium of glomerular capillaries, allowing plasma proteins to filter out into the urine. The presence of protein in the urine—typically an abnormal finding—is called **proteinuria**. Proteinuria may also occur following intense physical exercise. In this instance, researchers think the proteinuria may result because hormones released during exercise temporarily alter the permeability of the filtration membrane.*

Life lesson: Hypertension and kidney damage

A common cause of kidney damage and kidney failure is uncontrolled hypertension. Systemic hypertension pushes the normally high glomerular pressure even higher. As a result, the glomerular capillaries can burst, causing scarring. Hypertension also causes atherosclerosis in blood vessels throughout the body, including those in the kidneys. This decreases blood flow to the kidneys, leading to further damage.

Regulation of the Glomerular Filtration Rate

For the body to maintain fluid and electrolyte balance, glomerular filtration should continue at a fairly constant rate despite periodic changes in blood pressure. If the flow rate is too high, the body will lose excessive amounts of water and nutrients; if it's too slow, the tubules may reabsorb toxins that should be excreted.

The kidneys employ various mechanisms to control blood flow and ensure a steady glomerular filtration rate. For example, rising blood pressure stimulates the afferent arterioles to contract, preventing a surge of blood into the glomerulus. (The opposite is also true: falling blood pressure causes the afferent arterioles to relax.) In addition, specialized cells in the distal convoluted tubule monitor the flow rate and composition of filtrate, allowing the renal tubules to make adjustments to alter flow as needed.

Finally, a key mechanism for maintaining blood pressure and, therefore, a steady glomerular filtration rate, is the **renin-angiotensin-aldosterone system.** The chain of events that occur in this system is outlined below. (See the section "Hormones Affecting the Urinary System" for more information on aldosterone.)

ANIMATION

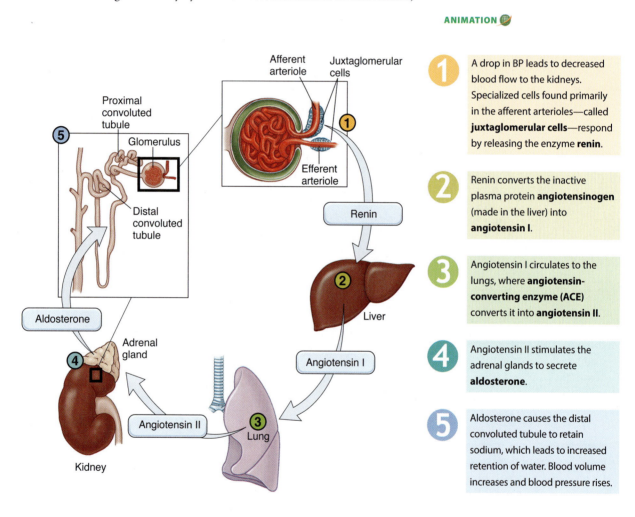

1 A drop in BP leads to decreased blood flow to the kidneys. Specialized cells found primarily in the afferent arterioles—called **juxtaglomerular cells**—respond by releasing the enzyme **renin.**

2 Renin converts the inactive plasma protein **angiotensinogen** (made in the liver) into **angiotensin I.**

3 Angiotensin I circulates to the lungs, where **angiotensin-converting enzyme (ACE)** converts it into **angiotensin II.**

4 Angiotensin II stimulates the adrenal glands to secrete **aldosterone.**

5 Aldosterone causes the distal convoluted tubule to retain sodium, which leads to increased retention of water. Blood volume increases and blood pressure rises.

FAST FACT

During circulatory shock, the sympathetic nervous system constricts the afferent arterioles to divert blood from the kidneys to the heart and brain. In this situation, the glomerular filtration rate may slow to only a few milliliters per minute.

Tubular Reabsorption and Secretion

After the filtrate leaves the glomerulus, it enters the renal tubules. Here, additional chemicals are removed from the filtrate and returned to the blood **(tubular reabsorption)** while other chemicals are added **(tubular secretion)**. Most of the water, electrolytes, and nutrients are reabsorbed in the proximal convoluted tubules by active and passive transport.

1 Sodium moves by active transport out of the proximal convoluted tubule and into the bloodstream of the peritubular capillaries. Water follows sodium, diffusing rapidly from the tubular fluid into the blood. Glucose, amino acids, chloride, potassium, and bicarbonate follow suit, passing out of the tubules and into the blood. About half of the nitrogenous waste urea is also reabsorbed.

Simultaneously, wastes such as ammonia (NH_3) and uric acid, as well as drugs (such as aspirin and penicillin), are secreted out of the blood and into the tubules. Tubular secretion of hydrogen ions also occurs, helping to regulate the body's pH.

ANIMATION 🌐

4 The distal convoluted tubule and collecting ducts reabsorb variable amounts of water and salts. Specialized cells within this part of the nephron play a role in acid-base balance, reabsorbing potassium and secreting hydrogen into the tubule. Several different hormones help regulate reabsorption by the cells in the distal convoluted tubule. (These hormones are discussed in the next section, "Hormones Affecting the Urinary System.")

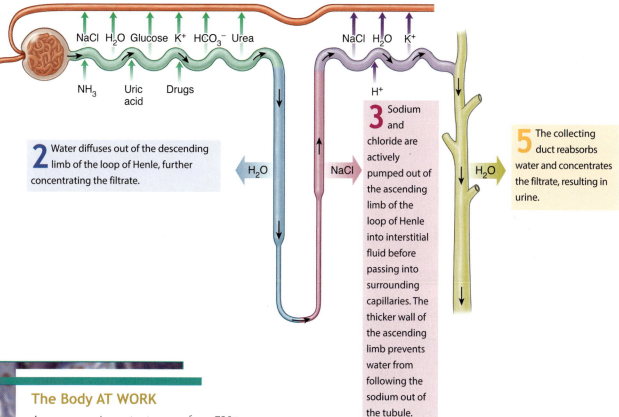

NaCl H_2O Glucose K^+ HCO_3^- Urea

NH_3 Uric acid   Drugs

NaCl H_2O K^+

H^+

2 Water diffuses out of the descending limb of the loop of Henle, further concentrating the filtrate.

H_2O

NaCl

3 Sodium and chloride are actively pumped out of the ascending limb of the loop of Henle into interstitial fluid before passing into surrounding capillaries. The thicker wall of the ascending limb prevents water from following the sodium out of the tubule.

H_2O

5 The collecting duct reabsorbs water and concentrates the filtrate, resulting in urine.

The Body AT WORK

An average urine output ranges from 720 to 2400 ml daily. However, that amount varies with fluid intake. Drinking a large volume of fluid causes urine output to increase. Conversely, restricting fluid intake leads to a diminished urine output. Other common causes of a diminished urine output include excessive perspiration or a diet high in sodium (which causes the body to retain water).

FAST FACT

Glucose is one of the body's most valuable nutrients; consequently, the tubules normally reabsorb all glucose so that none remains in the urine.

Hormones Affecting the Urinary System

Several different hormones act on the distal convoluted tubule and collecting duct to help regulate the amount of water, salt, and even calcium absorbed by this part of the nephron.

Hormone	Actions	Effects on Kidney	Effects on Blood Volume and Pressure
Aldosterone	When blood levels of Na$^+$ fall, or when the concentration of K$^+$ rises, the adrenal cortex secretes aldosterone. Called the "salt-retaining hormone," aldosterone prompts the distal convoluted tubule to absorb more Na$^+$ and secrete more K$^+$. Water and Cl$^-$ naturally follow Na$^+$, with the end result being that the body retains NaCl and water. Blood volume increases, causing blood pressure (BP) to rise.	Reabsorbs NaCl and H$_2$O Excretes K$^+$	↑ Blood volume ↑ BP
Atrial natriuretic peptide (ANP)	When blood pressure rises, the atria of the heart secrete ANP, which, in turn, inhibits the secretion of aldosterone and antidiuretic hormone. As a result, the distal convoluted tubule excretes more NaCl and water, thereby reducing blood volume and pressure.	Excretes NaCl and H$_2$O	↓ Blood volume ↓ BP
Antidiuretic hormone (ADH)	Secreted by the posterior pituitary gland (neurohypophysis), ADH causes the cells of the collecting duct to become more permeable to water. Water flows out of the tubule and into capillaries, causing urine volume to fall and blood volume to increase.	Reabsorbs H$_2$O	↑ Blood volume ↑ BP
Parathyroid hormone (PTH)	Secreted by the parathyroid glands in response to low blood calcium levels, PTH prompts the renal tubules to reabsorb more calcium and excrete more phosphate. (If the blood were to retain its phosphate levels, the reabsorbed calcium would be deposited in the bone rather than remain in circulation.)	Reabsorbs calcium Excretes phosphate	No effect on blood volume or pressure

Life lesson: Diuretics

Drugs called *diuretics* are frequently administered to increase urine volume. Increased urine volume leads to decreased blood volume *and* blood pressure, making diuretics useful in the treatment of hypertension and congestive heart failure.

Many diuretics work by blocking tubular reabsorption of sodium, which also blocks the reabsorption of water. Other drugs, such as caffeine, promote diuresis by dilating the afferent arteriole, which increases glomerular filtration rate.

That Makes Sense

The term **diuresis** means the passage of large amounts of urine. The name anti-*diuretic* means against *diuresis*. Therefore, antidiuretic hormone (ADH) prevents the passage of large amounts of urine.

Composition of Urine

Urine consists of 95% water and 5% dissolved substances. The dissolved substances include nitrogenous wastes—such as urea, uric acid, ammonia, and creatinine—as well as other solutes, such as sodium, potassium, and sulfates.

The components of urine reveal a great deal about the health of the kidneys as well as other organs of the body. That's why a **urinalysis** (an examination of the characteristics of urine) is one of the most frequently prescribed medical tests.

The following table lists the normal characteristics of urine along with the possible implications of some common abnormalities. *Note:* Glucose, blood, free hemoglobin, albumin, ketones, and bile pigments are not normally found in urine; their presence indicates a disease process.

Characteristic	Normal Finding	Possible Abnormalities
Color	Transparent pale yellow to amber	• Darker urine usually results from poor hydration. • Cloudy urine may result from bacteria, indicating an infection.
Odor	Mild	• A pungent smell (such as in a stale diaper) results when urine is allowed to stand: bacteria multiplies and converts urea into ammonia. • A sweet, fruity odor (acetone) often occurs in diabetes. • A rotten odor may indicate a urinary tract infection.
Specific gravity (Indicates the amount of solid matter in a liquid)	1.001–1.035	• A high specific gravity could result from dehydration (reflecting a low volume of water in relation to the amount of solids).
pH	Average of 6.0	• A high pH reflects alkalosis. • A low pH indicates acidosis.

FAST FACT

Comparing the amount of creatinine in the urine against the level of creatinine in the blood reflects the GFR; in turn, this reflects kidney function. A high serum creatinine indicates a low GFR and poor kidney function.

FAST FACT

Urine's yellow color results from the pigment **urochrome**, a by-product of the breakdown of hemoglobin in worn-out red blood cells.

The Body AT WORK

Most adults produce 1 to 2 liters of urine a day. A urine output of less than 400 ml/day (called **oliguria***) is insufficient for clearing waste products from the body.*

Some diseases, particularly diabetes mellitus, cause urine output to increase significantly. In this instance, high levels of glucose oppose the reabsorption of water, causing more water to pass through the kidneys and exit the body as urine. Another disorder that produces large volumes of urine is diabetes insipidus. This disorder results from hyposecretion of ADH. Without an adequate supply of ADH, the collecting duct doesn't reabsorb much water and large volumes of water pass out of the body as urine.

Storage and Elimination of Urine

The remaining structures of the urinary system are the ureters, urinary bladder, and urethra. The ureters and urethra serve as passageways for conducting urine away from the kidneys and out of the body while the bladder stores urine until it can be eliminated.

Ureters

Connecting the renal pelvis of each kidney with the bladder are slender, muscular tubes called **ureters.** Each ureter measures about 25 cm (9.8 inches) in length and has a very narrow diameter. Peristaltic waves help propel urine from the renal pelvis toward the bladder.

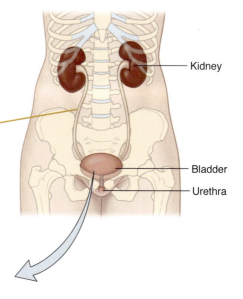

Kidney

Bladder

Urethra

FAST FACT

Because the ureter is so narrow, kidney stones can easily become lodged and obstruct the flow of urine.

Urinary Bladder

A collapsible muscular sac, the urinary bladder sits behind the symphysis pubis and below the peritoneal membrane. In women, it resides in front of the vagina and uterus; in men, it rests on top of the prostate gland.

The wall of the bladder, called the **detrusor muscle**, consists of three layers of smooth muscle.

Mucous transitional epithelium lines the bladder. When the bladder is relaxed, this layer of tissue forms folds called **rugae**. As urine fills the bladder, the rugae flatten and the epithelium thins, allowing the bladder to expand. (Considered moderately full when it contains 500 ml of urine, the bladder has a maximum capacity of about 800 ml.)

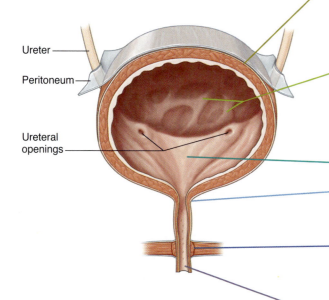

Ureter

Peritoneum

Ureteral openings

The floor of the bladder has three openings: two from the ureters (which pass behind the bladder to enter from below) and one from the urethra. Together they form a triangular-shaped, smooth area on the floor of the bladder called the **trigone**. Infections commonly attack this area of the bladder.

At the point where the urethra leaves the bladder, a ring of smooth muscle forms the **internal urethral sphincter**. This sphincter contracts involuntarily to retain urine in the bladder.

A second sphincter, called the **external urinary sphincter**, exists where the urethra passes through the pelvic floor. This sphincter consists of skeletal muscle and is, therefore, under voluntary control.

The **urethra** is a small tube that conveys urine away from the bladder and out of the body. The opening of the urethra leading to the outside of the body is called the **external urinary meatus**.

Urethra

The structure of the urethra varies between males and females.

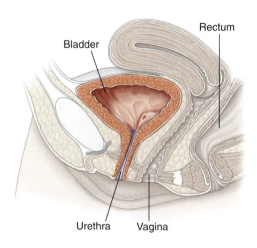

Bladder — Rectum — Urethra — Vagina

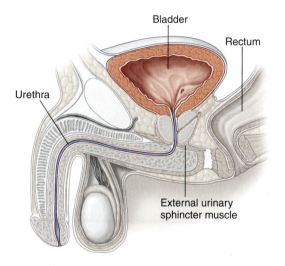

Bladder — Rectum — Urethra — External urinary sphincter muscle

Female urethra

In women, the urethra is 3 cm (1.2 inches) long and exits the body just in front of the vaginal orifice.

Male urethra

In males, the urethra is much longer, measuring about 20 cm (7.9 inches). From the bladder, the urethra passes through the center of the prostate gland, curves around to enter the penis, and then exits the body at the tip of the penis. In men, the urethra performs a dual role. Besides conveying urine, it also conveys semen. (For more information on the male reproductive system, see Chapter 23, *Reproductive Systems*.)

FAST FACT

Females are particularly prone to urinary tract infections because bacteria such as *Escherichia coli* (found in the lower digestive tract) can easily migrate up the short urethra and infect the bladder.

Life lesson: Kidney stones

Kidney stones, or *renal calculi*, result when minerals (such as calcium, phosphate, uric acid, or protein) crystallize in the renal pelvis. Many times these calculi are small enough to travel through the urinary tract and out of the body unnoticed. Sometimes, though, the stones become large enough to block the renal pelvis or ureter. When this occurs, excruciating pain results as the ureter contracts violently as it attempts to dislodge the stone. If the stone remains lodged, urine may back up to the kidney, resulting in *hydronephrosis*.

Doctors often treat renal calculi with a technique called *lithotripsy*. This technique uses ultrasound to disintegrate the stone into particles small enough to pass through the urinary tract.

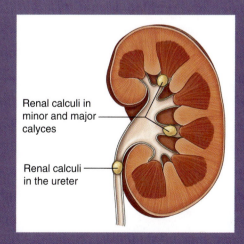

Renal calculi in minor and major calyces

Renal calculi in the ureter

Urination

Also called **micturition** or voiding, **urination** begins when the external sphincter muscle of the bladder voluntarily relaxes and the detrusor muscle of the bladder contracts. The entire process involves several steps requiring input from the central nervous system.

ANIMATION 🌐

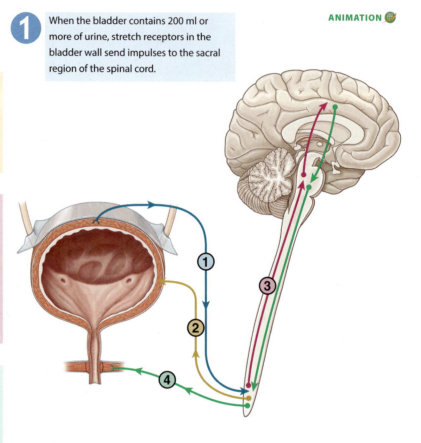

1 When the bladder contains 200 ml or more of urine, stretch receptors in the bladder wall send impulses to the sacral region of the spinal cord.

2 The spinal cord then sends motor impulses to the bladder wall to contract and to the internal sphincter to relax. When this happens, voiding will occur involuntarily *unless* the brain overrides the impulse.

3 The brain has the ability to override the impulse to void because the stretch receptors in the bladder also send impulses to the micturition center in the pons. The pons integrates information from the stretch receptors with information from other parts of the brain, such as the cerebrum, and evaluates whether the time is appropriate to urinate.

4 If the time to urinate is not appropriate, the brain sends impulses to inhibit urination and to keep the external urinary sphincter contracted. If the time to urinate is appropriate, the brain sends signals to the bladder wall to contract and to the external urethral sphincter to relax, at which point voluntary urination occurs.

Life lesson: Renal insufficiency and dialysis

Renal insufficiency (also called *renal failure*) results when an extensive number of nephrons have been destroyed through disease or injury, impairing the ability of the kidneys to function. Loss of function may occur suddenly—as in *acute renal failure*—or over time—as in *chronic renal insufficiency*.

In acute renal failure, the kidneys often stop functioning as the result of an infection, drugs, or an injury. After the cause of the renal failure is treated, kidney function may return to normal.

In contrast, chronic renal insufficiency develops over years, perhaps even decades. Typically, a disease (such as diabetes, hypertension, glomerulonephritis, or an autoimmune disorder) gradually destroys the nephrons. Eventually, damage becomes so extensive that the kidneys can no longer effectively clear blood plasma of waste. In this instance, the damage is irreversible. A variety of symptoms develop as wastes accumulate in the blood, making a kidney transplant or dialysis necessary.

There are two forms of dialysis: hemodialysis and peritoneal dialysis. In *hemodialysis*, blood is pumped from the patient's radial artery to a dialysis machine (which is sometimes called an artificial kidney). In the machine, the blood flows through a series of semi-permeable tubes immersed in dialysis fluid. Waste products such as urea, potassium, and creatinine, as well as excess water, diffuse out of the blood and into the dialysis fluid. The dialysis fluid is then discarded.

In *peritoneal dialysis*, the peritoneum serves as the semi-permeable membrane. In this procedure, dialysis fluid is introduced into the peritoneal cavity through a catheter. The fluid is left in the body cavity for a few minutes to an hour, during which time waste products diffuse out of the blood and into the dialysate. At the end of the specified time, the fluid is drained and discarded.

Review of Key Terms

Aldosterone: Hormone that causes the distal convoluted tubule to retain sodium, which leads to the retention of water, resulting in increased blood pressure

Angiotensin: A plasma protein produced when renin is released from the kidney; angiotensin II stimulates the adrenal glands to secrete aldosterone

Antidiuretic hormone: Hormone that inhibits diuresis by stimulating the kidneys to conserve water

Bowman's capsule: Two layers of epithelial cells that envelop the glomerulus in an open-ended covering; also called a glomerular capsule

Calyx: A cup-like structure that collects urine leaving the papilla of the kidney

Collecting duct: Receives drainage from the distal convoluted tubules of several different nephrons; eventually drains into a minor calyx

Detrusor muscle: Wall of the bladder

Diuresis: The secretion of large amounts of urine

Glomerulus: Cluster of capillaries that are part of the renal corpuscles in the nephrons

Hilum: Concave notch on medial side of kidney; where blood vessels, the ureters, and nerves enter and leave the kidney

Loop of Henle: U-shaped portion of the renal tubule

Micturition: Urination

Nephrons: The filtration units of the kidney

Peritubular capillaries: Network of capillaries surrounding the renal tubules

Renal corpuscles: One of the main components of nephrons, consisting of a glomerulus and Bowman's capsule, that filters blood plasma

Renal cortex: Outer region of the kidney; site of urine production

Renal medulla: Inner region of the kidney; site of urine collection

Renal tubules: Series of tube-like structures within the nephron; where urine is formed

Renin: Enzyme released by the kidneys in response to a drop in blood pressure that causes the conversion of angiotensinogen into angiotensin I

Specific gravity: Measurement that indicates the amount of solid matter in a liquid

Tubular resorption: Process whereby chemicals are removed from filtrate in the renal tubules and returned to the blood

Tubular secretion: Process whereby chemicals are added to the filtrate in the renal tubules

Ureters: Muscular tubes connecting the renal pelvis of each kidney with the bladder

Urethra: Small tube that conveys urine away from the bladder and out of the body

Urinary bladder: Collapsible muscular sac that stores urine

Own the Information

To make the information in this chapter part of your working memory, take some time to reflect on what you've learned. On a separate sheet of paper, write down everything you recall from the chapter. After you're done, log on to the DavisPlus website, and check out the Study Group podcast and Study Group Questions for the chapter.

Key Topics for Chapter 18:
- Location of the kidney
- The internal and external structures of the kidney
- Blood flow through the kidney
- Nerve supply to the kidney
- Structure and function of the nephron
- Structure and function of the renal tubule
- Process of glomerular filtration
- Regulation of the glomerular filtration rate
- The renin-angiotensin-aldosterone system
- Tubular reabsorption and secretion occurring in the different parts of the renal tubule
- Hormones affecting the urinary system
- The composition of urine
- The structure and function of the ureters, urinary bladder, and urethra
- The process of urination

Test Your Knowledge

1. The cluster of capillaries in the nephron is the:
   a. renal corpuscle.
   b. loop of Henle.
   c. proximal convoluted tubule.
   d. glomerulus.

2. The location where blood vessels, nerves, and the ureter enter and leave the kidney is the:
   a. renal pelvis.
   b. hilum.
   c. calyx.
   d. renal pyramid.

3. The portion of the nephron in charge of making urine is the:
   a. renal corpuscle.
   b. renal tubule.
   c. Bowman's capsule.
   d. afferent arteriole.

4. Most sodium is reabsorbed from the glomerular filtrate in the:
   a. proximal convoluted tubule.
   b. distal convoluted tubule.
   c. collecting duct.
   d. glomerulus.

5. Which of the following substances should never be found in urine?
   a. Sodium
   b. Urea
   c. Glucose
   d. Potassium

6. The hormone aldosterone:
   a. causes the distal convoluted tubule to reabsorb more sodium, which leads to water retention and a rise in blood pressure.
   b. causes the distal convoluted tubule to excrete more sodium and water, thereby reducing blood pressure.
   c. causes the distal and collecting tubules to become more permeable to water.
   d. prompts the renal tubules to reabsorb more calcium and excrete more phosphate.

7. Many diuretics work by blocking tubular reabsorption of:
   a. water.
   b. glucose.
   c. sodium.
   d. potassium.

Answers: Chapter 18

1. *Correct answer:* **d.** The renal corpuscle consists of a glomerulus and Bowman's capsule. The loop of Henle is the hairpin turn taken by the renal tubule between the proximal and distal convoluted tubule. The proximal convoluted tubule is a winding portion of the renal tubule arising from Bowman's capsule.

2. *Correct answer:* **b.** The renal pelvis, formed by the convergence of the major calyces, channels urine out of the kidney. The calyx collects urine leaving the papilla. Renal pyramids are the cone-shaped sections in the kidney.

3. *Correct answer:* **b.** The renal corpuscle filters blood plasma. Bowman's capsule is part of the renal corpuscle. An afferent arteriole supplies blood to a nephron.

4. *Correct answer:* **a.** The distal convoluted tubule and collecting ducts reabsorb variable amounts of water and salt. In the glomerulus, water and small solutes filter out of the blood and into the surrounding space of Bowman's capsule.

5. *Correct answer:* **c.** The other substances are all normal constituents of urine.

6. *Correct answer:* **a.** Atrial natriuretic peptide (ANP) causes the distal convoluted tubule to excrete more sodium and water, thereby reducing blood pressure. Antidiuretic hormone (ADH) causes the distal and collecting tubules to become more permeable to water. Parathyroid hormone (PTH) prompts the renal tubules to reabsorb more calcium and excrete more phosphate.

7. *Correct answer:* **c.** None of the other answers is correct.

8. *Correct answer:* **d.** In women, the urethra is much shorter than it is in men; therefore, bacteria from the nearby rectal area can easily migrate up the short tube to the bladder. The other structures are similar in both men and women.

9. *Correct answer:* **c.** None of the other answers is correct.

10. *Correct answer:* **d.** Rugae are folds of tissue on the inside of the bladder. Papillae are the blunt points of the renal pyramids. The cortex is the outer zone of the kidney.

8. In women, the _____ is shorter than it is in men, which contributes to the higher incidence of urinary tract infections in women.
   a. urinary sphincter
   b. loop of Henle
   c. ureter
   d. urethra

9. Urination occurs when:
   a. the bladder and internal urethral sphincter relax.
   b. the bladder and external urethral sphincter contract.
   c. the bladder contracts and the external urethral sphincter relaxes.
   d. the bladder relaxes and the external urethral sphincter contracts.

10. A triangular-shaped smooth area on the floor of the bladder is called the:
   a. rugae.
   b. papilla.
   c. cortex.
   d. trigone.

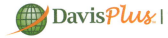

Go to **http://davisplus.fadavis.com** Keyword: Thompson to see all of the resources available with this chapter.

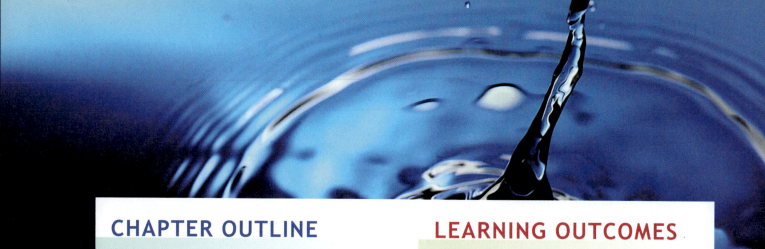

CHAPTER OUTLINE

Water Balance

Electrolyte Balance

Acid-Base Balance

Acid-Base Imbalances

LEARNING OUTCOMES

1. Name the major fluid compartments.

2. Explain how fluid moves from one compartment to another.

3. Identify the means by which the body normally gains and loses fluid.

4. Describe the mechanisms for regulating intake and output.

5. Differentiate between volume depletion and dehydration.

6. Discuss the fluid shifts that occur in dehydration.

7. Explain the physiological consequences of fluid excess.

8. Explain how edema occurs.

9. Identify the main electrolytes found in intracellular and extracellular fluid.

10. Explain the roles of sodium in the body.

11. Describe the mechanisms used by the body to regulate the levels of sodium.

12. Identify common causes and consequences of sodium, potassium, and calcium imbalances.

13. Define *buffer*.

14. Explain how chemical buffers can alter pH in the body.

15. Explain how the respiratory system can alter the pH in the body.

16. Describe how the kidneys help control pH.

17. Pinpoint the timeframe during which each buffer system responds.

18. Identify the causes of respiratory acidosis and alkalosis.

19. Identify the causes of metabolic acidosis and alkalosis.

20. Describe how the lungs and kidneys compensate for acid-base imbalances.

chapter

19

FLUID, ELECTROLYTE, & ACID-BASE BALANCE

Approximately two-thirds of the body—or about 50% to 70% of an adult's weight—consists of water.

The body is awash in fluid: it surrounds cells, fills tissues, and, of course, is the main component of blood and lymph. While this fluid is primarily water, it also contains thousands of dissolved substances, such as electrolytes, that are used in the body's biochemical reactions. If the quantity of fluid, the concentration of electrolytes, or the pH strays outside precise boundaries, life-threatening disorders may occur. In other words, homeostasis depends upon *balance*—of water, electrolytes, and pH.

Water Balance

The maintenance of water balance involves more than the total volume of fluid within the body. How that fluid is divided among the various fluid compartments is also important.

Fluid Compartments

Most of the body's water (about 65%) resides inside cells; this is called **intracellular fluid (ICF)**. The remaining 35% of the body's water resides outside cells: this is called **extracellular fluid (ECF)**. Extracellular fluid includes the fluid between the cells inside tissue, called **interstitial fluid**, as well as the fluid within vessels as blood plasma and lymph. Various other extracellular fluids—such as cerebrospinal fluid, synovial fluid in the joints, vitreous and aqueous humors of the eye, and digestive secretions—are called **transcellular fluid**.

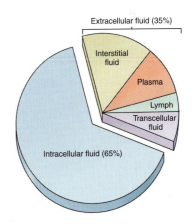

Extracellular fluid (35%)

Interstitial fluid

Plasma

Lymph

Transcellular fluid

Intracellular fluid (65%)

That Makes Sense

To remember the names for the various body fluids, keep this in mind: the prefix intra- *means "within" (as in intravenous fluids) while the prefix* extra- *means "outside of" (as in extracurricular activities). Therefore, intracellular means "within the cell," while extracellular means "outside of the cell."*

Furthermore, the prefix inter- *means "between." (For example, the word* intercede *means "to come between two parties.") Therefore, interstitial fluid refers to fluid between cells.*

FAST FACT

A man's body weight is about 55% to 60% water, while women average slightly less because of an increased amount of body fat. (Adipose tissue contains less water than muscle. In fact, the weight of an obese person may be only 45% water.) In contrast, the weight of a newborn infant is as much as 75% water.

The Body AT WORK

Fluid doesn't remain locked within a single compartment. Rather, ICF and ECF continually mingle, as the fluid easily passes through the semipermeable membrane surrounding each compartment. The concentration of solutes (particularly electrolytes) within each compartment determines the amount and direction of flow. For example:

- *If the concentration of electrolytes (and therefore the osmolarity) of tissue fluid rises, water moves out of the cells and into the tissues.*

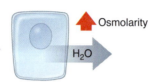

Osmolarity

H_2O

- *If the osmolarity of tissue fluid falls, water moves out of the tissues and into the cells. The passage of fluid happens within seconds so as to maintain equilibrium. (The various electrolytes and their role in water balance are discussed later in this chapter.)*

Osmolarity

H_2O

FAST FACT

Water loss varies considerably with environmental temperature as well as physical activity. For example, cold, dry air increases respiratory loss while hot, humid air increases the loss through perspiration. Also, heavy physical exercise increases fluid loss through perspiration.

Balancing Water Gain and Loss

Normally, the amount of water gained and lost by the body through the course of a day is equal. Specifically, an adult gains and loses about 2500 ml of fluid each day. Most fluid intake occurs through eating and drinking; however, the cells themselves produce a fair amount of water as a by-product of metabolic reactions. (This is called *metabolic* water.) Fluid is lost through the kidneys (as urine), the intestines (as feces), the skin (by sweat as well as diffusion), and the lungs (through expired air).

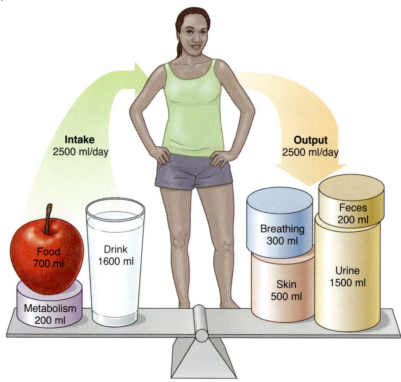

Intake 2500 ml/day

Food 700 ml

Drink 1600 ml

Metabolism 200 ml

Output 2500 ml/day

Feces 200 ml

Breathing 300 ml

Skin 500 ml

Urine 1500 ml

Regulation of Intake and Output

To keep the total volume of water in the body in balance, the body uses mechanisms that adjust fluid intake as well as urine output.

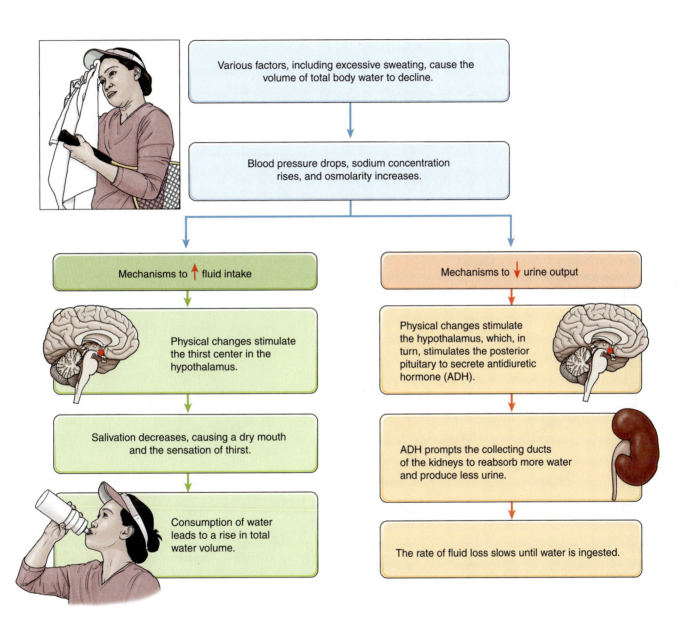

Various factors, including excessive sweating, cause the volume of total body water to decline.

Blood pressure drops, sodium concentration rises, and osmolarity increases.

Mechanisms to ↑ fluid intake

Physical changes stimulate the thirst center in the hypothalamus.

Salivation decreases, causing a dry mouth and the sensation of thirst.

Consumption of water leads to a rise in total water volume.

Mechanisms to ↓ urine output

Physical changes stimulate the hypothalamus, which, in turn, stimulates the posterior pituitary to secrete antidiuretic hormone (ADH).

ADH prompts the collecting ducts of the kidneys to reabsorb more water and produce less urine.

The rate of fluid loss slows until water is ingested.

FAST FACT

Elderly adults have a diminished sensation of thirst, placing them at risk for dehydration.

The Body AT WORK

When blood volume and pressure are too high, or blood osmolarity is too low, the hypothalamus inhibits the release of ADH. This causes the renal tubules to reabsorb less water, leading to an increased urine output and a decline in total body water.

Disorders of Water Balance

A water imbalance can result from an abnormality in any of the following: fluid volume, fluid concentration, or the distribution of fluid between compartments.

Fluid Deficiency

A fluid deficiency occurs when output exceeds intake over a period of time. There are two types of fluid deficiency: volume depletion (**hypovolemia**) and dehydration.

- **Volume depletion** results from blood loss or when both sodium and water are lost, such as from diarrhea.
- **Dehydration** results when the body eliminates more water than sodium. Not only is there a loss of fluid, the concentration of sodium (and the osmolarity) of the extracellular fluid (ECF) also rises. The increase in osmolarity prompts the shifting of fluid from one compartment to another in an effort to balance the concentration of sodium. (See "Life Lesson: Dehydration" on this page.) Basically, dehydration results from consuming an inadequate amount of water to cover the amount of water lost. Other causes include diabetes mellitus and the use of diuretics.

When severe, fluid deficiency can lead to circulatory collapse (**hypovolemic shock**) due to loss of blood volume.

The Body AT WORK

*The fluid within tissues—interstitial fluid—is a ready source of fluid to help maintain blood volume during the early stages of fluid loss. As tissue loses fluid, it also loses elasticity, or **turgor**. A common test to evaluate hydration status involves lightly pinching the skin on the back of the hand, lower arm, or abdomen. When hydration is normal, the skin will spring back to its normal shape when released. During dehydration, the skin remains peaked, flattening slowly. The persistence of pinched skin after release resembles a tent, which is why this finding is called **tenting**.*

FAST FACT

Infants are more prone to dehydration than adults are. That's because their immature kidneys don't concentrate urine effectively, they have a high metabolism that requires more water to flush out toxins, and they have a large surface area in relationship to their volume, meaning they lose more water to evaporation.

Life lesson: Dehydration

Dehydration affects all fluid compartments. For example, if you exercise strenuously on a hot day, you will lose a significant amount of water through sweat. The water in sweat comes from the bloodstream. As water shifts out of the bloodstream, the osmolarity of the blood rises. To compensate, fluid moves from the tissues into the bloodstream. The loss of fluid from the tissues causes the osmolarity of the fluid in this space to rise. If the imbalance continues, fluid will shift out of the cells and into the tissues, resulting in a depletion of intracellular fluid. Consequently, dehydration affects the bloodstream, tissues, and cells.

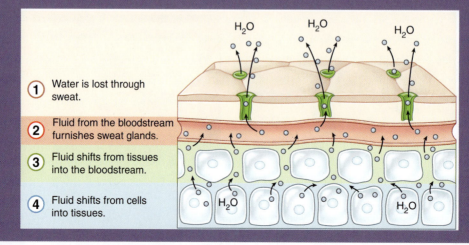

1. Water is lost through sweat.
2. Fluid from the bloodstream furnishes sweat glands.
3. Fluid shifts from tissues into the bloodstream.
4. Fluid shifts from cells into tissues.

Fluid Excess

The kidneys usually compensate for excessive fluid intake by producing more urine; consequently, fluid excess occurs less commonly than fluid deficit. However, when a fluid excess does occur, it can be life-threatening.

One cause of fluid excess is renal failure. (In this instance, both sodium and water are retained, and the ECF remains isotonic.) Another type of fluid excess is called **water intoxication**. Water intoxication can occur if someone consumes an excessive amount of water or if someone replaces heavy losses of water and sodium (such as from profuse sweating) with just water. When this occurs, the amount of sodium in the ECF drops. Water moves into the cells, causing them to swell. Possible complications of either type of fluid excess include pulmonary or cerebral edema.

Fluid Accumulation

Another type of water imbalance involves the accumulation of fluid within a body compartment. For example, **edema** occurs when fluid accumulates in interstitial spaces, causing tissues to swell. Even though fluid can accumulate in any organ or tissue in the body, it typically affects the lungs, brain, and dependent areas (such as the legs). A disturbance in any of the factors regulating the movement of fluid between blood plasma and the interstitial compartment—such as electrolyte imbalances, increased capillary pressure, and decreased concentration of plasma proteins—can trigger edema.

Electrolyte Balance

Electrolytes are substances that break up into electrically charged particles called ions when dissolved in water. For example, sodium chloride (NaCl) breaks up into Na^+, a cation carrying a positive charge, and Cl^-, an anion carrying a negative charge. A balance of electrolytes is crucial for the body to function properly: electrolytes drive chemical reactions, affect distribution of the body's water content, and determine a cell's electrical potential.

The major cations of the body are sodium (Na^+), potassium (K^+), calcium (Ca^{2+}), and hydrogen (H^+). The major anions are chloride (Cl^-), bicarbonate (HCO_3^-), and phosphates (P_i). The following table shows the chief electrolytes, their concentration in blood plasma, and the terms used to describe imbalances. (Of the electrolytes listed, the body can tolerate broad variations in phosphate, making homeostasis of this substance not as crucial as that of sodium, potassium, calcium, and chloride.)

> **FAST FACT**
>
> Although sodium (Na^+), potassium (K^+), calcium (Ca^{2+}) and chloride (Cl^-) are really ions, they are commonly referred to as electrolytes.

Electrolyte Concentrations

Electrolyte	Plasma Level	Term for Imbalances	
		Deficiency	Excess
Sodium (Na^+)	136 to 146 mEq/l	Hyponatremia	Hypernatremia
Potassium (K^+)	3.6 to 5.0 mEq/l	Hypokalemia	Hyperkalemia
Calcium (Ca^{2+})	8.8 to 10.3 mEq/l	Hypocalcemia	Hypercalcemia
Chloride (Cl^-)	96 to 106 mEq/l	Hypochloremia	Hyperchloremia
Phosphate (PO_4^{3-})	2.4 to 4.1 mEq/l	Hypophosphatemia	Hyperphosphatemia

> **FAST FACT**
>
> *Remember:* Cations refer to ions with a positive charge; anions refer to ions with a negative charge.

Sodium

Sodium is the main electrolyte in extracellular fluid, accounting for 90% of its osmolarity. Sodium not only determines the volume of total body water but also influences how body water is distributed between fluid compartments. Furthermore, sodium plays a key role in depolarization, making it crucial for proper nerve and muscle function.

Sodium levels are primarily regulated by aldosterone and ADH: aldosterone adjusts the excretion of sodium while ADH adjusts the excretion of water, as described below.

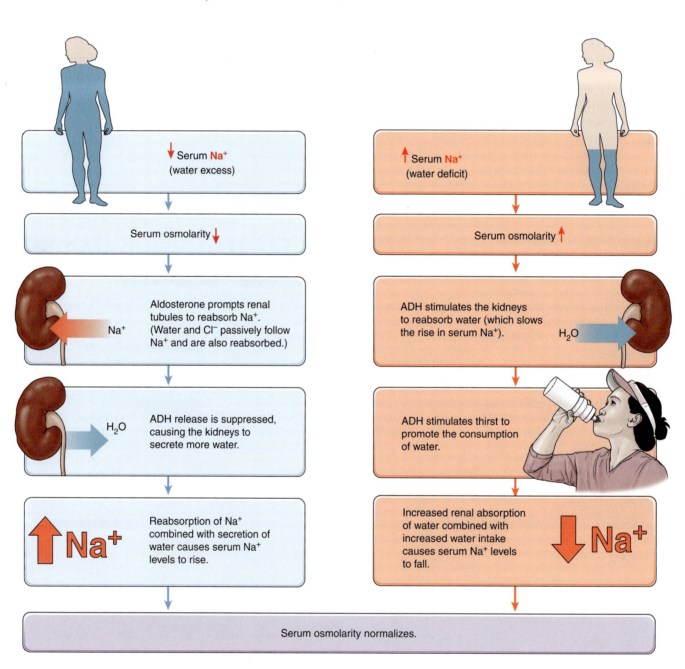

↓ Serum Na⁺ (water excess)

↑ Serum Na⁺ (water deficit)

Serum osmolarity ↓

Serum osmolarity ↑

Na⁺ — Aldosterone prompts renal tubules to reabsorb Na⁺. (Water and Cl⁻ passively follow Na⁺ and are also reabsorbed.)

ADH stimulates the kidneys to reabsorb water (which slows the rise in serum Na⁺). — H₂O

H₂O — ADH release is suppressed, causing the kidneys to secrete more water.

ADH stimulates thirst to promote the consumption of water.

↑Na⁺ — Reabsorption of Na⁺ combined with secretion of water causes serum Na⁺ levels to rise.

Increased renal absorption of water combined with increased water intake causes serum Na⁺ levels to fall. — ↓Na⁺

Serum osmolarity normalizes.

Sodium Imbalances

Imbalances in sodium—the chief cation in **extracellular** fluid—affects total body water, the distribution of water between compartments, and nerve and muscle function.

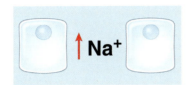

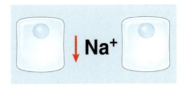

Hypernatremia

- **Hypernatremia** refers to a plasma sodium concentration greater than 146 mEq/l.
- It usually indicates a water deficit (such as from a lack of fluid intake).
- Other possible causes include an excessive loss of body water, such as from severe diarrhea or the use of certain types of diuretics.
- Hypernatremia usually self-corrects because even a small rise in sodium triggers thirst. (An exception is elderly adults, who tend to have an impaired thirst mechanism.)
- If uncorrected, hypernatremia can cause edema, lethargy, and weakness.

Hyponatremia

- **Hyponatremia** refers to a plasma sodium concentration of less than 139 mEq/l.
- It usually results from an excess of body water, such as when someone drinks only water to replace heavy losses of sodium and water through perspiration.
- Hyponatremia is usually corrected by excretion of excess water.
- Uncorrected, hyponatremia can result in pulmonary or cerebral edema as fluid moves into cells.

Potassium

Potassium is the chief cation of intracellular fluid, just as sodium is the chief cation of extracellular fluid. Potassium works hand-in-hand with sodium. For example, potassium is crucial for proper nerve and muscle function (which also depends upon adequate levels of sodium). Furthermore, aldosterone regulates serum levels of potassium, just as it does sodium. Rising potassium levels stimulate the adrenal cortex to secrete aldosterone; aldosterone causes the kidneys to excrete potassium as they reabsorb sodium.

> **FAST FACT**
>
> Potassium imbalances are the most dangerous of any electrolyte imbalance: very high levels are considered a medical emergency.

Potassium Imbalances

Imbalances in potassium—the chief electrolyte of intracellular fluid—can develop suddenly or over a long period of time. Either way, imbalances can cause life-threatening cardiac arrhythmias.

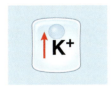

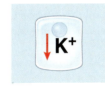

Hyperkalemia

- **Hyperkalemia** refers to a plasma concentration of K^+ above 5.0 mEq/l.
- It may develop suddenly following a crush injury or severe burn (as damaged cells release large amounts of K^+ into the bloodstream).
- It may also develop gradually from the use of potassium-sparing diuretics or renal insufficiency.
- Hyperkalemia makes nerve and muscle cells irritable, leading to potentially fatal cardiac arrhythmias.

Hypokalemia

- **Hypokalemia** refers to a plasma concentration of K^+ less than 3.5 mEq/l.
- It often results from prolonged use of potassium-wasting diuretics.
- It may also result from chronic vomiting or diarrhea.
- Hypokalemia causes K^+ to move out of cells into plasma, making cells less excitable.
- Hypokalemia results in muscle weakness, depressed reflexes, and cardiac arrhythmias.

Calcium

Besides strengthening bones, calcium plays a key role in muscle contraction, nerve transmission, and blood clotting. Plasma calcium levels are regulated by parathyroid hormone, which affects intestinal absorption of calcium and enhances the release of calcium from bones.

Calcium Imbalances

Calcium is a cation that exists mostly outside the cell.

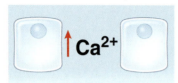

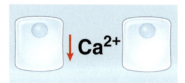

Hypercalcemia

- **Hypercalcemia** refers to a plasma concentration above 5.8 mEq/l.
- It may result from hyperparathyroidism, hypothyroidism, or alkalosis.
- Hypercalcemia inhibits depolarization of nerve and muscles cells, leading to muscle weakness, depressed reflexes, and cardiac arrhythmia.

Hypocalcemia

- **Hypocalcemia** refers to a plasma concentration below 4.5 mEq/l.
- It may result from hypoparathyroidism, hyperthyroidism, acidosis, or diarrhea.
- Hypocalcemia increases excitation of nerves and muscles, leading to muscle spasms and tetany.

Chloride and Phosphate

Chloride, the most abundant extracellular anion, is strongly linked to sodium. As sodium is retained or excreted, so is chloride. Therefore, chloride balance occurs along with sodium balance. Chloride contributes to the formation of stomach acid and also helps regulate fluid balance and pH. Phosphate participates in carbohydrate metabolism, bone formation, and acid-base balance.

Acid-Base Balance

One of the most important factors influencing homeostasis is the body's balance between acids and bases. Even slight deviations in pH can have profound, even fatal, consequences. Most enzymes used in the body's metabolic reactions are very sensitive to pH; the slightest change can dramatically slow, or even halt, metabolic activity. Electrolyte activity, too, can be profoundly affected by changes in pH, as can that of hormones.

Acids and Bases

The pH of a solution is determined by its concentration of hydrogen (H^+) ions.
- An acid is any chemical that *releases* H^+ in solution.
  - Strong acids dissociate freely in solution, releasing most of their H^+ ions and can, consequently, markedly lower the pH of a solution.
  - Weak acids release few H^+ ions in solution; consequently, they don't affect pH.

- A base is any chemical that *accepts* H^+.
  - A strong base has a strong tendency to bind H^+, removing the H^+ out of a solution and raising the pH.
  - A weak base binds few of the available H ions and has less of an effect on pH.

(For further review of acids, bases, and pH, see Chapter 2, *Chemistry of Life*.)

FAST FACT

As the concentration of H^+ ions increases, the pH decreases and the solution becomes more acidic.

The Body AT WORK

The pH of blood and tissue fluid ranges from 7.35 to 7.45. Maintaining the pH within this very narrow range is no small feat. Not only do we introduce acids into our bodies through food, the body's metabolic processes also continually produce acids. For example, anaerobic metabolism produces lactic acid; the catabolism of nucleic acids produces phosphoric acids; and the catabolism of fat produces fatty acids and ketones.

Buffers

The body employs various mechanisms, called **buffers,** to keep acids and bases in balance. A buffer is any mechanism that resists changes in pH by converting a strong acid or base into a weak one. There are two categories of buffers: chemical buffers and physiological buffers.

Chemical Buffers

Chemical buffers use a chemical to bind H^+ and remove it from solution when levels rise too high and to release H^+ when levels fall. The three main chemical buffer systems are the **bicarbonate buffer system**, the **phosphate buffer system**, and the **protein buffer system**. Each system uses a pair of chemicals: a weak base to bind H^+ ions and a weak acid to release them. The bicarbonate buffer system—the main buffering system of extracellular fluid—uses bicarbonate and carbonic acid. This reaction is detailed in the figure below. Note that this reaction is *reversible:* it proceeds to the right when the body needs to lower pH, and it proceeds to the left when pH needs to be raised.

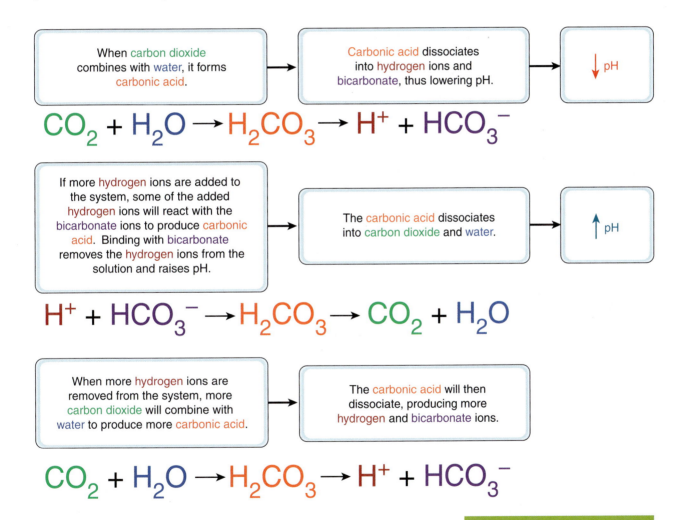

When carbon dioxide combines with water, it forms carbonic acid.

Carbonic acid dissociates into hydrogen ions and bicarbonate, thus lowering pH.

↓ pH

$$CO_2 + H_2O \rightarrow H_2CO_3 \rightarrow H^+ + HCO_3^-$$

If more hydrogen ions are added to the system, some of the added hydrogen ions will react with the bicarbonate ions to produce carbonic acid. Binding with bicarbonate removes the hydrogen ions from the solution and raises pH.

The carbonic acid dissociates into carbon dioxide and water.

↑ pH

$$H^+ + HCO_3^- \rightarrow H_2CO_3 \rightarrow CO_2 + H_2O$$

When more hydrogen ions are removed from the system, more carbon dioxide will combine with water to produce more carbonic acid.

The carbonic acid will then dissociate, producing more hydrogen and bicarbonate ions.

$$CO_2 + H_2O \rightarrow H_2CO_3 \rightarrow H^+ + HCO_3^-$$

FAST FACT

In the kidneys and red blood cells, the enzyme *carbonic anhydrase* accelerates the reactions of the bicarbonate buffer system, allowing them to occur at lightning speed.

Physiological Buffers

Physiological buffers use the respiratory and urinary systems to alter the output of acids, bases, or CO_2. In turn, this stabilizes pH.

Respiratory Control of pH

The metabolism of food constantly produces CO_2 as a byproduct. When CO_2 increases, so does the concentration of H^+ ions. (Recall the equation for the bicarbonate buffer system: when CO_2 reacts with water, H^+ ions result.) Normally, the lungs expel CO_2 at the same rate that metabolic processes produce it, keeping pH in balance. If CO_2 begins to accumulate in the bloodstream, the respiratory physiological buffer system begins to act.

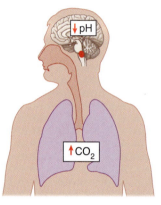

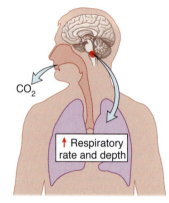

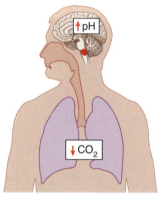

1 Central chemoreceptors in the brainstem detect a fall in pH resulting from an accumulation of CO_2.

2 The central chemoreceptors signal the respiratory centers to increase the rate and depth of breathing, resulting in the expulsion of more CO_2.

3 Since less CO_2 is available to combine with water to form carbonic acid, the concentration of H^+ ions falls and pH rises.

The opposite is also true. When pH rises, the respiratory rate slows, which allows CO_2 to accumulate. The concentration of H^+ ions increases and pH drops.

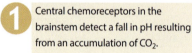

The Body AT WORK

Not all the buffer systems begin work at the same time. Chemical buffers respond first, followed by the respiratory system and, finally, the renal system.

- *When blood plasma pH rises above or falls below normal, chemical buffers respond instantaneously. Chemical buffers often restore blood plasma to a normal pH within a fraction of a second.*
- *If pH remains outside the normal range for more than 1 to 2 minutes, the respiratory system changes the rate and depth of breathing. This adjusts the amount of CO_2, which, in turn, alters H^+ ion concentration and helps stabilize pH.*
- *If the pH continues outside the normal range despite the involvement of chemical buffers and the respiratory system, the renal physiological buffer system becomes involved. The renal system can neutralize more acids or bases than either of the other systems; however, it's the slowest to respond, taking as long as 24 hours to be initiated.*

FAST FACT

Death occurs when pH falls below 6.8 or rises above 8.0.

Renal Control of pH

The kidneys are the only buffer system that actually expels H^+ ions from the body. At the same time, they also reabsorb bicarbonate, the predominant buffer in extracellular fluid. This double effect makes the renal system the most powerful of all the buffer systems. The following figure details how the kidneys help control pH.

ANIMATION

Peritubular capillary | Renal tubular cells | Tubular fluid

1 Carbon dioxide leaves the blood and enters into cells along the distal kidney tubules.

CO_2

2 In these cells, CO_2 combines with water to form carbonic acid (H_2CO_3).

$CO_2 + H_2O$

H_2CO_3

3 The carbonic acid immediately dissociates to yield hydrogen ions and bicarbonate ions.
  • The hydrogen ions diffuse out of the cell and into the tubular fluid, where they displace sodium.
  • The displaced sodium diffuses into the tubular cell, where it combines with the bicarbonate to form sodium bicarbonate.

H^+ ----→ H^+

H_2CO_3

$(Na)HCO_3^-$

Na^+

4 Sodium bicarbonate is then reabsorbed into the blood.

$NaHCO_3$

5 The end result is that H^+ ions are excreted into the urine (making the urine acidic) while sodium bicarbonate is reabsorbed into the blood. Both actions help raise plasma pH.

H^+

↓

Urine

That Makes Sense

The key to understanding the acid-base buffer system is to realize that the body operates within a very narrow pH range. Fighting against this are the body's own cells. Cells constantly produce CO_2 as a by-product of metabolic reactions. In turn, CO_2 reacts with water to produce H^+ (an acid). The body combats this continual production of acid by:

- *Binding with and "disguising" the acid (by way of the chemical buffer system)*
- *Expelling CO_2 (through the respiratory system)*
- *Excreting H^+ ions (through the renal system)*

FAST FACT

The brush border of the renal tubule cells contain the enzyme carbonic anhydrase, which accelerates the breakdown of H_2CO_3 into CO_2 and H_2O.

Acid-Base Imbalances

Maintaining the body's normal pH range of 7.35 to 7.45 depends on a precise ratio of bicarbonate ions to carbonic acid.

An excess of carbonic acid (resulting in a gain in acid) causes the scale to dip toward acidosis.

An excess of bicarbonate (resulting in a loss of acid) causes the scale to dip toward alkalosis.

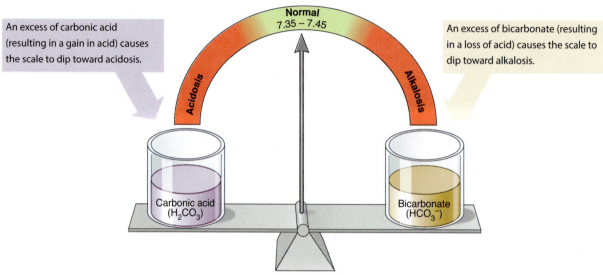

Depending upon the type of disturbance causing the change in acid concentration, the imbalance is classified as either **respiratory** or **metabolic.** Respiratory imbalances result from either an excess or deficiency of CO_2. (*Remember:* CO_2 combines with water to produce carbonic acid, which quickly dissociates to produce H^+. So, an excess of CO_2 results in acidosis while a deficiency results in alkalosis.) On the other hand, metabolic imbalances result from an excess or deficiency of bicarbonate. (*Remember:* Bicarbonate is a buffer that helps bind H^+.) Keep in mind that a deficiency of bicarbonate may also result from a generation of acids that would use up the bicarbonate.

Either way, the end result is a gain or loss of acid, which affects pH. The following table outlines some of the chief causes of acid gains and losses.

Causes of Acid Gain and Losses

Reaction	Causes of Acid Gain (Acidosis)	Causes of Acid Loss (Alkalosis)
Respiratory	• Retention of CO_2 (hypoventilation—such as from emphysema or pneumonia—as well as apnea)	• Loss of CO_2 (hyperventilation)
Metabolic	• Increased production of acids (such as ketone bodies in diabetes mellitus or lactic acid in anaerobic metabolism)	• Loss of gastric juices (such as through vomiting or suctioning)
	• Consumption of acidic drugs (such as aspirin)	• Excessive ingestion of bicarbonates (such as antacids)
	• Inability of the kidneys to excrete H^+ ions	
	• Loss of bicarbonate (such as chronic diarrhea or overuse of laxatives)	

The Body AT WORK

Acid-base imbalances directly effect blood potassium levels. As discussed previously, potassium imbalances can cause life-threatening cardiac arrhythmias.

ACIDOSIS → HYPERKALEMIA

In acidosis, plasma contains an excess concentration of H^+. As the body tries to achieve acid-base balance, H^+ moves out of the plasma and into the cells. The gain of cations inside the cell changes the polarity of the cell. So, to restore polarity, K^+ moves out of the cell as H^+ moves in. The movement of K^+ into plasma results in hyperkalemia.

ALKALOSIS → HYPOKALEMIA

Just the opposite occurs in alkalosis. Because plasma contains a low concentration of H^+, H^+ moves out of cells and into plasma; at the same time, K^+ moves out of the plasma and into the cells. The movement of K^+ out of plasma results in hypokalemia.

Compensation for Acid-Base Imbalances

In general, the body uses the respiratory system to compensate for metabolic pH imbalances and the kidneys to compensate for respiratory pH imbalances.

Respiratory Compensation

Changing the rate of ventilation alters the concentration of CO_2 in the plasma and, therefore, alters pH. Obviously, the respiratory system can't compensate for acid-base imbalances caused by a respiratory disturbance, but for imbalances with a metabolic cause, the respiratory system is the quickest means of raising or lowering pH.

- If the pH is too low, as in metabolic acidosis, the respiratory center increases the rate of respirations. The increased respiratory rate "blows off" CO_2, which raises pH.

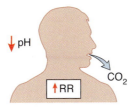

- In metabolic alkalosis, the pH is too high. Breathing slows, allowing CO_2 to accumulate, and pH drops.

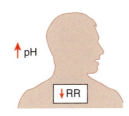

Renal Compensation

Although the kidneys are the most effective regulators of pH, they take hours or even days to respond to an acid-base imbalance. The kidneys alter pH by adjusting the rate of H^+ ion excretion.

- In response to acidosis, the kidneys eliminate H^+ and reabsorb more bicarbonate.

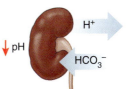

- In response to alkalosis, the kidneys conserve H^+ and excrete more bicarbonate.

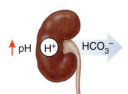

The Body AT WORK

High H^+ ion concentration depresses the central nervous system, which is why acidosis causes symptoms such as disorientation, confusion, and coma. Alkalosis, on the other hand, makes the nervous system more excitable, resulting in symptoms such as tetany and convulsions.

FAST FACT

Although respiratory compensation is powerful, it doesn't eliminate fixed acids, like lactic acid or ketone bodies. To restore balance in those situations, renal compensation is also necessary.

Review of Key Terms

Acidosis: A decrease in the pH of the blood due to an accumulation of acids; may result from respiratory or metabolic disturbances

Alkalosis: An increase in the pH of the blood due to a loss of acid; may result from respiratory or metabolic disturbances

Anion: Ion with a negative charge

Buffers: Mechanisms employed by the body to keep acids and bases in balance

Cation: Ion with a positive charge

Dehydration: A fluid deficiency resulting from the loss of more water than sodium

Edema: Accumulation of fluid in interstitial spaces

Electrolytes: Substances that break up into electrically charged particles called ions when dissolved in water

Extracellular fluid: Body fluid residing outside of cells

Hypercalcemia: An excessive concentration of calcium in the blood

Hyperkalemia: An excessive concentration of potassium in the blood

Hypernatremia: An excessive concentration of sodium in the blood

Hypocalcemia: Abnormally low blood calcium

Hypokalemia: Abnormally low blood potassium

Hyponatremia: Abnormally low blood sodium

Hypovolemia: Decreased blood volume

Interstitial fluid: Fluid residing between cells inside tissues; a component of extracellular fluid

Intracellular fluid: Body fluid residing inside of cells

Transcellular fluid: Miscellaneous extracellular fluid that includes cerebrospinal fluid, synovial fluid in the joints, vitreous and aqueous humors of the eye, and digestive secretions

Turgor: Elasticity of the skin

Own the Information

To make the information in this chapter part of your working memory, take some time to reflect on what you've learned. On a separate sheet of paper, write down everything you recall from the chapter. After you're done, log on to the Davis*Plus* website, and check out the Study Group podcast and Study Group Questions for the chapter.

Key Topics for Chapter 19:
- Body fluid compartments and the movement of fluid between compartments
- Balancing water gain and loss
- Mechanisms for regulating intake and output
- Disorders of water balance

- The major cations and anions of the body
- Mechanisms for balancing the level of sodium in the body
- The causes and consequences of imbalances of sodium, potassium, calcium, and chloride
- Acid-base balance
- How chemical buffers serve to stabilize pH
- How physiological buffers help to stabilize pH
- The time frame during which each buffer system responds
- Types of acid-base imbalances
- Respiratory and renal compensation for acid-base imbalances

Test Your Knowledge

1. Most of the body's water resides:
   a. inside cells.
   b. outside of cells.
   c. between tissue cells.
   d. in blood plasma.

2. Which factor determines the amount and direction of fluid that flows between body compartments?
   a. The volume of fluid in one of the compartments
   b. The concentration of solutes
   c. The pH of the fluid
   d. The concentration of hydrogen ions in the fluid

3. Antidiuretic hormone is excreted in response to:
   a. a rise in pH.
   b. an increase in fluid volume.
   c. a decrease in serum sodium and a decrease in osmolarity.
   d. an increased serum sodium concentration and an increased osmolarity.

4. Which finding would you expect to find in someone with dehydration?
   a. Edema
   b. Increased skin turgor
   c. Tenting
   d. Cerebral edema

5. What is the main cation in extracellular fluid?
   a. Potassium
   b. Sodium
   c. Chloride
   d. Calcium

6. An excess concentration of potassium in the blood may cause:
   a. muscle weakness.
   b. tetany.
   c. shifting of fluid from tissues into the bloodstream.
   d. potentially fatal cardiac arrhythmias.

7. When the body's pH rises above normal, which possible response would occur first?
   a. The respiratory rate would increase.
   b. The kidneys would excrete H^+ ions.
   c. Hydrogen would bind with bicarbonate to produce carbonic acid.
   d. Hydrogen would bind with carbonic acid to form bicarbonate.

8. A deficiency of sodium ions in the blood is called:
   a. hyponatremia.
   b. hypernatremia.
   c. hypokalemia.
   d. hyperkalemia.

9. Retention of CO_2 from hypoventilation would cause:
   a. respiratory alkalosis.
   b. respiratory acidosis.
   c. metabolic acidosis.
   d. metabolic alkalosis.

10. Which electrolyte disturbance would result from acidosis?
    a. Hypernatremia
    b. Hyponatremia
    c. Hyperkalemia
    d. Hypokalemia

Answers: Chapter 19

1. *Correct answer:* **a.** Only 35% of the body's water resides outside of cells, which includes the fluid between tissue cells as well as the fluid within blood vessels (such as plasma).

2. *Correct answer:* **b.** None of the other factors influence fluid shifts between body compartments.

3. *Correct answer:* **d.** ADH is secreted in response to increased serum sodium and increased osmolarity. pH does not affect ADH secretion.

4. *Correct answer:* **c.** Edema involves the accumulation of fluid within a body compartment. Skin turgor would be decreased in dehydration and would cause tenting. Cerebral edema does not result from dehydration.

5. *Correct answer:* **b.** Potassium is the main cation in intracellular fluid. Chloride is the most abundant extracellular anion and is strongly linked to sodium. Calcium exists mostly outside the cell, but it is not the chief extracellular cation.

6. *Correct answer:* **d.** Muscle weakness results from hypokalemia. Tetany may result from hypocalcemia. Shifting of fluid from tissues into the bloodstream would result from hypernatremia (such as from dehydration).

7. *Correct answer:* **c.** While both an increase in respiratory rate and the excretion of H^+ ions from the kidneys help lower pH, neither would be the body's first response. Hydrogen does not bind with carbonic acid.

8. *Correct answer:* **a.** Hypernatremia is an increased concentration of sodium in the blood. Hypokalemia is a decreased concentration of potassium, while hyperkalemia is an increased concentration of potassium.

9. *Correct answer:* **b.** Respiratory alkalosis would result from hyperventilation. Metabolic imbalances result from an excess or deficiency of bicarbonate, not from respiratory dysfunction.

10. *Correct answer:* **c.** Acidosis does not affect the concentration of sodium in the blood, so neither hyponatremia nor hypernatremia would result from acidosis. Hypokalemia would result from alkalosis, caused as potassium moves into the cell to balance the movement of hydrogen ions out of the cell.

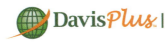

CHAPTER OUTLINE

Overview of the Digestive System

Mouth

Pharynx

Esophagus

Stomach

Liver, Gallbladder, and Pancreas

Small Intestine

Chemical Digestion and Absorption

Large Intestine

LEARNING OUTCOMES

1. Differentiate between mechanical and chemical digestion.

2. Describe the tissue layers of the digestive tract.

3. Explain the role of the enteric nervous system.

4. Describe the structure and role of the peritoneum.

5. Describe the anatomy of the mouth.

6. Explain the composition and function of saliva.

7. Describe the path that food takes as it travels from the mouth to the stomach.

8. Describe the structure and function of the stomach.

9. Identify the secretions of the stomach and state the functions of each.

10. Describe the three phases of stimulating gastric secretion.

11. Describe the anatomy of the liver, gallbladder, and pancreas.

12. Identify and explain the function of the digestive secretions of the liver, gallbladder, and pancreas.

13. Name the divisions of the small intestine.

14. Describe the two types of movements that occur in the small intestine.

15. Describe the lining of the small intestine and explain the purpose it serves.

16. Explain the process of digestion for carbohydrates, proteins, and fats.

17. Define *contact digestion* and explain where this occurs.

18. Describe the anatomy of the large intestine.

19. Describe the types of contractions that occur in the large intestine.

20. Explain the function of the bacteria found in the large intestine.

20

DIGESTIVE SYSTEM

The bowel has been called the second brain. Not only does it contain more neurons than the spinal cord, it secretes neurotransmitters and hormones similar to those of the brain.

The digestive system performs the vital task of transforming food into chemicals that cells can absorb and use for energy. It breaks down food into its simplest components, after which it absorbs the components so they can be distributed throughout the body. Converting food into fuel requires a dozen organs, a vast array of enzymes, and thousands of chemical reactions.

Overview of the Digestive System

The digestive system consists of the **digestive tract** (also called the *alimentary canal*) as well as **accessory organs**. The digestive tract is basically a tube that extends from the mouth to the anus; it contains several distinct sections, as shown below. The accessory organs are separate organs that aid digestion.

The **digestive tract** includes the:

- Mouth
- Pharynx
- Esophagus
- Stomach
- Large intestine
- Small intestine
- Rectum
- Anus

The **accessory organs** include the:

- Teeth
- Tongue
- Salivary glands
- Liver
- Pancreas
- Gallbladder

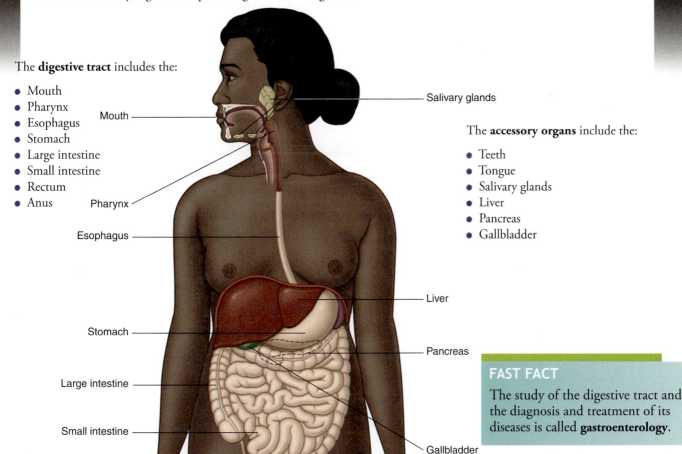

Salivary glands
Mouth
Pharynx
Esophagus
Stomach
Large intestine
Small intestine
Rectum
Anus
Liver
Pancreas
Gallbladder

FAST FACT

The study of the digestive tract and the diagnosis and treatment of its diseases is called **gastroenterology**.

PART IV Maintenance of the Body

The Body AT WORK

Digestion breaks down food—both physically and chemically—and transforms it into a substance that cells can use. Mechanical digestion and chemical digestion are two distinct phases of this process.

- *Mechanical digestion:* This is the first phase of digestion. It involves physically breaking down food into smaller pieces, beginning with chewing in the mouth and continuing with contractions and churning in the stomach and small intestine.
- *Chemical digestion:* The second phase of digestion uses digestive enzymes produced in the salivary glands, stomach, pancreas, and small intestines to break down food particles into nutrients (such as glucose, amino acids, and fatty acids) that cells can use.

Once nutrients are released from food, they move into the epithelial cells lining the digestive tract before passing into the bloodstream for distribution throughout the body. Food that isn't digested or absorbed becomes waste (feces) and is eliminated from the body.

Food material inside the digestive tract is considered to be *external* to the body.

Tissue Layers of the Digestive Tract

Four layers of tissue make up the walls of the digestive tract: the mucosa, the submucosa, the muscularis, and the serosa.

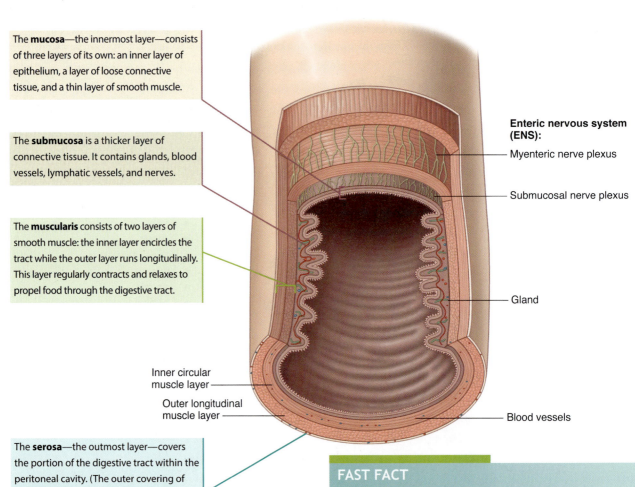

The **mucosa**—the innermost layer—consists of three layers of its own: an inner layer of epithelium, a layer of loose connective tissue, and a thin layer of smooth muscle.

The **submucosa** is a thicker layer of connective tissue. It contains glands, blood vessels, lymphatic vessels, and nerves.

The **muscularis** consists of two layers of smooth muscle: the inner layer encircles the tract while the outer layer runs longitudinally. This layer regularly contracts and relaxes to propel food through the digestive tract.

Inner circular muscle layer

Outer longitudinal muscle layer

The **serosa**—the outmost layer—covers the portion of the digestive tract within the peritoneal cavity. (The outer covering of the esophagus and rectum is called the *adventitia*.)

Enteric nervous system (ENS):

Myenteric nerve plexus

Submucosal nerve plexus

Gland

Blood vessels

The serosa is actually the visceral layer of the peritoneum. As you may recall, the *visceral layer* of the peritoneum covers the organs in the abdominopelvic cavity; the *parietal layer* of the peritoneum attaches to the walls of the cavity.

The Body AT WORK

*A network of nerves called the **enteric nervous system (ENS)** innervates the digestive system. Consisting of 100 million neurons, the enteric nervous system—a part of the autonomic nervous system—regulates digestive tract motility, secretion, and blood flow. One portion of the ENS (the submucosal plexus) is embedded in the submucosa; another portion (the myenteric plexus) resides between the two layers of the muscularis.*

The enteric nervous system usually communicates with the central nervous system (CNS). However, even if contact between the two systems is severed, the ENS will continue to function. This amazing, self-contained nervous system contains sensory neurons that monitor mechanical and chemical conditions within the digestive tract, motor neurons that control the churning and movement of the intestines, and still other neurons that control the secretion of enzymes. It also contains support cells similar to the astroglia of the brain and, finally, it uses more than 30 neurotransmitters, most of which are identical to those found in the CNS.

FAST FACT

Organs like the stomach and liver are enclosed by mesentery (or serosa) on both sides, placing them within the peritoneal cavity (**intraperitoneal**). Organs such as the duodenum and most of the pancreas lie against the dorsal abdominal wall; mesentery covers only their ventral sides, so they are outside the peritoneal cavity (**retroperitoneal**).

Peritoneum

Because the stomach and intestines vigorously contract as they digest, they need to be free to move. At the same time, they need to be anchored enough so that the intestines don't twist or kink when the body changes position. Layers of visceral peritoneum called **mesenteries** suspend the digestive organs within the abdominal cavity while anchoring them loosely to the abdominal wall. Mesenteries also contain blood vessels, nerves, lymphatic vessels, and lymph nodes that supply the digestive tract. (Although this figure shows the intestines separated from each other, in actuality, they are closely packed.)

FAST FACT

Because the peritoneal cavity contains empty space, it can fill with fluid from disease or trauma. The accumulation of fluid in the peritoneal cavity is called **ascites**.

Extending from the greater curvature of the stomach and hanging down over the small intestines like an apron is a portion of the mesentery called the **greater omentum**. Deposits of fat scattered throughout the omentum give it a lacy appearance. Besides helping to prevent friction, the omentum also helps localize infection. If areas of inflammation develop in the stomach or intestines, the omenta adheres to the area to keep the infection from spreading to the rest of the abdomen.

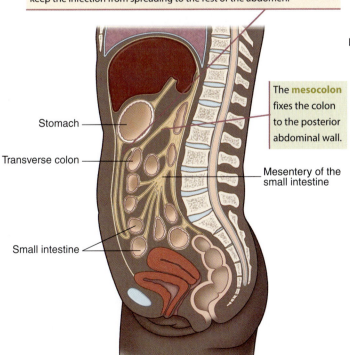

Stomach

Transverse colon

Small intestine

The **mesocolon** fixes the colon to the posterior abdominal wall.

Mesentery of the small intestine

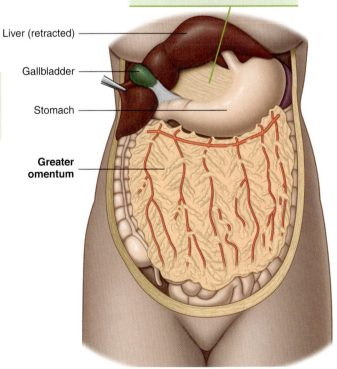

The **lesser omentum** extends from the lesser curve of the stomach to the liver.

Liver (retracted)

Gallbladder

Stomach

Greater omentum

Mouth

The mouth is also called the **oral**, or **buccal**, **cavity**. It's surrounded by lips and bordered on each side by the cheeks. The palate forms the roof of the mouth while the tongue and its muscles form the floor. The mouth is the entryway to the digestive tract; it's also where digestion begins.

Palatine tonsil

Upper lip

The **hard palate**—formed by portions of the maxillae and palatine bones—separates the mouth from the nasal cavity.

The **tongue** is a skeletal muscle covered by a mucous membrane. It repositions food in the mouth during chewing; it also contains taste buds within projections called **lingual papillae**. (For more information on taste buds, see Chapter 11, *Sense Organs*.)

The **soft palate**, which consists of mostly skeletal muscle, forms an arch between the mouth and nasopharynx.

A fold of mucous membrane called the **lingual frenulum** anchors the tongue to the floor of the mouth. Numerous superficial blood vessels populate the floor of the mouth, making this an ideal site for soluble drugs (such as nitroglycerine) to be absorbed quickly into the circulation.

Sublingual salivary duct orifice

Submandibular salivary duct orifice

Lower lip

A cone-shaped process called the **uvula** hangs downward from the soft palate.

Salivary Glands

Salivary glands secrete **saliva**, a clear fluid consisting mostly of water, but also containing mucus, an enzyme that kills bacteria, antibacterial compounds, electrolytes, and two digestive enzymes. Besides the major salivary glands shown in the figure below, the mouth also contains minor salivary glands in the tongue, inside the lips, and on the inside of the cheeks.

The Body AT WORK

*Saliva moistens the mouth and lubricates and protects the teeth. It also plays an important role in taste. One of its main roles, though, is to moisten food and transform it into a mass called a **bolus** that can be swallowed easily. Enzymes contained in saliva begin the digestion process: **amylase** breaks down starch while **lipase** begins the digestion of fat.*

Salivary glands secrete about 1 liter of saliva daily. The pressure and taste of food in the mouth stimulates the secretion of saliva. The smell or sight of food—or even just the thought of food—also stimulates salivation. On the other hand, stimulation of the sympathetic nervous system, such as through fear, inhibits the secretion of saliva, causing the mouth to feel dry.

The **parotid gland** lies just underneath the skin anterior to the ear. Its duct drains saliva to an area near the second upper molar. The mumps virus causes swelling and inflammation of the parotid gland.

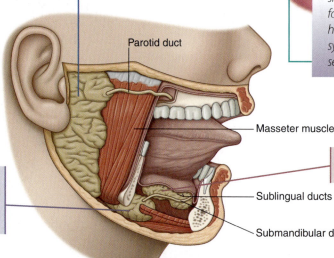

Parotid duct

Masseter muscle

The **sublingual gland** drains through multiple ducts onto the floor of the mouth.

The **submandibular gland** empties into the mouth on either side of the lingual frenulum.

Sublingual ducts

Submandibular duct

Teeth

Digestion begins when food enters the mouth and is chewed: a process called **mastication**. Besides breaking food into pieces small enough to be swallowed, chewing allows food to become moistened with saliva. The adult mouth contains 32 permanent teeth designed to cut, tear, and grind food.

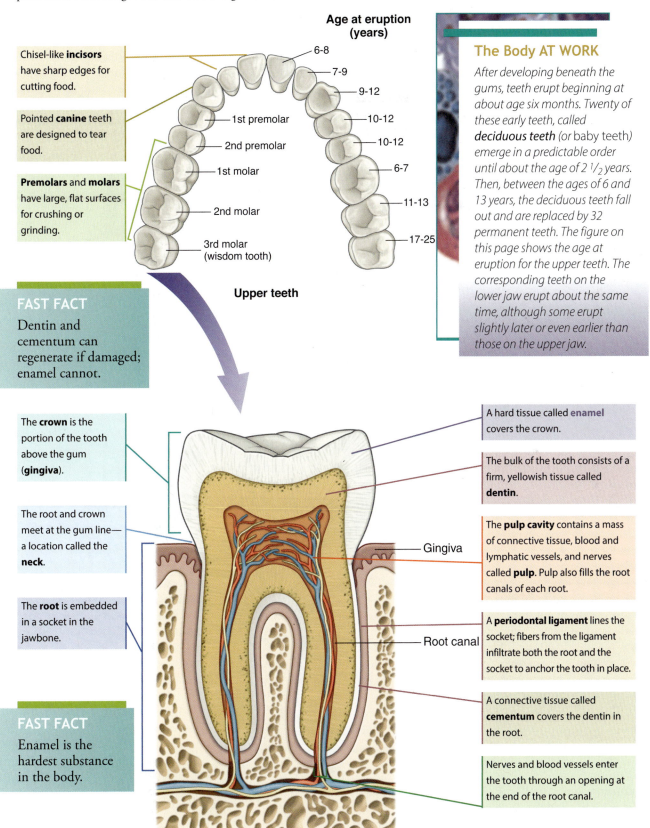

Age at eruption (years)

- 6-8
- 7-9
- 9-12
- 10-12
- 10-12
- 6-7
- 11-13
- 17-25

- 1st premolar
- 2nd premolar
- 1st molar
- 2nd molar
- 3rd molar (wisdom tooth)

Upper teeth

Chisel-like **incisors** have sharp edges for cutting food.

Pointed **canine** teeth are designed to tear food.

Premolars and **molars** have large, flat surfaces for crushing or grinding.

FAST FACT

Dentin and cementum can regenerate if damaged; enamel cannot.

The Body AT WORK

After developing beneath the gums, teeth erupt beginning at about age six months. Twenty of these early teeth, called **deciduous teeth** *(or baby teeth) emerge in a predictable order until about the age of 2 ½ years. Then, between the ages of 6 and 13 years, the deciduous teeth fall out and are replaced by 32 permanent teeth. The figure on this page shows the age at eruption for the upper teeth. The corresponding teeth on the lower jaw erupt about the same time, although some erupt slightly later or even earlier than those on the upper jaw.*

The **crown** is the portion of the tooth above the gum (**gingiva**).

The root and crown meet at the gum line—a location called the **neck**.

The **root** is embedded in a socket in the jawbone.

FAST FACT

Enamel is the hardest substance in the body.

A hard tissue called **enamel** covers the crown.

The bulk of the tooth consists of a firm, yellowish tissue called **dentin**.

The **pulp cavity** contains a mass of connective tissue, blood and lymphatic vessels, and nerves called **pulp**. Pulp also fills the root canals of each root.

Gingiva

Root canal

A **periodontal ligament** lines the socket; fibers from the ligament infiltrate both the root and the socket to anchor the tooth in place.

A connective tissue called **cementum** covers the dentin in the root.

Nerves and blood vessels enter the tooth through an opening at the end of the root canal.

Pharynx

After food leaves the oral cavity, it moves into the pharynx. (For detailed information about the pharynx, see Chapter 17, *Respiratory System.*) While air moves through all three divisions of the pharynx (the nasopharynx, oropharynx, and laryngopharynx), food moves through only the last two of those divisions.

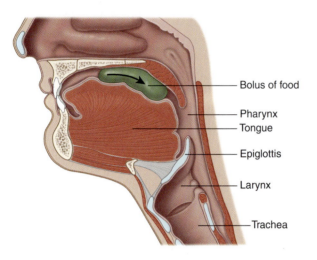

Bolus of food

Pharynx
Tongue

Epiglottis

Larynx

Trachea

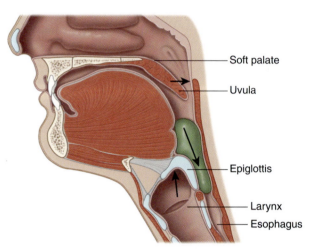

Soft palate

Uvula

Epiglottis

Larynx

Esophagus

1 After food has been broken down by the teeth and moistened by saliva, the tongue manipulates the bolus to the back of the oral cavity.

2 At this point, the soft palate lifts (closing off the nasopharynx) while the larynx rises (forcing the epiglottis over the entrance to the trachea) and food moves through the oropharynx and laryngopharynx on its way to the esophagus.

Esophagus

Connecting the pharynx to the stomach is the **esophagus**: a muscular tube about 10 inches (25 cm) long.

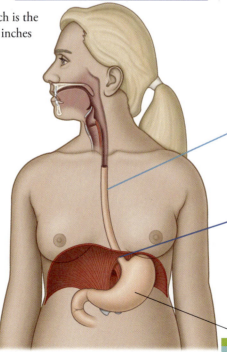

Lying posterior to the trachea, the esophagus travels through the mediastinum, penetrates the diaphragm, and enters the stomach.

A muscular sphincter called the **lower esophageal sphincter (LES)** helps prevent the backflow of stomach acid into the esophagus.

Stomach

FAST FACT

Swallowing requires the coordination of 22 muscles in the mouth, pharynx, and esophagus, all controlled by nerve impulses sent from the medulla oblongata and pons.

Glands within the wall of the esophagus secrete mucus that helps lubricate the food bolus as it passes through. When a bolus enters the esophagus, it triggers wave-like muscular contractions (**peristalsis**) that propel the food toward the stomach.

FAST FACT

"Heartburn," or indigestion, is a burning sensation that results from the regurgitation of acidic stomach contents into the esophagus.

Stomach

Just below the diaphragm, the digestive tube expands to form the stomach, a muscular sac whose primary function is to store food. The stomach also prepares food for digestion (most of which occurs in the intestines). Specifically, the muscles of the stomach contract and churn to break food into small particles and to mix it with gastric juice. What results is a semi-fluid mixture called **chyme**. Chyme leaves the stomach and enters the duodenum by passing through the **pyloric sphincter**.

The normal curvature of the stomach creates two anatomical landmarks: the **lesser curvature** (along the upper surface of the stomach) and the **greater curvature** (along the lower surface). The stomach itself is divided into four regions, as shown in the figure below.

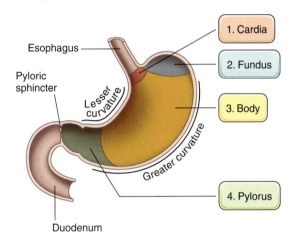

Esophagus
Pyloric sphincter
Lesser curvature
Greater curvature
Duodenum

1. Cardia
2. Fundus
3. Body
4. Pylorus

The Body AT WORK

While enzymes in the stomach partially digest protein as well as small amounts of starch and fat, most of the digestion process, and the absorption of nutrients, takes place in the intestine. Alcohol is also absorbed mostly by the small intestine. However, the rate at which alcohol is absorbed depends on how quickly the stomach empties its contents into the intestine (which is why eating before consuming alcohol slows the effect of the alcohol).

The stomach contains the same layers as the rest of the digestive tract (mucosa, submucosa, muscularis, and serosa). However, the muscularis layer of the stomach has an extra layer of oblique muscle in addition to longitudinal and circular layers.

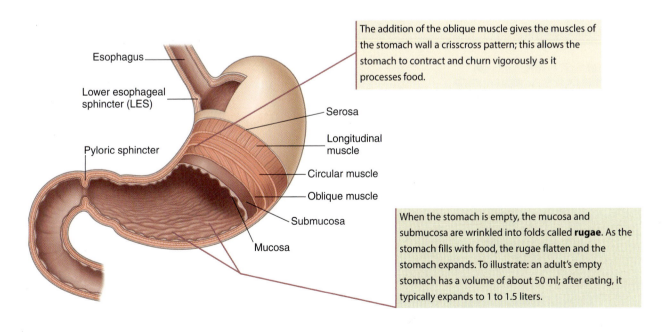

Esophagus
Lower esophageal sphincter (LES)
Pyloric sphincter
Serosa
Longitudinal muscle
Circular muscle
Oblique muscle
Submucosa
Mucosa

The addition of the oblique muscle gives the muscles of the stomach wall a crisscross pattern; this allows the stomach to contract and churn vigorously as it processes food.

When the stomach is empty, the mucosa and submucosa are wrinkled into folds called **rugae**. As the stomach fills with food, the rugae flatten and the stomach expands. To illustrate: an adult's empty stomach has a volume of about 50 ml; after eating, it typically expands to 1 to 1.5 liters.

The gastric mucosa contains depressions called **gastric pits**. Several different glands (called **gastric glands**) open into the bottom of each gastric pit. These glands secrete the various components of **gastric juice**.

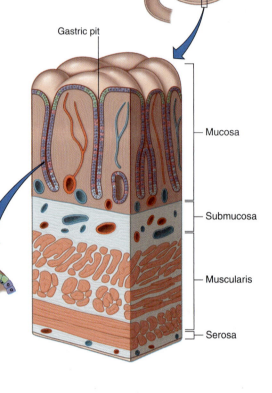

Gastric pit

Mucosa

Submucosa

Muscularis

Serosa

FAST FACT

Gastric glands produce up to 3 liters of gastric juice each day.

Mucous cells secrete mucus, which protects the stomach lining and keeps the stomach from digesting itself.

Parietal cells secrete hydrochloric acid and intrinsic factor (which is necessary for the absorption of vitamin B_{12}). Hydrochloric acid helps kill microbes in swallowed food.

Chief cells secrete digestive enzymes, such as pepsinogen.

Enteroendocrine cells secrete the hormone *ghrelin* (which stimulates the hypothalamus to increase appetite) and *gastrin* (which influences digestive function).

FAST FACT

The stomach empties in less than 4 hours following a liquid meal, or it may take as long as 6 hours to empty following a meal high in fat.

The Body AT WORK

Swallowing signals the stomach to relax so as to allow food to enter. Once the food has entered, the stomach goes to work, mixing the food with gastric juices and propelling it toward the duodenum.

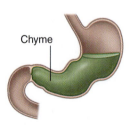

Chyme

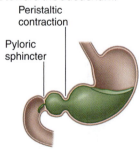

Peristaltic contraction

Pyloric sphincter

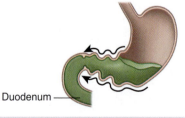

Duodenum

1 Contractions originate in the fundus and move toward the pyloric region. Starting out gently and growing progressively stronger, wave-like peristaltic contractions break down food and mix it with gastric juices to form chyme.

2 Chyme moves toward the pyloric sphincter, propelled by the rhythm of the contractions. Under the pressure of a contraction, about 30 ml of chyme squirts into the duodenum.

3 The stomach continues to churn and mix its contents as it gradually releases chyme into the duodenum. This continues until the stomach empties, which takes about 4 hours following a typical meal.

The Body AT WORK

The stimulation of gastric secretion occurs in three phases. Each phase (the cephalic phase, gastric phase, and intestinal phase) is activated by a different part of the body (the brain, the stomach, and the intestine, respectively).

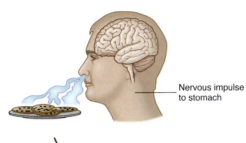

Nervous impulse to stomach

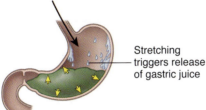

Stretching triggers release of gastric juice

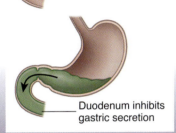

Duodenum inhibits gastric secretion

1. *The mere thought of food—as well as its sight, smell, or taste—creates neural impulses that are relayed to the brainstem. The parasympathetic nervous system then signals the stomach to secrete gastric juice as well as gastrin. Gastrin further stimulates gastric secretion. Because the brain controls this phase of gastric secretion, it's called the* **cephalic phase***.*

2. *The next phase—the* **gastric phase***—begins when food enters the stomach. The stretching of the stomach as it fills with food triggers nerve reflexes that increase the secretion of gastric juice and gastrin.*

3. *As chyme moves into the duodenum, the* **intestinal phase** *begins. At this point, the duodenum triggers nerve impulses and secretes hormones, both of which inhibit gastric secretion.*

Life lesson: Peptic ulcer

Crater-like sores, or ulcerations, in the lining of the stomach or duodenum are called *peptic ulcers*. Typical symptoms include gnawing or burning pain in the middle or upper stomach between meals or at night, bloating, and heartburn. Untreated, ulcers can erode through the organ wall, resulting in a potentially fatal hemorrhage.

While there is no single cause of ulcers, an acid-resistant bacterium called *Helicobacter pylori* (*H. pylori*) is often implicated. By invading the mucosa of the stomach and duodenum, the bacterium causes chronic inflammation that often leads to the development of an ulcer. Another common cause of peptic ulcers is the use of nonsteroidal anti-inflammatory drugs (NSAIDs); these drugs interfere with the production of mucus that protects the lining of the stomach and duodenum, thus opening the door to chemical damage.

Ulcers caused by *H. pylori* are usually successfully treated with antibiotics.

The Body AT WORK

Vomiting may result from a variety of stimuli: overstretching of the stomach, chemical irritants (such as alcohol or toxins), or even pain or fear. When these types of stimuli occur, the emetic center of the medulla oblongata sends two types of impulses: one to the upper esophageal sphincter to open and one to the esophagus and body of the stomach to relax. As this is happening, the abdominal muscles forcefully contract to force chyme out of the stomach and mouth.

Liver, Gallbladder, and Pancreas

Although the liver, gallbladder, and pancreas are accessory organs of the digestive system, they play a crucial role in the digestive process. Each of these organs secretes digestive fluids or enzymes into the digestive tract at the junction of the stomach and small intestine.

Liver

The body's largest gland, the liver fills the upper right abdomen below the diaphragm. Even more impressive than its size is its function: the liver performs over 250 tasks, including storing and releasing glucose, processing vitamins and minerals, filtering toxins, and recycling old blood cells. This chapter focuses on the liver's role in digestion. (More of the liver's functions will be discussed in Chapter 21, *Nutrition & Metabolism*.)

The liver has four lobes. Two of the lobes (the **right** and **left lobes**) are visible from an anterior view.

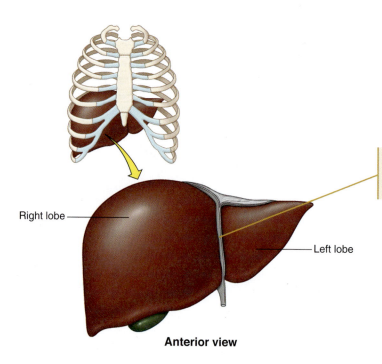

FAST FACT
The term **hepatic** refers to the liver.

The right and left lobes are separated by the **falciform ligament**, which also serves to anchor the liver to the abdominal wall.

Right lobe

Left lobe

Anterior view

FAST FACT
Swelling and inflammation of the liver is called **hepatitis**. Hepatitis is a symptom, rather than a condition, although the term is often used to refer to a viral infection of the liver.

Two additional lobes—the **caudate lobe** (near the inferior vena cava) and the **quadrate lobe** (next to the gallbladder)—are visible from behind.

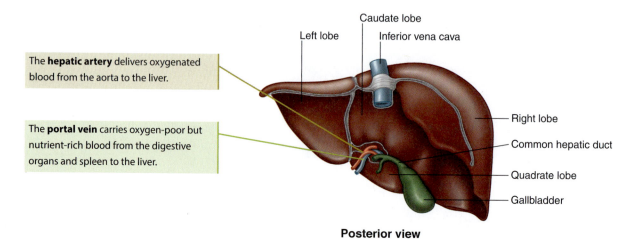

The **hepatic artery** delivers oxygenated blood from the aorta to the liver.

The **portal vein** carries oxygen-poor but nutrient-rich blood from the digestive organs and spleen to the liver.

Caudate lobe

Left lobe

Inferior vena cava

Right lobe

Common hepatic duct

Quadrate lobe

Gallbladder

Posterior view

Liver Lobules

Tiny, six-sided cylinders called **hepatic lobules** fill the interior of the liver. These are the functional units of the liver.

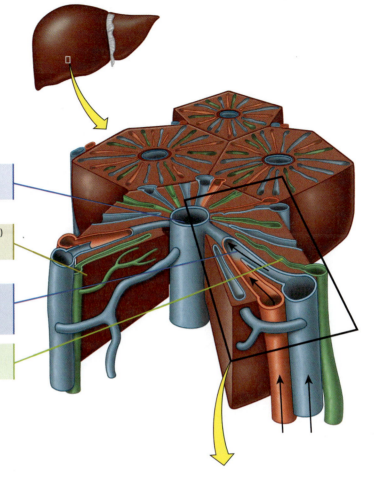

A **central vein** passes through the core of each lobule.

Sheets of hepatic cells (called **hepatocytes**) fan out from the center of the lobule.

In between the sheets of cells are passageways filled with blood called **sinusoids**.

Tiny canals called **canaliculi** carry bile secreted by hepatocytes.

Blood Flow Through the Liver

Each liver lobule receives nutrient-rich venous blood from the intestines as well as oxygenated blood from the celiac trunk.

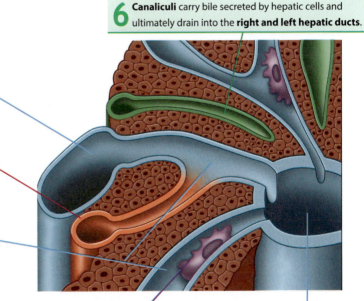

1 Nutrient-rich blood from the stomach and intestine enters the lobule through small branches of the **portal vein**.

2 Oxygen-rich blood enters the lobule through small branches of the **hepatic artery**.

3 The blood filters through the **sinusoids**, allowing the cells to remove nutrients (such as glucose, amino acids, iron, and vitamins) as well as hormones, toxins, and drugs. At the same time, the liver secretes substances—such as clotting factors, albumin, angiotensinogen, and glucose—into the blood for distribution throughout the body.

4 Also, phagocytic cells called *Kupffer cells* remove bacteria, worn-out red blood cells, and debris from the bloodstream.

5 The **central vein** carries the processed blood out of the liver.

6 **Canaliculi** carry bile secreted by hepatic cells and ultimately drain into the **right and left hepatic ducts**.

Gallbladder

A sac attached to the underside of the liver, the gallbladder stores and concentrates bile. The gallbladder is about 3 to 4 inches (7 to 10 cm) long and holds 30 to 50 ml of bile.

Bile reaches the gallbladder through a series of ducts. It leaves the liver by the **right and left hepatic ducts**. These two ducts converge to form the **common hepatic duct**, which goes on to become the **common bile duct**. Bile from the liver first fills the common bile duct before backing up into the gallbladder through the **cystic duct**.

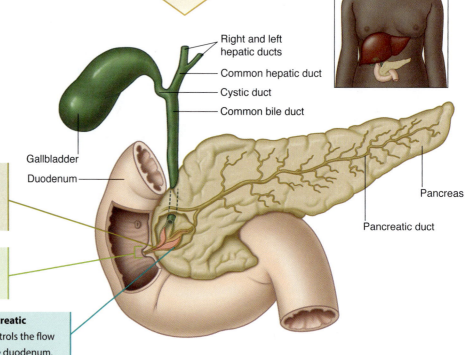

Right and left hepatic ducts

Common hepatic duct

Cystic duct

Common bile duct

Gallbladder

Duodenum

Pancreas

Pancreatic duct

The bile duct merges with the duct of the pancreas to form the **hepatopancreatic ampulla (ampulla of Vater)**.

The ampulla enters the duodenum at a raised area called the **major duodenal papilla**.

A sphincter called the **hepatopancreatic sphincter (sphincter of Oddi)** controls the flow of bile and pancreatic juice into the duodenum.

The Body AT WORK

Each day, the liver secretes up to 1 liter of **bile***: a yellow-green fluid containing minerals, cholesterol, phospholipids, bile salts, bile pigments, and cholesterol. The main bile pigment is* **bilirubin***, which results from the breakdown of hemoglobin. However, the most important component of bile is* **bile salts***. Formed in the liver from cholesterol, bile salts aid in the digestion and absorption of fat in the small intestine. After secretion, 80% of bile salts are reabsorbed in the final section of the small intestine (the ileum). It is then returned to the liver, where hepatocytes absorb and then secrete the bile once again. The 20% of bile not reabsorbed is excreted in feces. In fact, bile is responsible for giving feces its brown color. If bile isn't being secreted, or if the flow of bile is obstructed, feces become grayish-white in color.*

Life lesson: Gallstones

Hard masses, called *gallstones*, can form inside the gallbladder, often because of excessive cholesterol in the bile. Gallstones may cause no signs or symptoms. However, if a gallstone lodges within a duct, excruciating pain may occur. If the gallstone blocks the flow of bile into the duodenum, bile will back up to the liver and be absorbed into the bloodstream, resulting in jaundice (a yellow discoloration of the skin, mucous, membranes, and sclerae). Treatment of symptomatic gallstones includes surgery to remove the gallbladder or medications to dissolve the gallstones.

Pancreas

The pancreas lies behind the stomach; its head is nestled in the curve of the duodenum while its tapered tail sits below the spleen and above the left kidney.

The pancreas is both an endocrine and exocrine gland. Its endocrine function centers on pancreatic islets that secrete insulin and glucagon. (For more information on the endocrine function of the pancreas, see Chapter 12, *Endocrine System*.)

Most of the pancreas, though, consists of exocrine tissue. Each day, the pancreas secretes about 1.5 liters of pancreatic juice—essentially digestive enzymes and an alkaline fluid—into the small intestine.

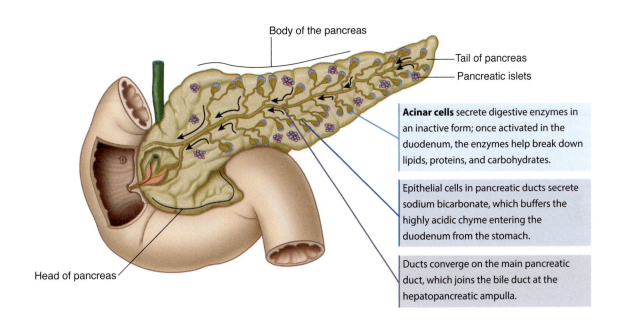

Body of the pancreas

Tail of pancreas

Pancreatic islets

Acinar cells secrete digestive enzymes in an inactive form; once activated in the duodenum, the enzymes help break down lipids, proteins, and carbohydrates.

Epithelial cells in pancreatic ducts secrete sodium bicarbonate, which buffers the highly acidic chyme entering the duodenum from the stomach.

Ducts converge on the main pancreatic duct, which joins the bile duct at the hepatopancreatic ampulla.

Head of pancreas

The Body AT WORK

The vagus nerve and the hormones cholecystokinin, gastrin, and secretin stimulate the secretion of bile and pancreatic juice.

- *Cholecystokinin (CCK): The arrival of chyme in the duodenum stimulates the duodenum to secrete the hormone CCK. CCK causes gallbladder contraction—forcing bile into the bile duct— and the release of pancreatic enzymes. At the same time, it prompts the hepatopancreatic sphincter to relax, which allows bile and pancreatic juice to enter the duodenum.*
- *Gastrin: This hormone from the stomach and duodenum triggers both gallbladder contraction and pancreatic enzyme secretion. However, it exerts a much less powerful effect than does CCK.*
- *Secretin: The acid in chyme also triggers the duodenum to release secretin. Secretin causes the bile and pancreatic ducts to release bicarbonate, which helps neutralize the stomach acid entering the duodenum.*

Small Intestine

Most chemical digestion, and most nutrient absorption, occurs in the small intestine. Filling most of the abdominal cavity below the stomach, and held in place by mesentery, the small intestine consists of three divisions: the duodenum, the jejunum, and the ilium.

The **duodenum** is the first 10 inches (25 cm) of small intestine. (The name *duodenum* is Latin for "twelve"; the duodenum is about 12 finger breadths long.) It begins at the pyloric valve and ends as the intestine turns abruptly downward. The duodenum receives chyme from the stomach as well as pancreatic juice and bile. This is where stomach acid is neutralized and pancreatic enzymes begin the task of chemical digestion. More digestive processes occur here than in any other part of the intestine.

The **jejunum** constitutes the next 8 feet (2.4 m) of small intestine. Many large, closely spaced folds and millions of microscopic projections give the jejunum an enormous surface area, making it an ideal location for nutrient absorption. The wall of the jejunum is thick and muscular with a rich blood supply, which imparts a red color to this part of the intestine.

FAST FACT

The term *small* intestine refers to its diameter, not its length. The small intestine is much longer than the large intestine—the small intestine is about 20 feet long whereas the large intestine is about 5 feet long—but its diameter is smaller.

The **ileum** is the last 12 feet (3.6 m) of intestine. The wall of the ileum is thinner and has less blood supply than does the wall of the jejunum. Clusters of lymphatic nodules called **Peyer's patches** are scattered throughout the ileum.

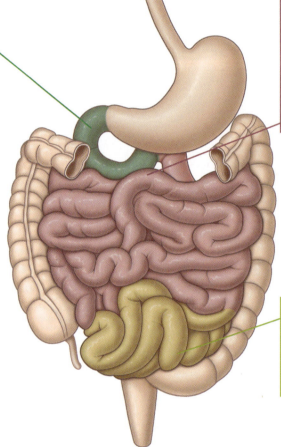

The Body AT WORK

Contractions in the small intestine help break down food particles, mix food with digestive juices, and bring digested food in contact with the intestinal mucosa to facilitate absorption. Contractions also propel food residue toward the large intestine. The two types of intestinal contractions are segmentation and peristalsis.

Segmentation involves ring-like constrictions that occur at intervals along the small intestine. When the first contracted areas relax, new contractions occur in other locations. This back-and-forth movement breaks up food particles and kneads the contents of the intestines, thoroughly mixing it with digestive juices.

Segmentation

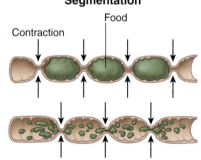

Food

Contraction

Peristalsis

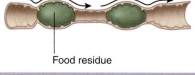

Food residue

Peristalsis begins when most of the nutrients have been absorbed and undigested residue remains. With this type of contraction, successive, wave-like ripples move the digested material along the GI tract.

The intestinal lining contains multiple projections that increase its surface area and enhance the absorption of nutrients.

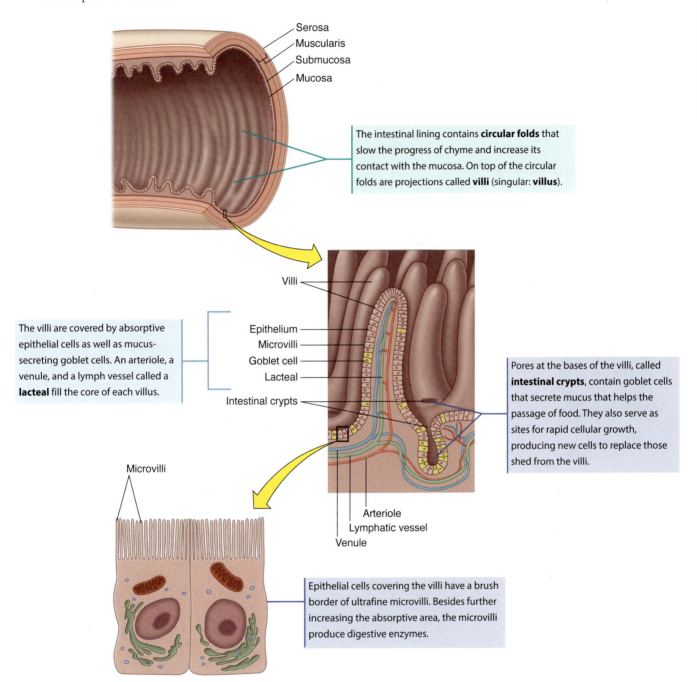

Serosa
Muscularis
Submucosa
Mucosa

The intestinal lining contains **circular folds** that slow the progress of chyme and increase its contact with the mucosa. On top of the circular folds are projections called **villi** (singular: **villus**).

Villi

The villi are covered by absorptive epithelial cells as well as mucus-secreting goblet cells. An arteriole, a venule, and a lymph vessel called a **lacteal** fill the core of each villus.

Epithelium
Microvilli
Goblet cell
Lacteal
Intestinal crypts

Pores at the bases of the villi, called **intestinal crypts**, contain goblet cells that secrete mucus that helps the passage of food. They also serve as sites for rapid cellular growth, producing new cells to replace those shed from the villi.

Microvilli

Arteriole
Lymphatic vessel
Venule

Epithelial cells covering the villi have a brush border of ultrafine microvilli. Besides further increasing the absorptive area, the microvilli produce digestive enzymes.

FAST FACT
The folds, villi, and microvilli increase the surface area of the small intestine more than 500 times.

The Body AT WORK
Most nutrients pass into the bloodstream through capillaries, and then travel to the liver. Most fat, however, is absorbed by the lacteal.

Chemical Digestion and Absorption

Once food has been mechanically broken down into minute particles, chemical digestion takes control. Using digestive enzymes, chemical digestion transforms food molecules into particles that can be absorbed into the bloodstream. By the time food residue leaves the small intestine, most nutrients have been absorbed. The process of digestion and absorption varies between classes of nutrients, with the major classes being carbohydrates, proteins, and fats.

Carbohydrates

Carbohydrates consist of sugars called saccharides:

- **Polysaccharides** contain many saccharide groups linked together; these include starches and glycogen.
- **Disaccharides** contain two groups linked together; these include sucrose, lactose, and maltose.
- **Monosaccharides** contain only one saccharide group; these include glucose, fructose, and galactose.

Most foods contain polysaccharides, which must be broken into smaller particles (namely, disaccharides and monosaccharides). To do so, the digestive system uses enzymes.

FAST FACT

Cellulose is an indigestible carbohydrate found in the diet. Even though cellulose doesn't provide the body with nutrients, it is an important source of dietary fiber. (Cellulose will be discussed further in Chapter 21, *Nutrition & Metabolism*.)

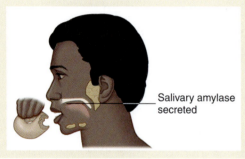

Salivary amylase secreted

The process begins in the mouth, where salivary glands secrete the enzyme **amylase**. Salivary amylase works to hydrolyze polysaccharides into disaccharides.

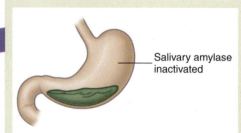

Salivary amylase inactivated

Once the food is swallowed, the low pH of stomach acid inactivates the salivary amylase. By this point, though, about 50% of the starch has already been digested.

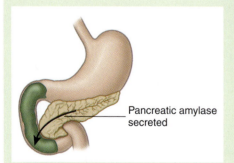

Pancreatic amylase secreted

When the resultant chyme reaches the small intestine, it mixes with **pancreatic amylase**, and the process of starch digestion resumes.

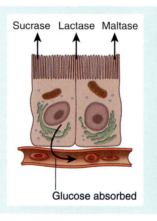

Sucrase   Lactase   Maltase

Glucose absorbed

The final steps in carbohydrate digestion take place at the level of the villi. The membranes of the epithelial cells covering the villi contain the enzymes sucrase, lactase, and maltase. As the chyme slides against the brush border of the epithelial cells, the enzymes bind with the disaccharides. (This is called **contact digestion**.) This final step in the digestion process produces glucose, which is immediately absorbed.

Proteins

Proteins are complex molecules made up of folded and twisted chains of amino acids linked together by peptide bonds. Before the body can absorb amino acids, it must break the peptide bonds. To do so, it uses enzymes called **proteases**. Absent from saliva, proteases work in the stomach and small intestine.

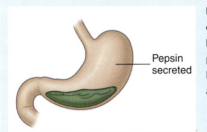

Pepsin secreted

In the stomach, the enzyme **pepsin** hydrolyzes the peptide bonds between certain amino acids.

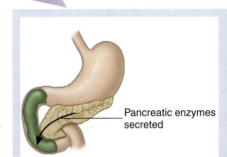

Pancreatic enzymes secreted

As soon as the chyme enters the duodenum, pepsin is inactivated. At that point, the pancreatic enzymes **trypsin** and **chymotrypsin** assume the task of breaking the peptide bonds.

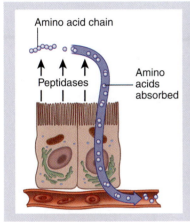

Amino acid chain

Peptidases

Amino acids absorbed

Finally, brush border enzymes called **peptidases** break the remaining chains into individual amino acids, which are then absorbed into the bloodstream.

FAST FACT

Amino acids arrange themselves in a wide variety of combinations, with each combination employing a slightly different peptide bond. As a result, the body calls upon a vast array of proteases to digest protein.

Fats

Although fat digestion begins in the mouth, most fat digestion occurs in the small intestine. Because fat doesn't dissolve in water, it enters the duodenum as a congealed mass. To facilitate digestion, the fat must first be broken into small droplets, a process called **emulsification**.

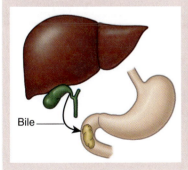

Bile

When a fat globule enters the duodenum, two substances in bile (lecithin and bile salts) break up the fat into small droplets.

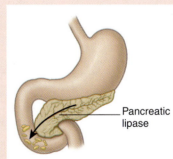

Pancreatic lipase

Once the fat is emulsified, pancreatic **lipase** (the main fat-digesting enzyme) begins to digest the fat. In the process, fats are broken down into a mixture of glycerol, short-chain fatty acids, long-chain fatty acids, and monoglycerides.

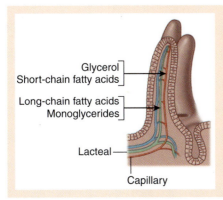

Glycerol
Short-chain fatty acids

Long-chain fatty acids
Monoglycerides

Lacteal

Capillary

Glycerol and short-chain fatty acids are absorbed into the bloodstream of the villi. Long-chain fatty acids and monoglycerides, which are too large to be absorbed by the capillaries, are absorbed into the walls of the villi. There, they are changed into triglycerides, which eventually enter the lacteal of the villi. After travelling through the lymphatic system, the triglycerides enter the bloodstream at the left subclavian vein.

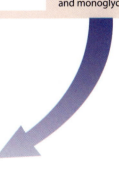

Large Intestine

Once the food has been processed and its nutrients absorbed, the remaining residue is ready to leave the small intestine for the large intestine. In fact, about 500 ml of residue—consisting of undigested food, sloughed off epithelial cells, minerals, salts, and bacteria—enter the large intestine each day. The large intestine absorbs large amounts of water from the residue before passing the resulting waste material (**feces**) out of the body.

The following figure shows the regions of the colon, beginning with the cecum, where food residue enters the colon, and ending with the anal canal, through which waste material leaves the body. All along the way are pouches called **haustra**, which result from the increased tone of the smooth muscle of the muscularis layer.

ANIMATION 🌐

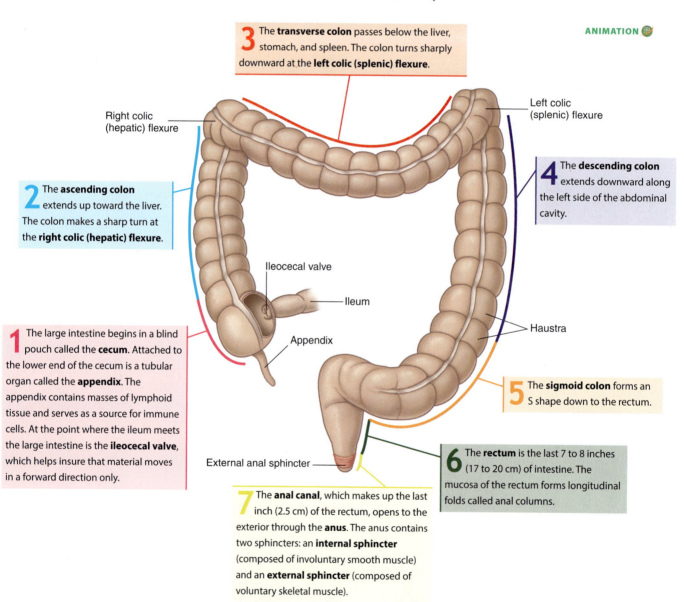

3 The **transverse colon** passes below the liver, stomach, and spleen. The colon turns sharply downward at the **left colic (splenic) flexure**.

Right colic (hepatic) flexure

Left colic (splenic) flexure

2 The **ascending colon** extends up toward the liver. The colon makes a sharp turn at the **right colic (hepatic) flexure**.

4 The **descending colon** extends downward along the left side of the abdominal cavity.

Ileocecal valve

Ileum

Haustra

1 The large intestine begins in a blind pouch called the **cecum**. Attached to the lower end of the cecum is a tubular organ called the **appendix**. The appendix contains masses of lymphoid tissue and serves as a source for immune cells. At the point where the ileum meets the large intestine is the **ileocecal valve**, which helps insure that material moves in a forward direction only.

Appendix

5 The **sigmoid colon** forms an S shape down to the rectum.

External anal sphincter

6 The **rectum** is the last 7 to 8 inches (17 to 20 cm) of intestine. The mucosa of the rectum forms longitudinal folds called anal columns.

7 The **anal canal**, which makes up the last inch (2.5 cm) of the rectum, opens to the exterior through the **anus**. The anus contains two sphincters: an **internal sphincter** (composed of involuntary smooth muscle) and an **external sphincter** (composed of voluntary skeletal muscle).

FAST FACT

Appendicitis, an inflammation of the appendix, results when a blockage traps infectious material inside the appendix. Surgical removal of the appendix (**appendectomy**) is one of the most commonly performed emergency surgeries.

The Body AT WORK

The large intestine houses over 700 species of bacteria; these are called **bacterial flora**. These bacterial flora, also called the normal flora, perform a variety of functions beneficial to the body's health. For example, some of the bacteria digest cellulose and other materials for which we have no digestive enzymes. Other bacteria produce significant amounts of vitamins, particularly vitamin K and a B vitamin.

One of the products of bacterial action is intestinal gas, or **flatus**. Although flatus partially results from swallowed air, it also results from bacterial fermentation of undigested polysaccharides. Flatus mainly consists of nitrogen and carbon dioxide, although it also contains hydrogen, methane, and hydrogen sulfide. When a large amount of undigested nutrients pass into the colon, painful cramping can result as the bacterial action produces an increased volume of intestinal gas.

The Body AT WORK

Intestinal contractions move feces through the colon and toward the rectum.

- **Haustral contractions**: As a haustrum fills with residue, it becomes distended, which stimulates the haustrum to contract. Besides mixing the residue, the contraction pushes the residue into the next haustrum. Haustral contractions generally occur every 30 minutes.
- Stronger peristaltic contractions called **mass movements**, move larger amounts of material several inches at a time along the colon. In particular, these movements are triggered by the filling of the stomach or duodenum.

The mass movement of feces into the rectum stimulates the defecation reflex: the rectum contracts and the internal anal sphincter relaxes. When the external anal sphincter relaxes (which is under voluntary control to prevent the uncontrolled release of feces), feces is expelled from the body (**defecation**).

Key Digestive Enzymes

Organ	Enzyme	Substance Digested
Salivary glands	Amylase Lipase	Starch Fat
Stomach	Pepsin	Protein
Pancreas	• Proteases (trypsin, chymotrypsin) • Lipase • Amylase	• Protein • Fats • Starch
Intestine	• Peptidases • Sucrase • Lactase • Maltase	• Peptides • Sucrose (cane sugar) • Lactose (milk sugar) • Maltose (malt sugar)

FAST FACT

Hemorrhoids are swollen, engorged veins in the anal canal.

Life lesson: Changes with Aging

Efficiency of the digestive system decreases with age. Over time, the muscular wall of the digestive tract weakens and intestinal peristalsis slows, often resulting in constipation and hemorrhoids. Peristalsis also slows in the esophagus, making swallowing more difficult. The cardiac sphincter—the sphincter that regulates the flow of food from the esophagus into the stomach—also weakens, often leading to esophageal reflux and "heartburn." Tooth loss is common, making eating difficult. Factoring in diminished sensations of smell and taste, it's easy to understand why many elderly individuals have poor appetites.

Aging also interferes with the absorption of nutrients. Specifically, the stomach has decreased production of hydrochloric acid and other digestive enzymes, leading to poor absorption of vitamin B$_{12}$. Efficiency of the liver also declines, slowing an elderly individual's ability to metabolize drugs, placing them at greater risk for drug overdose.

Review of Key Terms

Amylase: Enzyme contained in saliva that breaks down starch

Appendix: Tubular organ attached to the lower end of the cecum; serves as a source for immune cells

Bile: Yellow-green fluid secreted by the liver that aids in digestion

Cecum: Blind pouch that serves as the beginning of the large intestine

Chief cells: Cells in the gastric mucosa that secrete digestive enzymes

Chyme: Semi-fluid mixture consisting of particles of food mixed with digestive juices

Dentin: Firm, yellowish tissue forming the bulk of a tooth

Duodenum: The first 10 inches of small intestine; the portion of intestine that performs most digestive processes

Enteric nervous system: Network of nerves innervating the digestive system

Enteroendocrine cells: Cells in the gastric mucosa that secrete the hormone ghrelin

Esophagus: Muscular tube connecting the pharynx to the stomach

Gallbladder: Sac attached to the liver that stores and concentrates bile

Gastric pits: Depressions within the gastric mucosa containing glands that secrete components of gastric juice

Gingiva: Tissue surrounding the necks of teeth; the gums

Hard palate: Bony structure that separates the mouth from the nasal cavity

Haustra: Pouches along the length of the large intestine

Ileum: The third and last portion of the small intestine

Jejunum: The second portion of the small intestine; location where many nutrients are absorbed

Lacteal: Lymph vessel found inside the villi of the small intestine

Lipase: Enzyme that digests fat

Mastication: Process of chewing, which begins the digestion of food

Mesentery: Sheet of connective tissue that suspends the digestive organs within the abdominal cavity

Parotid gland: Salivary gland located just underneath the skin anterior to the ear

Peristalsis: Wave-like muscular contractions that propel food along the digestive tract

Proteases: Enzymes working in the stomach and small intestine to break peptide bonds

Rugae: Folds of mucosa and submucosa in the stomach

Salivary glands: Glands in the oral cavity that secrete saliva

Segmentation: Type of contraction in the small intestine that involves ring-like constrictions

Soft palate: Structure consisting mostly of skeletal muscle that forms an arch between the mouth and nasopharynx

Own the Information

To make the information in this chapter part of your working memory, take some time to reflect on what you've learned. On a separate sheet of paper, write down everything you recall from the chapter. After you're done, log on to the Davis*Plus* website, and check out the Study Group podcast and Study Group Questions for the chapter.

Key Topics for Chapter 20:
• Mechanical and chemical digestion
• Tissue layers of the digestive tract
• Role of the enteric nervous system
• Structure and function of the peritoneum and mesenteries

• Anatomy of the mouth, teeth, pharynx, and esophagus
• Composition and function of saliva
• Structure and function of the stomach
• Anatomy and physiology of gastric pits
• Three phases of gastric secretion
• Structure and function of the liver, gallbladder, and pancreas
• Structure and function of the small intestine
• Chemical digestion and absorption of carbohydrates, proteins, and fats
• Structure and function of the large intestine

Test Your Knowledge

1. In which phase of digestion do enzymes break down food into particles cells can absorb?
   a. Mechanical digestion
   b. Absorption
   c. Chemical digestion
   d. Ingestion

2. The layer of the digestive tract that contracts and relaxes to propel food forward is the:
   a. mucosa.
   b. muscularis.
   c. submucosa.
   d. serosa.

3. Which mesentery hangs over the small intestine like an apron?
   a. Greater omentum
   b. Lesser omentum
   c. Mesocolon
   d. Jejunum

4. Which enzyme acts in the mouth to begin the breakdown of starch?
   a. Amylase
   b. Pepsin
   c. Trypsin
   d. Sucrase

5. The muscular tube that connects the pharynx to the stomach is the:
   a. duodenum.
   b. ileum.
   c. sigmoid colon.
   d. esophagus.

6. How do triglycerides enter the bloodstream?
   a. They pass directly into the bloodstream after passing through the intestinal brush border.
   b. They enter the lacteal and travel through the lymphatic system to enter the bloodstream.

   c. They are absorbed into the wall of the villi, after which they pass into the bloodstream.
   d. Triglycerides don't enter the bloodstream.

7. What is the purpose of rugae?
   a. Secrete gastric juice
   b. Propel food residue through the small intestine.
   c. Allow the stomach to expand.
   d. Help break food into small particles.

8. Which of the following acts as an initial trigger to the stomach to begin secreting gastric juice?
   a. The smell of food
   b. The stretching of the stomach as it fills with food
   c. The movement of chyme into the duodenum
   d. Contractions within the stomach

9. Which pancreatic cells secrete digestive enzymes?
   a. Acinar cells
   b. Islets of Langerhans
   c. Duct cells
   d. Kupffer cells

10. Most nutrients are absorbed in the:
    a. stomach.
    b. small intestine.
    c. large intestine.
    d. mouth.

11. Where is most fat digested?
    a. Mouth
    b. Stomach
    c. Duodenum
    d. Large intestine

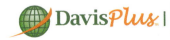 DavisPlus | Go to **http://davisplus.fadavis.com** Keyword: Thompson to see all of the resources available with this chapter.

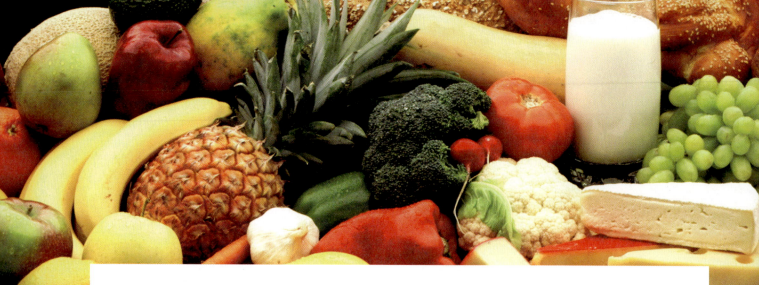

CHAPTER OUTLINE

Units of Energy

Hunger and Satiety

Nutrients

Metabolism

Thermoregulation

LEARNING OUTCOMES

1. Define *metabolism* and *calorie*.

2. Explain basal metabolic rate and identify the factors that influence it.

3. Discuss the five hormones that affect hunger and satiety.

4. Define *nutrient* and identify the five categories of nutrients.

5. Name the three forms of dietary carbohydrates.

6. Describe three roles of fat in the body.

7. Differentiate between saturated and unsaturated fats.

8. Differentiate between complete and incomplete proteins.

9. Name the fat-soluble and water-soluble vitamins, and explain the difference between them.

10. Identify the major minerals in the body and describe their functions.

11. Summarize the process of carbohydrate metabolism, including glycolysis, anaerobic fermentation, and aerobic fermentation.

12. Explain what occurs in glycogenesis, glycogenolysis, and gluconeogenesis.

13. Describe the process of lipid metabolism.

14. Describe the process of protein metabolism.

15. Explain what is meant by protein balance, differentiating between negative and positive nitrogen balance.

16. Identify the three means by which the body loses heat.

17. Explain the negative feedback mechanisms that help regulate the body's temperature.

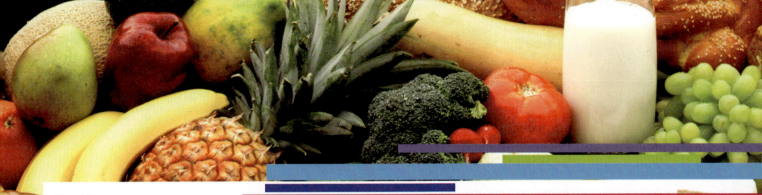

21

NUTRITION & METABOLISM

About two-thirds of an adult's energy expenditure is used simply to maintain normal body function.

The body—even at rest—consumes a tremendous amount of energy. Obviously, walking across a room or even picking up a book requires energy, but so does the beating of the heart, the conduction of nervous impulses, the movement of the lungs during respiration, and even the manufacture of new blood cells. In fact, the body needs a steady supply of fuel just to survive.

As was discussed in the previous chapter, the body's source of fuel is food. Once consumed, the digestive system breaks food into usable food components (called **nutrients**), which are then absorbed into the bloodstream. That's just the beginning, however. The nutrients then enter the cells and undergo further chemical reactions, called **metabolism.** It's through the process of metabolism that nutrients are transformed into energy or materials the body can either use or store.

As shown in the figure below, some body systems demand a greater supply of energy than others.

Percentage of energy expended by various organs

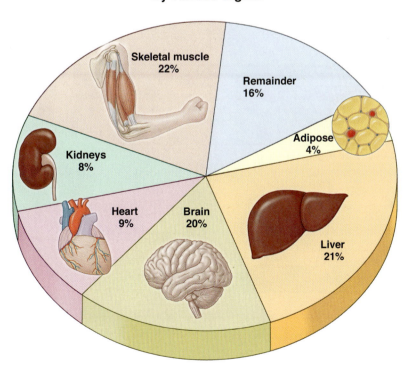

Units of Energy

Energy expenditure is measured by the output of heat from the body. In nutrition, the unit of heat often used is the **calorie:** the amount of heat (or energy) needed to raise the temperature of 1 gram of water by 1 degree Celsius. One thousand calories is called a Calorie (with a capital C) or a kilocalorie. In other words, calories are *energy* that the body uses as fuel.

People obtain dietary calories through the consumption of carbohydrates, proteins, and fats. The number of calories in food is a measure of the potential energy contained in that food. Not all food groups furnish the same number of calories. For example, carbohydrates and proteins both yield 4 Calories/gram, while fats yield 9 Calories/gram. For optimal nutrition, energy needs should be supplied by a balance of carbohydrates, proteins, and fats as well as vitamins and other nutrients.

The Body AT WORK

The amount of energy the body needs at rest (such as that required for the heart to beat, the lungs to breathe, and the kidneys to function) is called the **basal metabolic rate (BMR).** *The BMR for adults is about 2000 Calories/day for males and slightly less for females. Factors that increase metabolic rate include anxiety, fever, eating (the metabolic rate increases as the body processes the ingested food), and thyroid hormones. A number of factors influence the number of calories each person needs. (See "Key Factors Affecting Metabolic Rate" on this page.)*

The next factor affecting caloric need is physical activity. Physical activity includes everything from brushing your teeth to jogging. The number of calories burned during a physical activity varies according to a person's body weight as well as the intensity of the activity.

To maintain weight, calorie intake must equal output. If you consume a greater number of calories than your body expends, you will gain weight. The opposite is also true: consuming fewer calories than your body expends will result in weight loss.

FAST FACT

It takes an excess of 3500 Calories to gain 1 pound of fat.

Key Factors Affecting Metabolic Rate

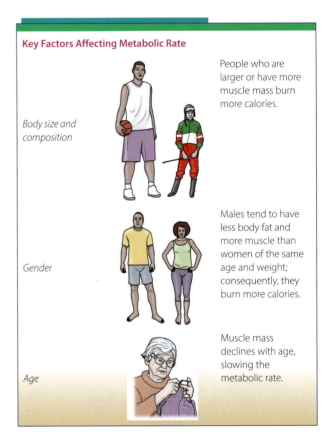

Body size and composition — People who are larger or have more muscle mass burn more calories.

Gender — Males tend to have less body fat and more muscle than women of the same age and weight; consequently, they burn more calories.

Age — Muscle mass declines with age, slowing the metabolic rate.

FAST FACT

Some foods, such as alcohol and those high in sugar, provide what's called "empty calories." That's because these types of foods contain a large number of calories but relatively few nutrients.

Hunger and Satiety

The hypothalamus contains control centers for both hunger and satiety (the feeling of being satisfied after eating). Recent research has identified a number of hormones that profoundly affect these centers. The following figure illustrates five key hormones affecting appetite: one of the hormones—ghrelin—stimulates appetite while the other four suppress it.

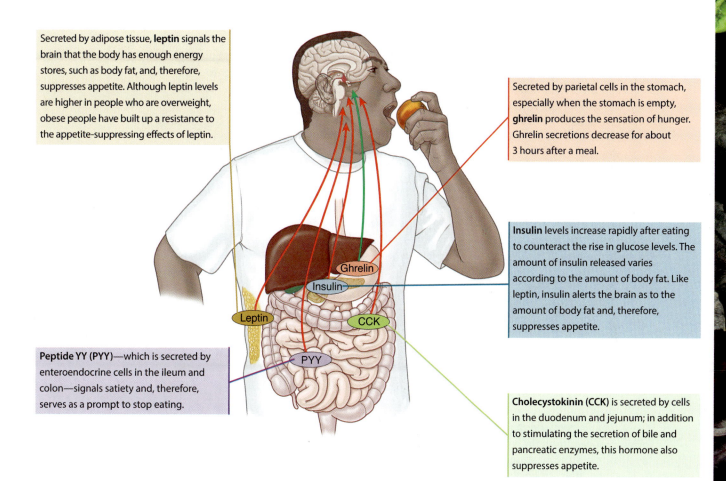

Secreted by adipose tissue, **leptin** signals the brain that the body has enough energy stores, such as body fat, and, therefore, suppresses appetite. Although leptin levels are higher in people who are overweight, obese people have built up a resistance to the appetite-suppressing effects of leptin.

Secreted by parietal cells in the stomach, especially when the stomach is empty, **ghrelin** produces the sensation of hunger. Ghrelin secretions decrease for about 3 hours after a meal.

Insulin levels increase rapidly after eating to counteract the rise in glucose levels. The amount of insulin released varies according to the amount of body fat. Like leptin, insulin alerts the brain as to the amount of body fat and, therefore, suppresses appetite.

Peptide YY (PYY)—which is secreted by enteroendocrine cells in the ileum and colon—signals satiety and, therefore, serves as a prompt to stop eating.

Cholecystokinin (CCK) is secreted by cells in the duodenum and jejunum; in addition to stimulating the secretion of bile and pancreatic enzymes, this hormone also suppresses appetite.

FAST FACT
Ghrelin levels fall dramatically following gastric bypass surgery, suggesting that this may be one of the factors contributing to weight loss after the procedure.

Nutrients

Nutrients used by the body for growth, repair, and maintenance include carbohydrates, lipids, proteins, and water as well as vitamins and minerals. Because the body requires fairly large amounts of carbohydrates, lipids, proteins, and water, these are called **macronutrients.** On the other hand, the body needs only small quantities of vitamins and minerals; therefore, these are called **micronutrients.**

The body must obtain most of its nutrients—including most vitamins, minerals, eight amino acids, and some fatty acids—through diet. These are called **essential nutrients** because they're essential in the diet. Some nutrients, however, the body can synthesize; because they're not essential in the diet, these nutrients are called **nonessential nutrients.**

(Basic concepts of nutrition and metabolism were discussed in Chapter 2, *Chemistry of Life.* It may be helpful to review these topics before proceeding with this chapter.)

Carbohydrates

Carbohydrates are the body's primary energy source. We obtain carbohydrates by eating foods (particularly plants) that contain them. In plants, carbohydrates result from photosynthesis: the process by which plants use energy from sunlight to take up carbon dioxide and release oxygen. In essence, the carbohydrates in plants represent stored energy. By consuming carbohydrates, the body has access to that energy.

Dietary carbohydrates occur in three forms: monosaccharides, disaccharides, and polysaccharides.

Monosaccharides

- Known as **simple sugars**
- Taste sweet
- Absorbed through the small intestine without being broken down
- Examples include glucose, fructose (fruit sugar), and galactose

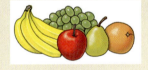

Disaccharides

- Also called simple sugars
- Broken down into monosaccharides during the digestive process
- Examples include sucrose (table sugar), lactose (milk sugar), and maltose (a sugar found in germinating cereals, such as barley)

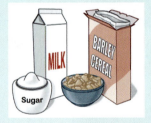

Polysaccharides

- Known as **complex carbohydrates**
- Consist of the starches found in vegetables, grains, potatoes, rice, and legumes
- Includes cellulose as an important polysaccharide (See "The Body at Work" on this page)

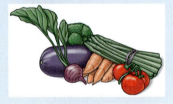

Because the body continually burns carbohydrates for fuel, they should form the greatest percentage of the diet. Specifically, average adults should obtain 40% to 50% of their calories from carbohydrates; very active people may need to obtain up to 60% of their calories from carbohydrates.

Most of the carbohydrates consumed should be complex carbohydrates. That's because these foods contain other vital nutrients in addition to carbohydrates. Also, the body absorbs complex carbohydrates more slowly than simple sugars, which helps prevent unhealthy spikes in blood glucose levels.

The Body AT WORK

Because the body can't digest cellulose, it's not considered a nutrient. Nevertheless, cellulose still makes an important contribution to the diet in the form of dietary fiber. A major component of plant tissues, cellulose absorbs water in the intestines and swells. This adds bulk to the stool, which stretches the colon and increases peristalsis. In turn, this allows stool to pass more quickly out of the body.

Lipids

Lipids, or fats, act as a reservoir of excess energy. Specifically, excess carbohydrates are converted to fat. Then, during periods of decreased food intake, fat reserves can be mobilized and broken down to release energy.

Fat is an ideal substance for storing energy: not only is it more compact than carbohydrates, it's also more energy dense. Each gram of fat contains 9 Calories per gram, compared to 4 Calories for each gram of carbohydrate. Fat fulfills other key roles in the body as well. For example:

- **Fat enables absorption of certain vitamins.** Vitamins A, D, E, and K are fat-soluble, meaning that they depend on dietary fat to be absorbed by the intestine.

- **Fat contributes to cellular structure.** Dietary fats can be converted to other lipids (such as phospholipids and cholesterol), which are major structural components of cell membranes and myelin. Cholesterol also acts as a precursor to steroid hormones, bile acids, and vitamin D.

- **Fat insulates and protects the body.** Besides insulating the body to conserve heat, fat also surrounds delicate internal organs to protect them from damage.

As was discussed in Chapter 2, fats can be saturated or unsaturated depending on the structure of their carbon chains.

> **FAST FACT**
>
> Excessive consumption of saturated fat has been linked to arteriosclerosis, heart disease, diabetes mellitus, and even breast and colon cancers.

Saturated fats

- Derived mainly from animals
- Tend to be solid at room temperature
- Found in meat, egg yolks, and dairy products
- Include hydrogenated oils (oils that are processed so as to make them solid at room temperature), such as vegetable shortening and margarine

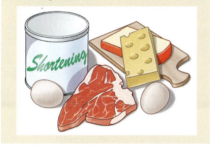

Unsaturated fats

- Occur in nuts, seeds, and vegetable oils
- Tend to be in liquid form at room temperature

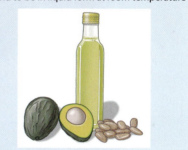

Ideally, fat should comprise no more than 30% of an adult's daily intake, with no more than 20% being saturated fat. For example, based on a 2000-calorie-a-day diet, fat intake should be limited to 400 to 700 calories, or 44 to 78 grams. Of that, less than 10% should be saturated fat.

A specific type of saturated fat commonly found in commercial baked goods and snack foods is trans fat. Trans fat results when hydrogen is added to liquid vegetable shortening during food processing to make it more solid. Trans fat increases the risk for heart attack and stroke, which is why the American Heart Association recommends limiting trans fat consumption to no more than 1% of daily calorie intake.

The body can synthesize most of the fatty acids it needs. However, there are a few (such as linolenic acid, which is a necessary part of the cell membrane) it cannot synthesize. Called **essential fatty acids,** these fats must be obtained through the diet. They are found in such foods as vegetable oils, whole grains, and vegetables.

> **FAST FACT**
>
> Processed foods typically contain saturated fats because they resist becoming rancid and because they tend to remain solid at room temperature.

Protein

Proteins fulfill a vast array of functions in the body. For example, proteins are a major component of all cellular membranes. In addition, they make up much of the structure of bone, cartilage, tendons, ligaments, skin, hair, and nails. Antibodies, hormones, and hemoglobin—as well as about 2000 different enzymes—also consist of proteins. In fact, about 12% to 15% of the body's mass is made of protein.

The body contains over 100,000 different proteins. Each of these proteins consists of various combinations of just 20 different amino acids. (See "The Body at Work" on this page.)

During the process of digestion, proteins are broken down into their individual amino acids. Once absorbed, the body recombines the amino acids to create a new protein for a specific purpose. Foods that supply all the essential amino acids are called **complete proteins.** Foods that lack one or more essential amino acids are called **incomplete proteins.** Nutritionists once thought that, for the body to create new proteins, all amino acids needed to be present simultaneously. In other words, they felt it was necessary to consume all 9 essential amino acids at each meal. Recent studies have shown, however, that the body can combine complementary proteins that are consumed over the course of a day.

Complete proteins

- Mainly come from animal sources
- Include meat, fish, eggs, and dairy

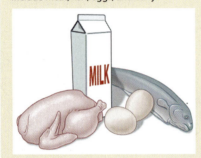

Incomplete proteins

- Come from plant sources
- Include nuts, grains, and legumes

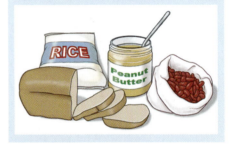

FAST FACT

It's possible to obtain all the essential amino acids from plant sources by combining a food deficient in one amino acid with another food containing that amino acid. For example, combining beans, which are deficient in the amino acid lysine, with rice, which is rich in lysine, forms a complete protein.

The Body AT WORK

The body can synthesize 11 of its 20 amino acids. Because it's not necessary to consume them through the diet, they're called **nonessential amino acids.** (Keep in mind that these amino acids are still essential in the body.) The remaining 9 amino acids are called **essential amino acids** because they must be obtained through food. The following table lists the names of the body's 20 amino acids.

The Human Body's 20 Amino Acids

Essential Amino Acids	Nonessential Amino Acids
Histidine	Alanine
Isoleucine	Arginine
Leucine	Asparagine
Lysine	Aspartic acid
Methionine	Cysteine
Phenylalanine	Glutamic acid
Threonine	Glutamine
Tryptophan	Glycine
Valine	Proline
	Serine
	Tyrosine

Vitamins

Besides carbohydrates, lipids, and proteins, the body also requires small amounts of organic compounds called vitamins. Vitamins are mostly incorporated into coenzymes: molecules that support enzymes in metabolic processes. Other than vitamin D (which can be formed by exposure of the skin to the sun), the body cannot manufacture vitamins. Therefore, vitamins must be obtained regularly through food.

Vitamins are classified as either water-soluble or fat-soluble. **Water-soluble vitamins** are absorbed with water in the small intestine, after which they are dissolved in body fluids and then excreted by the kidneys. Because water-soluble vitamins aren't stored in the body, the risk of toxicity (*hypervitaminosis*) is slight. (However, toxicity can still occur from megadoses of water-soluble vitamins, such as vitamin C.)

Fat-soluble vitamins are absorbed with dietary fat, after which they are stored in the liver and fat tissues of the body until needed. Consequently, megadosing may lead to toxicity. Vitamins A, D, E, and K are fat-soluble vitamins. The following table outlines the major vitamins along with their dietary sources, their function, and the symptoms of deficiency.

Major Vitamins

Vitamin	Dietary Source	Functions	Deficiency Symptoms
Water-Soluble Vitamins			
Ascorbic acid (C)	Citrus fruits, green vegetables	Synthesis of collagen, antioxidant, red blood cell formation, wound healing, aids in iron absorption	Scurvy; degeneration of skin, bone, and blood vessels
Thiamine (B_1)	Red meat, eggs, legumes	Carbohydrate metabolism, blood formation, circulation, central nervous system maintenance	Beriberi (nervous system disorder), edema
Riboflavin (B_2)	Meat, eggs, whole grains, legumes	Energy metabolism; cell respiration; epithelial, eye, and mucosal tissue maintenance	Dry, scaly skin; corneal opacities; keratitis
Niacin (B_3)	Meat, fish, legumes, grains	Circulation; cholesterol level reduction; growth; stimulates central nervous system; metabolism of carbohydrate; protein, and fat	Dermatitis, dementia, diarrhea
Pyridoxine (B_6)	Red meat, fish, green vegetables, whole grains	Helps in metabolism of amino acids and unsaturated fatty acids, antibody formation, DNA and RNA synthesis	Dermatitis, anemia, muscle weakness
Folic acid (B_9)	Vegetables, liver	Synthesis of DNA, catabolism of lipids and amino acids, cell growth and reproduction, red blood cell formation	Anemia
Cyanocobalamin (B_{12})	Red meat, eggs, milk	Formation and maturation of red blood cells, nerve cell maintenance	Pernicious anemia
Biotin	Raw egg yolks, liver, peanuts, tomatoes	Necessary for cell growth, the production of fatty acids, and the metabolism of fats and amino acids	Dermatitis, hair loss, neurological symptoms
Fat-Soluble Vitamins			
Vitamin A (retinol)	Fish oil, eggs, green and yellow vegetables	Growth, night vision, maintenance of epithelial tissue	Night blindness; dry, scaly skin
Vitamin D (calciferol)	Fish oils, eggs, milk, liver	Calcium and phosphorus absorption and metabolism, development of bones and teeth, normal blood clotting	Rickets (in children), osteomalacia (in adults)
Vitamin E (tocopherol)	Fish oils, eggs, milk, seed oils (such as corn and soybean oil)	Antioxidant, normal muscle function, fetal development, myocardial perfusion	Reproductive disorders
Vitamin K	Vegetables such as cabbage, spinach, and tomatoes	Essential for normal blood clotting	Blood coagulation disorders, hemorrhage

FAST FACT

Vitamins were originally named with letters according to the order of their discovery. However, vitamins also have chemically derived names, such as ascorbic acid for vitamin C.

Minerals

The body also needs various inorganic substances called minerals. Minerals are needed for numerous vital functions, including nerve conduction, brain function, heart contraction, and red blood cell formation. Good sources of minerals include vegetables, legumes, milk, eggs, fish, shellfish, and some meats. Most cereals and grains are a poor source of minerals (although minerals are typically added to processed cereals).

Major & Trace Minerals

Minerals	Dietary Source	Functions	Deficiency Symptoms
Major Minerals			
Calcium	Milk and other dairy products, greens, legumes, sardines	Formation of bones and teeth, blood clotting, muscle contraction and relaxation, nerve function	Numbness and tingling, muscle spasms, arrhythmias
Phosphorus	Meat, fish, poultry, eggs, milk, grains	Formation of bones and teeth, cell growth and repair, aids in acid-base balance	Bone degeneration
Magnesium	Meat, seafood, nuts, legumes, grains	Muscle relaxation and nerve impulse transmission, protein synthesis	Nerve disorders, heart arrhythmias
Sodium	Table salt, meat, seafood, milk	Fluid balance, nerve and muscle function, cell permeability	Weakness
Potassium	Potatoes, melons, citrus fruit, bananas, meat, most fruits and vegetables	Nerve and muscle function, acid-base balance, cardiac rhythm	Muscle weakness, nerve disorders
Trace Minerals			
Iron	Liver, red meat, egg yolks, nuts, legumes	Hemoglobin production	Anemia, fatigue
Iodine	Seafood, iodized salt	Thyroid hormone production, physical and mental development	Goiter, hypothyroidism
Selenium	Grains, meat, fish, dairy products	Antioxidant, immune mechanisms	Anemia
Zinc	Meat, seafood, whole grains	Wound healing, nutrient metabolism, carbohydrate digestion	Delayed growth, rough skin, poor appetite
Copper	Legumes, grains, nuts, organ meats	Component of many enzymes	Fatigue, anemia
Fluoride	Fluoridated drinking water, seafood, seaweed	Formation of bones and teeth	Dental caries
Manganese	Greens, legumes, grains	Formation of bone, activation of some enzymes	Delayed wound healing, dizziness, menstrual disorders

FAST FACT

About 4% of the body's mass consists of minerals. Of this, three-quarters is calcium and phosphorus, which are found in the bones and teeth.

Metabolism

Once inside the cell, nutrients are transformed through metabolism into energy that the body can use immediately or store for later use. Metabolism involves two processes:

- **Catabolism:** Used in the metabolism of carbohydrates and lipids, this process breaks down complex substances into simpler ones or into energy.
- **Anabolism:** Used in protein metabolism, this process forms complex substances out of simpler ones.

Carbohydrate Metabolism

All ingested carbohydrates are converted to glucose, most of which is immediately burned as energy. If the body doesn't need the glucose for immediate energy, it stores it as glycogen or converts it to lipids.

The primary goal of glucose catabolism is to generate adenosine triphosphate (ATP), which cells use for energy. This crucial task occurs in three distinct phases: glycolysis, anaerobic fermentation, and aerobic respiration.

> **FAST FACT**
>
> Processes that occur without oxygen are called **anaerobic** processes; those that require oxygen are called **aerobic.**

Glycolysis

Taking place without oxygen, glycolysis splits one glucose molecule into two molecules of pyruvic acid. Glycolysis releases only a fraction of the available energy; further reactions are needed to release the rest of the energy. Which reactions occur depend upon whether oxygen is available. When oxygen is *not* available—such as during intense exercise when the demand for energy exceeds the supply of oxygen—**anaerobic fermentation** occurs. Most ATP, however, is generated in mitochondria, which require oxygen. So, when oxygen is available, **aerobic respiration** is the pathway of choice.

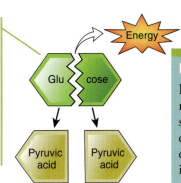

> **FAST FACT**
>
> Because glycolysis doesn't require oxygen, it can supply the cell with energy (although limited energy) even when oxygen is absent.

Anaerobic Fermentation

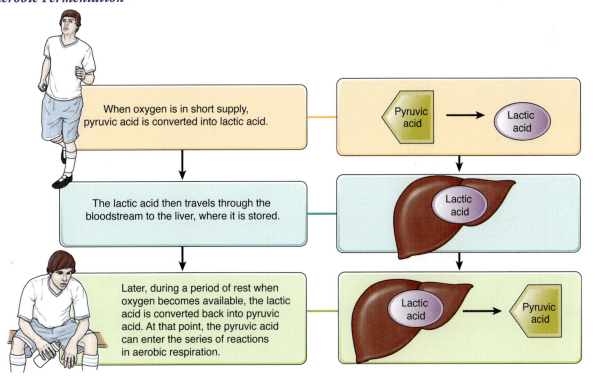

When oxygen is in short supply, pyruvic acid is converted into lactic acid.

The lactic acid then travels through the bloodstream to the liver, where it is stored.

Later, during a period of rest when oxygen becomes available, the lactic acid is converted back into pyruvic acid. At that point, the pyruvic acid can enter the series of reactions in aerobic respiration.

Aerobic Respiration

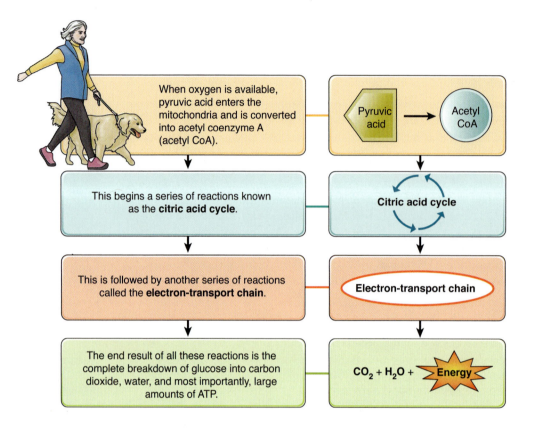

When oxygen is available, pyruvic acid enters the mitochondria and is converted into acetyl coenzyme A (acetyl CoA).

Pyruvic acid → Acetyl CoA

This begins a series of reactions known as the **citric acid cycle**.

Citric acid cycle

This is followed by another series of reactions called the **electron-transport chain**.

Electron-transport chain

The end result of all these reactions is the complete breakdown of glucose into carbon dioxide, water, and most importantly, large amounts of ATP.

$CO_2 + H_2O +$ Energy

The Body AT WORK

Because most cells depend on a steady supply of glucose for fuel, the body uses several mechanisms to maintain a consistent level of glucose in the blood. These mechanisms include glycogenesis, glycogenolysis, and gluconeogenesis.

- *Glycogenesis: When the amount of glucose in the blood exceeds the body's needs, hormones stimulate the liver to convert glucose into glycogen, which is then stored in the liver.*
- *Glycogenolysis: When blood glucose levels fall, such as between meals, glycogen stored in the liver is broken down into glucose. The glucose diffuses into the bloodstream for use by the body's cells.*
- *Gluconeogenesis: The body also has the ability to create glucose from noncarbohydrates, such as fats and amino acids. This mainly occurs in the liver.*

That Makes Sense

To remember the terms related for the formation and breakdown of glycogen and glucose, keep the following in mind:

- *Genesis means "to create."*
- *Lysis means "to break down."*
- *Neo- means "new."*

Therefore, glycogenesis means "the creation of glycogen." Glyconeogenesis means "the creation of new glycogen." Glycogenolysis means "the breakdown of glycogen."

Lipid Metabolism

Fats account for most of the body's stored energy. The breakdown of fat produces more than twice as much energy as the breakdown of carbohydrates.

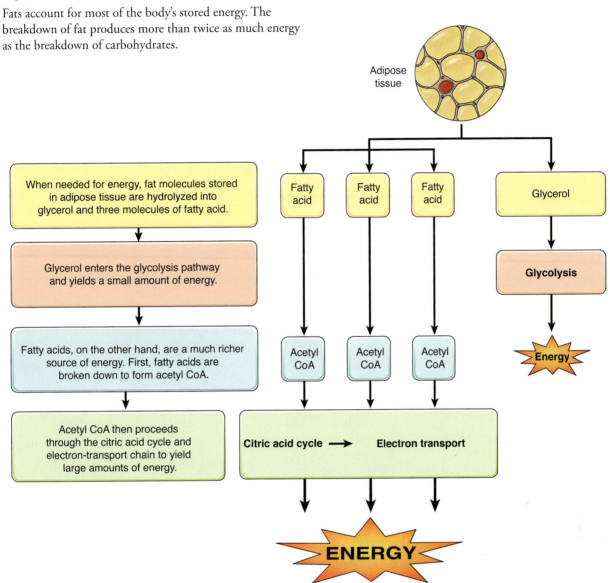

Adipose tissue

When needed for energy, fat molecules stored in adipose tissue are hydrolyzed into glycerol and three molecules of fatty acid.

Glycerol enters the glycolysis pathway and yields a small amount of energy.

Fatty acids, on the other hand, are a much richer source of energy. First, fatty acids are broken down to form acetyl CoA.

Acetyl CoA then proceeds through the citric acid cycle and electron-transport chain to yield large amounts of energy.

Fatty acid   Fatty acid   Fatty acid   Glycerol

Glycolysis

Acetyl CoA   Acetyl CoA   Acetyl CoA   Energy

Citric acid cycle → Electron transport

ENERGY

The Body AT WORK

When the body rapidly metabolizes fat, an excessive number of acetyl CoA units are formed. (A particular instance in which the body rapidly metabolizes fat is in diabetes mellitus. In this situation, the lack of insulin keeps glucose from entering cells, forcing the cells to burn fat for energy.) The liver handles the large supply of acetyl CoA by grouping some of the units together to form ketone bodies. If fat catabolism continues, the ketone bodies will begin to accumulate, resulting in a pH imbalance known as **ketoacidosis.**

FAST FACT

Although lipid catabolism follows the same pathway as carbohydrate catabolism, 1 gram of fat produces 9 Calories of energy, as opposed to carbohydrates, which yield about 4 Calories for the same amount.

Protein Metabolism

Whereas carbohydrates and fat are mainly used to supply energy, proteins are primarily used to build tissue. Protein anabolism plays a significant role in the growth and maintenance of the body: new proteins are used to repair tissue, replace worn-out cells (including red blood cells), create enzymes, grow muscle, and synthesize antibodies, among many other things.

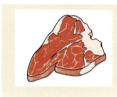

When food containing protein is digested...

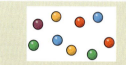

...the proteins are broken down into individual amino acids to create a pool of amino acids.

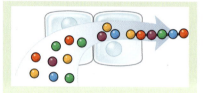

Within the cells, ribosomes pull amino acids from the amino acid pool and recombine them to form new proteins.

Proteins may also be catabolized: converted to glucose and fat or used directly as fuel. Before that happens, however, the amino acids must be altered in the liver.

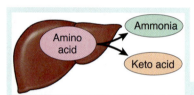

The liver splits an amino group (NH_2) from an amino acid (called **deamination**), forming a molecule of ammonia and a molecule of keto acid.

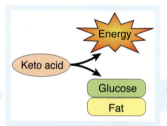

The keto acid may then enter the citric acid cycle, where it is oxidized for energy; it may also be converted to glucose or fat.

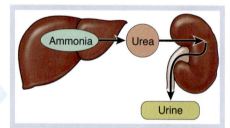

The liver converts the ammonia, which is toxic to cells, to urea, a nitrogenous waste product that is excreted through urine by the kidneys.

The Body AT WORK

The body doesn't store amino acids or proteins like it does fat or carbohydrates; therefore, protein turnover must occur continually. Remarkably, in healthy adults, the amount of protein being broken down equals the amount of protein being created. This state—in which the rate of protein anabolism equals the rate of protein catabolism—is called **protein balance.**

Recall that the catabolism of protein yields nitrogenous waste products. Therefore, if the body is in protein balance, it's also in nitrogen balance: the amount of nitrogen being consumed in the form of protein-containing foods equals the amount of nitrogen being excreted in urine, feces, and sweat as a waste product.

When more proteins are being catabolized than are being created—such as during starvation or a wasting illness—the amount of nitrogen in the urine exceeds the amount of nitrogen in the protein foods ingested. In this instance, the body is said to be in a state of **negative nitrogen balance.**

On the other hand, if the amount of nitrogen being consumed through foods is greater than the nitrogen output in urine, the body is in a state of **positive nitrogen balance.** *This situation—in which protein anabolism outpaces protein catabolism—occurs when large amounts of tissue are being synthesized, such as during periods of growth, during pregnancy, or when recovering from a wasting illness.*

FAST FACT

Ammonia is so toxic that, if a diseased liver fails to remove this nitrogenous waste product, coma and death will soon result.

Thermoregulation

A key factor in homeostasis is the maintenance of body temperature within a narrow range. For this to occur, heat production must balance heat loss. This is known as **thermoregulation.**

Normal body temperature is not static. Rather, it fluctuates about 1.8° F (1° C) through the course of a day, being lowest in the early morning and highest in the late afternoon. Body temperature also varies from one region of the body to another. Specifically, temperature of the deeper body regions—such as that of organs in the cranial, thoracic, and abdominal cavities—ranges from 99° F to 99.7° F (37.2° C to 37.6° C). Temperature closer to the body's surface—such as that of the skin and mouth—ranges from 97.9° F to 98.6° F (36.6° C to 37° C). The temperature of the body's deeper regions, known as **core temperature,** is obtained with a rectal thermometer. The temperature near the surface, called the **shell temperature,** is obtained with an oral thermometer.

Heat Production and Loss

Most of the body's heat results as a by-product of the chemical reactions occurring in cells. The cells of the muscles, brain, liver, and endocrine glands provide the greatest portion of heat when the body is at rest. While skeletal muscles provide 20% to 30% of the heat when the body is at rest, this percentage increases dramatically during vigorous exercise.

To balance the production of heat, the body loses heat by three means: radiation, conduction, and evaporation.

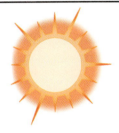

Radiation involves the transfer of heat through the air by electromagnetic heat waves. An example of gaining heat by radiation would be standing in bright sunlight. Because our bodies are typically warmer than the air around us, we tend to lose heat through radiation.

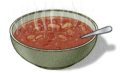

Conduction involves the transfer of heat between two materials that touch each other. In other words, heat passes out of our bodies and into objects that we touch, such as our clothes. (The reason a chair is warm immediately after someone has been sitting in it is because conduction has caused heat to pass out of the body and into the chair.) A practical example is a spoon placed in a bowl of hot soup; after a while, the spoon will become hot through the process of conduction. Conductive heat loss can be accelerated by **convection,** which is the transfer of heat by the actual movement of the warmed matter. For example, heat rises from the body just as steam rises from hot coffee. As the hot air rises, it is replaced by cooler air.

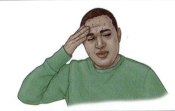

Evaporation requires heat to change water into a gas. That's why perspiration can effectively cool the body. Sweat causes the skin to become wet; then, as evaporation occurs, heat is drawn from the body.

Regulation of Body Temperature

Several negative feedback mechanisms regulate the body's temperature.

When the body temperature rises too high, the hypothalamus signals cutaneous blood vessels to dilate. More warm blood flows close to the body's surface, and heat is lost through the skin.

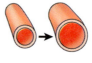

If the temperature remains high, sweat glands produce sweat, and the evaporation of sweat produces cooling.

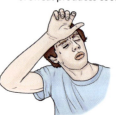

The hypothalamus acts as the body's thermostat: it monitors the temperature of the blood and sends signals to blood vessels and sweat glands.

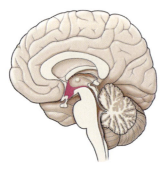

When the body temperature falls below normal, the hypothalamus signals cutaneous blood vessels to constrict. Instead of flowing to the skin, warm blood remains confined deep in the body. As a result, less heat is lost through the skin.

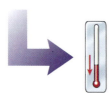

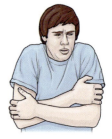

If the temperature remains below normal, the body begins to shiver. Muscle contractions associated with shivering release heat and raise the body's temperature.

The Body AT WORK

Because newborn infants don't have the ability to shiver, their bodies use a mechanism called **nonshivering thermogenesis** *to produce heat. A type of adipose tissue called brown fat makes up about 5% of a newborn's body mass. If a newborn's temperature drops too low, the newborn's body breaks down brown fat to release a considerable amount of heat.*

FAST FACT

Both muscle mass and the number of superficial blood vessels decline with age, making thermoregulation less efficient in elderly individuals. This places them at greater risk for developing hypothermia during cold weather and heat-related disorders during hot weather.

Life lesson: Heat-related disorders

Exposure to extreme heat can produce several disorders, including heat cramps, heat exhaustion, and heat stroke.

- *Heat cramps* are painful muscle spasms resulting from an excessive loss of electrolytes through sweat, usually following strenuous exercise.
- *Heat exhaustion* may develop following prolonged exposure to high temperatures without adequate fluid replacement. Symptoms include dizziness, headache, muscle cramps, nausea or vomiting, and fainting. People prone to heat exhaustion include the elderly, people with high blood pressure, and people working or exercising in a hot environment.
- *Heat stroke* is a life-threatening condition that occurs when the body's temperature reaches 104° F (40° C) or higher. Caused by high environmental temperatures or strenuous physical activity, heat stroke requires immediate medical attention to avoid brain damage, organ failure, or death. Symptoms include hot, dry, flushed skin; headache; rapid heart rate; and muscle cramps or weakness. Seizures, hallucinations, or unconsciousness may also occur.
- *Hypothermia* occurs when the body's temperature falls below 95° F (35° C). Typically caused by exposure to cold weather or immersion in cold water, symptoms include shivering, lack of coordination, slurred speech, confusion, and drowsiness. The confused thinking associated with hypothermia usually keeps the person from being aware of his condition. If body temperature drops below 90° F (32.2° C), death usually occurs.

Review of Key Terms

Aerobic: Processes that require oxygen

Anaerobic: Processes occurring without oxygen

Basal metabolic rate: The amount of energy the body needs at rest

Calorie: The amount of heat needed to raise the temperature of 1 gram of water by 1° Celsius

Carbohydrates: The body's primary energy source

Complete protein: Foods that supply all the essential amino acids

Essential fatty acid: Fat that must be obtained through the diet

Essential nutrients: Nutrients essential in the diet because they cannot be synthesized by the body

Ghrelin: Hormone secreted by cells in the stomach that stimulates appetite.

Glycolysis: The breakdown of carbohydrates for energy

Incomplete proteins: Foods that lack one or more essential amino acids

Lipids: Fats that act as a reservoir of excess energy

Metabolism: Chemical processes occurring in cells that transform nutrients into energy or into materials the body can use or store

Mineral: An inorganic element or compound needed for numerous vital functions

Nonessential amino acids: Amino acids the body can synthesize, making them nonessential in the diet

Nutrients: Usable food components that supply the body with chemicals necessary for energy

Vitamins: Vital nutrients, obtained mostly through food and needed for metabolism

Own the Information

To make the information in this chapter part of your working memory, take some time to reflect on what you've learned. On a separate sheet of paper, write down everything you recall from the chapter. After you're done, log on to the Davis*Plus* website, and check out the Study Group podcast and Study Group Questions for the chapter.

Key Topics for Chapter 21:

- Units of energy
- Hunger and satiety
- Nutrients
- Metabolism of carbohydrates, lipids, and proteins
- Thermoregulation

Test Your Knowledge

1. Which statement about basal metabolic (BMR) rate is accurate?
   a. BMR is fixed at birth.
   b. BMR tends to be higher in females.
   c. A person's size affects his BMR.
   d. Eating a large meal temporarily slows BMR.

2. Which hormone stimulates the appetite?
   a. Ghrelin
   b. Leptin
   c. Peptide YY
   d. Cholecystokinin

3. In the body, what stores the greatest amount of energy in the smallest amount of space?
   a. Vitamins
   b. Protein
   c. Fat
   d. Glucose

4. Nonessential amino acids are:
   a. not necessary for metabolic processes.
   b. synthesized by the body.
   c. not necessary for the synthesis of new proteins.
   d. unavailable in most foods.

5. Which of the following is a digestible polysaccharide?
   a. Starch
   b. Glucose
   c. Cellulose
   d. Maltose

6. An incomplete protein is one that:
   a. cannot be broken down completely.
   b. lacks one or more essential amino acids.
   c. comes mainly from animal sources.
   d. is manufactured by the body and, therefore, not necessary in the diet.

7. The major nitrogenous waste resulting from protein metabolism is:
   a. carbon dioxide.
   b. keto acid.
   c. fluoride.
   d. urea.

Answers: Chapter 21

1. *Correct answer:* **c.** BMR is higher in those who are larger or have more muscle mass. It is not fixed at birth. BMR is higher in males. Eating increases BMR as the body processes the ingested food.

2. *Correct answer:* **a.** All the other hormones listed suppress the appetite.

3. *Correct answer:* **c.** All of the other answers are incorrect.

4. *Correct answer:* **b.** Nonessential amino acids are necessary for metabolic processes, but because they are synthesized by the body, they are not necessary in the diet. Nonessential amino acids are necessary for the synthesis of new proteins.

5. *Correct answer:* **a.** Glucose is a monosaccharide. Cellulose is a polysaccharide, but it is not digestible by humans. Maltose is a disaccharide.

6. *Correct answer:* **b.** Incomplete proteins are broken down into individual amino acids, just like complete proteins. Incomplete proteins are mainly found in plant sources. Incomplete proteins are obtained through food, as opposed to being manufactured by the body.

7. *Correct answer:* **d.** Carbon dioxide results from protein metabolism; however, it is not a nitrogenous waste. Keto acid results (along with ammonia) when the liver splits an amino group from an amino acid during protein catabolism. Fluoride is a mineral found in the diet.

8. *Correct answer:* **c.** All of the other statements pertain to fat-soluble vitamins.

9. *Correct answer:* **c.** Convection is the transfer of heat by the actual movement of the warmed matter, such as heat rising from the body. Heat loss through radiation occurs as we lose warmth to the air around us. Evaporation involves the evaporation of water, which carries heat with it.

10. *Correct answer:* **a.** Starches are complex carbohydrates and are obtained through food. Carbohydrates are not converted to proteins. Excess carbohydrates are stored in the body as fat.

8. Which statement about water-soluble vitamins is true?
   a. A deficiency may result from a very-low-fat diet.
   b. They include the vitamins A, D, E, and K.
   c. They are excreted by the kidney through urine and must be replaced daily.
   d. They are stored in the liver and fat tissues of the body.

9. Sitting on the cold ground causes heat loss through:
   a. convection.
   b. radiation.
   c. conduction.
   d. evaporation.

10. All ingested carbohydrates are first converted to:
   a. glucose.
   b. starch.
   c. protein.
   d. fat.

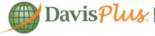 Go to **http://davisplus.fadavis.com** Keyword: Thompson to see all of the resources available with this chapter.

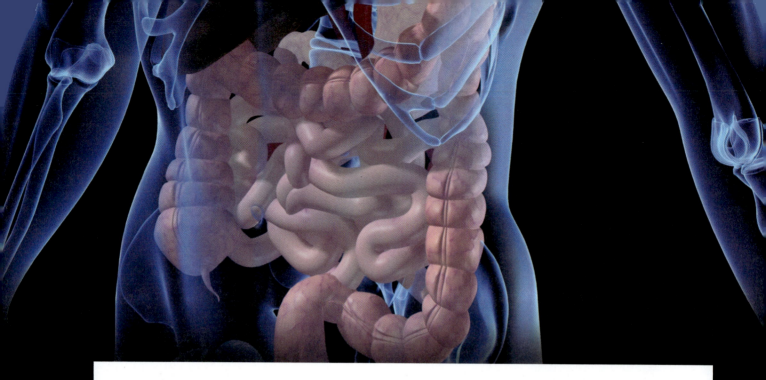

CHAPTER OUTLINE

Building a Microbiome

Components of the Microbiome

LEARNING OUTCOMES

1. Describe the findings of the Human Microbiome Project.

2. Explain how an individual acquires a microbiome.

3. Describe the components of a microbiome, including how microbiomes differ across sites on the body as well as between individuals.

4. Identify the structural components of bacteria.

5. Identify the structural components of viruses.

6. Explain how a disruption in the microbiome can occur.

7. Describe some of the ways a disruption in the microbiome can affect health.

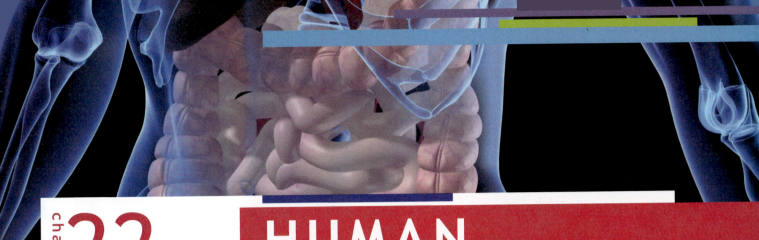

chapter 22

HUMAN MICROBIOME

Ninety percent of the cells in the human body are bacterial,

fungal, or otherwise nonhuman.

For decades, bacteria have been viewed as forerunners of disease, something to be avoided or eradicated. In actuality, every healthy adult houses more than 100 trillion microorganisms. In other words, microbes outnumber human cells by 10 to 1. This community of microbes—known as the **human microbiome**—is essential for human life, so much so that many experts say it should be considered an organ system in its own right.

Although scientists have long been aware that bacteria live on the human body, many of these microbes resist being cultured and grown in a laboratory. It wasn't until the advent of sophisticated DNA sequencing technology, and the subsequent completion of the Human Microbiome Project, that scientists caught a glimpse of this unseen world. (See "Life lesson: The Human Microbiome Project" on the next page.)

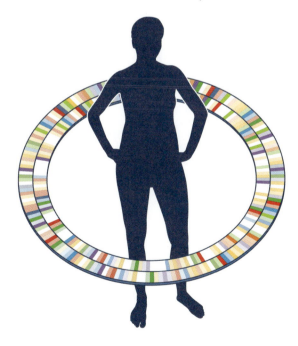

The individual microorganisms found within the microbiome work constantly on our behalf: They digest food, synthesize vitamins, and form a barricade against disease-causing bacteria. Recent research suggests that bacteria even alter brain chemistry, which could affect mood and behavior.

Furthermore, when the composition of the microbiome is disrupted, such as by an excess of a specific bacteria or, more often, through the use of broad-spectrum antibiotics, disease can result. In fact, imbalances in the microbiome are being linked to such disorders as diabetes, heart disease, asthma, multiple sclerosis, and even obesity.

This view of the body as a vast, changeable ecosystem is gradually altering how medicine is practiced. Instead of simply combating bacteria, practitioners are recognizing the need to cultivate and nurture the bacterial communities within our bodies.

FAST FACT

If gathered together, the microorganisms that inhabit the human body would occupy a space about the size of the liver and weigh approximately 3 pounds.

Life lesson: The Human Microbiome Project

After successful completion of the Human Genome Project, the National Institutes of Health decided to use DNA sequencing technology to study the microbial population of healthy adults. So, for 5 years, scientists followed 242 healthy adults, periodically sampling bacteria from 15 or more sites on the subjects' bodies, including their mouths, nasal passages, skin, stool, and, in women, vaginas. The study, known as the Human Microbiome Project, was completed in 2012, and scientists are still coming to terms with the results.

Specifically, the study revealed the existence of a vast, organized system of microbes within healthy adults. This system, known as a *microbiome*, consists of more than 100 trillion microscopic life-forms. Most appear to be bacteria, although viruses and even fungi are included. The diversity of bacteria within the microbiome is staggering; thus far, more than 10,000 species have been identified, and scientists are still analyzing microorganisms that have never before been successfully cultured or identified. One surprising finding was that nearly everyone carried bacteria known to cause disease. However, instead of causing illness, they coexisted peacefully with the rest of the microbiome, prompting scientists to rethink current concepts of how disease occurs.

What is clear is that every person's body contains numerous microbial communities. Each community seems to be charged with a distinct set of metabolic tasks, such as the digestion of sugars in the mouth or of complex carbohydrates in the intestines. The components of each community vary widely across locations. For example, the mouth contains a rich diversity of bacteria, whereas the microbiome in the vagina contains far fewer species.

Adding complexity, the specific inhabitants of each community vary between individuals: Bacteria found in abundant numbers in one person's mouth, for example, may be scarce in another person's. Even more interesting, different microbes appear to perform the same tasks in different individuals. In other words, the intestines need a population of bacteria to digest fat; however, the specific species of bacteria performing that job can vary between persons.

Although researchers are just beginning to understand what all of these microbes do, it is certain they play an important role in maintaining human health. Preliminary evidence suggests that when we eradicate a certain species of bacteria or alter its relative population, we can open the door to the development of any number of diseases, ranging from asthma to obesity.

The Body AT WORK

Each person carries a unique mix of pathogens. Consider this: A study analyzed bacteria on the hands of 51 undergraduate students leaving an examination room. Each student carried approximately 3200 bacteria from 150 species on his or her hands. However, only five species were found on all students' hands; in addition, any two hands (even those belonging to the same person) had only 13% of their bacteria in common.

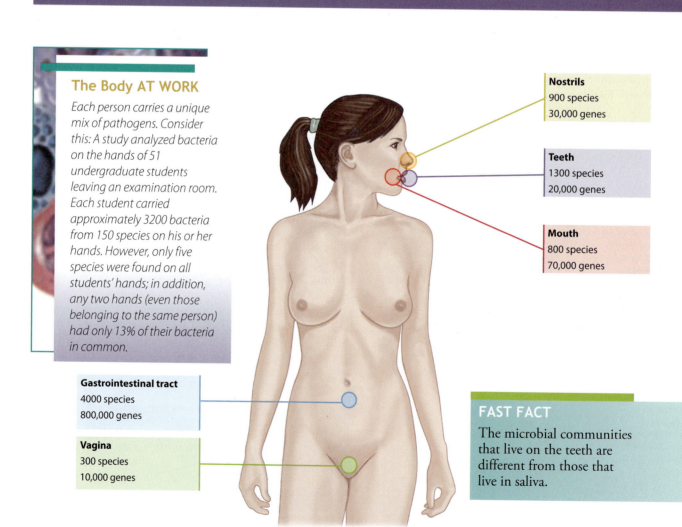

Nostrils
900 species
30,000 genes

Teeth
1300 species
20,000 genes

Mouth
800 species
70,000 genes

Gastrointestinal tract
4000 species
800,000 genes

Vagina
300 species
10,000 genes

FAST FACT

The microbial communities that live on the teeth are different from those that live in saliva.

Microbial species and genes inhabiting the body

Building a Microbiome

The first, crucial step in the development of a microbiome occurs when a newborn passes through the birth canal. The newborn leaves the womb without a single microbe. Then, during the birth process, bacteria from the mother's vagina coat the newborn. This allows microbes to pass from mother to child, forming the basis of the newborn's microbiome. (See "The Body at Work" on the next page.)

After birth, the microbiome expands as the newborn picks up bacteria from his or her immediate environment—other people, food, clothing, furniture, pets, and even the air. As the child grows, the microbiome becomes more complex. At the same time, the microbiome seems to boost development of the immune system. If something disrupts the vibrancy of the microbiome, such as the use of broad-spectrum antibiotics, health seems to suffer. According to researchers, children who take high levels of antibiotics have a higher risk for the development of allergies and asthma.

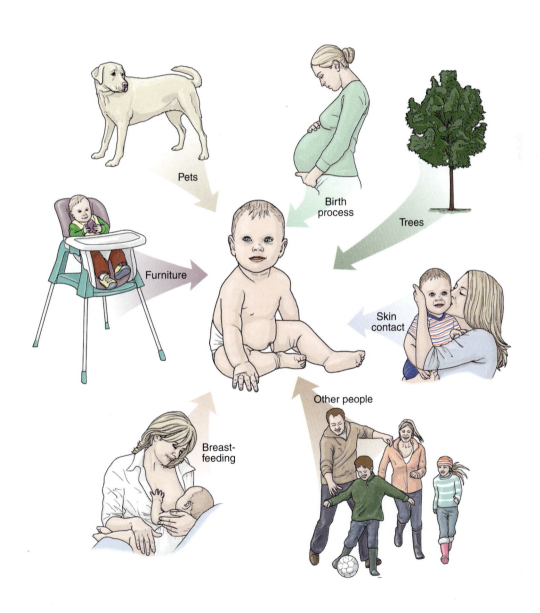

The Body AT WORK

During pregnancy, the bacterial community within a woman's vagina changes significantly as it prepares for the newborn's passage. Normally abundant species become rare, while once-rare species begin to proliferate. Bacteria not normally found in the vagina also take up residence.

For example, one recent study discovered a sizable population of a bacterium called Lactobacillus johnsonii. *This bacterium normally resides in the gut, where it produces enzymes that digest milk. Its appearance in the vagina seemed unusual until researchers considered that the neonate would be coated with, and ingest, the bacteria during the birth process. They then concluded that the* L. johnsonii *would inoculate the newborn and prepare him or her to digest milk.*

Mothers further contribute to their children's microbiomes when they breastfeed. A recent study of lactating women showed that the subjects' breast milk contained 1600 species of bacteria along with sugars (oligosaccharides) that infants cannot digest. The sugar nourishes beneficial gut bacteria, helping good bacteria proliferate, which, in turn, inhibits the growth of harmful bacterial species.

FAST FACT

Infants delivered by cesarean section—and who, therefore, lack many microbes routinely passed from mother to child—have a much higher incidence of allergies and asthma than do children delivered by vaginal birth.

Life lesson: Bacteria may prevent sinusitis

The sinus passages of a person with sinusitis are typically inhabited by some 900 strains of bacteria. Remarkably, a healthy person has even more—1200 species. Experts think that the other members of the bacterial community help keep the infection in check.

Specifically, one study found that the bacterium *Lactobacillus sakei* may be a key player in warding off the condition: Persons with this particular microbe had a far lower incidence of sinusitis. Unfortunately, *L. sakei* is destroyed by antibiotics, leading some to speculate that frequent antibiotic use may actually set the stage for the development of sinusitis.

FAST FACT

Because children acquire significant components of their microbiomes from their mothers, some experts theorize that diseases that appear to be genetic, but whose causative genes can't be located, really are heritable; it's just that the genes causing the disease are bacterial.

FAST FACT

By the age of 18 years, the average American child has received from 10 to 20 courses of antibiotics.

Components of the Microbiome

Bacteria make up the bulk of the human microbiome, although viruses and fungi have also been identified. We also know that bacteria, viruses, and fungi can cause illness. Currently, scientists don't clearly understand how the body determines which microbes to kill and which microbes to nourish.

Bacteria

Bacteria—the chief inhabitants of the microbiome—are single-celled microscopic organisms. They come in a variety of shapes and sizes and are found practically everywhere on earth. Indeed, bacteria can be found in such extreme environments as volcanic vents and Antarctic ice.

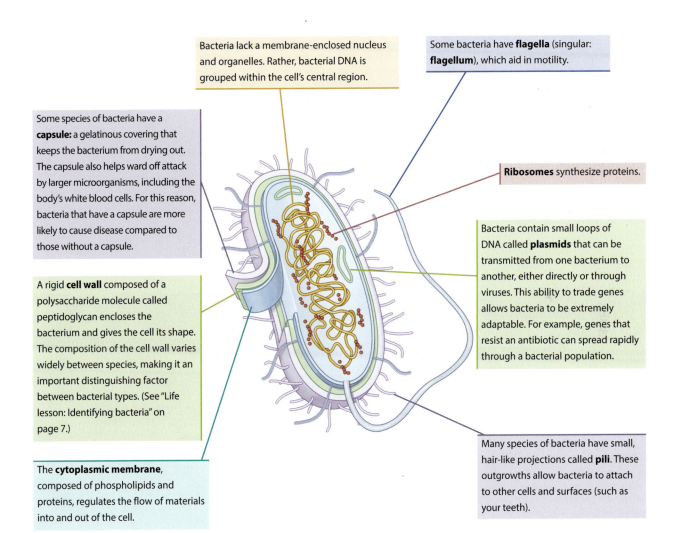

Bacteria lack a membrane-enclosed nucleus and organelles. Rather, bacterial DNA is grouped within the cell's central region.

Some bacteria have **flagella** (singular: **flagellum**), which aid in motility.

Some species of bacteria have a **capsule:** a gelatinous covering that keeps the bacterium from drying out. The capsule also helps ward off attack by larger microorganisms, including the body's white blood cells. For this reason, bacteria that have a capsule are more likely to cause disease compared to those without a capsule.

Ribosomes synthesize proteins.

Bacteria contain small loops of DNA called **plasmids** that can be transmitted from one bacterium to another, either directly or through viruses. This ability to trade genes allows bacteria to be extremely adaptable. For example, genes that resist an antibiotic can spread rapidly through a bacterial population.

A rigid **cell wall** composed of a polysaccharide molecule called peptidoglycan encloses the bacterium and gives the cell its shape. The composition of the cell wall varies widely between species, making it an important distinguishing factor between bacterial types. (See "Life lesson: Identifying bacteria" on page 7.)

The **cytoplasmic membrane**, composed of phospholipids and proteins, regulates the flow of materials into and out of the cell.

Many species of bacteria have small, hair-like projections called **pili**. These outgrowths allow bacteria to attach to other cells and surfaces (such as your teeth).

Bacterial Shapes

Most bacteria have one of three shapes:

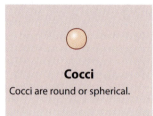

Cocci
Cocci are round or spherical.

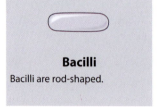

Bacilli
Bacilli are rod-shaped.

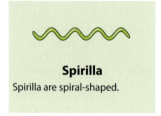

Spirilla
Spirilla are spiral-shaped.

Some bacteria live singly; others exist in aggregates or clusters.

Diplococci
Diplococci are cocci that exist in sets of two, whereas monococci live singly.

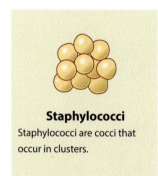

Staphylococci
Staphylococci are cocci that occur in clusters.

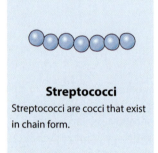

Streptococci
Streptococci are cocci that exist in chain form.

Life lesson: Bacterial transplants

Broad-spectrum antibiotics can be lifesavers. Unfortunately, they also annihilate good bacteria along with the bad. Once treatment stops, there is no guarantee that the microbiome will return to normal. The disrupted bacterial ecosystem then allows harmful bacteria to invade. Once in place, they can proliferate with abandon, unchecked by the good bacteria.

One particularly vicious bacterium that may invade a person's gut following a course of antibiotics is *Clostridium difficile*. According to the Centers for Disease Control and Prevention, *C. difficile* afflicts more than 330,000 persons in the United States each year and results in 14,000 deaths. The infection, which usually afflicts hospitalized patients, is very difficult to treat, and patients are left to suffer from intense diarrhea and abdominal pain.

A major breakthrough in the treatment of this serious infection recently occurred when researchers transplanted feces from a healthy individual into the intestines of patients with *C. difficile*. Once delivered (by way of an enema or colonoscopy), the good bacteria multiplied rapidly, squeezing out the *C. difficile*. Most patients felt significant improvement almost immediately. In fact, one recent study involving 77 patients had an initial success rate of 91%. When the seven who didn't respond the first time were given a second transplant, six were cured.

The Body AT WORK

The organisms gathered during the Human Microbiome Project contained about 8 million genes; this dwarfs the 22,000 contained in the human genome. Put another way, for every human gene in your body, you also have 360 microbial genes.

The function of half the microbial genes remains a mystery. What is certain, though, is that microbial genes have just as great an influence on health and the development of disease as human genes do.

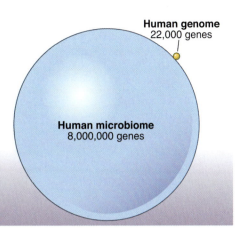

Human genome
22,000 genes

Human microbiome
8,000,000 genes

Life lesson: Identifying bacteria

Gram staining—which involves applying dye to a bacterial sample—is almost always the first step in identifying the bacterial cause of an illness. Whether or not the bacteria retain the dye determines whether the bacteria will be classified as *gram negative* or *gram positive.* Although the technique can't identify the species of bacteria causing an illness, the fact that it provides immediate results can be useful when making treatment decisions.

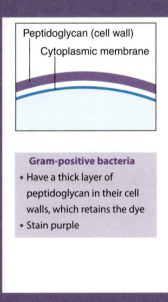

Peptidoglycan (cell wall)
Cytoplasmic membrane

Gram-positive bacteria
• Have a thick layer of peptidoglycan in their cell walls, which retains the dye
• Stain purple

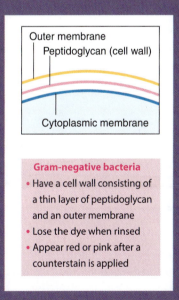

Outer membrane
Peptidoglycan (cell wall)
Cytoplasmic membrane

Gram-negative bacteria
• Have a cell wall consisting of a thin layer of peptidoglycan and an outer membrane
• Lose the dye when rinsed
• Appear red or pink after a counterstain is applied

Because antibiotics such as penicillin work by attacking the peptidoglycan in the bacterial cell wall, they are more effective against Gram-positive bacteria.

FAST FACT

Penicillin interferes with a bacterium's ability to manufacture peptidoglycan. As a result, the cell wall becomes fragile and bursts, killing the bacterium. Because human cells don't contain peptidoglycan, they are not harmed.

Viruses

Viruses are extremely small infectious agents, too small in most cases even to be seen under a light microscope. Unlike bacteria, viruses are *not* cells. They can't metabolize nutrients, produce or excrete wastes, or move around independently. They can't even reproduce on their own; to do so, they must be inside a host cell. Even so, viruses spark many human diseases, including smallpox, AIDS, influenza, certain types of cancer, and the common cold.

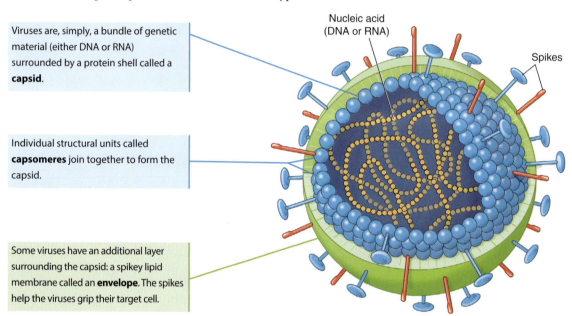

Viruses are, simply, a bundle of genetic material (either DNA or RNA) surrounded by a protein shell called a **capsid**.

Individual structural units called **capsomeres** join together to form the capsid.

Some viruses have an additional layer surrounding the capsid: a spikey lipid membrane called an **envelope**. The spikes help the viruses grip their target cell.

Nucleic acid (DNA or RNA)

Spikes

Viral Shapes

The capsid may assume one of three basic shapes: helical, polyhedral, or complex. In each case, an envelope may, or may not, surround the capsid.

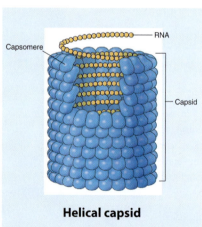

Capsomere

RNA

Capsid

Helical capsid

Helical viruses consist of a strand of RNA spiraled within a protein cylinder. The rabies virus and Ebola virus are both helical viruses. The influenza virus is a helical virus with an envelope.

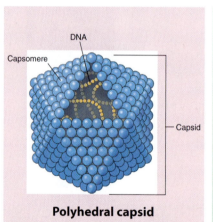

DNA

Capsomere

Capsid

Polyhedral capsid

In polyhedral viruses, the capsid consists of many triangular faces that surround a strand of DNA. Adenovirus is a polyhedral virus. Herpes virus is a polyhedral virus with an envelope.

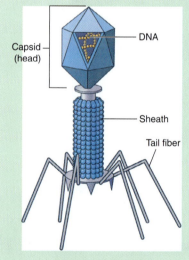

DNA

Capsid (head)

Sheath

Tail fiber

Complex capsid

Complex viruses are neither helical nor polyhedral. **Bacteriophages** (which infect bacterial cells) are complex viruses, consisting of a helical sheath and a complex head containing DNA or RNA. A bacteriophage uses the tail fibers to attach to the surface of its host. It then uses the sheath like a syringe to inject its nucleic acid into the target cell.

Viral Replication

Left to themselves, viruses are inert. To replicate, they must invade a host cell and hijack that cell's metabolic chemicals and ribosomes.

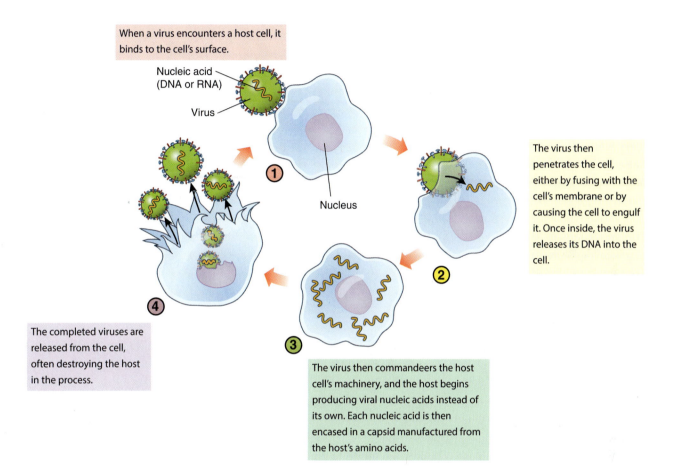

When a virus encounters a host cell, it binds to the cell's surface.

Nucleic acid (DNA or RNA)

Virus

Nucleus

①

The virus then penetrates the cell, either by fusing with the cell's membrane or by causing the cell to engulf it. Once inside, the virus releases its DNA into the cell.

②

The virus then commandeers the host cell's machinery, and the host begins producing viral nucleic acids instead of its own. Each nucleic acid is then encased in a capsid manufactured from the host's amino acids.

③

The completed viruses are released from the cell, often destroying the host in the process.

④

FAST FACT

A single cell may produce from 10,000 to 50,000 new viruses in as little as 48 hours.

FAST FACT

Viruses can mutate rapidly. These frequent changes make it difficult to create effective vaccines to protect humans against infection.

Fungi

Fungi, which include molds and yeasts, live in the soil, on plants, and even in the air. Some fungi reproduce through tiny spores in the air, making it possible to inhale the spores or for them to land on your skin. Consequently, many fungal infections begin on the skin or in the lungs.

Persons most likely to experience fungal infections include those with weakened immune systems or those taking antibiotics. For example, when the microbiome becomes disrupted by a course of antibiotics, a yeast-like fungus called *Candida albicans*—which normally resides on the skin as well as in the mouth, intestines, and vagina—can overgrow, resulting in vaginitis or oral thrush. Athlete's foot and ringworm are also fungal infections.

The Body AT WORK

Bacteria are microscopic, ranging in size from 1 to 10 micrometers. In contrast, viruses are ultramicroscopic; they are measured in nanometers (nm). In fact, 2000 bacteriophages would fit into a single bacterial cell.

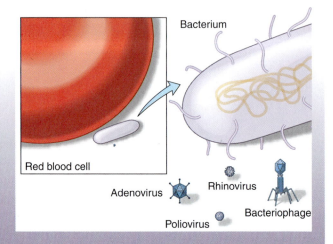

Life lesson: A bacterial link to obesity

The incidence of obesity has become epidemic in the United States, particularly among children. Recent scientific findings suggest that in some instances, obesity may result from disruption of the microbiome in the gut. One study, for example, found that mice gained weight rapidly after their intestinal microbiomes were disrupted by antibiotic medication. Given in doses comparable to those used to treat children with ear infections, the antibiotics eradicated bacteria needed to metabolize calories efficiently. Without the microbes, the mice absorbed more calories from the same amount of food and gained weight.

The link between antibiotic ingestion and weight gain has been a well-known fact in the ranching community for years. In fact, approximately three quarters of antibiotics consumed in the United States are given to livestock, not to treat illness but rather to promote rapid growth and weight gain.

Although antibiotics save lives and are a key weapon against bacterial infections, it is becoming evident that antibiotics also disrupt the microbiome in ways still not completely understood.

The Body AT WORK

*Experts have long maintained that infectious disease occurs when a microorganism known to cause disease (called a **pathogen**) invades the human body through a **portal of entry** (such as a break in the skin or the respiratory, gastrointestinal, or genitourinary tract). However, the focus on one pathogen as the cause of a particular disease is beginning to change.*

It's now clear that nearly everyone carries pathogens within the mix of the microbiome. In healthy individuals, potential pathogens coexist peacefully within the microbiome and produce no ill effects. Research is ongoing as scientists seek to discover why, and under what conditions, some pathogens trigger illness. Findings are beginning to show that what matters is not a particular bacterium, but the function of the microbiome as a whole.

Review of Key Terms

Bacilli: Rod-shaped bacteria

Bacteria: Single-celled microscopic organisms that are the chief inhabitants of the microbiome

Capsid: Protein shell that surrounds viral genetic material

Capsomeres: Individual structural units forming the viral capsid

Capsule: Gelatinous covering that keeps the bacterium from drying out

Cocci: Round- or spherical-shaped bacteria

Gram stain: Staining technique used to classify bacteria into one of two groups

Human microbiome: Microbial makeup of healthy humans

Microbe: Microscopic organism, including bacteria, viruses, and fungi

Pathogen: Disease-causing microorganism

Plasmids: Small loops of DNA contained within bacteria that allow them to transmit DNA from one cell to another

Portal of entry: Pathway by which infectious organisms gain access to the body

Spirilla: Spiral-shaped bacteria

Virus: Ultramicroscopic pathogen consisting of a nucleic acid within a protein shell

Own the Information

To make the information in this chapter part of your working memory, take some time to reflect on what you've learned. On a separate sheet of paper, write down everything you recall from the chapter. After you're done, log on to the Davis*Plus* website, and check out the Study Group podcast and Study Group Questions for the chapter.

Key Topics for Chapter 22:
- Findings of the Human Microbiome Project
- How individuals acquire their microbiomes
- Role of the microbiome in health and disease
- Components of the microbiome
- Effect of antibiotics on the microbiome
- Structural components of bacteria
- Structural components of viruses
- How viruses replicate

Test Your Knowledge

1. What was the goal of the Human Microbiome Project?
   a. To sequence the human genome
   b. To identify disease-causing microorganisms
   c. To identify microorganisms residing within and on healthy adults
   d. To discover whether bacteria contain DNA

2. The Human Microbiome Project discovered that healthy adults:
   a. harbor more bacterial cells than they have human cells.
   b. harbor a significant number of bacterial cells but still have more human cells than bacterial cells.
   c. have no bacterial cells, confirming that bacteria cause disease.
   d. harbor very few bacterial cells.

3. How does a person's microbiome normally develop?
   a. The microbiome begins to develop in the womb, as bacterial cells cross the placenta.
   b. The microbiome begins to develop at age 3 months.
   c. Immunizations are necessary to trigger the development of the microbiome.
   d. The microbiome begins to develop as the infant passes through the birth canal.

4. Which statement about the human microbiome is most accurate?
   a. Every healthy adult carries a mix of microorganisms that is basically similar, except for a few minor variations.
   b. The components of the microbiome are basically the same from one part of the body to another.
   c. The components of the microbiome vary considerably between sites on the body and between individuals.
   d. A healthy microbiome should be free from any disease-causing bacteria.

5. Which statement about bacteria is most accurate?
   a. Bacteria are microscopic cells that contain a nucleus and organelles.
   b. The one consistent feature among all bacterial species is the composition of the cell wall.
   c. Bacteria have the ability to transmit DNA from one bacterium to another.
   d. All bacteria have the same basic shape.

6. What effect do bacterial genes have on human health?
   a. Bacterial genes exert some effect, although human DNA exerts a greater effect.
   b. Bacterial genes have just as great an influence on human health as human genes do.
   c. Bacteria within the microbiome stay within their own community; therefore, their genes do not influence health.
   d. Bacteria do not have genes.

Answers: Chapter 22

1. *Correct answer:* **c.** The Human Genome Project sequenced the human genome. Scientists have been aware of bacteria that cause disease for some time, and that was not the goal of this project. Scientists already knew that bacteria contain DNA.

2. *Correct answer:* **a.** The Human Microbiome Project discovered that healthy adults house more than 100 trillion microorganisms, most of which are bacteria. This means that microbes outnumber human cells by 10 to 1. Although bacteria can cause disease, these adults were healthy, which showed that bacteria play a beneficial role within the body.

3. *Correct answer:* **d.** The newborn leaves the womb without a single microbe. The microbiome begins to develop during the birth process, as the newborn is exposed first to bacteria within the vagina and later to microbes within the environment. Immunizations protect newborns against certain diseases; they do not trigger development of the microbiome.

4. *Correct answer:* **c.** The components of the microbiome vary considerably between sites on the body and between individuals. The Human Microbiome Project also discovered that nearly everyone in the study carried known disease-causing bacteria despite being healthy.

5. *Correct answer:* **c.** Bacteria are microscopic cells, but they have neither a nucleus nor organelles. The composition of the cell wall varies widely among species of bacteria, making it an important distinguishing factor. Bacteria occur in a variety of shapes, the most common of which are round (cocci), rod-shaped (bacilli), or spiral-shaped (spirilla).

6. *Correct answer:* **b.** Microbial genes outnumber human genes 360 to 1; therefore, they exert a greater influence on human health. Bacteria do not isolate themselves within a particular community. Bacteria contain DNA, so, therefore, they contain genes.

7. *Correct answer:* **d.** The cell wall gives the cell its shape. The cytoplasmic membrane regulates the flow of materials into and out of the cell. Ribosomes synthesize proteins.

8. *Correct answer:* **a.** All of the other answers describe bacteria.

9. *Correct answer:* **d.** An excess of a specific bacteria can disrupt the composition of the microbiome; however, the most common way it is disrupted is through the use of broad-spectrum antibiotics. A viral infection has not been shown to disrupt the microbiome, and neither has the ingestion of alcohol.

10. *Correct answer:* **d.** Imbalances in the microbiome have been linked to a number of disorders, including asthma, heart disease, and obesity.

---

7. What purpose does the capsule serve in bacteria?
   a. It gives the cell its shape.
   b. It regulates the flow of materials into and out of the cell.
   c. It synthesizes proteins.
   d. It helps ward off attack by larger microorganisms.

8. Which statement most accurately describes viruses?
   a. Viruses are not cells but, rather, are a bundle of genetic material surrounded by a protein shell.
   b. Viruses are single-celled microscopic organisms that inhabit almost every environment on earth.
   c. Viruses are often categorized through Gram staining.
   d. Viruses have a cell wall that consists of peptidoglycan.

9. What is the most common way a person's microbiome can become disrupted?
   a. Acquisition of a bacterial infection
   b. Acquisition of a viral infection
   c. Ingestion of alcohol
   d. Use of broad-spectrum antibiotics

10. Imbalances in the microbiome have been linked to which of the following disorders?
    a. Asthma
    b. Heart disease
    c. Obesity
    d. All of the above

DavisPlus | Go to http://davisplus.fadavis.com Keyword: Thompson to see all of the resources available with this chapter.

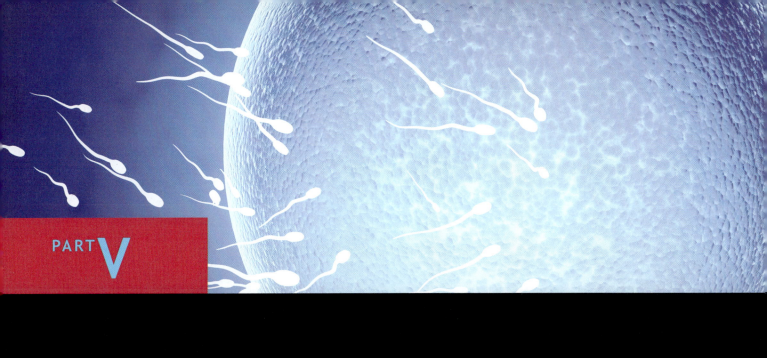

PART V

CONTINUITY

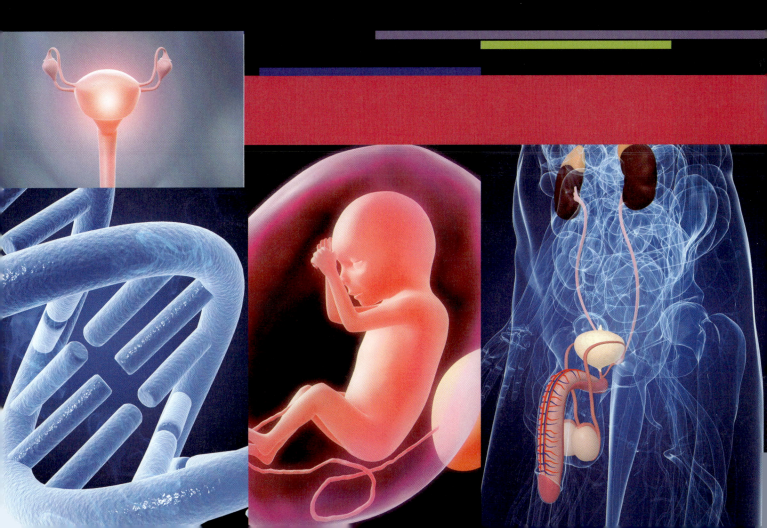

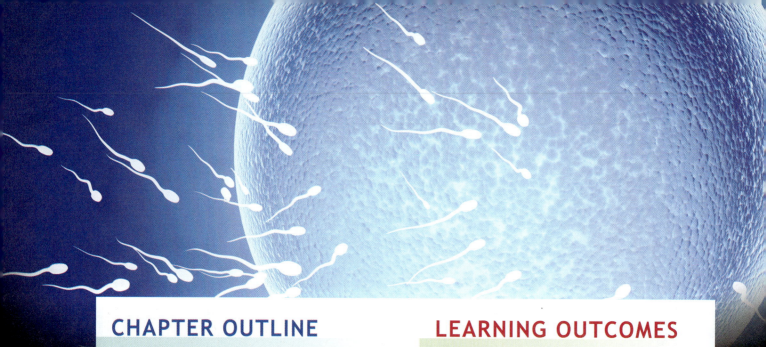

CHAPTER OUTLINE

Overview of the Reproductive System

Male Reproductive System

Female Reproductive System

Methods of Birth Control

LEARNING OUTCOMES

1. Differentiate between primary and secondary sex organs.

2. Describe the structure and function of the testes and the male accessory glands.

3. Describe the structure and function of the penis.

4. Explain the process of male puberty and identify the hormones that play a role in puberty.

5. Explain the process of spermatogenesis.

6. Describe the components of semen.

7. Trace the path taken by sperm from formation to ejaculation.

8. Describe the four phases of the male sexual response.

9. Describe the structure and function of the ovaries.

10. Describe the structure and function of the fallopian tubes, uterus, and vagina.

11. Identify the structures of the female external genitalia.

12. Describe the structures of the female breast.

13. Explain the process of female puberty and identify the hormones that play a role in puberty.

14. Identify the two interrelated cycles of the female reproductive cycle.

15. Discuss the events of the ovarian cycle.

16. Discuss the phases of the menstrual cycle.

17. Describe the four phases of the female sexual response.

23

REPRODUCTIVE SYSTEMS

The reproductive system is the only body system that doesn't become fully functional until puberty.

Obviously, the survival of any species depends upon its ability to reproduce. Some organisms replicate by simply splitting in two. With humans, though, it's a bit more complicated. As opposed to the asexual reproduction of some organisms, human reproduction is sexual, meaning that it requires both a male and a female to reproduce. In this process, sex cells from the male and female fuse together to form an offspring having genes contributed by each parent. In other words, each human offspring is genetically different from his or her parents.

Structurally, the reproductive systems of males and females differ significantly from each other. Regardless, both systems are designed for a specific series of events that range from the genesis of sex cells to the birth of a baby.

Overview of the Reproductive System

The reproductive system consists of both primary and secondary organs. Basically, primary sex organs produce and house sex cells, while secondary sex organs provide the route by which sex cells unite.

Primary sex organs

- Primary sex organs are called **gonads**; they include:
  - testes in males
  - ovaries in females
- The gonads produce sex cells (**gametes**); these include:
  - sperm in males
  - eggs (ova) in females

Secondary sex organs

- Secondary sex organs encompass all other organs necessary for reproduction.
- In males, this includes a system of ducts, glands, and the penis, all of which are charged with storing and transporting sperm.
- In females, the secondary sex organs are concerned with providing a location for the uniting of egg and sperm as well as the environment for nourishing a fertilized egg.

FAST FACT

The sexual and parenting instincts are among the most powerful of all human drives.

Male Reproductive System

The male reproductive system serves to produce, transport, and introduce mature sperm into the female reproductive tract, which is where fertilization occurs.

Testes

The penis and the scrotum (a tissue sac hanging behind the penis) are the external portions of the male reproductive system. Inside the scrotum reside two testes, the organs that generate sperm and secrete the male sex hormone testosterone.

Extending from the abdomen to each testicle is a strand of connective tissue and muscle called the **spermatic cord**; it contains the sperm duct (vas deferens), blood and lymphatic vessels, and nerves.

Two small, oval **testes** lie suspended in a sac of tissue called the **scrotum**.

The **median septum** divides the scrotum, isolating each testicle. This helps prevent any infection from spreading from one testicle to the other.

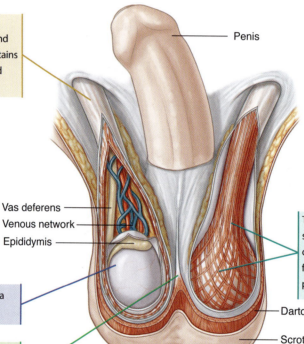

Penis

Vas deferens

Venous network

Epididymis

The **cremaster muscle** surrounds the spermatic cord and testes. In cold weather, it contracts to draw the testes closer to the body for warmth. (See "The Body at Work" on this page.)

Dartos fascia

Scrotal skin

Life lesson: Undescended testicle

In utero, the testes begin development near the kidneys. Then, through the course of fetal development, the testes descend into the scrotum. A small percentage of boys, however, are born with undescended testes, a condition called *cryptorchidism*. If the testes don't descend on their own during the first year of life, a surgical procedure, which involves pulling the testis into the scrotum, is typically done. Alternatively, it may sometimes be corrected through an injection of testosterone. Regardless, if left untreated, the condition will lead to sterility or, possibly, testicular cancer.

The Body AT WORK

*A key reason the testes reside outside the body is because the temperature inside the body is too warm for sperm to develop. (The temperature inside the scrotum is 5° F [3° C] cooler than the temperature inside the body.) Muscles within the scrotum help the testes maintain an ideal temperature for sperm production. For example, in warm temperatures, the cremaster muscle relaxes, allowing the testes to drop further away from the body so as to avoid becoming too warm. In cold weather, it contracts to draw the testes closer to the body for warmth. A layer of smooth muscular fiber (**dartos fascia**) in the scrotum also contracts when it's cold, drawing the testes closer to the body. This gives the scrotum a wrinkled appearance.*

Inside the Testes

Underneath its fibrous capsule covering, the testes contain a vast length of tubules and a series of **spermatic ducts**.

Spermatic ducts

Sperm continue to mature as they follow a specific path through the spermatic ducts.

1 A network of vessels called the **rete testis** leads away from the seminiferous tubules; these vessels provide a location in which sperm partially mature.

2 **Efferent ductules** conduct immature sperm away from the testis to the epididymis.

3 Sperm pass into the **epididymis**, which is attached to the posterior side of the testis. (Note that the epididymis is outside of the testis but still inside the scrotum.) Sperm move from the head of the epididymis to the tail, maturing as they go. They are then stored in the tail of the epididymis, where they remain fertile for 40 to 60 days. After that, unless they are ejaculated, the aging sperm disintegrate and are reabsorbed by the epididymis.

4 Sperm leave the tail of the epididymis and pass into the **vas deferens**.

5 The vas deferens travels up the spermatic cord, through the inguinal canal, and into the pelvic cavity. It loops over the ureter and descends along the posterior bladder wall.

6 As the vas deferens turns downward, it widens into an ampulla and ends by joining the **seminal vesicle** to form the **ejaculatory duct**. (Remember that there are two ejaculatory ducts: one for each testis.) The ejaculatory ducts pass through the prostate and empty into the urethra.

Tubules

The tubules continuously generate sperm.

Fibrous tissue separates each testis into over 200 **lobules**.

Coiled within each lobule are one to three **seminiferous tubules**: tiny tubes in which sperm are produced. Several layers of cells line the walls of the tubules, with each layer containing **germ cells** in the process of becoming sperm. (A germ cell is a cell that gives rise to gametes.) Also contained in the wall of the tubule are cylindrical cells called **Sertoli cells**. These cells promote the development of sperm by supplying nutrients, removing waste, and secreting the hormone *inhibin*, which plays a role in the maturation and release of sperm.

Lying between the seminiferous tubules are clusters of **interstitial cells**—also called **Leydig cells**—that produce testosterone.

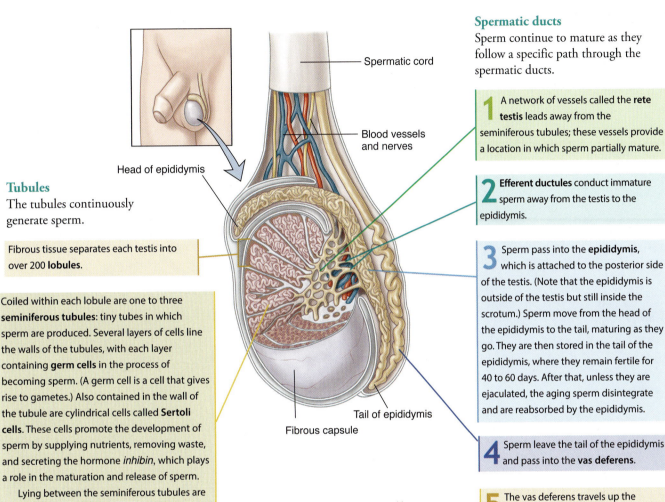

Spermatic cord

Blood vessels and nerves

Head of epididymis

Tail of epididymis

Fibrous capsule

Seminal vesicle

Ejaculatory duct

Prostate gland

Urethra

Testis

Accessory Glands

The male reproductive system includes three sets of accessory glands: the seminal vesicles, prostate gland, and bulbourethral glands.

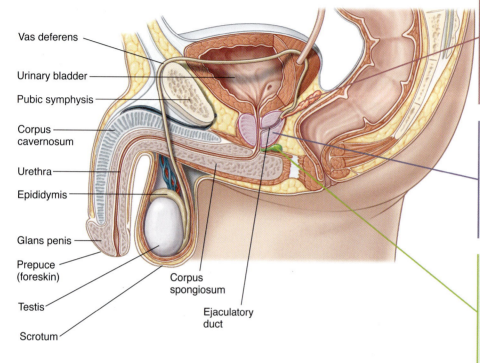

Vas deferens

Urinary bladder

Pubic symphysis

Corpus cavernosum

Urethra

Epididymis

Glans penis

Prepuce (foreskin)

Testis

Scrotum

Corpus spongiosum

Ejaculatory duct

Located at the base of the bladder, a pair of **seminal vesicles** (one for each vas deferens) secretes a thick, yellowish fluid into the ejaculatory duct. The fluid—which comprises about 60% of semen—contains fructose (an energy source for sperm motility) as well as other substances that nourish and ensure sperm motility.

The **prostate gland** sits just below the bladder, where it encircles both the urethra and ejaculatory duct. It secretes a thin, milky, alkaline fluid into the urethra; besides adding volume to semen (it comprises about 30% of the fluid portion of semen), the fluid also enhances sperm motility.

Two pea-shaped **bulbourethral glands** (also called **Cowper's glands**) secrete a clear fluid into the penile portion of the urethra during sexual arousal. Besides serving as a lubricant for sexual intercourse, the fluid also neutralizes the acidity of residual urine in the urethra, which would harm the sperm.

Life lesson: Prostate disorders

The prostate gland is about the size of a walnut in a young man. By about the age of 45, however, the gland begins to enlarge slowly. This noncancerous enlargement resulting from normal aging is called *benign prostatic hyperplasia (BPH)*. As the prostate enlarges, it squeezes the urethra and obstructs the flow of urine. Symptoms include difficulty urinating, slowing of the urine stream, and frequent urination, particularly at night.

Prostate cancer, on the other hand, involves the growth of a malignant tumor within the prostate gland. These types of tumors usually grow slowly and, because they tend to develop outside of the gland, don't obstruct urine flow. As a result, they often go unnoticed. Eventually, the tumor can spread beyond the prostate gland and metastasize to surrounding tissues as well as the lungs and other organs.

Prostate cancer is the most common cancer in American men and the second leading cause of death from cancer (after lung cancer). It is diagnosed by digital rectal examination as well as by blood tests for prostate-specific antigen (PSA) and acid phosphatase (a prostatic enzyme). When detected and treated early, prostate cancer has a high survival rate; however, the survival rate falls dramatically if the cancer has spread beyond the prostate gland.

Penis

The purpose of the penis in the reproductive system is to deposit sperm in the female vagina.

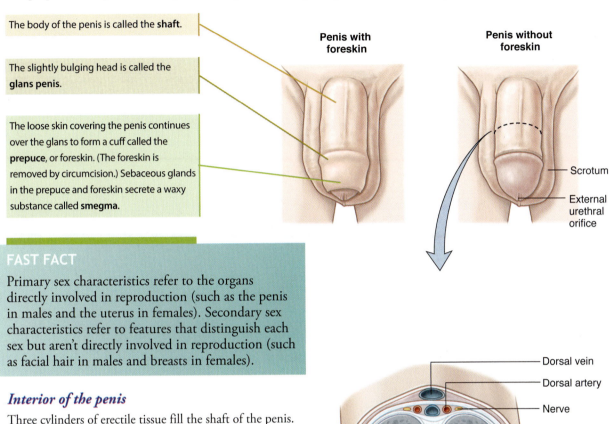

The body of the penis is called the **shaft**.

The slightly bulging head is called the **glans penis**.

The loose skin covering the penis continues over the glans to form a cuff called the **prepuce**, or foreskin. (The foreskin is removed by circumcision.) Sebaceous glands in the prepuce and foreskin secrete a waxy substance called **smegma**.

Penis with foreskin

Penis without foreskin

Scrotum

External urethral orifice

FAST FACT

Primary sex characteristics refer to the organs directly involved in reproduction (such as the penis in males and the uterus in females). Secondary sex characteristics refer to features that distinguish each sex but aren't directly involved in reproduction (such as facial hair in males and breasts in females).

Interior of the penis

Three cylinders of erectile tissue fill the shaft of the penis. During sexual arousal, the tissues fill with blood, causing the penis to enlarge and become erect.

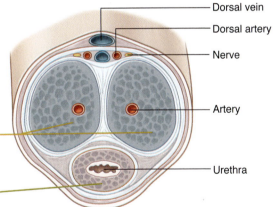

Dorsal vein

Dorsal artery

Nerve

Artery

Urethra

The two larger cylinders of tissue are called the **corpus cavernosa**.

The smaller cylinder of tissue, called the **corpus spongiosum**, encircles the urethra.

The Body AT WORK

During the first trimester of male fetal development, the testes secrete a significant amount of testosterone. After birth, testosterone levels continue to rise for several weeks before falling dramatically, becoming barely detectable by age 4 to 6 months. Low levels of testosterone continue through childhood until, at about age 13, puberty begins; this is the period in which the child's body begins to transform into an adult capable of reproduction.

*The onset of puberty is marked by the secretion of **gonadotropin-releasing hormone (GnRH)** by the hypothalamus. This triggers the secretion of two gonadotropins: **follicle-stimulating hormone (FSH)** and **luteinizing hormone (LH)**. These hormones promote enlargement of the testes, which is the first sign of puberty. LH—also called interstitial cell-stimulating hormone (ICSH) in males—prompts the interstitial cells to begin secreting testosterone. FSH primes the spermatogenic cells to respond to testosterone, and sperm production begins.*

The increased production of testosterone also stimulates the development of such secondary sex characteristics as:

- *Pubic, axillary, and facial hair*
- *Darker and thicker skin*
- *Increased activity of oil and sweat glands, leading to body odor*
- *Increased growth along with an increase in muscle mass*
- *Deepening of the voice due to a larger larynx*

Sperm

The ability of the male's reproductive system to manufacture sperm begins at puberty and continues throughout life.

The Body AT WORK

Reproduction obviously requires a steady supply of gametes. While most cells reproduce through the process of mitosis (as was discussed in Chapter 3), the development of gametes involves a process called **meiosis**.

As you may recall, the process of mitosis equally distributes chromosomes between two daughter cells, resulting in two genetically identical cells: each with 46 chromosomes identical to those of the parent.

In contrast, germ cells (which develop into gametes) divide through **meiosis**. *In this process, the parent cell splits its supply of 46 chromosomes to form two daughter cells with 23 chromosomes each. (This way, when a sperm having 23 chromosomes unites with an egg having 23 chromosomes, the resulting cell has 46 chromosomes.) What's more, the daughter cells are genetically unique. That's because, before separating, homologous chromosomes in the parent cell come together to exchange genetic information. This ensures that the chromosomes we pass on to our children are unique: they aren't identical to our chromosomes or those of our parents. Finally, while mitosis yields only two daughter cells, meiosis produces four. In other words, in males, each germ cell produces four sperm.*

Spermatogenesis

Sperm formation—called **spermatogenesis**—begins when a male reaches puberty and usually continues throughout life.

FAST FACT

Sperm—thousands of which are produced each second—take over two months to mature.

ANIMATION 🌐

1 Sperm begin as **spermatogonia**, primitive sex cells with 46 chromosomes located in the walls of the seminiferous tubules.

2 Spermatogonia divide by mitosis to produce two daughter cells, each with 46 chromosomes.

3 These cells then differentiate into slightly larger cells called **primary spermatocytes**, which move toward the lumen of the seminiferous tubule.

4 Through meiosis, the primary spermatocyte yields two genetically unique **secondary spermatocytes**, each with 23 chromosomes.

5 Each secondary spermatocyte divides again to form two **spermatids**.

6 Spermatids differentiate to form heads and tails and eventually transform into mature **spermatozoa** (sperm), each with 23 chromosomes.

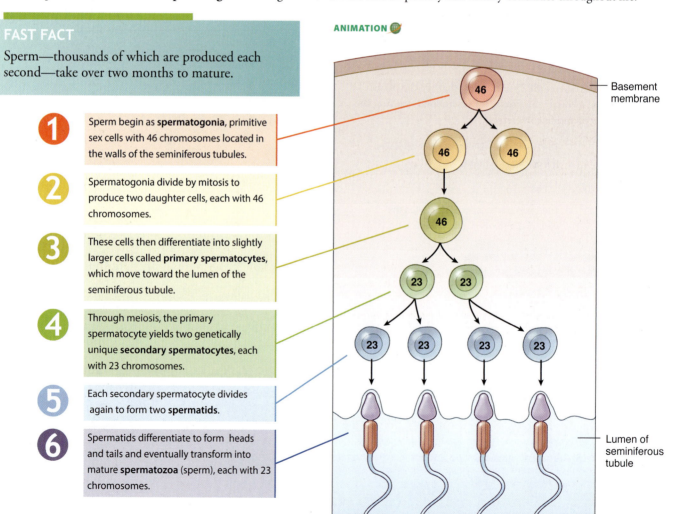

Spermatozoa

The mature sperm consists of a head, a middle piece, and a long, whip-like tail.

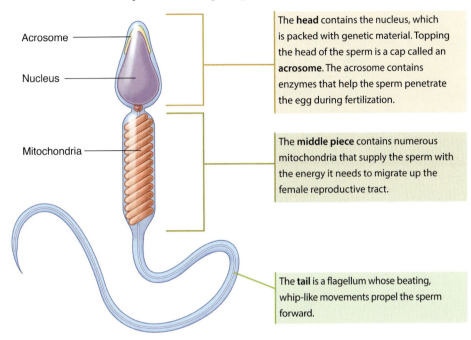

The **head** contains the nucleus, which is packed with genetic material. Topping the head of the sperm is a cap called an **acrosome**. The acrosome contains enzymes that help the sperm penetrate the egg during fertilization.

The **middle piece** contains numerous mitochondria that supply the sperm with the energy it needs to migrate up the female reproductive tract.

The **tail** is a flagellum whose beating, whip-like movements propel the sperm forward.

The Body AT WORK

After puberty, testosterone is continually secreted throughout the life of the male. Testosterone controls spermatogenesis and supports the male sex drive. Blood levels of testosterone are controlled through a negative feedback loop:

- *High levels of testosterone inhibit secretion of GnRH by the hypothalamus. This depresses secretion of LH by the anterior pituitary, and testosterone production declines.*
- *Low testosterone levels stimulate the anterior pituitary to increase secretion of LH, which triggers the interstitial cells to step up testosterone secretion.*

Semen

Emitted during the ejaculation that accompanies orgasm, **semen** is a whitish fluid containing both sperm and the fluid secretions of the accessory glands. About 65% of the fluid volume of semen comes from the seminal vesicles, about 30% comes from the prostate gland, and about 5% comes from the bulbourethral gland. Each ejaculation expels between 2 and 5 ml of semen containing between 40 and 100 million sperm.

Two key qualities of semen include its stickiness and its alkalinity. Immediately after ejaculation, semen becomes sticky and jelly-like. This characteristic promotes fertilization by allowing the semen to stick to the walls of the vagina and cervix instead of immediately draining out. The alkalinity of semen counteracts the acidity of the vagina; this is important because sperm become immobile in an acidic environment.

Life lesson: Male infertility

Over 2 million couples in the United States suffer from infertility. About half of those cases are due to male infertility. The most common form of male infertility is a low sperm count; even so, a number of other factors—including the size, shape, and motility of sperm—also influence male fertility. The World Health Organization provides a number of characteristics of a "normal" sperm sample. For example, the total volume of semen per ejaculate should be at least 2 ml and contain at least 40 million sperm. Of the total spermatozoa in the ejaculate:

- At least 75% should be alive (it is normal for up to 25% to be dead)
- At least 30% should have a normal shape
- At least 25% should be swimming with rapid forward movement
- At least 50% should be swimming forward, if only sluggishly

A sperm count lower than 20 million indicates **infertility**.

Male Sexual Response

The male sexual response can be divided into four phases: excitement, plateau, orgasm, and resolution.

Excitement

- Visual, mental, or physical stimulation causes sexual excitement.
- Parasympathetic nerves cause the arteries in the penis to relax and fill with blood.
- As tissues within the penis become engorged with blood, the penis enlarges and becomes rigid and erect so as to allow it to enter the female reproductive tract.

Plateau

- The urethral sphincter contracts to prevent urine from mixing with semen.
- Heart rate, blood pressure, and respirations remain elevated.

Orgasm

- This brief, intense reaction involves the **ejaculation** of semen.
- Ejaculation occurs in two stages: **emission** and **expulsion**.
  - In emission, the sympathetic nervous system stimulates peristalsis in the vas deferens to propel sperm to the urethra; it also triggers the release of fluids from the prostate gland and seminal vesicles.
  - Semen in the urethra activates somatic and sympathetic reflexes that result in the expulsion of semen.

Resolution

- Immediately following orgasm, sympathetic signals cause the arteries in the penis to constrict, reducing blood flow.
- Muscles between the erectile tissues contract to squeeze blood out of the erectile tissues.
- The penis becomes flaccid.

Female Reproductive System

The female's reproductive system does more than produce gametes. It is also charged with carrying, nourishing, and giving birth to infants.

Unlike the male, the organs of the female reproductive system are housed within the abdominal cavity. The female's primary reproductive organs (gonads) are the ovaries. The ovaries produce ova, the female gametes. The accessory organs—which include the fallopian tubes, uterus, and vagina—extend from near the ovary to outside the body.

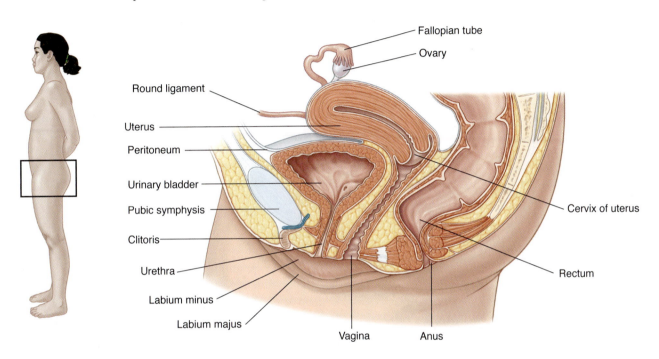

Ovaries

Two ovaries—about the size and shape of almonds—sit on each side of the uterus, where they produce both egg cells (**ova**) and sex hormones. Several ligaments, including the ovarian ligament and a sheet of peritoneum called the broad ligament, hold the ovaries in place.

Each ovary contains thousands of **ovarian follicles** that consist of an immature egg, or **oocyte**, surrounded by **follicular cells**. The follicles evolve during the fetal period, during which time they undergo mitotic division and the first phase of meiosis; at that point, development halts until puberty.

During a menstrual cycle, the hormone FSH prompts several follicles to resume meiosis. As the follicles develop, they migrate toward the surface of the ovary. (The stages of development are shown in the figure to the right.) Usually only one follicle fully matures and reaches the surface. There, it forms a fluid-filled blister called a **graafian follicle**. The follicle bursts and releases the egg contained inside. (This process, called **ovulation**, is discussed in greater detail later in this chapter.)

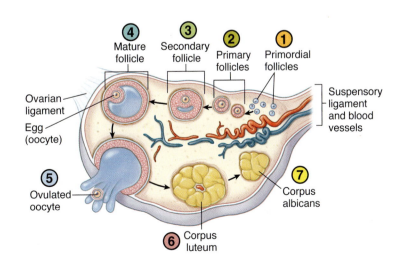

Internal Genitalia

The female reproductive system includes both internal and external genitalia. The internal genitalia include the fallopian tubes, uterus, and vagina. Because the fallopian tubes do not attach to the ovaries, the female reproductive tract is essentially an "open" system in which infection can spread from the reproductive tract into the peritoneal cavity.

Fallopian Tubes

The **fallopian tubes** (also called **uterine tubes**), are about 4 inches (10 cm) long and extend from the ovary to the uterus.

Uterus

A muscular chamber called the **uterus** houses and nurtures a growing embryo. The uterus sits between the urinary bladder and the rectum, held in place by the broad ligament. Usually, the uterus tilts forward over the bladder.

A narrow **isthmus** is the portion of the fallopian tube closest to the uterus.

The middle portion of the tube, called the **ampulla**, is the usual site of egg fertilization. Cilia line the inside of the tube. Their beating movements, combined with peristaltic contractions of the tube, propel an egg toward the uterus.

The distal funnel-shaped end of the fallopian tube is called the **infundibulum**. The fallopian tube does not attach directly to the ovary. Instead, finger-like projections called **fimbriae** fan over the ovary.

The curved upper portion of the uterus is called the **fundus**. The upper two corners of the uterus connect with the fallopian tubes.

The central region of the uterus is the **body**.

The inferior end is the **cervix**. A passageway through the cervix, called the **cervical canal**, links the uterus to the vagina. Glands within the cervical canal secrete thick mucus; during ovulation, the mucus thins to allow sperm to pass.

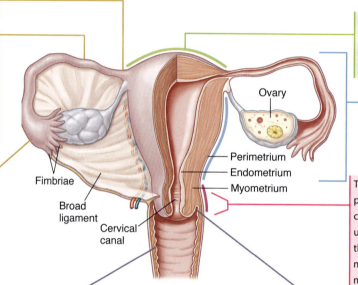

Ovary

Fimbriae

Broad ligament

Cervical canal

Perimetrium
Endometrium
Myometrium

Vagina

A muscular tube about 3 inches (8 cm) long, the **vagina** serves as a receptacle for the penis and sperm, a route for the discharge of menstrual blood, and the passageway for the birth of a baby. The smooth muscle walls of the vagina can expand greatly, such as during childbirth.

The lower end of the vagina contains ridges (**vaginal rugae**) that help stimulate the penis during intercourse and allow for expansion during childbirth.

A fold of mucous membrane called the **hymen** partially covers the entrance to the vagina. During the first intercourse, the hymen ruptures, sometimes producing blood. However, a number of things can tear the hymen before that time, including the use of tampons, vigorous exercise, and medical examinations.

The vagina extends slightly beyond the cervix, creating pockets called **fornices**.

The Body AT WORK

The wall of the uterus has two key roles: housing and nourishing a growing fetus and expelling the fetus from the body during delivery. The uterine wall consists of three layers that aid in those tasks:
- The outer layer—called the **perimetrium**—is a serous membrane.
- A thick middle layer—called the **myometrium**—consists of smooth muscle that contracts during labor to expel the fetus from the uterus.
- The innermost layer—the **endometrium**—is where an embryo attaches. The upper two-thirds portion (called the **stratum functionalis**) thickens each month in anticipation of receiving a fertilized egg. If this doesn't occur, this layer sloughs off, resulting in menstruation. The layer underneath—**the stratum basalis**—attaches the endometrium to the myometrium. It does not slough off; rather, it helps the functionalis layer regenerate each month.

External Genitalia

The external genitals, which include the mons pubis, labia majora (singular: labium majus), labia minora (singular: labium minus), clitoris, and accessory glands, are collectively called the **vulva.**

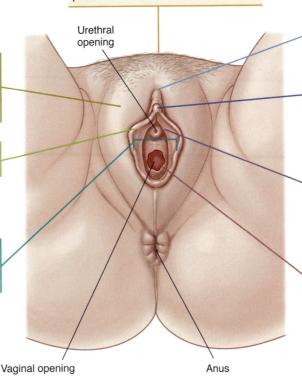

The **mons pubis** is a mound of hair-covered adipose tissue overlying the symphysis pubis.

Urethral opening

The **labium majus** is one of two thick folds of skin and adipose tissue; hair grows on the lateral surfaces of the labia majora while the inner surfaces are hairless.

The **labium minus** is a thinner, hairless fold of skin just inside each labium majus.

The area inside the labia is called the **vestibule**; it contains the urethral and vaginal openings.

The labia minora meet to form a hood of tissue called the **prepuce** over the clitoris.

The **clitoris** is small mound of erectile tissue that resembles a penis. Its role is strictly sensory, providing a source of sexual stimulation.

A pair of mucous glands, called the **lesser vestibular glands** (or **Skene's glands**), open into the vestibule near the urinary meatus, providing lubrication.

Two pea-sized glands called **greater vestibular glands** (or **Bartholin's glands**) sit on either side of the vaginal opening; their secretions help keep the vulva moist and provide lubrication during sexual intercourse.

Vaginal opening   Anus

Breasts

Developing during puberty (as a result of stimulation by estrogen and progesterone), the **breasts** lie over the pectoralis major muscle.

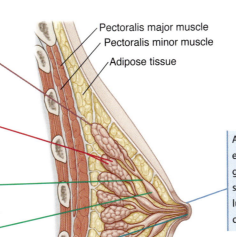

Each breast contains 15 to 20 **lobules** separated by fibrous tissue and adipose tissue.

Each lobule consists of clusters of tiny, sac-like **acini** that secrete milk during lactation. Minute ducts drain the acini, merging to form larger ducts as they travel toward the nipple.

The ducts unite to form a single **lactiferous duct** for each lobe. Before reaching the nipple, the ducts enlarge slightly to form **lactiferous sinuses**.

Each duct ends in a tiny opening on the surface of the nipple.

Pectoralis major muscle
Pectoralis minor muscle
Adipose tissue

FAST FACT

The amount of adipose tissue—not the size of the mammary glands—determines breast size; therefore, breast size has no relationship to the amount of milk breasts can produce.

A pigmented area called the **areola** encircles the nipple. Numerous sebaceous glands (that look like small bumps) dot the surface. Sebum from these glands lubricates the areola, helping prevent dryness and cracking during nursing.

Suspensory ligaments help support the breasts and also serve to attach the breasts to the underlying pectoralis muscles.

The Body AT WORK

Just as in males, female puberty is triggered by rising levels of gonadotropin-releasing hormone (GnRH). GnRH stimulates the anterior lobe of the pituitary to secrete follicle-stimulating hormone (FSH) and luteinizing hormone (LH). FSH stimulates the development of ovarian follicles; in turn, ovarian follicles secrete estrogen and progesterone. Estrogen is the hormone responsible for producing the feminine physical changes that occur during puberty, such as the development of breasts; the deposition of fat beneath the skin of the hips, thighs, and buttocks; and the widening of the pelvis.

*Puberty tends to begin earlier in females than in males, at about age 9 or 10 as opposed to age 13. The first sign of puberty in girls is breast development. This is followed by the growth of pubic and axillary hair. Finally, at about age 12 or 13, the first menstrual period (**menarche**) arrives, although ovulation doesn't begin for another year. In other words, menstruation doesn't indicate fertility.*

FAST FACT

In 1860, most girls began to menstruate at age 16; today, the average age is 12 or 13.

Female Reproductive Cycle

Beginning in adolescence and extending until menopause, a woman's reproductive system undergoes cyclical changes each month as it prepares for the possibility of pregnancy. These changes, called the reproductive cycle, consist of two interrelated cycles: the **ovarian cycle,** which centers on changes in the ovaries, and the **menstrual cycle,** which focuses on changes in the uterus.

Controlled by varying patterns of hormone secretion, the reproductive cycle averages 28 days in length; however, the length of the cycle can range from 20 to 45 days, depending upon the individual. Both cycles are controlled by the cyclical secretion of hormones: the ovarian cycle is governed by the hormones FSH and LH, while the menstrual cycle is under the influence of estrogen and progesterone.

FAST FACT

The process through which a mature ovum is formed is called **oogenesis.**

Life lesson: Breast cancer

Breast cancer affects one out of eight women and is one of the leading causes of cancer-related death. Most breast cancers begin in the ducts and, from there, can spread to other organs by way of the lymphatic system. Symptoms of breast cancer include a lump in the breast or armpit; redness, dimpling, or puckering of the skin of the breast; or drainage from the nipple.

About 20% to 30% of women with breast cancer have a family history of the disease. Scientists have recently discovered defects in the *BRCA1* and *BRCA2* genes that increase the risk for developing breast cancer. Because many breast tumors are stimulated by estrogen, women who begin menstruating before age 12, as well as those who go through menopause after age 55, have an increased risk for the developing breast cancer. Women who have never had children or who had them only after age 30 also have an increased risk. Other risk factors include aging, excessive alcohol use, and exposure to radiation.

The Ovarian Cycle

At birth, a female's ovaries contain about 2 million eggs, or **oocytes.** Each oocyte (which is surrounded by follicular cells) reaches an early stage of meiosis before halting development. Many of these oocytes—also called **primary follicles**—degenerate during childhood. By the time puberty arrives, only 400,000 oocytes remain. (Considering that most women ovulate fewer than 500 times during the course of their reproductive lives, the supply of oocytes is more than adequate.)

The ovarian cycle, as described in the table below, begins on the first day of menstruation as the ovaries prepare to release an egg.

Phases of the Ovarian Cycle
ANIMATION 🌐

LAST DAYS OF MENSTRUATION	Low levels of estrogen and progesterone stimulate the hypothalamus to release GnRH.
	GnRH stimulates the anterior pituitary to release FSH and LH.
FOLLICULAR PHASE	FSH triggers several of the follicles in the ovary to resume development, beginning what is known as the **follicular phase.** Usually, only one follicle will make it to maturity. As the follicle develops, it secretes estrogen (which stimulates the thickening of the endometrium in the menstrual cycle) as well as small amounts of progesterone.
	As the follicle matures, it migrates to the surface of the ovary. The mature follicle is called a **graafian follicle.** In the mid-point of the cycle, estrogen levels peak, triggering a spike in LH.
OVULATION	The sudden spike in LH causes the follicle to rupture and release the ovum—a process called **ovulation.** The fimbriae of the fallopian tube sweep across the top of the ovary to catch the emerging oocyte.
LUTEAL PHASE	Meanwhile, the remnants of the follicle remain on the ovary and form the **corpus luteum,** which marks the beginning of the **luteal phase.** The corpus luteum secretes large amounts of progesterone and small amounts of estrogen. The progesterone causes the endometrium to continue to thicken and become more vascular, preparing it for pregnancy. High levels of progesterone and estrogen also inhibit the pituitary from producing FSH and LH, so no other follicles develop.
	If fertilization doesn't occur, the corpus luteum degenerates into inactive scar tissue called the **corpus albicans.**
MENSTRUATION	Estrogen and progesterone levels plummet, causing the endometrium to slough off, resulting in menstruation. With the decline in ovarian hormones, the pituitary gland is no longer inhibited; FSH levels begin to rise, and a new cycle begins.

The Menstrual Cycle

The hormones estrogen and progesterone—which are secreted by the ovaries—drive the menstrual cycle. This cycle involves the buildup of the endometrium (which occurs through most of the ovarian cycle) followed by its breakdown and discharge. The menstrual cycle is divided into four phases: the menstrual phase, proliferative phase, secretory phase, and premenstrual phase.

Phases of the Menstrual Cycle

Phase	Days	Activity	
Menstrual	1 to 5		The first day of noticeable vaginal bleeding is the first day of the menstrual cycle. Lasting from 3 to 5 days, menstruation occurs as the endometrium sheds its functional layer (the stratum functionalis).
Proliferative	6 to 14	↑estrogen → growth of blood vessels	When menstruation ceases (about day 5 of the cycle), only the base layer (stratum basalis) remains in the uterus. About day 6, rising levels of estrogen (secreted by the ovaries) stimulates the repair of the base layer as well as the growth of blood vessels. During this stage, the endometrium thickens to 2 to 3 mm.

·········· OVULATION ··········

Phase	Days	Activity	
Secretory	15 to 26	↑progesterone → ↑endometrial thickening	After ovulation (about day 14), increased progesterone from the corpus luteum causes the functional layer to thicken even more, this time as a result of secretion and fluid accumulation. During this phase, the endometrium develops into a nutritious bed about 5 to 6 mm thick, just right for a fertilized ovum.
Premenstrual	26 to 28	↓ progesterone → ischemic endometrium	If fertilization doesn't occur, the corpus luteum atrophies and progesterone levels plummet. Blood vessels nourishing the endometrium spasm, interrupting blood flow. The endometrium becomes ischemic and necrotic, causing it to slough off the uterine wall. This forms the menstrual flow.

Interrelationship between the Ovarian Cycle and the Menstrual Cycle

As previously discussed, the ovarian and menstrual cycles are interrelated, with activities in both cycles occurring simultaneously. Study the chart below to tie the activities of the two cycles together and to link each to the fluctuations in hormone levels.

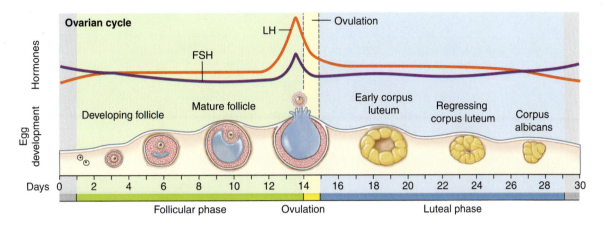

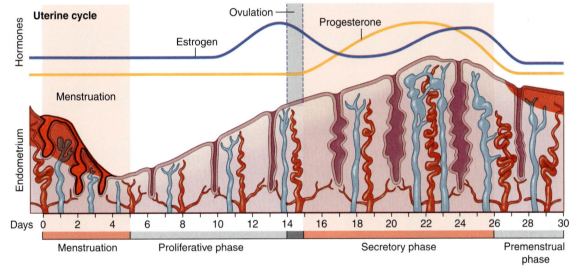

Life lesson: Menopause

Menstruation continues from puberty until about the age of 45 or 50, when it ceases. Called *menopause*, this stage of life is associated with declining estrogen and progesterone levels (as the remaining ovarian follicles are less responsive to gonadotropins). As a result of the declining hormone levels, the uterus, vagina, and breasts atrophy. Vaginal dryness can make intercourse uncomfortable and vaginal infections more common. Symptoms of menopause vary, although common symptoms include hot flashes and mood changes.

Female Sexual Response

The female sexual response can be divided into the same four phases as that of a male: excitement, plateau, orgasm, and resolution.

Excitement

- Blood flow to the genitals increases, causing the labia minora and majora to swell with blood.
- The clitoris becomes engorged and swollen.
- The breasts swell and the nipples become erect and harden.
- The vaginal wall becomes purple from increased blood flow, and the greater vestibular glands produce secretions to lubricate the vagina.
- The uterus stands more erect.

Plateau

- The outer third of the vagina swells.
- The clitoris becomes highly sensitive and retracts beneath its prepuce.

Orgasm

- Muscles in the outer third of the vagina contract rapidly in a series of pulses.
- The muscles in the uterus also contract.
- The skin may appear red or flushed.

Resolution

- The clitoris and nipples soften.
- The vagina and genitals return to normal size and color.
- The uterus drops forward to its usual position.

Methods of Birth Control

Any method used to prevent pregnancy is called **contraception,** or birth control. The following table summarizes some of the most common methods of contraception, beginning with the most effective methods and ending with the least effective.

Method	Characteristics
Surgical Sterilization 	• Sterilization involves cutting or tying the fallopian tubes or vas deferens to block passage of the egg or sperm.
Preventing Implantation 	• An intrauterine device (IUD) is a plastic device inserted into the uterus to prevent fertilization and implantation of a fertilized egg. There are two types of IUDs: one contains a copper wire, and the other contains the hormone progestin. Both types trigger inflammation in the uterus that interferes with a sperm's ability to reach an egg. The progestin IUD also thickens cervical mucus, which further blocks sperm. • Emergency contraceptive pills (ECPs), or "morning after pills," provide a high dose of estrogen and progesterone; taken within 72 hours after intercourse, ECPs prevent pregnancy by inhibiting ovulation or by preventing fertilization.
Hormonal Methods 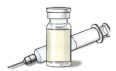	• Birth control pills consist of estrogen and progesterone, which inhibit FSH secretion and, as a result, prevent follicle development and ovulation. • Depo-Provera is a synthetic progesterone that can be injected 2 to 4 times a year to halt ovulation.
Barrier Methods 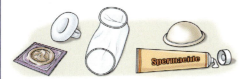	• This form of contraceptive blocks sperm from entering or proceeding past the vagina. • Male and female condoms are the only contraceptives that help prevent the transmission of disease. • Using a chemical spermicide, such as foams, creams, and jellies, greatly improves the effectiveness of barrier methods.
Behavioral Methods Rhythm method 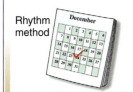	• The rhythm method involves refraining from intercourse during the time the female is most fertile, which is from at least 7 days before ovulation until at least 2 days after ovulation. Because it is difficult to predict the time of ovulation, this method has a 25% failure rate. • Withdrawal (coitus interruptus) requires the male to withdraw his penis before ejaculation. This method also has a high failure rate, both due to a lack of control as well as the fact the some sperm are present in pre-ejaculatory fluids.

Review of Key Terms

Ampulla: Middle portion of the fallopian tube

Cervix: Inferior end of the uterus

Corpus albicans: Inactive scar tissue that results when the corpus luteum degenerates

Corpus luteum: Remnants of the ovarian follicle after ovulation that secretes large amounts of progesterone and small amounts of estrogen

Endometrium: Vascular mucous membrane lining the uterus; thickens each cycle in anticipation of receiving a fertilized egg

Epididymis: Convoluted tube resting on the side of the testes in which sperm mature

Estrogen: Hormone secreted by the ovaries that is responsible for stimulating development of female secondary sex characteristics; it also plays a role in triggering ovulation

Fallopian tubes: Tubes extending from near the ovary to the uterus

Gametes: Sex cells, which include the sperm in males and eggs in females

Gonad: Primary sex organs; includes the testes in males and the ovaries in females

Graafian follicle: A mature follicle of the ovary

Infundibulum: Funnel-shaped, distal end of the fallopian tube

Isthmus: Portion of the fallopian tube closest to the uterus

Meiosis: Process of cell division producing cells (eggs or sperm) that contain half the number of chromosomes found in somatic cells

Menopause: The period that marks the permanent cessation of menstruation

Menstruation: Cyclical shedding of uterine endometrium

Myometrium: Smooth muscle layer of the uterus; contracts during delivery

Oocyte: Immature egg

Oogenesis: Process whereby a mature ovum is formed

Ovarian follicle: Oocyte and surrounding follicular cells

Perimetrium: Outer serous layer of uterine wall

Prostate gland: Gland that surrounds the neck of the bladder and urethra in males; secretes alkaline fluid that forms part of semen

Scrotum: Sac of tissue surrounding the testes

Semen: Whitish fluid containing sperm emitted during ejaculation

Seminiferous tubules: Tiny ducts in the testes in which sperm are produced

Spermatogenesis: Sperm formation that takes place in the seminiferous tubules of the testicles

Testes: Male organs that manufacture sperm and produce the male hormone testosterone

Testosterone: Primary male sex hormone; secreted by the testes

Uterus: Muscular chamber that houses and nurtures a growing embryo and fetus

Vas deferens: Tube that carries sperm out of the epididymis to the ejaculatory duct

Own the Information

To make the information in this chapter part of your working memory, take some time to reflect on what you've learned. On a separate sheet of paper, write down everything you recall from the chapter. After you're done, log on to the Davis*Plus* website, and check out the Study Group podcast and Study Group Questions for the chapter.

Key Topics for Chapter 23:
- Primary and secondary sex organs
- Structure and function of the testes
- Structure and function of the male accessory glands
- Structure and function of the penis

- Process of male puberty
- Formation of sperm
- Components of semen
- Male sexual response
- Structure and function of the ovaries, fallopian tubes, uterus, and vagina
- Female external genitalia
- Structure of the female breast
- Process of female puberty
- Female reproductive cycle
- Female sexual response

Test Your Knowledge

1. The first hormone secreted at the onset of puberty in both males and females is:
   a. testosterone.
   b. follicle-stimulating hormone.
   c. gonadotropin-releasing hormone.
   d. progesterone.

2. Gametes are:
   a. primary sex organs.
   b. sex cells.
   c. immature sperm.
   d. immature ova.

3. Until ejaculation, sperm are stored in the:
   a. vas deferens.
   b. seminiferous tubules.
   c. seminal vesicle.
   d. epididymis.

4. Where is testosterone produced?
   a. Seminiferous tubules
   b. Interstitial cells of the testes
   c. Epididymis
   d. Sustentacular (Sertoli) cells

5. Which organ supplies most of the fluid volume of semen?
   a. Bulbourethral gland
   b. Penis
   c. Seminal vesicles
   d. Prostate

6. The surge in which hormone causes ovulation?
   a. Follicle-stimulating hormone
   b. Luteinizing hormone
   c. Estrogen
   d. Progesterone

7. An embryo attaches to which layer of the uterine wall?
   a. Perimetrium
   b. Endometrium
   c. Myometrium
   d. Vestibule

8. Falling levels of which two hormones trigger menstruation?
   a. FSH and LH
   b. Estrogen and progesterone
   c. GnRH and FSH
   d. Estrogen and testosterone

9. The structure that secretes progesterone during the last half of the ovarian cycle is the:
   a. corpus albicans.
   b. ovarian follicle.
   c. acini.
   d. corpus luteum.

10. Birth control pills prevent pregnancy by:
    a. preventing implantation of a fertilized egg.
    b. changing the acidity of the vagina to kill sperm.
    c. interfering with follicular development and ovulation.
    d. blocking the passage of an egg through the fallopian tube.

DavisPlus | Go to **http://davisplus.fadavis.com** Keyword: Thompson to see all of the resources available with this chapter.

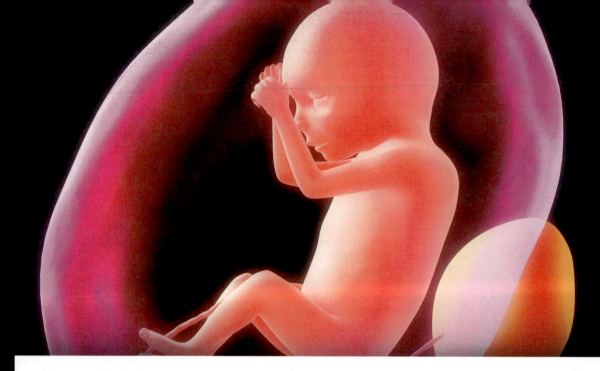

CHAPTER OUTLINE

LEARNING OUTCOMES

1. Discuss the process of fertilization, including when and where it occurs and how the egg prevents fertilization by more than one sperm.

2. Describe the events of the preembryonic stage of development.

3. Summarize the process of implantation and the changes that occur in the blastocyst.

4. Name the three germ layers and identify the major organs and tissues arising from each.

5. Identify the four extraembryonic membranes and describe the functions of each.

6. Describe the structure and functions of the placenta.

7. Trace the path of the fetal circulatory system.

8. Describe the major events of fetal development.

9. List the key physical changes that occur during pregnancy.

10. Identify three factors thought to trigger labor.

11. Identify the three stages of labor and describe the actions, as well as the duration, of each stage.

12. Name the hormones that promote development of the mammary glands for lactation.

13. Describe the process of milk production and milk secretion.

14. Discuss some of the changes experienced by a neonate immediately after delivery.

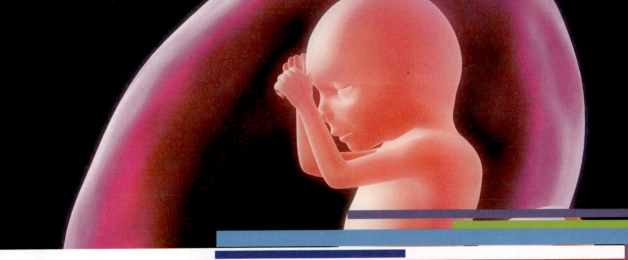

24

PREGNANCY & HUMAN DEVELOPMENT

The human body—which contains 100 trillion cells and thousands of organs—begins as a single cell.

For new life to begin, an egg and a sperm must meet and fuse together. The instant that occurs, the fertilized egg begins a series of changes that, amazingly, transforms a single cell into a fully developed human being. Consider: from that one cell come 100 trillion cells—cells that, in turn, evolve into tissues as diverse as skin, nerves, and blood, and organs as varied as the kidneys, brain, and heart. Indeed, from one cell come not just your physical body but also your mind, your emotions, and your intellect. The process of human development, from conception until birth, is perhaps the most fascinating and miraculous aspect of human life.

Fertilization

Sperm enter the female reproductive tract when the male ejaculates, releasing approximately 100 million sperm into the vagina. Once there, the sperm actively swim toward the fallopian tubes, drawn forward on a mission to fertilize an egg. Only a precious few thousand make it that far, however. The acidity of the vagina destroys many of the sperm; others fail to make it through the cervical mucus; finally, white blood cells in the uterus destroy still more.

Only a few hundred sperm make it through these hazards. Even then, despite being able to reach the egg within minutes of ejaculation, fertilization doesn't occur instantly.

Sperm can remain viable within the female reproductive tract for as long as six days. On the other hand, the egg is only viable for 24 hours. Because it takes 72 hours for the egg to reach the uterus, fertilization typically occurs in the distal third of the fallopian tube.

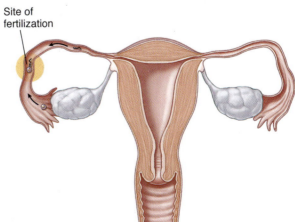

Site of fertilization

FAST FACT

A woman is most fertile during a period of time ranging from a few days before to 14 hours after ovulation.

Even though only one sperm actually fertilizes the egg, a team of sperm helps make fertilization possible by clearing a path through the layer of cells and glycoprotein membrane (the **zona pellucida**) encasing the ovum. The following figure describes this process. Keep in mind that this is a "time lapse" view of fertilization: although many sperm assist with fertilization, only one sperm actually enters the egg.

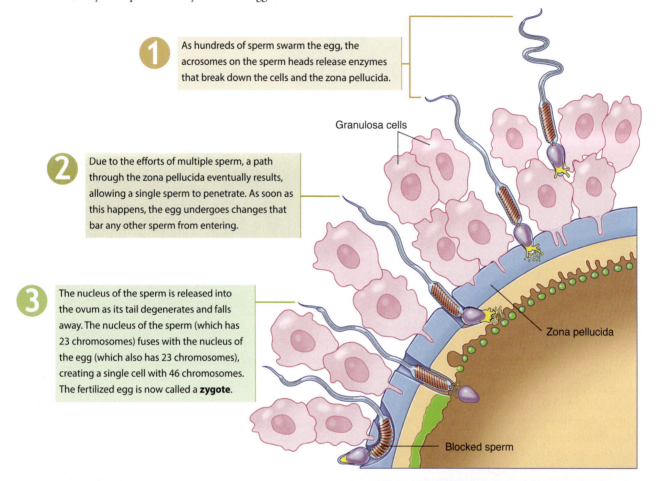

1 As hundreds of sperm swarm the egg, the acrosomes on the sperm heads release enzymes that break down the cells and the zona pellucida.

Granulosa cells

2 Due to the efforts of multiple sperm, a path through the zona pellucida eventually results, allowing a single sperm to penetrate. As soon as this happens, the egg undergoes changes that bar any other sperm from entering.

Zona pellucida

3 The nucleus of the sperm is released into the ovum as its tail degenerates and falls away. The nucleus of the sperm (which has 23 chromosomes) fuses with the nucleus of the egg (which also has 23 chromosomes), creating a single cell with 46 chromosomes. The fertilized egg is now called a **zygote**.

Blocked sperm

The Body AT WORK

*Pregnancy, or **gestation**, ranges from conception until birth and lasts about 266 days. (Typically, gestation is measured from the first day of the last menstrual period, making the time until birth about 40 weeks or 280 days.)*

- *The duration of pregnancy is divided into three-month periods called **trimesters**.*
- *The **first trimester** lasts from conception through the first 12 weeks. (During this period of time, the developing embryo is most susceptible to toxins, stress, drugs, and nutritional deficiencies.)*
- *The **second trimester** ranges from week 13 through week 24. (Most of the organs are developed during this phase.)*
- *The **third trimester** lasts from week 25 until birth. Most infants are viable after about 35 weeks.*

Life lesson: In vitro fertilization

Couples experiencing infertility, particularly women with blocked or damaged fallopian tubes, may choose to undergo in vitro fertilization (IVF) in an effort to conceive. To perform the procedure, a doctor retrieves eggs from the woman's ovary using a needle inserted through the vagina. At the same time, the man provides a semen sample. The active sperm are then combined with the retrieved eggs in a laboratory dish. After about 18 hours in a temperature-controlled environment, the eggs are examined. If fertilization has occurred, the eggs are kept in an incubator for 2 or 3 more days to allow them to grow into the 8- or 16-cell stage. At that point, the doctor transfers the developing embryos into the woman's uterus by way of a catheter inserted through the woman's vagina and cervix. If implantation occurs, the pregnancy test is positive and the pregnancy proceeds.

It's estimated that since 1981 (when IVF was used for the first time), 5 million babies have been born as a result of this procedure. Even so, a normal term birth occurs only about 30% of the time following IVF.

Stages of Prenatal Development

The union of egg and sperm ignites a period of development that ends with the birth of a baby. This period of growth before birth is called the **prenatal** period. During this time, the fetus undergoes three major stages of development:

- The **preembryonic stage,** which begins at fertilization and lasts for 16 days
- The **embryonic stage,** which begins after the sixteenth day and lasts until the eighth week
- The **fetal stage,** which begins the eighth week and lasts until birth

Preembryonic Stage

Shortly after fertilization, the fertilized cell divides by mitosis—a process called **cleavage**—to produce two identical daughter cells. The mitotic divisions continue, with each division doubling the number of cells, until the **zygote** arrives at the uterus. The following illustration portrays this sequence of events, beginning with ovulation and ending with implantation of a fertilized egg.

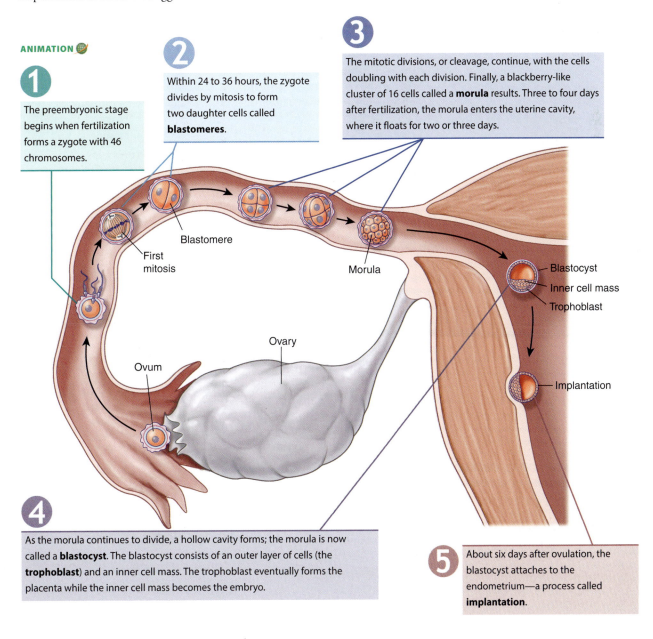

ANIMATION

1 The preembryonic stage begins when fertilization forms a zygote with 46 chromosomes.

2 Within 24 to 36 hours, the zygote divides by mitosis to form two daughter cells called **blastomeres**.

3 The mitotic divisions, or cleavage, continue, with the cells doubling with each division. Finally, a blackberry-like cluster of 16 cells called a **morula** results. Three to four days after fertilization, the morula enters the uterine cavity, where it floats for two or three days.

First mitosis

Blastomere

Morula

Ovum

Ovary

Blastocyst
Inner cell mass
Trophoblast

Implantation

4 As the morula continues to divide, a hollow cavity forms; the morula is now called a **blastocyst**. The blastocyst consists of an outer layer of cells (the **trophoblast**) and an inner cell mass. The trophoblast eventually forms the placenta while the inner cell mass becomes the embryo.

5 About six days after ovulation, the blastocyst attaches to the endometrium—a process called **implantation**.

Implantation

The process of implantation takes about a week, being completed about the time the next menstrual period would have occurred if the woman had not become pregnant. As the blastocyst attaches to the endometrium, it continues to change rapidly as it moves toward becoming an embryo.

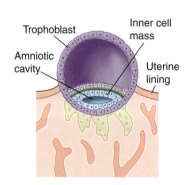
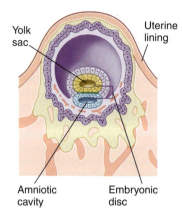
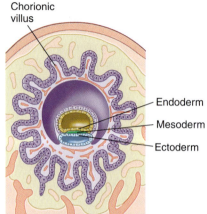

When the blastocyst attaches to the endometrium, the trophoblast cells on the side of the endometrium divide to produce two layers of cells. The outer layer secretes enzymes that erode a gap in the endometrium. As these outer cells penetrate the endometrium, the inner cell mass separates from the trophoblast, creating a narrow space called the **amniotic cavity**.

The inner cell mass flattens to form the **embryonic disc**. Some of the cells on the interior portion of the embryonic disc multiply to form another cavity, called the **yolk sac**. Meanwhile, the rapidly growing endometrium covers the top of the blastocyst, burying it completely.

The embryonic disc gives rise to three layers, called **germ layers**, which produce all the organs and tissues of the body. The three germ layers are the **ectoderm**, **mesoderm**, and **endoderm**.

Germ layers: Each germ layer gives rise to specific organs, a process called **organogenesis**.

Ectoderm	Develops into the epidermis, nervous system, pituitary gland, optic lens, and salivary glands.
Mesoderm	Develops into bones, muscle, cartilage, blood, and the kidneys.
Endoderm	Develops into the epithelial lining of the digestive and respiratory tracts, parts of the bladder and urethra, thyroid and parathyroid glands, liver, and thymus.

The Body AT WORK

*The trophoblast plays a key role in ensuring the continuation of an early pregnancy. These cells secrete **human chorionic gonadotropin (HCG)**, a hormone that prompts the corpus luteum to secrete estrogen and progesterone. In turn, progesterone stimulates endometrial growth and prevents menstruation.*

For the first two months of a pregnancy, levels of HCG in the mother's blood rise. By that time, the placenta begins to secrete large amounts of estrogen and progesterone—effectively taking over the role of the corpus luteum—and the levels of HCG decline.

FAST FACT

The detection of HCG in the mother's blood or urine forms the basis for pregnancy tests. In fact, HCG may be detectable within 8 to 10 days following fertilization.

Embryonic Stage

Once the germ layers are formed—a mere 16 days after conception—the blastocyst enters the embryonic stage and is now called an **embryo.** Two key events occur during the next six weeks: the germ layers differentiate into organs and organ systems, and several accessory organs emerge to aid the developing embryo. The accessory organs include four extraembryonic membranes—the amnion, chorion, allantois, and yolk sac—as well as the placenta and umbilical cord.

Extraembryonic Membranes

The **amnion** is a transparent sac that completely envelops the embryo. The amnion is filled with amniotic fluid, which protects the embryo from trauma as well as changes in temperature. Later, the fetus will "breathe" the fluid and also swallow it. The volume remains stable because the fetus also regularly urinates into the amniotic sac.

The **chorion**—the outermost membrane—surrounds the other membranes. Finger-like projections from the chorion penetrate the uterus. In the area of the umbilical cord, the chorion forms what will become the fetal side of the placenta.

The **allantois** serves as the foundation for the developing umbilical cord. Later, it becomes part of the urinary bladder.

The **yolk sac** produces red blood cells until the sixth week, after which this task is taken over by the embryonic liver. Besides contributing to the formation of the digestive tract, the yolk sac provides nutrients and handles waste disposal.

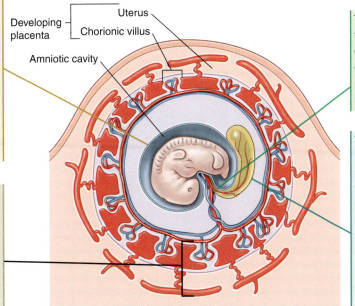

Developing placenta — Uterus
Chorionic villus
Amniotic cavity

Placenta and Umbilical Cord

About 11 days after conception, the embryo develops a disc-shaped, pancake-like organ called the **placenta.** The placenta plays a dual role: it secretes hormones necessary to maintain the pregnancy; it also becomes increasingly important in supplying the embryo, and later the fetus, with oxygen and nutrition. (See "The Body at Work" on the following page.)

The placenta actually begins to form during implantation when specialized cells in the trophoblastic layer extend into the endometrium. As shown in the following figure, these extensions grow into the endometrium like the roots of a tree, forming early chorionic villi.

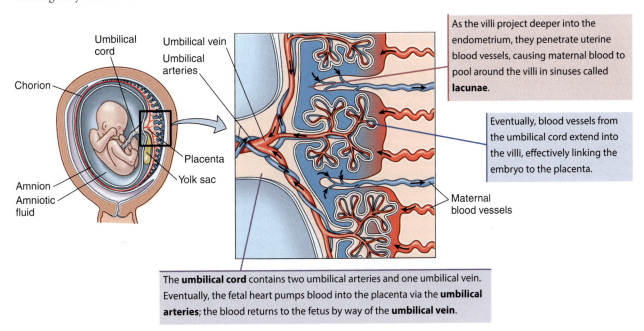

Umbilical cord
Umbilical vein
Umbilical arteries
Chorion
Placenta
Yolk sac
Amnion
Amniotic fluid
Maternal blood vessels

As the villi project deeper into the endometrium, they penetrate uterine blood vessels, causing maternal blood to pool around the villi in sinuses called **lacunae.**

Eventually, blood vessels from the umbilical cord extend into the villi, effectively linking the embryo to the placenta.

The **umbilical cord** contains two umbilical arteries and one umbilical vein. Eventually, the fetal heart pumps blood into the placenta via the **umbilical arteries**; the blood returns to the fetus by way of the **umbilical vein.**

The Body AT WORK

The fetal stage begins the eighth week, and, by the twelfth week, the placenta is the fetus' sole source of nutrition. Although the mother's blood furnishes the developing fetus with nutrients, maternal and fetal blood do not actually mix. Instead, the chorionic villi are filled with fetal blood and surrounded by maternal blood. A thin layer of placental cells separates the two blood systems.

Maternal artery
Maternal vein

Fetal waste products move from fetal blood in the umbilical arteries to the maternal blood; the maternal veins carry away the waste for disposal.

Oxygen, nutrients, and some antibodies pass from the maternal blood—which is pooled in the lacunae around the chorionic villi—to fetal blood in the umbilical veins of the placenta.

Umbilical vein
Umbilical artery

Unfortunately, some toxins such as nicotine, alcohol, and most drugs can also cross the placenta. When they do, they can have a devastating effect on embryonic development.

The placenta also serves an endocrine function, secreting hormones necessary for the continuation of the pregnancy. These hormones include estrogen, progesterone, and HCG.

FAST FACT

Aspirating and testing a sample of amniotic fluid, or testing a tissue sample of a chorionic villus, can reveal valuable genetic information about the developing fetus. The test carries certain risks, however, including miscarriage, infection, or the leakage of amniotic fluid.

Life lesson: Twins

Most twins result when two eggs are ovulated and then fertilized by separate sperm. These twins—called *dizygotic* or *fraternal twins*—do not have the same genetic information. They may be the same, or different, gender. Because they're formed from the union of different eggs and different sperm, they are no more similar than are siblings who are born on separate occasions. Each twin implants on a different part of the uterine wall, and each develops its own placenta.

Occasionally, twins result when a fertilized egg divides in two. In this instance, the twins are the same sex and carry identical genetic information; they are called *monozygotic* or *identical twins*. Monozygotic twins almost always share the same placenta, although each develops in a separate amniotic sac.

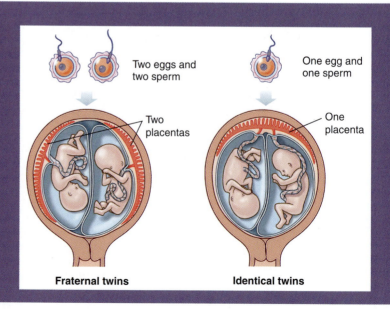

Two eggs and two sperm

One egg and one sperm

Two placentas

One placenta

Fraternal twins

Identical twins

Fetal Stage

The fetal stage, which is the final stage of prenatal development, encompasses the period from the eighth week until birth. This is primarily a stage of growth, as the organs that formed during the embryonic period grow and mature.

Because the fetus depends on the placenta for oxygen and nutrients as well as for the removal of waste products, the circulatory system of the fetus differs significantly from that of a newborn. In the fetus, neither the lungs nor the liver requires a great deal of blood: the lungs are nonfunctioning and the liver is still immature. Therefore, the fetus' circulatory system contains three shunts that allow blood to, for the most part, bypass these organs:

- The **ductus venosus** shunts blood around the liver.
- The **foramen ovale**, an opening between the two atria, shunts blood directly from the right atrium to the left.
- The **ductus arteriosus** diverts blood from right ventricle to the pulmonary artery, bypassing the lungs.

The following figure details circulation in the fetus.

1 Oxygen-rich blood enters the fetus through the vein in the umbilical cord.

2 Most of the blood bypasses the liver by flowing through the **ductus venosus** into the inferior vena cava (IVC). Placental blood from the umbilical vein then merges with fetal blood from the IVC as it flows to the heart.

3 Blood flows into the right atrium; most of the blood flows directly into the left atrium through the **foramen ovale**, bypassing the lungs.

4 The blood that does not flow through the foramen ovale flows into the right ventricle and then into the pulmonary trunk. From there, the blood flows through the **ductus arteriosus** and into the descending aorta, again bypassing the lungs.

5 Oxygen-depleted, waste-filled blood flows through two umbilical arteries to the placenta. The placenta then cleanses the blood—ridding it of carbon dioxide and waste products—reoxygenates it, and returns it to the fetus through the umbilical vein.

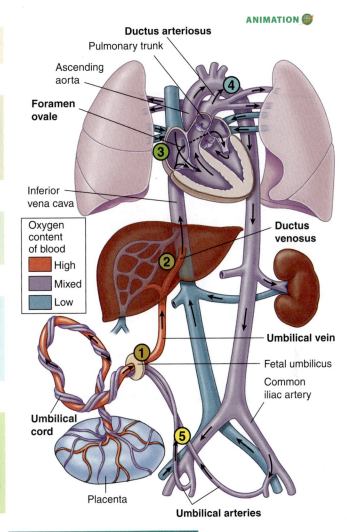

ANIMATION

That Makes Sense

When you think of the placenta as the center of the fetus' universe, the following makes more sense:

- Umbilical arteries pump oxygen-poor, waste-filled blood away from the fetus and toward the placenta.
- The umbilical vein carries oxygenated blood away from the placenta and toward the fetus.

However, much of the fetus' blood is a blend of oxygenated and unoxygenated blood.

The Body AT WORK

With the neonate's first breath, fetal circulation changes. As soon as the lungs are called upon to supply the fetus with oxygen, they demand a larger supply of blood. To meet this need, the ductus arteriosus closes so that blood no longer bypasses the lungs. Then, when blood flows into the left atrium after circulating through the lungs, the newly arriving blood increases the pressure in the left atrium. The increased pressure pushes back the flaps of the foramen ovale and closes the hole. Finally, the ductus venosus deteriorates, eventually becoming a ligament in the liver.

Fetal Development

During the first three months following conception, the outward appearance of the embryo changes rapidly as it develops into a fetus. During the last six months, the organs that formed during the embryonic stage mature and become functional. The fetus also continues to grow and accumulate fat stores.

Week 4

- The brain, spinal cord, and heart begin to develop.
- The gastrointestinal tract begins to form.
- The heart begins to beat about day 22.
- Tiny buds that will become arms and legs are visible.
- Length: 0.25 inch (0.6 cm)

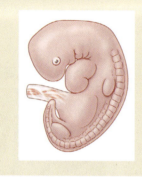

Week 12

- The face is well formed.
- The arms are long and thin.
- The sex is distinguishable.
- The liver produces bile.
- The fetus swallows amniotic fluid and produces urine.
- The eyes are well developed but the eyelids are fused shut.
- Length: 3.54 inches (9 cm)

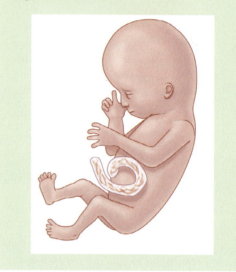

Week 8

- The embryo is now a fetus.
- Eyes, ears, nose, lips, tongue, and tooth buds take shape.
- Head is nearly as large as the rest of the body.
- Brain waves are detectable.
- The arms and legs are recognizable.
- Blood cells and major blood vessels form.
- Bone calcification begins.
- Genitals are present but gender is not distinguishable.
- Length: 1.2 inches (3 cm)

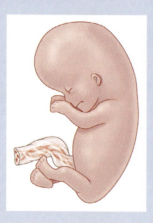

Week 16

- The scalp has hair.
- The lips begin sucking movements.
- The skeleton is visible.
- The heartbeat can be heard with a stethoscope.
- The kidneys are well formed.
- Length: 5.5 inches (14 cm)

FAST FACT

Between the fourteenth and twenty-second weeks of pregnancy, maternal blood is often screened for alpha-fetoprotein (AFP). AFP is a protein produced by the fetal yolk sac and, later, by the fetal liver. High levels of AFP suggest certain abnormalities, such as a neural tube defect in the developing fetus. Low levels suggest a chromosomal abnormality, such as Down syndrome.

Week 20

- A fine hair called **lanugo** covers the body, which, in turn is covered by a white cheese-like substance called **vernix caseosa**; both these substances protect the fetus' skin from amniotic fluid.
- Fetal movement (**quickening**) can be felt.
- Nails appear on fingers and toes.
- Length: 8 inches (20 cm)

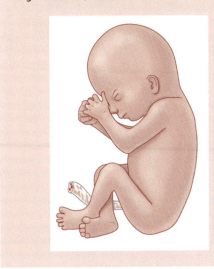

Week 24

- The fetus has a **startle reflex**.
- Lungs begin producing **surfactant**, a lipid and protein mixture that reduces alveolar surface tension.
- Skin is wrinkled and translucent.
- The fetus gains weight rapidly.
- Length: 11.8 inches (30 cm)

Life lesson: Respiratory distress syndrome

Because neonates born before 7 months lack pulmonary surfactant, they typically develop *respiratory distress syndrome (RDS)* after delivery. Surfactant serves to keep the alveoli from sticking together during exhalation. Without surfactant, the alveoli collapse every time the neonate exhales. As a result, he must work hard with every breath, exerting considerable energy just to reinflate the alveoli.

The condition is usually treated with mechanical ventilation that provides air at a positive pressure; this helps keep the alveoli inflated between breaths. Even so, RDS is the most common cause of neonatal death.

Week 28

- The eyes open and close.
- The respiratory system, although immature, is capable of gas exchange at 28 weeks.
- Testes begin to descend into the scrotum.
- The brain develops rapidly.
- Length: 14.8 inches (37.6 cm)

Week 32

- The amount of body fat increases rapidly.
- Rhythmic breathing movements begin, although lungs are still immature.
- The bones are fully formed, although they are still soft.
- Length: 16.7 inches (42 cm)

Week 36

- More subcutaneous fat is deposited.
- Lanugo has mostly disappeared, although it's still present on the upper arms and shoulders.
- Length: 18.5 inches (47 cm)

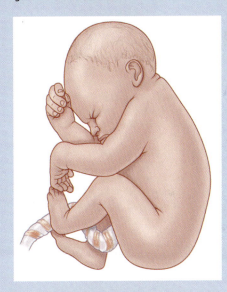

Weeks 39 and 40

- The fetus is considered full term.
- The average full-term infant measures approximately 20 inches (51 cm) long and weighs 7 to 7½ lbs (3.2 to 3.4 kg).

FAST FACT

Experts now define "full term" as being a two-week window starting at 39 weeks because those newborns tend to have the best health outcomes. Those born during a two-week window starting at 37 weeks are called "early term," whereas those born during a two-week window starting at 41 weeks are called "late term."

Physical Changes During Pregnancy

Pregnancy challenges almost every body system as the woman's body nourishes and carries the developing fetus. The following chart lists some of the key changes experienced by pregnant women.

Body System	Changes
Digestive system 	• Nausea and vomiting (morning sickness) commonly occur during the first three months; the cause is unknown. • Constipation often results from decreased intestinal motility. • Heartburn is a frequent occurrence later in the pregnancy as the enlarging uterus presses upward on the stomach. • The basal metabolic rate rises about 15% during the second half of the pregnancy, and the mother's appetite increases.
Circulatory system 	• The mother's blood volume increases by 30% to 50%. • Cardiac output increases 30% to 40% by week 27 as the uterus demands more of the blood supply; at the same time, heart rate also increases. • Later in the pregnancy, the uterus exerts pressure on the pelvic blood vessels, interfering with venous return; hemorrhoids, varicose veins, and swelling in the feet may result.
Respiratory system	• Ventilation increases about 50% to meet the increased demands for oxygen caused by the developing fetus. • Late in the pregnancy, the enlarged uterus pushes against the diaphragm, often causing shortness of breath. • Increased estrogen levels cause the nasal mucosa to swell, resulting in nasal stuffiness.
Urinary system	• An increase in aldosterone promotes water and salt retention by the kidneys. • The glomerular filtration rate increases to deal with the added burden of disposing of the fetus' waste; this leads to a slightly elevated urine output. • Later in the pregnancy, the enlarged uterus presses on the bladder and reduces its capacity; this leads to increased frequency of urination.
Integumentary system	• The skin of the abdomen grows and stretches to accommodate the expanding uterus; this often leads to stretch marks or striae. • Skin over the breasts also grows to accommodate the breasts, which enlarge in preparation for milk production.
Uterus 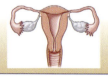	• The uterus enlarges dramatically during pregnancy. During the first 16 weeks of gestation, it grows from the size of a fist until it occupies most of the pelvic cavity. As pregnancy continues, the uterus expands until it reaches the level of the xiphoid process and fills most of the abdominal cavity. • The uterus increases from its nonpregnant weight of 0.1 lbs (50 g) to about 2 lbs (900 g) by the end of pregnancy.

FAST FACT

Even during the last trimester of pregnancy, pregnant women having a normal weight need to consume only an additional 300 kcal/day to give them the recommended weight gain of 24 lbs (11 kg).

Childbirth

At the end of a pregnancy, forceful contractions of the mother's uterine and abdominal muscles (called **labor contractions**) expel the fetus from the mother's body. The onset of labor is thought to result from several factors. These include:

- **A decline in progesterone:** Progesterone inhibits uterine contractions. After six months of gestation, the level of progesterone declines. Meanwhile, the level of estrogen, which stimulates uterine contractions, continues to rise. Falling levels of progesterone combined with rising levels of estrogen lead to uterine irritability.
- **The release of oxytocin (OT):** Toward the end of pregnancy, the posterior pituitary releases more oxytocin, a hormone that stimulates uterine contractions. At the same time, the uterus becomes increasingly sensitive to oxytocin, peaking just before the beginning of labor. In addition, oxytocin causes the fetal membranes to release prostaglandins, another substance that stimulates uterine contractions.
- **Uterine stretching:** As with any smooth muscle, stretching increases contractility.

FAST FACT

The process of giving birth is called **parturition.**

Stages of Labor

Labor occurs in three stages known as the dilation, expulsion, and placental stages.

Stage 1: Dilation of the Cervix

The first stage of labor is the longest stage. It lasts 6 to 18 hours in women giving birth for the first time (**primipara**); it's usually shorter in women who have previously given birth (**multipara**).

The key features of this stage are:

- Cervical **effacement:** the progressive thinning of the cervical walls
- Cervical **dilation:** the progressive widening of the cervix to allow for passage of the fetus

FAST FACT

Late in the pregnancy, the uterus normally exhibits weak, irregular **Braxton-Hicks contractions.** These are sometimes known as false labor.

The fetal membranes usually rupture during dilation, releasing amniotic fluid; this is often referred to as the water breaking.

When the cervix is fully dilated to approximately 4 inches (10 cm), the second stage of labor begins.

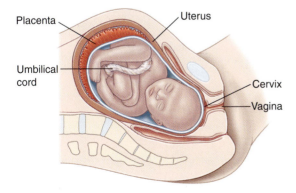

Beginning of dilation

Placenta · Uterus · Umbilical cord · Cervix · Vagina

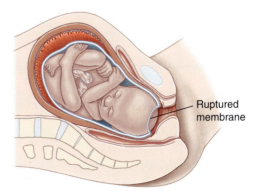

Fully effaced and dilated; membranes have ruptured

Ruptured membrane

Stage 2: Expulsion of the Baby

The second stage of labor—which begins with full dilation of the cervix and ends when the baby is born—lasts 30 to 60 minutes in primiparous women but can be much shorter in multiparous women.

Normally, the head of the baby is delivered first. (The first appearance of the top of the head is called **crowning.**) To facilitate the passage of the head, a surgical incision is sometimes made between the vagina and the anus to enlarge the vaginal opening; this is called an **episiotomy.**

As soon as the head emerges, mucus is cleared from the baby's mouth and nose so he can begin breathing. The umbilical cord is clamped and cut, and the third stage begins.

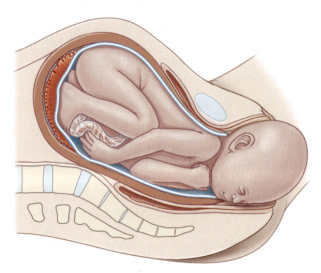

Expulsion of the fetus

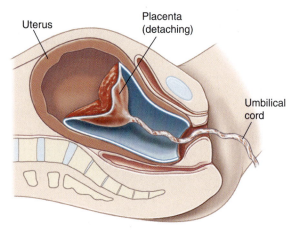

Uterus
Placenta (detaching)
Umbilical cord

Expulsion of the placenta

Stage 3: Delivery of the Placenta

The final stage involves delivery of the **afterbirth:** the placenta, amnion, and other fetal membranes. After delivery of the baby, the uterus continues to contract. These contractions cause the placenta to separate from the uterine wall; then, as they continue, they expel the fetal membranes from the body. The contractions also help seal any blood vessels that are still bleeding.

FAST FACT

Sometimes the baby fails to turn head-down in the uterus and the buttocks are delivered first; this is called a **breech** birth.

Lactation

Following childbirth, the mammary glands produce and secrete milk (called **lactation**) to nourish the newborn child (called a **neonate**). The process of preparing the mammary glands, as well as the process of producing and secreting milk, depends on the actions of various hormones. Specifically, development of the structure of the mammary glands depends on estrogen and progesterone, while the hormones prolactin and oxytocin control milk production and secretion.

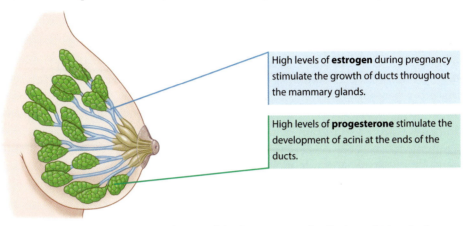

High levels of **estrogen** during pregnancy stimulate the growth of ducts throughout the mammary glands.

High levels of **progesterone** stimulate the development of acini at the ends of the ducts.

The production of milk depends on the hormone prolactin, while the secretion of milk through the nipple depends on the hormone oxytocin.

1. Suckling by the neonate sends nerve impulses to the anterior and posterior pituitary gland.

2. The anterior pituitary secretes prolactin, which initiates the production of milk. (Every time the neonate nurses, the mother's prolactin levels surge; this boosts milk production for the next feeding.)
Anterior pituitary → Prolactin → Milk production

3. The posterior pituitary secretes **oxytocin**. Oxytocin causes the lobules in the breast to contract, forcing milk into the ducts. (This is known as the **milk let-down reflex.**)
Posterior pituitary → Oxytocin → Milk secretion

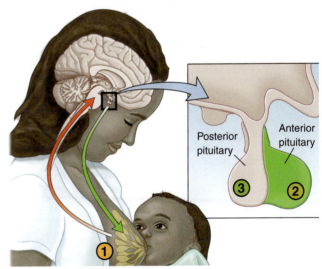

The Body AT WORK

During pregnancy, high levels of estrogen block the secretion of prolactin, keeping milk production at bay. As soon as the placenta is delivered, the levels of estrogen plummet: the anterior pituitary begins secreting prolactin and milk production begins. A lag of two to three days occurs, however, between the birth of the baby and the secretion of milk. In the interim, the breasts secrete a thin, yellowish fluid called **colostrum.** *Colostrum is rich in protein and immunoglobulins that provide the neonate with passive immunity.*

The composition of breast milk changes daily and even over the course of a feeding. The milk secreted at the beginning of a feeding (called foremilk) *is thin, bluish in color, low in fat, and high in carbohydrates. The milk secreted toward the end of a feeding (called* hindmilk) *is thicker, whiter, and much higher in fat.*

The World Health Organization recommends that women breastfeed exclusively for the first six months of life. Numerous studies show that breastfeeding lowers risks for sudden infant death syndrome (SIDS), infection, asthma, eczema, dental problems, and obesity. Breastfeeding also triggers uterine contractions that help reduce postpartum bleeding and also prompts the uterus' return to its pre-pregnancy size.

The Neonate

Immediately following birth, the neonate's body undergoes a number of changes as it adapts to life outside the mother's body. These changes affect most body systems.

- **Cardiovascular:** Pressure changes in the heart cause the foramen ovale to shut, while pressure changes in the pulmonary artery and aorta lead to the collapse of the ductus arteriosus. (The foramen ovale seals permanently during the first year of life, while the ductus arteriosus closes permanently about three months of age.)
- **Respiratory:** Although most neonates begin breathing spontaneously, the first few breaths require considerable effort as they work to inflate the collapsed alveoli.
- **Immune system:** Neonates have weak immune systems at birth, placing them at risk for infection.
- **Thermoregulation:** Neonates risk becoming hypothermic because their surface area, in relationship to their size, is larger than in an adult.
- **Fluid balance:** Neonates require a fairly high fluid intake because their immature kidneys do not concentrate urine adequately.

Life lesson: Apgar score

The first few minutes following birth are critical in the life of a neonate. With this in mind, a scoring system, called the *Apgar score,* is used to rate the neonate's condition and determine the need for respiratory support during this timeframe.

At 1 minute and 5 minutes following birth, the neonate is evaluated for heart rate, respiratory effort, skin color, muscle tone, and reflexes. Each criterion is scored 0, 1, or 2, with 0 being poor and 2 being excellent. The five values are then added together to give a total Apgar score. Scores 7 to 10 are normal; scores 4 to 6 are fairly low; scores 3 and below are critically low. A low Apgar score at 1 minute indicates that the neonate needs medical attention, but it does not necessarily mean that the child will suffer from long-term problems, particularly if the 5-minute score shows improvement.

Be aware that the Apgar score is used only to determine the neonate's immediate need for medical support. It is not designed to predict future health problems.

The Body AT WORK

Human development continues throughout the life span. Following the neonatal period (which encompasses the first four weeks of life), the developmental stages are:

- Infancy, *which lasts until the end of the first year*
- Childhood, *which lasts from the beginning of the second year until puberty*
- Adolescence, *which lasts from puberty until about age 19*
- Adulthood

Most body systems peak in development and efficiency during early adulthood. After that, a gradual but certain decline occurs. This process of degeneration is called **senescence**. The process of aging affects every organ system, with each experiencing a loss of reserve capacity, an impaired ability to repair damage, and an increased susceptibility to disease.

FAST FACT

Although some body systems (such as the cardiovascular, respiratory, and gastrointestinal systems) undergo significant change at birth, other systems take years to develop. For example, myelination of the nervous system isn't complete until adolescence.

Review of Key Terms

Amnion: Transparent sac enveloping the embryo and fetus; fills with amniotic fluid

Blastocyst: Cell cluster (forming at the end of preembryonic development) that implants in the endometrium

Chorion: Outermost fetal membrane that develops projections (chorionic villi) that penetrate the uterus

Colostrum: Thin, yellowish fluid rich in protein and immunoglobulins secreted by the mother's breast for the first few days following delivery

Ductus arteriosus: Shunt existing between the pulmonary artery and descending aorta that is present during fetal development

Ductus venosus: Shunt bypassing the fetal liver that is present during fetal development

Ectoderm: The outer germ layer in a developing embryo

Effacement: Progressive thinning of cervical walls during first stage of labor

Embryo: Stage of development beginning 16 days after conception and lasting until the eighth week

Endoderm: Innermost of the three germ layers in a developing embryo

Fertilization: The union of an egg and a sperm, which is the beginning of human development

Fetus: Stage of development beginning the eighth week and lasting until birth

Foramen ovale: Opening between the right and left atria present during fetal development; normally closes shortly after birth

Gestation: Length of time from conception until birth

Human chorionic gonadotropin (HCG): Hormone secreted during the early part of pregnancy that prompts the corpus luteum to secrete estrogen and progesterone; forms the basis for most pregnancy tests

Lactation: The process whereby the mammary glands secrete milk

Mesoderm: The middle germ layer in a developing embryo

Morula: Cluster of 16 cells resulting from cleavage of an ovum

Multipara: Woman who has previously given birth

Placenta: Pancake-shaped accessory organ that supplies the fetus with oxygen and nutrients and also secretes the hormones necessary to maintain the pregnancy

Primipara: Woman giving birth for the first time

Trophoblast: Outermost layer of the developing blastocyst

Umbilical cord: Cord containing two arteries and one vein that attach the developing fetus to the placenta

Zona pellucida: Gel-like membrane surrounding the ovum

Zygote: A fertilized egg

Own the Information

To make the information in this chapter part of your working memory, take some time to reflect on what you've learned. On a separate sheet of paper, write down everything you recall from the chapter. After you're done, log on to the *DavisPlus* website, and check out the Study Group podcast and Study Group Questions for the chapter.

Key Topics for Chapter 24:
- Process of fertilization
- Stages of prenatal development
- Implantation
- Development of germ layers
- Development of extraembryonic membranes
- Development of, and function of, the placenta and umbilical cord
- Fetal circulation
- Milestones in fetal development
- Physical changes during pregnancy
- Childbirth
- Lactation
- Physical changes in the neonate

Test Your Knowledge

1. The fertilized egg is at which stage when it implants in the uterus?
   a. Embryo
   b. Zygote
   c. Morula
   d. Blastocyst

2. How long can sperm remain viable within the female reproductive tract?
   a. As long as 72 hours
   b. As long as 6 days
   c. 24 hours
   d. 14 hours

3. What is the significance of the embryotic disc?
   a. It gives rise to the three germ layers.
   b. It develops into the amniotic cavity.
   c. It develops into the placenta.
   d. It develops into the yolk sac.

4. Which is a function of the yolk sac?
   a. Secrete HCG
   b. Supply the fetus with oxygen
   c. Supply the fetus with nutrients
   d. Secrete progesterone

5. During the first two months of pregnancy, what is the source of estrogen and progesterone?
   a. Placenta
   b. Chorion
   c. Allantois
   d. Corpus luteum

6. During which stage of pregnancy is the developing fetus most vulnerable to toxins, stress, drugs, and nutritional deficiencies?
   a. First trimester
   b. Second trimester
   c. Third trimester
   d. Throughout the entire pregnancy

7. What is the function of the foramen ovale?
   a. Divert blood from the right to the left atrium
   b. Divert blood from the umbilical vein to the inferior vena cava
   c. Divert blood from the pulmonary artery to the descending aorta
   d. Shunt blood from the umbilical artery to the umbilical vein

8. *Correct answer:* **d.** None of the other answers is correct.

9. *Correct answer:* **c.** The product of conception is known as an embryo once the germ layers are formed; it is known as a zygote at the moment of fertilization. The heart begins to beat on day 22; the product of conception isn't known as a fetus until the ninth week, which is after the organs are formed (which occurs in the embryonic stage).

10. *Correct answer:* **c.** Estrogen stimulates the growth of ducts throughout the mammary glands. Oxytocin is responsible for the secretion of milk. Progesterone stimulates the development of acini at the ends of the ducts.

8. Fertilization normally occurs in the:
   a. uterus.
   b. vagina.
   c. cervix.
   d. fallopian tube.

9. At which point is the product of conception called a fetus?
   a. Once the germ layers are formed
   b. At the moment of fertilization
   c. After the organs are formed
   d. When the heart begins to beat

10. Which hormone is responsible for the production of milk in the mammary glands?
   a. Estrogen
   b. Oxytocin
   c. Prolactin
   d. Progesterone

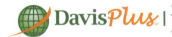 Go to **http://davisplus.fadavis.com** Keyword: Thompson to see all of the resources available with this chapter.

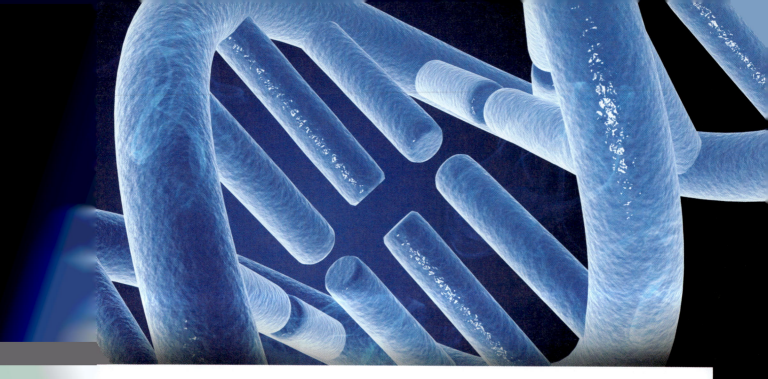

CHAPTER OUTLINE

Chromosomes

Genes

Sex-Linked Inheritance

Genetic Disorders

LEARNING OUTCOMES

1. Differentiate between heredity and genetics.

2. Explain the relationship between chromosomes, DNA, and genes.

3. Describe how chromosomes are paired in the human karyotype.

4. Explain how the gender of offspring is determined.

5. Define *allele* and describe how allele traits are expressed.

6. Discuss the process of sex-linked inheritance.

7. Explain autosomal dominant and autosomal recessive inheritance, and state the percentage chance that a disease will be expressed.

8. Explain what occurs in nondisjunction and identify a common disorder resulting from nondisjunction.

9. Discuss the interaction between heredity and the environment.

HEREDITY

Despite consisting of just four different building blocks, DNA contains all the information necessary to build a human being.

Contained within almost every human cell is a complete copy of a person's genetic blueprint. This blueprint dictates more than physical appearance; it also determines key physiological traits, such as athletic ability, as well as the tendency to develop certain diseases, such as heart disease and cancer. A person's genetic makeup is determined at the time of fertilization when an egg and sperm fuse, creating a new human being with a blend of traits from both parents. This process of passing traits from biological parents to children is called **heredity**, whereas the study of heredity or inheritance is called **genetics**.

A person's genetic information is carried in genes, which are segments along strands of DNA. In turn, DNA (and its accompanying genes) is packaged into chromosomes.

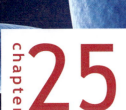

All human cells (except for germ cells) contain 23 *pairs*—a total of 46 individual—**chromosomes**.

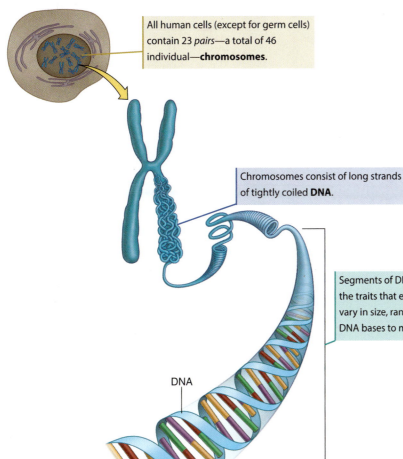

Chromosomes consist of long strands of tightly coiled **DNA**.

Segments of DNA, called **genes**, contain the traits that each person inherits. Genes vary in size, ranging from a few hundred DNA bases to more than 2 million.

DNA

Gene

FAST FACT

If it were to be unwound, the DNA contained within a single cell would measure 6 feet long.

FAST FACT

Each cell contains 25,000 to 35,000 genes.

Chromosomes

Of the 23 pairs of chromosomes contained within the cell's nucleus, 22 are matched with a similar-looking (**homologous**) chromosome. The following chart (called a **karyotype**) shows all the chromosomes, arranged in order by size and structure.

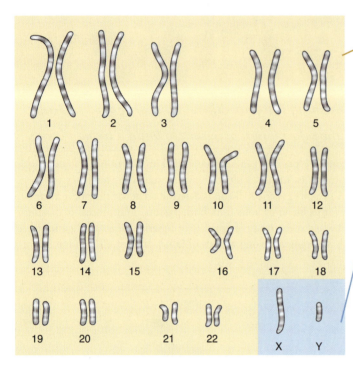

Each pair of chromosomes consists of a chromosome inherited from the mother and a chromosome inherited from the father. (See "The Body at Work" on this page.) These chromosomes are called **autosomes**.

The members of the last pair of chromosomes are known as the **sex chromosomes**. In females, both chromosomes are relatively large and are designated by the letter X. In males, one sex chromosome is an X chromosome and one is a smaller chromosome designated by the letter Y.

The Body AT WORK

Gametes (eggs and sperm) are the only cells that contain a single (unpaired) set of 23 chromosomes. At fertilization, the chromosomes from the father (contained in the sperm) align with similar chromosomes from the mother (contained in the egg) to create a set of 23 pairs, or 46 chromosomes. Consequently, the fertilized egg—as well as all the cells of the body that arise from it—contains genetic instructions from both the mother and the father.

The Body AT WORK

Each gamete produced by a female contains only an X chromosome, whereas the gametes produced by a male may contain either an X or a Y chromosome. When a sperm with an X chromosome fertilizes an egg, the offspring is female (two X chromosomes). When a sperm with a Y chromosome fertilizes an ovum, the offspring is male (one X and one Y chromosome).

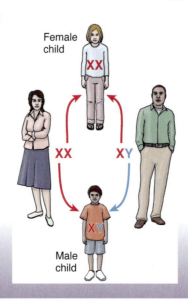

Female child

XX   XY

Male child

Each chromosome contains anywhere from a few hundred to several thousand genes.

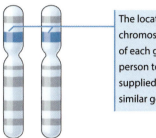

The location of a specific gene on a chromosome is called its **locus**. The locus of each gene does not vary from one person to another. (This allows the genes supplied by the egg to align with the similar genes supplied by the sperm.)

Homologous chromosomes

Even though homologous chromosomes carry the same gene at the same locus, they may carry an alternative form of that gene (called an **allele**). Alleles produce variations of a trait (such as brown versus blue eyes or curly versus straight hair). An individual may have two alleles that are the same or two alleles that are different.

If a person has two alleles that are the same, the person is said to be **homozygous** for that trait.

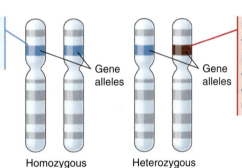

Gene alleles

Gene alleles

If the alleles are different, the person is said to be **heterozygous**. In heterozygous individuals, the trait that becomes detectable (called gene expression) depends on whether the allele is dominant or recessive.

Homozygous   Heterozygous

A **dominant allele** overshadows the effect of a **recessive** allele. Offspring express the trait of a dominant allele if both, or only one, chromosome in a pair carries it. For a recessive allele to be expressed, both chromosomes must carry identical alleles.

As an example, consider the allele for brown eyes (which is dominant) and blue eyes (which is recessive).

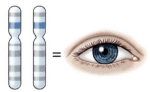 =

- When an allele for brown eyes is paired with an allele for blue eyes, the offspring (who is heterozygous for the trait) will have brown eyes.

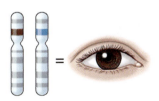 =

- When an allele with brown eyes is paired with another allele for brown eyes, the offspring (who is homozygous for that trait) will have brown eyes.

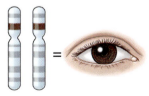 =

- When an allele with blue eyes is paired with another allele for blue eyes, the offspring (who is homozygous for that trait) will have blue eyes.

FAST FACT

A complete set of genetic information for one person (which is carried on the 23 pairs of chromosomes) is called a **genome**.

Some alleles are equally dominant (**codominant**). In this instance, both alleles are expressed. An example of codominance is the AB blood type.

The Body AT WORK

While it is generally true that genes for brown eyes are dominant over genes for green eyes, and genes for both brown and green eyes are dominant over genes for blue eyes, the expression of eye color is not that simple. Eye color results from the presence of melanin in the iris. The various combinations of yellow and black melanin produce the shades of eye color ranging between brown and blue, such as green and hazel. Many different genes participate in melanin production. If one of these genes contains a mutation, the eye color of the offspring will be affected. That's why it's possible for blue-eyed parents to give birth to a child with green or brown eyes. For example, if a blue-eyed man has a "brown-eye gene" because of a mutation, that gene would dominate the woman's "blue-eye gene," and the offspring would have brown eyes.

The phenomenon whereby genes at two or more loci contribute to the expression of a single trait is called polygenic inheritance. Skin color is another example of polygenic inheritance, as are certain diseases such as cancer, heart disease, asthma, and even some mood disorders.

FAST FACT

The genetic information stored at the locus of a gene, even if the trait is not expressed, constitutes a person's **genotype**. The detectable, outward manifestation of a genotype is called a **phenotype**.

Sex-Linked Inheritance

Some traits, called sex-linked traits, are carried on the sex chromosomes. Almost all of these traits, which are recessive, are carried on the X chromosome—mainly because the X chromosome has much more genetic material than does the Y. An example of a common sex-linked condition is red-green color deficit (color blindness).

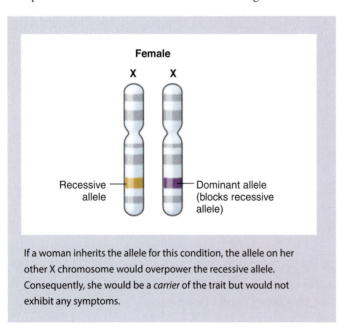

If a woman inherits the allele for this condition, the allele on her other X chromosome would overpower the recessive allele. Consequently, she would be a *carrier* of the trait but would not exhibit any symptoms.

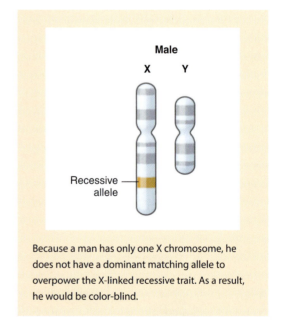

Because a man has only one X chromosome, he does not have a dominant matching allele to overpower the X-linked recessive trait. As a result, he would be color-blind.

FAST FACT

The X chromosome carries hundreds of genes, most of which have nothing to do with determining gender.

Genetic Disorders

Most of the time, DNA replicates smoothly; however, errors can occur. Such errors range from a mutation in a single gene to the addition or subtraction of an entire chromosome or set of chromosomes.

Single-Gene Disorders

A permanent change in genetic material is known as a **mutation**. Although mutations may occur spontaneously, they can also result from exposure to radiation, certain chemicals, or viruses. A variety of disorders result from inheriting defective genes. Ranging in severity from mild to fatal, some of these disorders become apparent soon after birth, while others don't reveal themselves for years. A few of the diseases that result from mutations include sickle cell disease, severe combined immunodeficiency syndrome (SCID), phenylketonuria (PKU), Huntington's disease, and cystic fibrosis. In some diseases (like Huntington's disease), the defective gene is dominant; in other diseases (like cystic fibrosis), it is recessive.

Autosomal Dominant Inheritance

When the defective allele is dominant, it overrides the normally functioning gene and the disorder results. The following diagram illustrates how disease occurs. Because each child receives one copy of the gene from the mother and one from the father, he or she has a 50% chance of inheriting the defective gene and developing the disorder.

Autosomal Recessive Inheritance

In autosomal recessive disorders, the offspring must inherit two copies of the defective allele before the disorder manifests itself. Children who inherit a single copy of the allele become carriers of the disorder. This means that they can pass the disorder on to their children, but they personally won't develop the disorder. A child has a 25% chance of inheriting the defective allele from both parents and, as a result, developing the disorder.

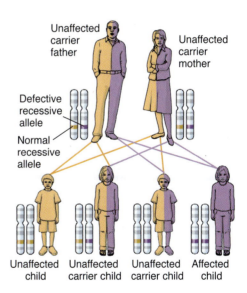

Life lesson: Cystic fibrosis

A defective gene on chromosome 7 causes a common and severe inherited disease called *cystic fibrosis*. The protein produced by this gene normally regulates the transfer of sodium into and out of cells. However, because of the mutation, the transfer is impaired; this causes exocrine cells to secrete profuse amounts of thick, sticky mucus. The excess mucus causes particular problems in the lungs and intestines, where it leads to complications such as infections, blockages, and difficulty digesting food. People with cystic fibrosis have a reduced life expectancy. Because this is a recessive disorder, the child must receive the defective gene from each parent to manifest the disease.

Chromosome Abnormalities

In these disorders, large segments of a chromosome, or even entire chromosomes, are missing, duplicated, or otherwise altered. The most common disorders result when homologous chromosomes fail to separate during meiosis. This is called **nondisjunction**.

Normal disjunction

Recall that, in meiosis, homologous chromosomes separate to produce two daughter cells with 23 chromosomes each. The separation process is called **disjunction.**

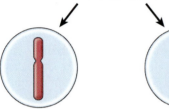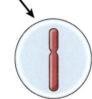

Fertilization supplies another 23 chromosomes, resulting in a complete set of 46 chromosomes.

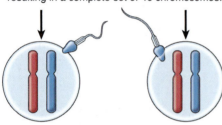

Nondisjunction

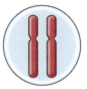

In **nondisjunction**, a pair of chromosomes fails to separate: both chromosomes go to the same daughter cell, while the other daughter cell doesn't receive a chromosome.

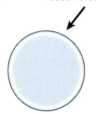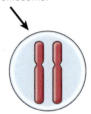

When fertilization adds the matching chromosome, one daughter cell has three of that particular chromosome (called **trisomy**), while the other daughter cell has one chromosome with no mate (called **monosomy**).

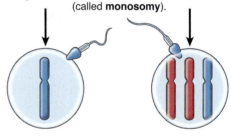

FAST FACT

Several tests, including chorionic villus sampling, amniocentesis, and umbilical blood sampling, can identify the presence of an extra chromosome 21 in a developing fetus.

Life lesson: Down syndrome

Most pregnancies involving extra or missing chromosomes end in miscarriage. The most survivable trisomy, and therefore the most common, is *Down syndrome* or *trisomy 21*. People with Down syndrome have distinctive physical features, including a round face, flattened nose, "Oriental" folds around the eyes, an enlarged tongue, and short fingers. Most have severe to profound mental retardation and also suffer from abnormalities of the heart and kidneys.

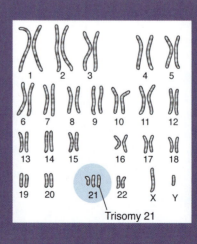

Trisomy 21

Nondisjunction of Sex Chromosomes

Nondisjunction can affect sex chromosomes as well as autosomal chromosomes. The effects from nondisjunction of a sex chromosome typically aren't as severe as nondisjunction of an autosomal chromosome. In fact, a boy with an extra Y chromosome or a girl with an extra X chromosome will usually have no symptoms. However, if a male inherits an extra X chromosome, or if a girl lacks an X chromosome, symptoms become apparent.

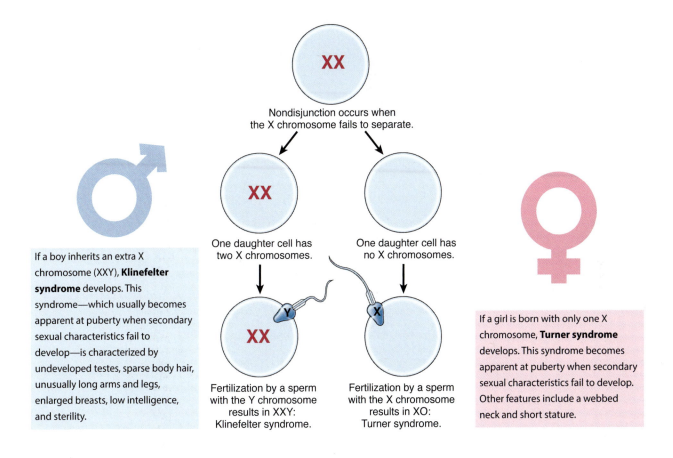

Nondisjunction occurs when the X chromosome fails to separate.

One daughter cell has two X chromosomes.

One daughter cell has no X chromosomes.

Fertilization by a sperm with the Y chromosome results in XXY: Klinefelter syndrome.

Fertilization by a sperm with the X chromosome results in XO: Turner syndrome.

If a boy inherits an extra X chromosome (XXY), **Klinefelter syndrome** develops. This syndrome—which usually becomes apparent at puberty when secondary sexual characteristics fail to develop—is characterized by undeveloped testes, sparse body hair, unusually long arms and legs, enlarged breasts, low intelligence, and sterility.

If a girl is born with only one X chromosome, **Turner syndrome** develops. This syndrome becomes apparent at puberty when secondary sexual characteristics fail to develop. Other features include a webbed neck and short stature.

Multifactorial Disorders

Many common diseases fall into a category called **multifactorial inheritance**. This means that environmental factors have a strong influence over genetic mutation, determining the progression of a disease or even whether the disease develops at all.

For example, heart disease tends to run in families, meaning it has a genetic link. Of course, environmental factors (such as diet, exercise, and whether or not a person smokes) also influence the onset and progression of heart disease. Other examples of multifactorial disorders include hypothyroidism, diabetes, and cancer.

FAST FACT

At least 10% of sperm and 25% of oocytes have extra, missing, or broken chromosomes; however, zygotes with extra or missing chromosomes don't usually survive more than a few days.

Life lesson: Human genome project

Beginning in 1990 and ending in 2003, a team of scientists studied the human genome to determine its entire sequence of DNA and the location and identity of all genes. Just one of the many fascinating findings is that all humans are 99.99% genetically identical. Even so, with just the .01% variation, over 3 million base pairs differ between individuals.

But perhaps the most exciting result of the project is the implication for medicine. Knowing the sequence of someone's genome could help doctors predict that person's risk for disease instead of just treating it once it develops. Other benefits include detecting a disease earlier and then fine-tuning treatment according to that individual's genetic makeup. New treatments, too, are evolving in which healthy genes are introduced into a person's body to replace the specific genes that are defective. This would allow more effective treatment of a variety of diseases and conditions, including cancer, Alzheimer's disease, Parkinson's disease, hemophilia, diabetes, and even high cholesterol levels.

FAST FACT

If the DNA sequence of the human genome were to be complied in books, it would fill 200 volumes having 1000 pages each.

Review of Key Terms

Allele: Alternative form of a gene

Autosomes: Non-sex chromosomes

Carrier: Someone who carries a normal gene along with its recessive allele

Chromosome: Long strand of DNA found in the cell's nucleus

Genes: Segments of DNA that contain the traits each person inherits

Genetics: The study of heredity or inheritance

Genome: A complete set of genetic information for one person

Genotype: The genetic information stored at the locus of a gene, even if those traits are not expressed

Heredity: The passing of traits from biological parents to children

Heterozygous: Possessing different alleles at a given locus

Homologous: Similar in structure, such as two similar chromosomes that are paired together

Homozygous: Possessing similar alleles at a given locus

Karyotype: A chart showing all the chromosomes arranged in order by size and structure

Locus: The location of a specific gene on a chromosome

Mutation: A permanent change in genetic material

Nondisjunction: When chromosomes fail to separate during meiosis

Phenotype: The detectable, outward manifestation of a genotype

Polygenic inheritance: Phenomenon whereby genes at two or more loci contribute to the expression of a single trait

Sex chromosomes: Chromosomes designated by the letters X and Y that determine gender

Own the Information

To make the information in this chapter part of your working memory, take some time to reflect on what you've learned. On a separate sheet of paper, write down everything you recall from the chapter. After you're done, log on to the Davis*Plus* website, and check out the Study Group podcast and Study Group Questions for the chapter.

Key Topics for Chapter 25:

- The difference between heredity and genetics
- Chromosomes and the human karyotype
- Genes
- Alleles and the expression of traits
- Sex-linked inheritance
- Single-gene genetic disorders
- Autosomal dominant and autosomal recessive inheritance
- Chromosome abnormalities
- Multifactorial disorders

Test Your Knowledge

1. Chromosomes consist of:
   a. pairs of nucleic acids.
   b. long strands of tightly coiled DNA.
   c. a single gene.
   d. autosomes.

2. The genetic information in male offspring is:
   a. inherited from both the father and the mother.
   b. inherited from only the father.
   c. inherited from only the mother.
   d. unique from that of either parent.

3. Female offspring result when:
   a. a sperm with a Y chromosome fertilizes the egg.
   b. a sperm with an X chromosome fertilizes the egg.
   c. an egg with a Y chromosome is fertilized by a sperm with an X chromosome.
   d. a sperm with two X chromosomes fertilizes the egg.

4. An alternative form of a gene is called:
   a. a locus.
   b. a genome.
   c. an allele.
   d. a karyotype.

5. Which of the following statements about alleles is correct?
   a. A dominant allele cancels out a recessive allele and the trait is suppressed.
   b. A recessive allele is expressed only when the corresponding allele is absent.
   c. If a person has two alleles that are the same, the person is said to be heterozygous.
   d. An individual may have two alleles that are the same or two alleles that are different.

6. Which of the following statements about sex-linked inheritance is correct?
   a. Almost all of the sex-linked traits are carried on the X chromosome and are recessive.
   b. Almost all of the sex-linked traits are carried on the X chromosome and are dominant.
   c. Almost all of the sex-linked traits are carried on the Y chromosome and are recessive.
   d. Almost all of the sex linked traits are carried on the Y chromosome and are dominant.

7. Most of the common chromosomal abnormalities result when:
   a. homologous chromosomes separate repeatedly.
   b. homologous chromosomes fail to separate during meiosis.
   c. an egg is fertilized by more than one sperm.
   d. a mutation occurs.

Answers: Chapter 25

1. *Correct answer:* **b.** Nucleic acids make up DNA. Chromosomes contain thousands of genes. Autosomes are any chromosomes other than the sex chromosomes.

2. *Correct answer:* **a.** Although the offspring is unique from either parent, he inherits half of his chromosomes from his mother and half from his father.

3. *Correct answer:* **b.** A male offspring results when a sperm with a Y chromosome fertilizes an egg. Eggs only have X chromosomes. A sperm with two X chromosomes would be considered abnormal.

4. *Correct answer:* **c.** A locus is the location of a specific gene on a chromosome. A genome is a complete set of genetic information for one person. A karyotype is a chart that shows all the chromosomes arranged in order by size and structure.

5. *Correct answer:* **d.** A dominant allele overrides a recessive allele and is expressed. A recessive allele is expressed when the corresponding allele is also recessive. A person who has two alleles that are the same is said to be homozygous for that trait.

6. *Correct answer:* **a.** All the other answers are incorrect.

7. *Correct answer:* **b.** All the other answers are incorrect.

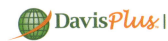 **DavisPlus** | Go to http://davisplus.fadavis.com Keyword: Thompson to see all of the resources available with this chapter.

Index

Capillaries, 293, 297–299
  peritubular, 359
Capillary beds, 297
Capillary exchange, 298–299
Capsid, 436
Capsomeres, 436
Capsule
  bacterial, 433
  joint, 120
Carbaminohemoglobin, 353
Carbohydrates, 29, 404, 414
  metabolism, 419–420
Carbon, 30
Carbon dioxide, 26, 381, 383, 385
  gas exchange and, 352
  respiration and, 345, 346
  transport, 353
Carbonic acid, 27, 381, 383
Carbonic anhydrase, 381, 383
Cardiac center, 180, 286–287
Cardiac conduction, 282–283
Cardiac cycle, 284
Cardiac muscle, 64, 131
Cardiac nerves, 286
Cardiac output (CO), 285–289
  blood pressure and, 307
Cardiology, 273
Cardiovascular system. *See also* Heart; Vascular system
  heat generation and, 12
  neonate, 478
Carina, 340
Carotene, 73
Carotid arteries, 303
Carotid body, 287
Carpal bones, 111
Carpal tunnel syndrome, 148
Carpopedal spasm, 240
Carrier, 45
Cartilage, 60, 62, 63
  articular, 120
  costal, 109
  disorders, 62
  exercise and, 126
Cartilaginous joints, 119
Catabolism, 23, 419
Catalysts, 24
Cataracts, 220
Catecholamines, 241
Categorical hemisphere, 187
Cations, 21
Cauda equina, 170
Caudate lobe, 398
Cavities
  body, 10
  joint, 120
CCK (cholecystokinin), 401, 413
Cecum, 406
Celiac trunk, 302
Cell body (soma), 163
Cell(s), 4
  aging, 50
  B, 328, 330
  chief, 396
  cycle, 50–51

cytoplasm and organelles, 40–42
  goblet, 58, 59
  growth and reproduction, 50–52
  layers in epithelial tissue, 58
  mast, 331
  movement through membranes of, 43–47
  nervous system, 161–164
  nucleus, 38, 40
  shape in epithelial tissue, 58
  stem, 57
  structure, 38–42
  T, 318, 327, 328, 329, 330
  variations, 37
Cellular (cell-mediated) immunity, 327, 329
Cellular respiration, 26
Cellulose, 29, 404, 414
Cell wall, 433, 435
Cementum, 393
Centers for ossification, 88
Central canal, 171
Central nervous system (CNS), 160. *See also* Nervous system; Spinal cord
  autonomic nervous system and, 191
  neuroglia of, 161
  pituitary secretions and, 235
Central obesity, 63
Central vein, 399
Centrioles, 41
Cephalic phase, 397
Cephalic vein, 304
Cerebellum, 176, 180
Cerebral cortex, 183, 345
  functions of, 184–187
Cerebral lateralization, 187
Cerebrospinal fluid (CSF), 178–179
Cerebrum, 176, 182–183, 210
Cerumen, 77
Ceruminous glands, 77
Cervical canal, 454
Cervical curve, 106
Cervical lymph nodes, 319
Cervical plexus, 174
Cervical vertebrae, 106
Cervix, 454
  dilation of, 475
Chambers, eye, 218
Chemical bonds, 20–22
  peptide, 32
Chemical buffers, 381, 382
Chemical digestion and absorption, 390, 404–405
Chemical reactions, 24
Chemicals
  atoms in, 19
  basic processes of life and, 23–24
  basic structures of life and, 18–22
  bonds, 20–22
  common elements and, 17
  compounds of life and, 25–33
  elements in, 18
  reactions, 24
Chemoreceptors, 206, 287
Chemotaxis, 323, 325
Chemotherapy, 52
Chewing muscles, 145
Cheyne-Stokes respirations, 350